D1558517

IMAGING PAINFUL SPINE DISORDERS

IMAGING PAINFUL SPINE DISORDERS

Leo F. Czervionke, M.D.
Associate Professor of Radiology
Mayo Medical School
Mayo Clinic Florida
Jacksonville, Florida

Douglas S. Fenton, M.D.
Assistant Professor of Radiology
Mayo Medical School
Mayo Clinic Florida
Jacksonville, Florida

ELSEVIER
SAUNDERS

1600 John F. Kennedy Blvd.
Ste 1800
Philadelphia, PA 19103-2899

IMAGING PAINFUL SPINE DISORDERS   ISBN: 978-1-4160-2904-5

Copyright © 2011 by Mayo Foundation for Medical Education and Research Published by Saunders, an imprint of Elsevier Inc. All rights reserved.

No part of this publication may be reproduced or transmitted in any form or by any means, electronic or mechanical, including photocopying, recording, or any information storage and retrieval system, without permission in writing from the publisher. Details on how to seek permission, further information about the Publisher's permissions policies and our arrangements with organizations such as the Copyright Clearance Center and the Copyright Licensing Agency, can be found at our website: www.elsevier.com/permissions.

This book and the individual contributions contained in it are protected under copyright by the Publisher (other than as may be noted herein).

Notices

Knowledge and best practice in this field are constantly changing. As new research and experience broaden our understanding, changes in research methods, professional practices, or medical treatment may become necessary.

Practitioners and researchers must always rely on their own experience and knowledge in evaluating and using any information, methods, compounds, or experiments described herein. In using such information or methods they should be mindful of their own safety and the safety of others, including parties for whom they have a professional responsibility.

With respect to any drug or pharmaceutical products identified, readers are advised to check the most current information provided (i) on procedures featured or (ii) by the manufacturer of each product to be administered, to verify the recommended dose or formula, the method and duration of administration, and contraindications. It is the responsibility of practitioners, relying on their own experience and knowledge of their patients, to make diagnoses, to determine dosages and the best treatment for each individual patient, and to take all appropriate safety precautions.

To the fullest extent of the law, neither the Publisher nor the authors, contributors, or editors, assume any liability for any injury and/or damage to persons or property as a matter of products liability, negligence or otherwise, or from any use or operation of any methods, products, instructions, or ideas contained in the material herein.

Library of Congress Cataloging-in-Publication Data
Czervionke, Leo F.
    Imaging painful spine disorders : expert consult / Leo F. Czervionke, Douglas S. Fenton.—1st ed.
        p. ; cm.
    Includes bibliographical references and index.
    ISBN 978-1-4160-2904-5 (hardcover : alk. paper)   1. Spine—Diseases—Imaging.   I. Fenton, Douglas S. (Douglas Scott)   II. Title.
    [DNLM: 1. Spinal Diseases—diagnosis.   2. Spinal Diseases—pathology.   3. Diagnosis, Differential.   4. Pain—diagnosis.   5. Pain—pathology. WE 725]
    RD768.C94 2011
    616.7'3—dc22

                                                                                        2010044384

Acquisitions Editor: Pamela Hetherington
Editorial Assistant: David Mack
Publishing Services Manager: Patricia Tannian
Team Manager: Radhika Pallamparthy
Senior Project Manager: Sharon Corell
Project Manager: Joanna Dhanabalan
Design Direction: Steven Stave

Working together to grow
libraries in developing countries

www.elsevier.com | www.bookaid.org | www.sabre.org

ELSEVIER | BOOK AID International | Sabre Foundation

Printed in the United States of America

Last digit is the print number: 9   8   7   6   5   4   3   2   1

To Jeanne, my loving wife and best friend, whose unwavering support, kindness, and understanding have helped to make this book possible … and to Zeus V.M., my loyal companion, who knows how to experience, enjoy, and accept each moment of life as it happens.

Thank you!

Leo C.

To my wonderful wife, Melissa (during the time I wrote this book, you got your Ph.D… you win!), my daughter, Brooke (the light to whom people are drawn), my son Derek (baseball's next Sultan of Swat), my son Mitchell (the happiest kid on Earth), and my four-legged friends, Dilly and Darla, who were literally there with me every step of the way, and Yogi, Prissy, and Tigger, who were with me in spirit (miss you so much).

All my love and gratitude,

Doug/Dad/Woof/Meow

PREFACE

Our primary goal in writing this book was to provide a readily accessible reference guide describing the imaging appearance of the major conditions that cause back pain. This book deals with common and some not so common disorders that cause back pain, with emphasis on the imaging appearance of disorders that are associated with spine pain.

The book is organized into two major sections: *Normal Computed Tomography and Magnetic Resonance Imaging Anatomy*, and *Painful Spine Disorders*. An illustrated chapter is also included on the nomenclature currently used to describe the various types of disc herniations. The anatomic sections of the book include normal CT and MR images of the cervical, thoracic, and lumbar spine as well as the sacrum. Representative cross-sectional images are presented in these anatomic areas in axial, sagittal, and coronal planes.

The clinical disorder section of the book is divided into chapters. Each chapter topic is introduced by an actual clinical case of a patient with a given disorder who presents with back pain. Each chapter includes a brief description of the clinical presentation, imaging findings, and clinical course when relevant. The case studies illustrate the imaging presentation of these patients with back pain. A detailed description of the disorder, including relevant clinical and pathologic information, follows. Also included in each chapter is specific information about the imaging appearance of the particular pain-producing condition, emphasizing the radiographic, CT, and MR appearance, and a differential diagnosis with imaging examples.

The images pertaining to the case presentations are the first set in each clinical disorder chapter. They are followed by additional relevant images of the same or other patients with the same condition. These additional images are used to emphasize the range of imaging features possible for the particular topic being discussed. Images of the disorders in the differential diagnosis are also included if available or relevant.

Following the imaging features in each chapter is a brief discussion or listing of the major treatment options currently available for the particular disorder being presented. This book is not intended to provide an exhaustive discussion of all treatment options for back pain but rather is a practical guide that can be used to aid in the diagnosis of pain-producing spine and paraspinal disorders. Hopefully this information will be helpful in formulating a treatment plan for the patient with back pain.

Carefully selected references are included at the end of each chapter. We have chosen these references because we believe they supplement the information presented in the chapter discussions and provide the reader with a starting point for more detailed investigation regarding a particular pathophysiologic feature, clinical presentation, or imaging finding mentioned in the chapter. References are also included for the disorders described in the differential diagnostic section of each chapter.

We have tried to include all the major categories of disorders that are associated with back pain and have recognizable imaging findings. However, not every disorder that can potentially produce back pain is discussed. We believe this book does provide a useful working reference guide for those physicians who diagnose and treat patients with back pain on a daily basis. Our hope is that this book will be a valuable resource for all physicians involved with the diagnosis and treatment of back pain.

Leo F. Czervionke

Douglas S. Fenton

CONTENTS

IMAGING PAINFUL SPINE DISORDERS

NORMAL COMPUTED TOMOGRAPHY AND MAGNETIC RESONANCE IMAGING ANATOMY

CERVICAL SPINE ANATOMY

Leo F. Czervionke, M.D.

COMPUTED TOMOGRAPHY (CT) CERVICAL AXIAL

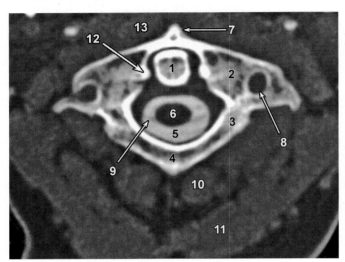

Figure 1-1 ▶ Axial CT Image. Odontoid process level. **1.** Odontoid process (dens) **2.** Lateral mass C1 **3.** Lateral arch C1 **4.** Posterior arch C1 **5.** Intrathecal contrast in subarachnoid space **6.** Cervical spinal cord **7.** Midline tubercle, anterior C1 arch **8.** Transverse foramen containing vertebral artery **9.** Dorsal rootlet **10.** Obliquus capitis inferior muscle **11.** Semispinalis capitis muscle **12.** Tubercle for transverse ligament attachment **13.** Longus coli (longus cervicis) muscle.

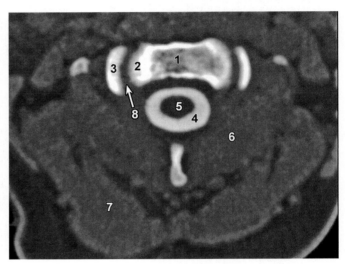

Figure 1-2 ▶ Axial CT Image. Base of odontoid level. **1.** Base of odontoid process **2.** Superior articular facet C2 **3.** Inferior articular facet C1 **4.** Intrathecal contrast in subarachnoid space **5.** Spinal cord **6.** Obliquus capitis inferior muscle **7.** Semispinalis capitis muscle **8.** Facet joint.

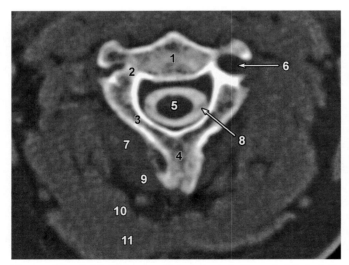

Figure 1-3 ▶ Axial CT Image. C2 body level. **1.** C2 vertebral body **2.** C2 pedicle **3.** C2 lamina **4.** C2 spinous process **5.** Spinal cord **6.** Vertebral artery in transverse foramen **7.** Obliquus capitis inferior muscle **8.** Dorsal rootlet **9.** Rectus capitis posterior minor muscle **10.** Semispinalis capitis muscle **11.** Splenius capitis muscle.

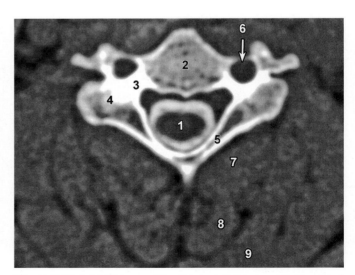

Figure 1-4 ▶ Axial CT Image. C4 pedicle level. **1.** Spinal cord **2.** C4 vertebral body **3.** C4 pedicle **4.** C4 articular pillar **5.** C4 lamina **6.** Transverse foramen containing vertebral artery **7.** Multifidus muscle **8.** Semispinalis capitis/cervicis muscle **9.** Splenius capitis/cervicis muscle.

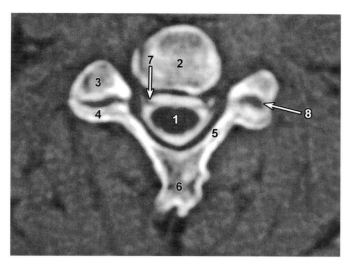

Figure 1-5 ▶ Axial CT Image. Superior C4-5 neural foramen. **1.** Spinal cord **2.** C4 vertebral body **3.** Superior articular process C5 **4.** Inferior articular process C4 **5.** C4 lamina **6.** C4 spinous process **7.** Ventral rootlet **8.** Facet joint.

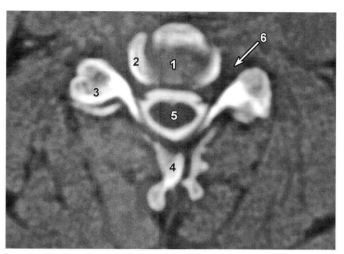

Figure 1-6 ▶ Axial CT Image. C4-5 intervertebral disc level. **1.** Intervertebral disc C4-5 **2.** Uncinate process C5 **3.** Superior articular facet C5 **4.** Spinous process C4 **5.** Spinal cord **6.** Neural foramen C4-5, inferior portion.

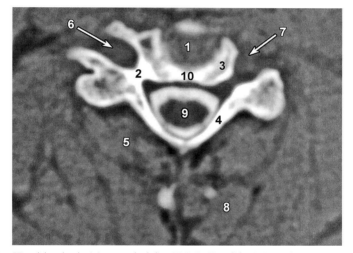

Figure 1-7 ▶ Axial CT Image. Superior C5 endplate level. **1.** Intervertebral disc C4-5 **2.** C5 pedicle **3.** C5 uncinate process **4.** C5 lamina **5.** Multifidus muscle **6.** Right vertebral artery **7.** Left vertebral artery **8.** Semispinalis cervicis muscle **9.** Spinal cord **10.** Posterosuperior C5 vertebral endplate.

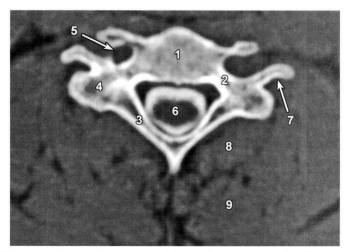

Figure 1-8 ▶ Axial CT Image. C5 pedicle level. **1.** C5 vertebral body **2.** C5 pedicle **3.** C5 lamina **4.** C5 articular pillar **5.** Transverse foramen containing vertebral artery **6.** Spinal cord **7.** C5 transverse process **8.** Multifidus muscle **9.** Semispinalis cervicis muscle.

MAGNETIC RESONANCE IMAGING (MRI) CERVICAL AXIAL

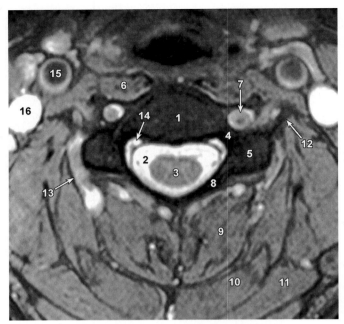

Figure 1-9 ▶ Axial Gradient-Recalled Echo (GRE) Image. C4 pedicle. **1.** C4 vertebral body **2.** CSF **3.** Cervical spinal cord **4.** C4 pedicle **5.** Articular pillar C4 **6.** Longus cervicis muscle **7.** Left vertebral artery **8.** Lamina **9.** Multifidus muscle **10.** Semispinalis cervicis muscle **11.** Splenius capitis muscle **12.** Lateral process C4 **13.** Paravertebral vein **14.** Epidural vein **15.** Right internal carotid artery **16.** Right internal jugular vein.

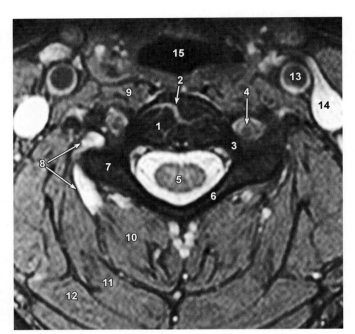

Figure 1-10 ▶ Axial Gradient-Recalled Echo (GRE) Image. Mid C4 vertebral body. **1.** C4 vertebral body **2.** Basivertebral vein **3.** Pedicle C4 **4.** Left vertebral artery **5.** Spinal cord **6.** Lamina C4 **7.** Articular pillar **8.** Paravertebral vein **9.** Longus cervicis muscle **10.** Multifidus muscle **11.** Semispinalis cervicis muscle **12.** Splenius cervicis muscle **13.** Left internal carotid artery **14.** Left internal jugular vein **15.** Cervical airway.

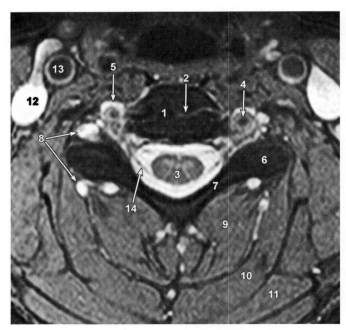

Figure 1-11 ▶ Axial Gradient-Recalled Echo (GRE) Image. Upper C4-5 neural foramen. **1.** C4 vertebral body **2.** Basivertebral vein C4 **3.** Spinal cord **4.** Left vertebral artery **5.** Venous plexus adjacent to vertebral artery **6.** Articular pillar C4 **7.** Lamina **8.** Paravertebral vein **9.** Multifidus muscle **10.** Semispinalis cervicis muscle **11.** Splenius cervicis muscle **12.** Right internal jugular vein **13.** Right internal carotid artery.

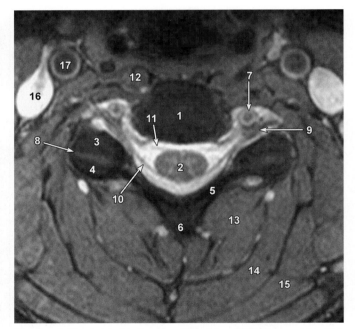

Figure 1-12 ▶ Axial Gradient-Recalled Echo (GRE) Image. Mid C4-5 foramen level. **1.** C4 vertebral body **2.** Spinal cord **3.** Superior articular process C5 **4.** Inferior articular process C4 **5.** Lamina **6.** Spinous process C4 **7.** Left vertebral artery **8.** Facet joint C4-5 **9.** Dorsal root ganglion C5 **10.** Dorsal rootlet **11.** Ventral rootlet **12.** Longus cervicis muscle **13.** Multifidus muscle **14.** Semispinalis cervicis muscle **15.** Splenius cervicis muscle **16.** Right internal jugular vein **17.** Right internal carotid artery.

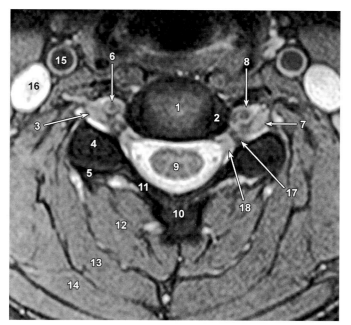

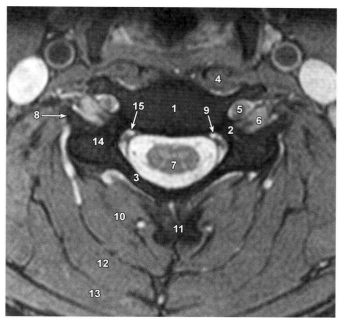

Figure 1-13 ▸ Axial Gradient-Recalled Echo (GRE) Image. Lower C4-5 foramen, intervertebral disc level. **1.** C4-5 intervertebral disc **2.** Uncinate process C5 **3.** Right dorsal root ganglion C5 **4.** Superior articular process C5 **5.** Inferior articular facet C4 **6.** Right vertebral artery **7.** Left dorsal root ganglion C5 **8.** Left vertebral artery **9.** Spinal cord **10.** Spinous process C4 **11.** C4 lamina, inferiorly **12.** Multifidus muscle **13.** Semispinalis cervicis muscle **14.** Splenius cervicis muscle **15.** Right internal carotid artery **16.** Right internal jugular vein **17.** Left C4-5 neural foramen **18.** Left C5 nerve root sheath.

Figure 1-14 ▸ Axial Gradient-Recalled Echo (GRE) Image. Upper C5 vertebral body level. **1.** C5 vertebral body **2.** Pedicle C5 **3.** Lamina C5 **4.** Longus cervicis muscle **5.** Left vertebral artery **6.** Left C5 spinal nerve **7.** Spinal cord, posterior funiculus **8.** Right C5 lateral process **9.** Left epidural venous plexus **10.** Multifidus muscle **11.** Spinous process C4 **12.** Semispinalis cervicis muscle **13.** Splenius cervicis muscle **14.** Articular pillar C5 **15.** Right epidural venous plexus.

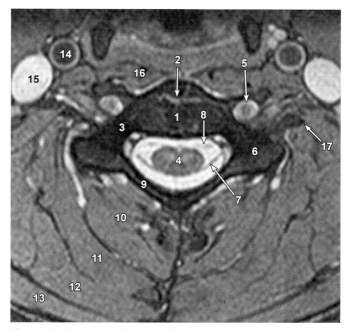

Figure 1-15 ▸ Axial Gradient-Recalled Echo (GRE) Image. Mid C5 vertebral body level. **1.** C5 vertebral body **2.** Basivertebral vein C5 **3.** C5 pedicle **4.** Spinal cord **5.** Left vertebral artery **6.** Articular pillar C5 **7.** Dorsal rootlet **8.** Ventral rootlet **9.** Lamina C5 **10.** Multifidus muscle **11.** Semispinalis cervicis muscle **12.** Splenius cervicis muscle **13.** Trapezius muscle **14.** Right internal carotid artery **15.** Right internal jugular vein **16.** Right longus cervicis muscle **17.** Left lateral process.

COMPUTED TOMOGRAPHY (CT) CERVICAL SAGITTAL

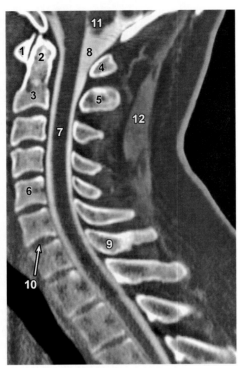

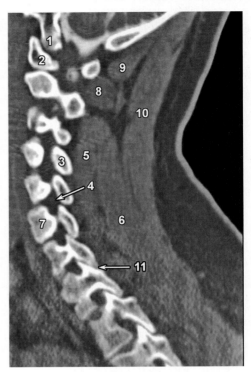

Figure 1-16 ►Midline Sagittal Postmyelogram CT Image. Spinal cord. **1.** Anterior arch C1 **2.** Odontoid process (dens) **3.** C2 vertebral body **4.** Posterior arch C1 **5.** Spinous process C2 **6.** C5 vertebral body **7.** Cervical spinal cord **8.** Opacified subarachnoid space **9.** C7 spinous process **10.** C6-7 intervertebral disc **11.** Cerebellar tonsil **12.** Semispinalis capitis muscle.

Figure 1-17 ►Sagittal Postmyelogram CT Image. Neural foramina. **1.** Occipital condyle **2.** Lateral mass C1 **3.** Lamina C4 **4.** C6 dorsal root ganglion in C5-6 neural foramen **5.** Multifidus muscle **6.** Semispinalis cervicis muscle **7.** C6 vertebral body **8.** Obliquus capitis inferior muscle **9.** Rectus capitis posterior major muscle **10.** Semispinalis capitis muscle **11.** C7-T2 facet joint.

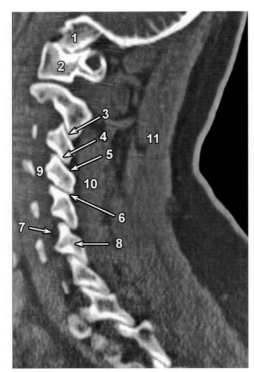

Figure 1-18 ►Sagittal Postmyelogram CT Image. Articular pillars/facet joints. **1.** Occipital condyle **2.** Lateral mass C1 **3.** C2-3 facet joint **4.** Inferior articular facet C3 **5.** Superior articular facet C4 **6.** Facet joint C4-5 **7.** Dorsal root ganglion C6 **8.** Articular pillar C6 **9.** Vertebral artery in transverse foramen **10.** Multifidus muscle **11.** Semispinalis capitis muscle.

MAGNETIC RESONANCE IMAGING (MRI) CERVICAL SAGITTAL

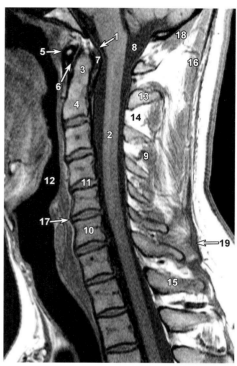

Figure 1-19 ► Sagittal T1-weighted MRI. Cervical spinal cord. 1. Tectorial membrane 2. Cervical spinal cord 3. Odontoid process (dens) 4. C2 vertebral body 5. Anterior arch C1 6. Midline anterior atlantoaxial joint 7. Transverse ligament of dens 8. CSF, subarachnoid space 9. Interspinous muscle C3-4 10. C6 vertebral body 11. C4-5 intervertebral disc 12. Supraglottic airway 13. C2 spinous process 14. C2-3 interspinous ligament, fat 15. T2 spinous process 16. Splenius capitis muscle 17. Anterior longitudinal ligament/disc anterior margin 18. Rectus capitis posterior minor muscle 19. Nuchal ligament.

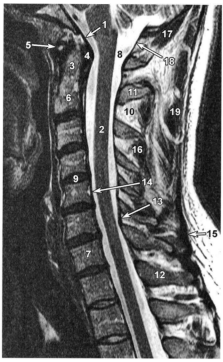

Figure 1-20 ► Sagittal T2-weighted MRI. Cervical spinal cord. 1. Tectorial membrane 2. Cervical spinal cord 3. Odontoid process (dens) 4. Transverse ligament of dens 5. Anterior arch C1 6. C2 vertebral body 7. C7 vertebral body 8. CSF in subarachnoid space 9. C4-5 intervertebral disc 10. Interspinous ligament/fat C2-3 11. C2 spinous process 12. T2 spinous process 13. Ligamentum flavum C6-7 14. Posterior longitudinal ligament 15. Nuchal ligament 16. Interspinous muscle C3-4 17. Rectus capitis posterior minor muscle 18. Occipitoatlantal membrane 19. Splenius capitis muscle.

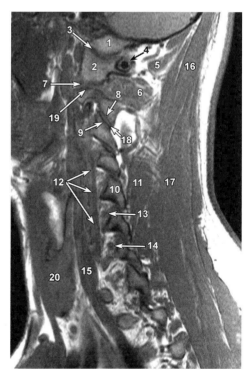

Figure 1-21 ► Sagittal T1-weighted MRI. Articular pillars. 1. Occipital condyle 2. Lateral mass C1 (atlas) 3. Occipitoatlantal joint 4. Vertebral artery C1 level 5. Rectus capitis posterior major muscle 6. Obliquus capitis inferior muscle 7. C1-2 facet joint (lateral atlantoaxial joint) 8. Inferior articular facet C2 9. Superior articular facet C3 10. Articular pillar C5 11. Multifidus muscle 12. Vertebral artery 13. C6 dorsal root ganglion 14. C7 dorsal root ganglion 15. Longus cervicis (coli) muscle 16. Splenius capitis muscle 17. Semispinalis cervicis muscle 18. C2-3 facet joint 19. Superior articular facet C3 20. Thyroid gland.

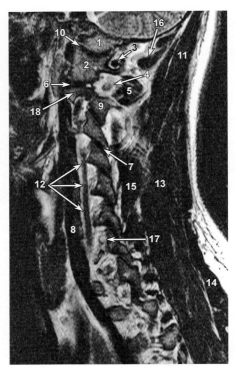

Figure 1-22 ▶ Sagittal T1-weighted MRI. Articular pillars. **1.** Occipital condyle **2.** Lateral mass C1 (atlas) **3.** Vertebral artery C1 level **4.** C2 dorsal root ganglion **5.** Obliquus capitis inferior muscle **6.** C1-2 facet joint (lateral atlantoaxial joint) **7.** C3-4 facet joint **8.** Longus cervicis (coli) muscle **9.** C2 Inferior articular process **10.** Occipitoatlantal joint **11.** Splenius capitis muscle **12.** Vertebral artery **13.** Semispinalis cervicis muscle **14.** Trapezius muscle **15.** Multifidus muscle **16.** Rectus capitis posterior major muscle **17.** C7 dorsal root ganglion **18.** Superior articular process C2.

COMPUTED TOMOGRAPHY (CT) CERVICAL CORONAL

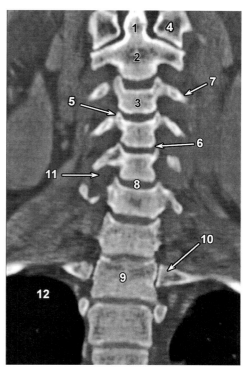

Figure 1-23 ▶ Coronal CT Image. Cervical vertebral bodies. **1.** Odontoid process (dens) **2.** C2 vertebral body **3.** C3 vertebral body **4.** C1 lateral mass **5.** Uncinate process C4 **6.** Uncovertebral joint C4-5 **7.** C3 transverse process **8.** C5-6 intervertebral disc **9.** T2 vertebral body **10.** First rib **11.** Nerve root C6 **12.** Lung apex.

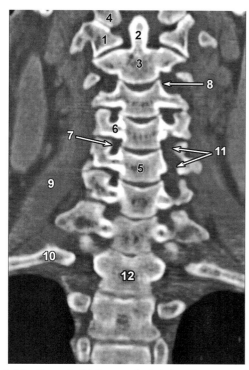

Figure 1-24 ▶ Coronal CT Image. Cervical foramina. **1.** Lateral mass C1 **2.** Odontoid process (dens) **3.** C2 vertebral body **4.** Occipital condyle **5.** C5 vertebral body **6.** C4 pedicle **7.** C4-5 neural foramen **8.** Uncinate process C3 **9.** Scalene muscle group **10.** 1st rib **11.** Vertebral artery in transverse foramina **12.** T2 vertebral body.

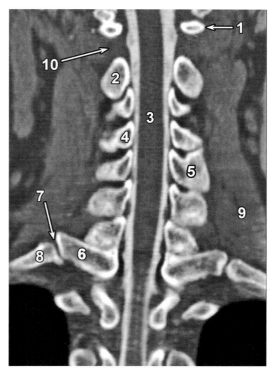

Figure 1-25 ▶ Coronal CT Image. Cervical spinal cord. **1.** Lateral arch C1 **2.** Pedicle C2 **3.** Cervical spinal cord **4.** Pedicle C4 **5.** Lateral mass C5 **6.** T2 transverse process **7.** 1st costotransverse joint **8.** First rib **9.** Scalene muscle group **10.** C1-2 neural foramen (contains C2 nerve root).

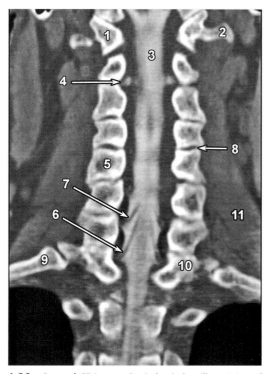

Figure 1-26 ▶ Coronal CT Image. Cervical articular pillars. **1.** Lateral mass C1 **2.** Transverse process C1 **3.** Contrast-opacified intrathecal subarachnoid space **4.** C3 nerve root in root sleeve **5.** C5 articular pillar **6.** T1 nerve root **7.** C8 nerve root **8.** C4-5 facet joint **9.** First rib **10.** T1 lateral mass/pars interarticularis **11.** Scalene muscle group.

MAGNETIC RESONANCE IMAGING (MRI AND SPICIMEN IMAGES) UPPER CERVICAL SPINE

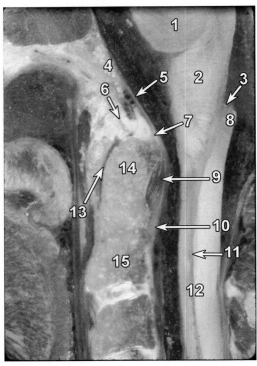

Figure 1-27 ► Midline Sagittal Cervical-Medullary Junction. Photograph of cadaver specimen following sagittal cryomicrotomographic sectioning. **1.** Pons **2.** Medulla **3.** Obex **4.** Clivus **5.** Tectorial membrane **6.** Apical ligament of dens **7.** Superior fasciculus of cruciform ligament **8.** Tuberculum gracile (clava) **9.** Transverse ligament of dens, part of cruciform ligament **10.** Inferior fasciculus of cruciform ligament **11.** Gray matter adjacent to central canal of cord **12.** Spinal cord **13.** Anterior atlantoaxial joint **14.** Odontoid process (dens) **15.** C2 vertebral body.

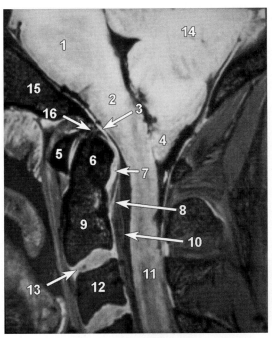

Figure 1-28 ► Midline Cervical-Medullary Junction. Sagittal gradient-recalled echo MRI. **1.** Pons **2.** Medulla **3.** Tectorial membrane **4.** Cerebellar tonsil, low-lying **5.** Anterior arch C1 **6.** Odontoid process (dens) **7.** Transverse ligament of dens, part of cruciform ligament **8.** Inferior fasciculus of cruciform ligament **9.** C2 body **10.** Posterior longitudinal ligament **11.** Spinal cord **12.** C3 vertebral body **13.** C2-3 intervertebral disc **14.** Cerebellum **15.** Clivus **16.** Apical ligament of dens.

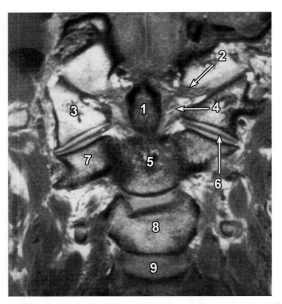

Figure 1-29 ► Coronal T1-weighted MRI. Through dens, cadaver. **1.** Odontoid process **2.** Left alar ligament of dens **3.** Right lateral mass of C1 (atlas) **4.** Left transverse ligament of dens, lateral portion **5.** C2 vertebral body **6.** Left C1-2 facet joint and adjacent articular cartilage **7.** Right lateral mass of C2 **8.** C3 vertebral body **9.** C2-3 intervertebral disc.

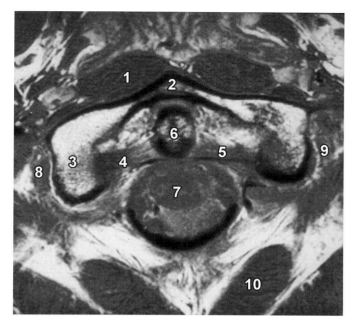

Figure 1-30 ▶ Axial T1-weighted MRI. Upper dens level, cadaver. **1.** Right longus coli muscle **2.** Anterior arch of C1 **3.** Right lateral mass of C1 **4.** Right alar ligament of dens **5.** Left alar ligament of dens **6.** Odontoid process (dens) **7.** Spinal cord **8.** Right vertebral artery, C1 level **9.** Left vertebral artery, C1 level **10.** Left rectus capitis posterior major muscle.

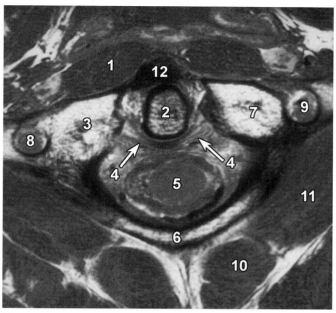

Figure 1-31 ▶ Axial T1-weighted MRI. Mid dens level, cadaver. **1.** Right longus coli muscle **2.** Dens **3.** Right lateral mass C1 **4.** Transverse ligament of dens (horizontal sling of cruciform ligament) **5.** Spinal cord **6.** Posterior arch of C1 **7.** Left lateral mass of C1 **8.** Right vertebral artery in right transverse foramen **9.** Left vertebral artery in left transverse foramen **10.** Left rectus capitis posterior major muscle **11.** Left obliquus capitis inferior muscle **12.** Anterior arch of C1.

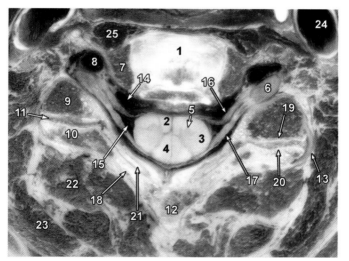

Figure 1-32 ▶ Axial C4-5 Intervertebral Disc Level. Photography of cadaver specimen following axial cryomicrotomographic sectioning. **1.** Intervertebral disc C4-5 **2.** Anterior funiculus, spinal cord **3.** Lateral funiculus, spinal cord **4.** Anterior motor horn, spinal cord **5.** Posterior funiculus, spinal cord **6.** C5 dorsal root ganglion **7.** Uncinate process **8.** Vertebral artery **9.** Superior articular process C5 **10.** Inferior articular process C4 **11.** C4-5 facet joint **12.** Spinous process C4 **13.** Lateral capsule, left C4-5 facet joint **14.** Anterior epidural vein **15.** Intrathecal subarachnoid space **16.** Ventral nerve root **17.** Dorsal nerve root **18.** C4 lamina, inferiorly **19.** Superior articular facet C5 **20.** Inferior articular facet C4 **21.** Ligamentum flavum **22.** Multifidus muscle **23.** Semispinalis cervicis muscle **24.** Left common carotid artery **25.** Longus cervicis muscle.

THORACIC SPINE ANATOMY

Douglas S. Fenton, M.D.

COMPUTED TOMOGRAPHY (CT)
AXIAL THORACIC

IMAGING SUPERIOR TO INFERIOR

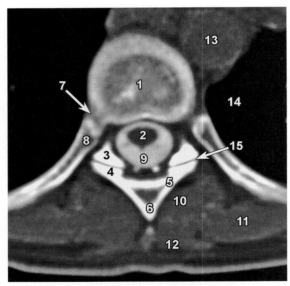

Figure 2-1 ▶ Axial CT Image. Disc level. **1.** Intervertebral disc T7-8 **2.** Spinal cord **3.** Superior articular process T8 **4.** Inferior articular process T7 **5.** Lamina T7 **6.** Spinous process T7 **7.** Costovertebral joint **8.** T8 rib head **9.** Myelographic contrast-filling thecal sac **10.** Multifidus muscle **11.** Longissimus dorsi muscle **12.** Trapezius muscle **13.** Aorta **14.** Lung **15.** Facet joint.

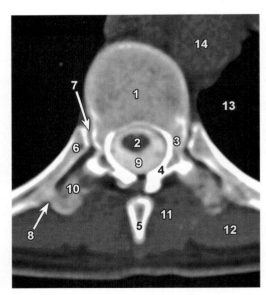

Figure 2-2 ▶ Axial CT Image. Upper pedicle level. **1.** T8 vertebral body **2.** Spinal cord **3.** Pedicle **4.** Lamina T8 **5.** Spinous process T7 **6.** T8 rib head **7.** Costovertebral joint **8.** Costotransverse joint **9.** Myelographic contrast-filling thecal sac **10.** Transverse process **11.** Multifidus muscle **12.** Longissimus dorsi muscle **13.** Lung **14.** Aorta.

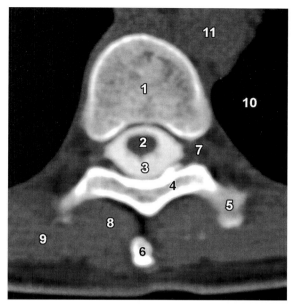

Figure 2-3 ▸ Axial CT Image. Mid pedicle level. **1.** T8 vertebral body **2.** Basivertebral vein **3.** Spinal cord **4.** Myelographic contrast-filling thecal sac **5.** Pedicle **6.** Lamina T8 **7.** Transverse process **8.** Spinous process T7 **9.** Multifidus muscle **10.** Longissimus dorsi muscle **11.** Lung **12.** Aorta **13.** Diaphragmatic crus.

Figure 2-4 ▸ Axial CT Image. Upper foraminal level. **1.** T8 vertebral body **2.** Spinal cord **3.** Myelographic contrast-filling thecal sac **4.** Lamina T8 **5.** Transverse process **6.** Spinous process T7 **7.** Neural foramen **8.** Multifidus muscle **9.** Longissimus dorsi muscle **10.** Lung **11.** Aorta.

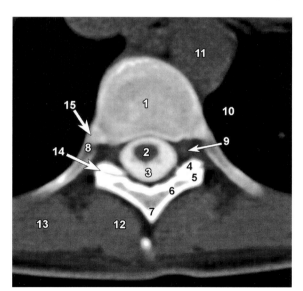

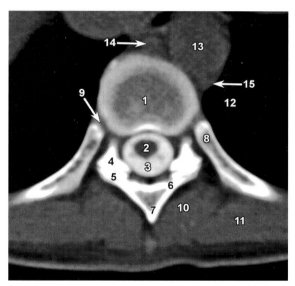

Figure 2-5 ▸ Axial CT Image. Lower foraminal level. **1.** Inferior T8 vertebral body **2.** Spinal cord **3.** Myelographic contrast-filling thecal sac **4.** Superior articular process T9 **5.** Inferior articular process T8 **6.** Lamina T8 **7.** Spinous process T8 **8.** Rib head T9 **9.** Left T8 nerve root in T8-9 neural foramen **10.** Lung **11.** Aorta **12.** Multifidus muscle **13.** Longissimus dorsi muscle **14.** T8-9 facet joint **15.** Costovertebral joint.

Figure 2-6 ▸ Axial CT Image. Disc level. **1.** Intervertebral disc T8-9 **2.** Spinal cord **3.** Myelographic contrast-filling thecal sac **4.** Superior articular process T9 **5.** Inferior articular process T8 **6.** Lamina T8 **7.** Spinous process T8 **8.** Rib head T9 **9.** Costovertebral joint **10.** Multifidus muscle **11.** Longissimus dorsi muscle **12.** Lung **13.** Aorta **14.** Azygos vein **15.** Hemiazygos vein.

IMAGING SUPERIOR TO INFERIOR

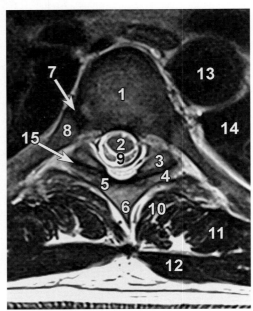

Figure 2-7 ▶ Axial MR T2-weighted Image. Disc level. **1.** Intervertebral disc T7-8 **2.** Spinal cord **3.** Superior articular process T8 **4.** Inferior articular process T7 **5.** Lamina T7 **6.** Spinous process T7 **7.** Costovertebral joint **8.** T8 rib head **9.** CSF in the thecal sac **10.** Multifidus muscle **11.** Longissimus dorsi muscle **12.** Trapezius muscle **13.** Aorta **14.** Lung **15.** Facet joint.

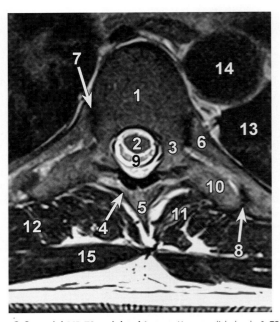

Figure 2-8 ▶ Axial MR T2-weighted Image. Upper pedicle level. **1.** T8 vertebral body **2.** Spinal cord **3.** Pedicle **4.** Lamina T8 **5.** Spinous process T7 **6.** T8 rib head **7.** Costovertebral joint **8.** Costotransverse joint **9.** CSF in the thecal sac **10.** Transverse process **11.** Multifidus muscle **12.** Longissimus dorsi muscle **13.** Lung **14.** Aorta **15.** Trapezius muscle.

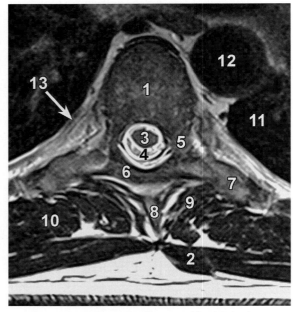

Figure 2-9 ▶ Axial MR T2-weighted Image. Mid pedicle level. **1.** T8 vertebral body **2.** Trapezius muscle **3.** Spinal cord **4.** CSF in the thecal sac **5.** Pedicle **6.** Lamina T8 **7.** Transverse process **8.** Spinous process T7 **9.** Multifidus muscle **10.** Longissimus dorsi muscle **11.** Lung **12.** Aorta **13.** Intercostal vein.

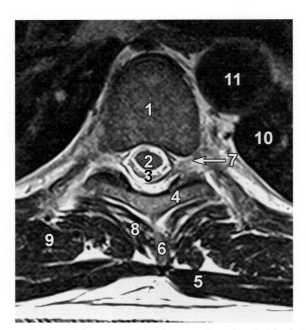

Figure 2-10 ▶ Axial MR T2-weighted Image. Upper foraminal level. **1.** T8 vertebral body **2.** Spinal cord **3.** CSF in the thecal sac **4.** Lamina T8 **5.** Trapezius muscle **6.** Spinous process T7 **7.** Neural foramen/T8 nerve root **8.** Multifidus muscle **9.** Longissimus dorsi muscle **10.** Lung **11.** Aorta.

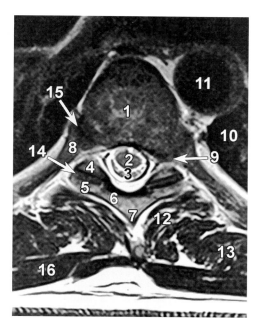

Figure 2-11 ▸ **Axial MR T2-weighted Image.** Lower foraminal level. **1.** Inferior T8 vertebral body **2.** Spinal cord **3.** CSF in the thecal sac **4.** Superior articular process T9 **5.** Inferior articular process T8 **6.** Lamina T8 **7.** Spinous process T8 **8.** Rib head T9 **9.** Inferior neural foramen **10.** Lung **11.** Aorta **12.** Multifidus muscle **13.** Longissimus dorsi muscle **14.** T8-9 facet joint **15.** Costovertebral joint.

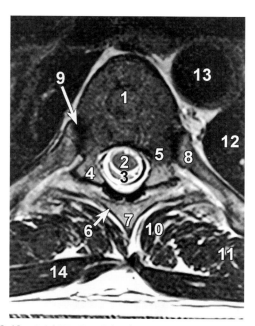

Figure 2-12 ▸ **Axial MR T2-weighted Image.** Disc level. **1.** Intervertebral disc T8-9 **2.** Spinal cord **3.** CSF in the thecal sac **4.** Superior articular process T9 **5.** Pedicle **6.** Lamina T8 **7.** Spinous process T8 **8.** Rib head T9 **9.** Costovertebral joint **10.** Multifidus muscle **11.** Longissimus dorsi muscle **12.** Lung **13.** Aorta **14.** Trapezius muscle.

COMPUTED TOMOGRAPHY (CT)
SAGITTAL THORACIC

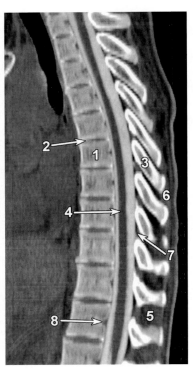

Figure 2-13 ▶ Midline Sagittal CT Image. 1. T7 vertebral body **2.** T6-7 intervertebral disc **3.** T7 spinous process **4.** Spinal cord **5.** Interspinous ligament **6.** Supraspinous ligament **7.** Ligamentum flavum **8.** Basivertebral vein.

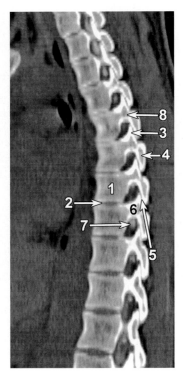

Figure 2-14 ▶ Off Midline Sagittal CT Image. Foraminal level. **1.** T8 vertebral body **2.** T8-9 intervertebral disc **3.** Superior articular process T7 **4.** Inferior articular process T7 **5.** Facet joint, T8-9 **6.** Pedicle **7.** Myelographic contrast-filled nerve root sleeve **8.** Pars interarticularis.

MAGNETIC RESONANCE IMAGING (MRI)
SAGITTAL THORACIC

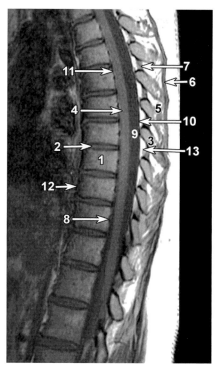

Figure 2-15 ▶ Mid Sagittal T1-weighted MRI. 1. Vertebral body **2.** Intervertebral disc **3.** Spinous process **4.** Spinal cord **5.** Interspinous ligament **6.** Supraspinous ligament **7.** Ligamentum flavum **8.** Basivertebral vein **9.** CSF in the thecal sac **10.** Posterior dura of the thecal sac **11.** Posterior longitudinal ligament **12.** Anterior longitudinal ligament **13.** Posterior epidural fat.

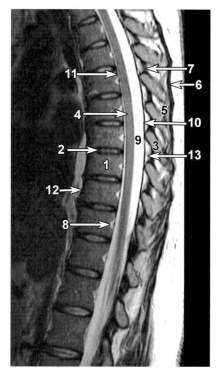

Figure 2-16 ▶ Mid Sagittal T2-weighted MRI. 1. Vertebral body **2.** Intervertebral disc **3.** Spinous process **4.** Spinal cord **5.** Interspinous ligament **6.** Supraspinous ligament **7.** Ligamentum flavum **8.** Basivertebral vein **9.** Cerebrospinal fluid in the thecal sac **10.** Posterior dura of the thecal sac **11.** Posterior longitudinal ligament **12.** Anterior longitudinal ligament **13.** Posterior epidural fat.

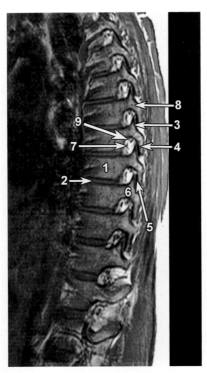

Figure 2-17 ► **Off Midline Sagittal T1-weighted MRI.** Foraminal level. **1.** Vertebral body **2.** Intervertebral disc **3.** Superior articular process **4.** Inferior articular process **5.** Facet joint **6.** Pedicle **7.** Neural foraminal vein **8.** Pars interarticularis **9.** Nerve root.

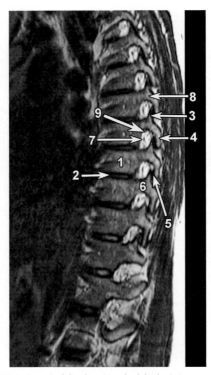

Figure 2-18 ► **Off Midline Sagittal T2-weighted MRI.** Foraminal level. **1.** Vertebral body **2.** Intervertebral disc **3.** Superior articular process **4.** Inferior articular process **5.** Facet joint **6.** Pedicle **7.** Neural foraminal vein **8.** Pars interarticularis **9.** Nerve root.

COMPUTED TOMOGRAPHY (CT) CORONAL THORACIC

IMAGING ANTERIOR TO POSTERIOR

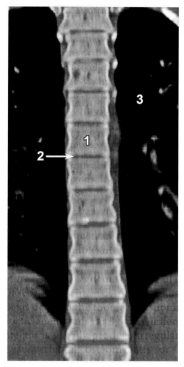

Figure 2-19 ▸ Coronal CT Image. Vertebral body level. **1.** Vertebral body **2.** Intervertebral disc **3.** Lung.

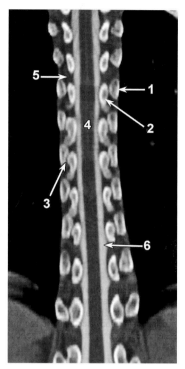

Figure 2-20 ▸ Coronal CT Image. Spinal cord level. **1.** Rib head **2.** Pedicle **3.** Costovertebral joint **4.** Spinal cord **5.** Neural foramen.

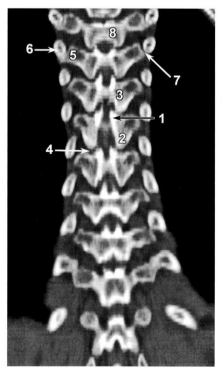

Figure 2-21 ▸ Coronal CT Image. Laminar level. **1.** Superior articular process **2.** Inferior articular process **3.** Pars interarticularis **4.** Facet joint **5.** Transverse process **6.** Rib **7.** Costotransverse joint **8.** Lamina.

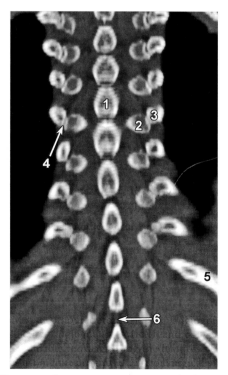

Figure 2-22 ▸ Coronal CT Image. Spinous process level. **1.** Spinous process **2.** Transverse process **3.** Rib, medial **4.** Costotransverse joint **5.** Rib, posterior. **6.**

LUMBAR SPINE ANATOMY

Leo F. Czervionke, M.D.

COMPUTED TOMOGRAPHY (CT) AXIAL LUMBAR

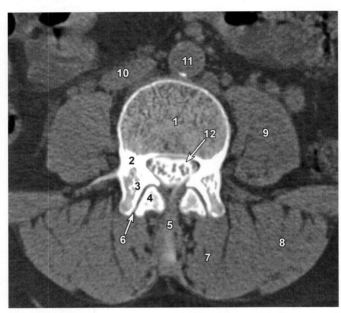

Figure 3-1 ▶ Axial CT Image. L4 pedicle level superiorly, lateral recess. **1.** L4 vertebral body **2.** L4 pedicle **3.** Superior articular process L4 **4.** Inferior articular process L3 **5.** Interspinous muscle/ligament L3-4 **6.** Facet joint L3-4 **7.** Multifidus muscle **8.** Erector spinae muscle **9.** Psoas muscle **10.** Inferior vena cava **11.** Abdominal aorta **12.** Cauda equina nerve roots.

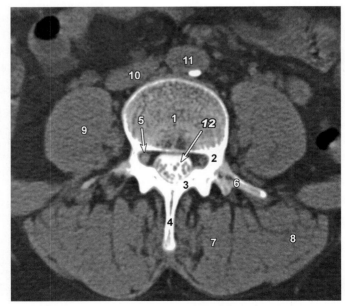

Figure 3-2 ▶ Axial CT Image. L4 pedicle inferiorly. **1.** L4 vertebral body **2.** L4 pedicle **3.** L4 lamina **4.** L4 spinous process **5.** L4 nerve root **6.** L4 transverse process **7.** Multifidus muscle **8.** Erector spinae muscle **9.** Psoas muscle **10.** Inferior vena cava **11.** Abdominal aorta **12.** Cauda equina nerve roots.

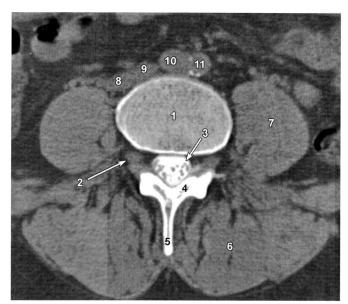

Figure 3-3 ▶ **Axial CT Image.** L4-5 neural foramen. **1.** L4 vertebral body **2.** L4 dorsal root ganglion **3.** Cauda equina nerve roots **4.** L4 lamina **5.** L4 spinous process **6.** Multifidus muscle **7.** Psoas muscle **8.** Right common iliac vein **9.** Left common iliac vein **10.** Right common iliac artery origin **11.** Left common iliac artery origin.

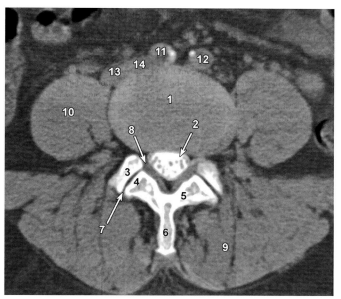

Figure 3-4 ▶ **Axial CT Image.** L4-5 intervertebral disc. **1.** Intervertebral disc L4-5 **2.** Cauda equina nerve roots **3.** L5 superior articular facet L5 **4.** L4 inferior articular facet L4 **5.** L4 lamina **6.** L4 spinous process **7.** L4-5 facet joint **8.** Ligamentum flavum **9.** Multifidus muscle **10.** Psoas muscle **11.** Right common iliac artery **12.** Left common iliac artery **13.** Right common iliac artery **14.** Left common iliac vein.

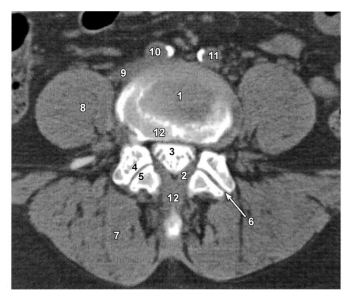

Figure 3-5 ▶ **Axial CT Image.** L4-5 intervertebral disc/superior L5 endplate. **1.** L4-5 intervertebral disc **2.** Ligamentum flavum **3.** Opacified CSF in thecal sac **4.** L5 superior articular facet **5.** L4 inferior articular facet **6.** Facet joint **7.** Multifidus muscle **8.** Psoas muscle **9.** Right common iliac vein **10.** Right common iliac artery **11.** Left common iliac artery **12.** Superior L4 vertebral endplate.

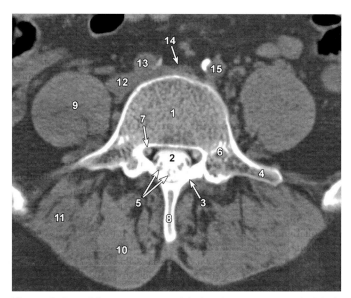

Figure 3-6 ▶ **Axial CT Image.** L5 pedicle, lateral recess. **1.** L5 vertebral body **2.** Opacified CSF in thecal sac **3.** L5 lamina, superior cortex **4.** L5 transverse process **5.** Cauda equina nerve roots **6.** L5 pedicle **7.** L5 nerve root/sheath in lateral recess **8.** L5 spinous process **9.** Psoas muscle **10.** Multifidus muscle **11.** Erector spinae muscle **12.** Right common iliac vein **13.** Right common iliac artery **14.** Left common iliac vein **15.** Left common iliac artery.

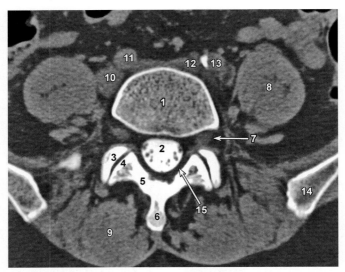

Figure 3-7 ▸ Axial CT Image. L5-S1 neural foramen. **1.** L5 vertebral body **2.** Opacified CSF in thecal sac **3.** S1 superior articular facet **4.** L5 inferior articular facet **5.** L5 lamina **6.** L5 spinous process **7.** L5 dorsal root ganglion **8.** Psoas muscle **9.** Multifidus muscle **10.** Right common iliac vein **11.** Right common iliac artery **12.** Left common iliac vein **13.** Left common iliac artery **14.** Iliac crest **15.** Ligamentum flavum.

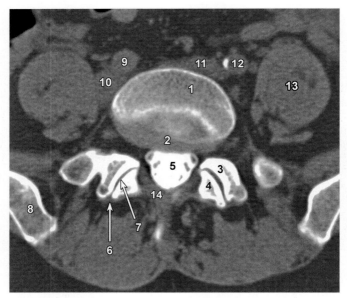

Figure 3-8 ▸ Axial CT Image. L5-S1 intervertebral disc level. **1.** L5 inferior vertebral body endplate **2.** Posterior L5-S1 intervertebral disc margin **3.** Superior articular process S1 **4.** Inferior articular process L5 **5.** Ligamentum flavum **6.** Posterior facet joint capsule **7.** Facet joint **8.** Iliac crest **9.** Right common iliac artery **10.** Right common iliac vein **11.** Left common iliac vein **12.** Left common iliac artery **13.** Psoas muscle **14.** Ligamentum flavum.

MAGNETIC RESONANCE IMAGING (MRI) AXIAL LUMBAR

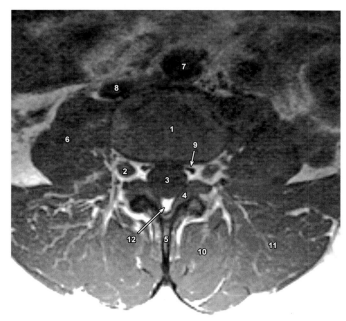

Figure 3-9 ► Axial T1-weighted MRI. L3-4 neural foramen level. **1.** Intervertebral disc **2.** L3 nerve root **3.** CSF in thecal sac **4.** Ligamentum flavum **5.** L3 spinous process **6.** Psoas muscle **7.** Aorta **8.** Inferior vena cava **9.** Anterior epidural vein **10.** Multifidus muscle **11.** Erector spinae muscle **12.** Posterior epidural fat.

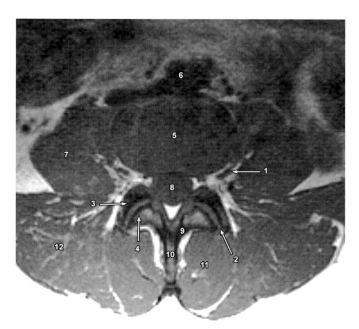

Figure 3-10 ► Axial T1-weighted MRI. L3-4 intervertebral disc level. **1.** Nerve root **2.** Facet joint **3.** Superior articular process L4 **4.** Inferior articular process L3 **5.** Intervertebral disc **6.** Aortic bifurcation **7.** Psoas muscle **8.** CSF in thecal sac **9.** Lamina **10.** Spinous process **11.** Multifidus muscle **12.** Erector spinae muscle.

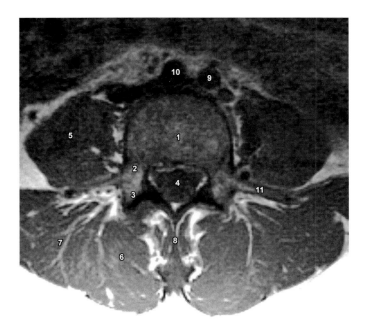

Figure 3-11 ► Axial T1-weighted MRI. L4 pedicle level. **1.** L4 vertebral body **2.** Pedicle **3.** Superior articular process L4 **4.** CSF in thecal sac **5.** Psoas muscle **6.** Multifidus muscle **7.** Erector spinae muscle **8.** Interspinous muscle/ligament **9.** Left common iliac artery **10.** Right common iliac artery **11.** Transverse process.

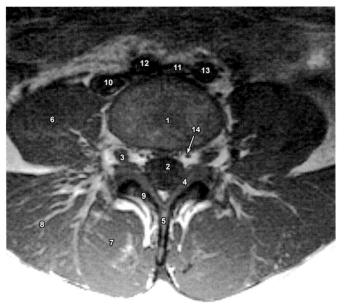

Figure 3-12 ► Axial T1-weighted MRI. Neural foramen level. **1.** L4 vertebra body **2.** CSF in thecal sac **3.** L4 dorsal root ganglion **4.** Ligamentum flavum **5.** L4 spinous process **6.** Psoas muscle **7.** Multifidus muscle **8.** Erector spinae muscle **9.** Lamina **10.** Right common iliac vein **11.** Left common iliac vein **12.** Right common iliac artery **13.** Left common iliac artery **14.** Anterior epidural vein.

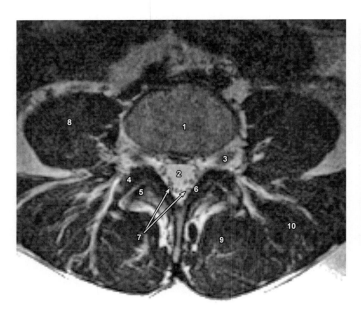

Figure 3-13 ▸ Axial T2-weighted MRI. L4-5 neural foramen level. **1.** L4 vertebral body **2.** CSF in thecal sac **3.** L4 dorsal root ganglion **4.** Superior articular process L5 **5.** Inferior articular process L4 **6.** Lamina **7.** Cauda equina nerve roots **8.** Psoas muscle **9.** Multifidus muscle **10.** Erector spinae muscle.

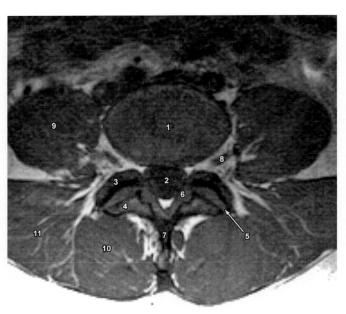

Figure 3-14 ▸ Axial T1-weighted MRI. L4-5 intervertebral disc level. **1.** L4-5 intervertebral disc **2.** CSF in thecal sac **3.** Superior articular process L5 **4.** Inferior articular process L4 **5.** Facet joint **6.** Ligamentum flavum **7.** Spinous process **8.** Nerve root **9.** Psoas muscle **10.** Multifidus muscle **11.** Erector spinae muscle.

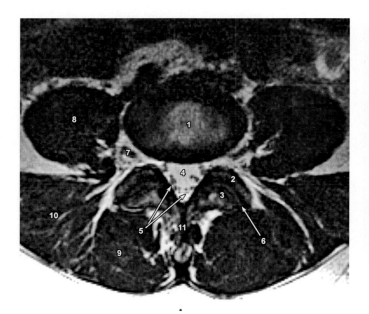

Figure 3-15 ▸ Axial T2-weighted MRI. L4-5 intervertebral disc level. **1.** L4-5 intervertebral disc **2.** Superior articular process L5 **3.** Inferior articular process L4 **4.** Facet joint **5.** Cauda equina nerve roots **6.** Facet joint **7.** Nerve root **8.** Psoas muscle **9.** Multifidus muscle **10.** Erector spinae muscle **11.** Spinous process.

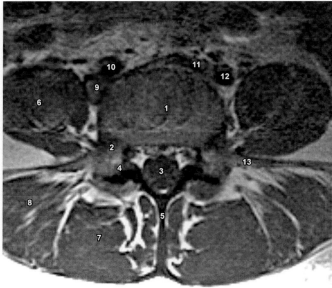

Figure 3-16 ▸ Axial T1-weighted MRI. L5 pedicle level. **1.** L5 vertebral body **2.** L5 pedicle **3.** CSF in thecal sac **4.** Superior articular process L5 **5.** Spinous process **6.** Psoas muscle **7.** Multifidus muscle **8.** Erector spinae muscle **9.** Right common iliac vein **10.** Right common iliac artery **11.** Left common iliac vein **12.** Left common iliac artery **13.** Left transverse process L5.

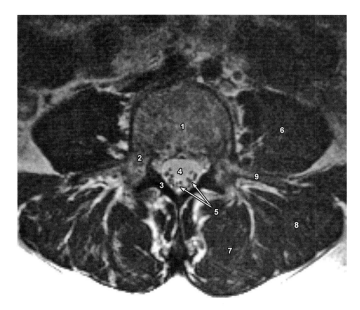

Figure 3-17 ▶ **Axial T2-weighted MRI.** L5 pedicle level. **1.** L5 vertebral body **2.** L5 pedicle **3.** Laminar cortex **4.** CSF in thecal sac **5.** Cauda equina nerve roots **6.** Psoas muscle **7.** Multifidus muscle **8.** Erector spinae muscle **9.** Left L5 transverse process.

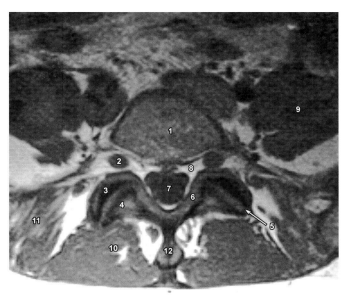

Figure 3-18 ▶ **Axial T1-weighted MRI.** L5-S1 neural foramen level. **1.** L5 vertebral body **2.** L5 nerve root **3.** Superior articular process S1 **4.** Inferior articular process L5 **5.** Facet joint **6.** Ligamentum flavum **7.** CSF in thecal sac **8.** Anterior epidural fat **9.** Psoas muscle **10.** Multifidus muscle **11.** Erector spinae muscle **12.** Spinous process.

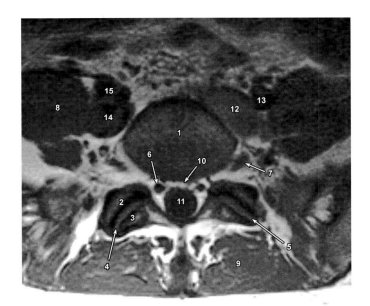

Figure 3-19 ▶ **Axial T1-weighted MRI.** L5-S1 intervertebral disc level. **1.** L5-S1 intervertebral disc **2.** Superior articular process S1 **3.** Inferior articular process L5 **4.** Right L5-S1 facet joint **5.** Left L5-S1 facet joint **6.** S1 nerve root/sheath **7.** L5 nerve root **8.** Psoas muscle **9.** Multifidus muscle **10.** Anterior epidural fat **11.** CSF in thecal sac **12.** Left common iliac vein **13.** Left common iliac artery **14.** Right common iliac vein **15.** Right common iliac artery.

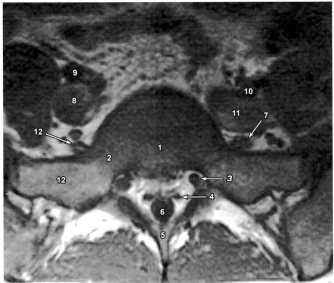

Figure 3-20 ▶ **Axial T1-weighted MRI.** Superior S1 vertebral level. **1.** S1 vertebral body **2.** S1 "pedicle." **3.** S1 nerve root/sheath **4.** S2 nerve root/sheath **5.** S1 spinous process **6.** CSF in thecal sac **7.** Left lumbosacral trunk (neural plexus) **8.** Right common iliac vein **9.** Right common iliac artery **10.** Left common iliac artery **11.** Left common iliac vein **12.** Right lumbosacral trunk (neural plexus).

COMPUTED TOMOGRAPHY (CT)
SAGITTAL LUMBAR

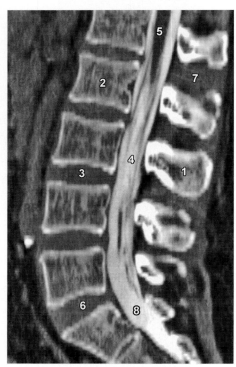

Figure 3-21 ▶ Mid Sagittal Post-myelogram CT Image. 1. L3 spinous process **2.** L2 vertebral body **3.** L3-4 intervertebral disc **4.** Cauda equina nerve roots **5.** conus medullaris **6.** L5-S1 intervertebral disc **7.** L1-2 interspinalis muscle/ligaments **8.** Contrast-filled thecal sac (subarachnoid space).

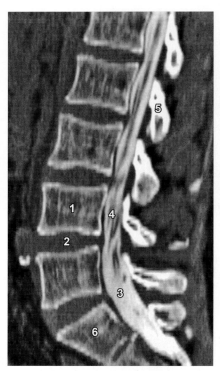

Figure 3-22 ▶ Left Paramidline Sagittal Post-myelogram CT Image. L4 vertebral body. **1.** L4-5 intervertebral disc **2.** Contrast in thecal sac (subarachnoid space) **3.** Cauda equina nerve roots **4.** L2 lamina **5.** S1 vertebral body.

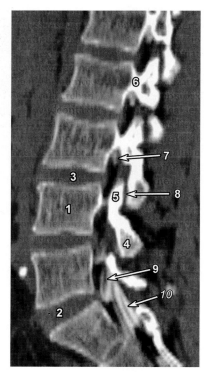

Figure 3-23 ▶ Left Sagittal Post-myelogram CT Image. Through neural foramina medially. **1.** L4 vertebral body **2.** L5-S1 intervertebral disc **3.** L3-4 intervertebral disc **4.** Inferior articular process L4 **5.** Superior articular process L4 **6.** L2 pedicle **7.** L3 nerve root **8.** L3-4 facet joint **9.** S1 nerve root in opacified sheath **10.** S2 and S2 nerve roots in opacified sheaths.

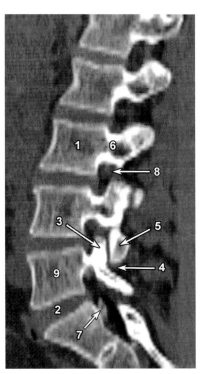

Figure 3-24 ▶ **Left Sagittal Post-myelogram CT Image.** Through mid neural foramina. **1.** L3 vertebral body **2.** L5-S1 intervertebral disc **3.** Superior articular process L5 **4.** Posteroinferior recess L4-5 facet joint **5.** Inferior articular process L4 **6.** L3 pedicle **7.** S1 nerve root in opacified sheath **8.** L3 nerve root **9.** L5 vertebral body.

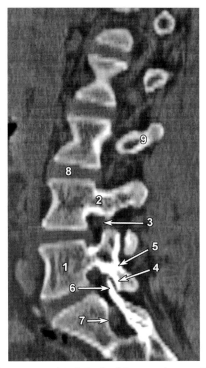

Figure 3-25 ▶ **Far Lateral Left Sagittal Post-myelogram CT Image. 1.** L5 vertebral body **2.** L4 pedicle **3.** L4 nerve root **4.** Inferior articular facet L5 **5.** Pars interarticularis L5 **6.** Superior articular facet S1 **7.** S1 nerve root in opacified sheath **8.** L3-4 intervertebral disc **9.** L3 lamina.

MAGNETIC RESONANCE IMAGING (MRI) SAGITTAL LUMBAR

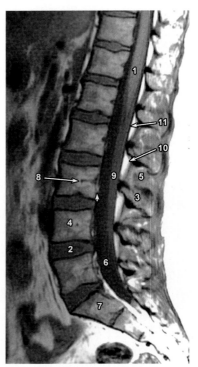

Figure 3-26 ▶ Mid Sagittal T1-weighted MRI. **1.** Conus medullaris **2.** L4-5 intervertebral disc **3.** L3 spinous process **4.** L4 vertebral body **5.** Interspinous lumborum muscle and ligaments **6.** Subarachnoid space **7.** S1 vertebral body **8.** Basivertebral vein L3 **9.** Cauda equina **10.** Posterior epidural fat **11.** Posterior thecal sac margin.

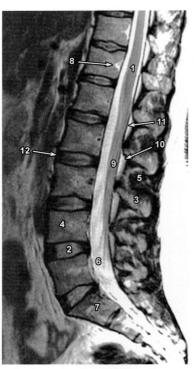

Figure 3-27 ▶ Mid Sagittal T2-weighted MRI. **1.** Conus medullaris **2.** L4-5 nucleus pulposus **3.** L3 spinous process **4.** L4 vertebral body **5.** Interspinous lumborum muscle and ligaments **6.** Subarachnoid space **7.** S1 vertebral body **8.** Basivertebral vein T12 **9.** Cauda equina **10.** Posterior epidural fat **11.** Posterior thecal sac margin **12.** Annulus fibrosus.

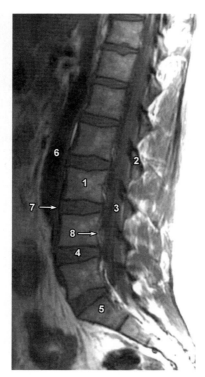

Figure 3-28 ▶ Left Paramidline Sagittal T1-weighted MRI. **1.** L3 vertebral body **2.** Left L2 lamina **3.** Cauda equina **4.** Intervertebral disc **5.** S1 vertebral body **6.** Aorta **7.** Anterior longitudinal ligament/anterior disc margin **8.** Anterior epidural space.

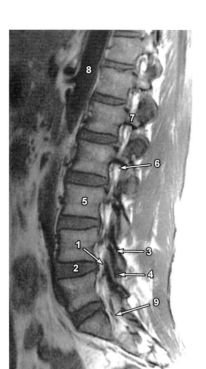

Figure 3-29 ▶ Left Parasagittal T1-weighted MRI. Medial neural foramen.
1. Superior articular process L5 **2.** L4-5 intervertebral disc **3.** L4 pars interarticularis
4. Inferior articular process L4 **5.** L3 vertebral body **6.** L2 nerve roots **7.** L1 pedicle
8. Aorta **9.** S1 nerve root.

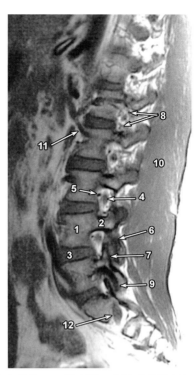

Figure 3-30 ▶ Left Parasagittal T1-weighted MRI. Lateral neural foramen
level. **1.** L4 vertebral body **2.** L4 pedicle **3.** L4-5 intervertebral disc **4.** L3 dorsal root
ganglion **5.** L3 intraforaminal vein **6.** L4 pars interarticularis **7.** L4-5 facet joint **8.** L1
superior and inferior foraminal veins **9.** Inferior articular process L5 **10.** Posterior
paraspinal muscles **11.** L2 lumbar vein.

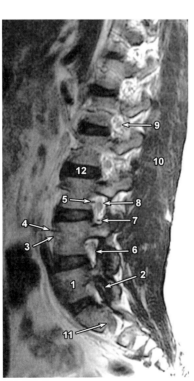

Figure 3-31 ▶ Left Parasagittal T2-weighted MRI. Lateral neural foramen
level. **1.** L5 vertebral body **2.** L5-S1 facet joint **3.** L4 lumbar artery **4.** L4 lumbar
vein **5.** Superior L3-4 intraforaminal vein **6.** L4-5 neural foramen **7.** Inferior L3-4
intraforaminal vein **8.** L3 nerve root **9.** L1 nerve root **10.** Posterior paraspinal
muscles **11.** Left S1 nerve root **12.** L2-3 intervertebral disc.

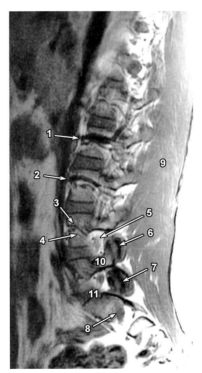

Figure 3-32 ▶ Right Paraspinal T1-weighted MRI. Far lateral level. **1.** L2
paravertebral venous plexus **2.** L3 paravertebral venous plexus **3.** L4 paravertebral
vein **4.** L4 lumbar artery **5.** L4 nerve root **6.** L4-5 facet joint **7.** L5-S1 facet joint
8. S1 nerve root **9.** Posterior paraspinal muscles **10.** L5 pedicle **11.** L5-S1 intervertebral disc.

COMPUTED TOMOGRAPHY (CT) CORONAL LUMBAR

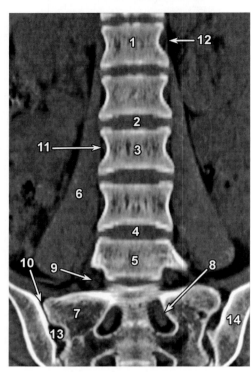

Figure 3-33 ▶ Coronal CT Image. Vertebral bodies. **1.** L1 vertebral body **2.** L2-3 intervertebral disc **3.** L3 vertebral body **4.** L4-5 intervertebral disc **5.** L5 vertebral body **6.** Psoas muscle **7.** Sacral wing (ala) **8.** S1 nerve root/sheath in S1 foramen **9.** L5 nerve root **10.** Sacroiliac joint, synovial-lined portion **11.** L3 lumbar vessels lateral to vertebral body **12.** Left crus of diaphragm **13.** Sacroiliac joint, fibrous portion **14.** Iliac wing.

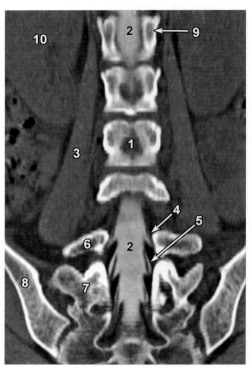

Figure 3-34 ▶ Coronal CT Image. L5 and S1 nerve roots. **1.** L3 vertebral body, posterior margin **2.** Contrast-opacified CSF, intrathecal subarachnoid space **3.** Psoas muscle **4.** Left L5 nerve root in opacified sleeve (pouch) **5.** Left S1 nerve root in opacified sleeve (pouch) **6.** Transverse process L5 **7.** Sacral wing (ala) **8.** Iliac wing **9.** L1 pedicle **10.** Right kidney.

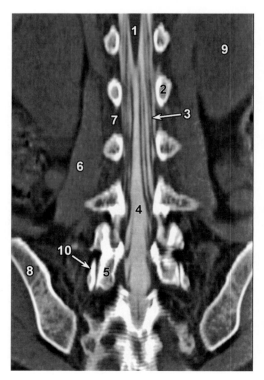

Figure 3-35 ▶ Coronal CT Image. Lumbar thecal sac. **1.** Conus medullaris **2.** L2 pedicle **3.** Cauda equina nerve roots in opacified cerebrospinal fluid (CSF) **4.** Contrast-opacified CSF, intrathecal subarachnoid space **5.** Inferior articular process L5 **6.** Psoas muscle **7.** L2-3 neural foramen **8.** Iliac wing **9.** Left kidney **10.** Superior articular process S1.

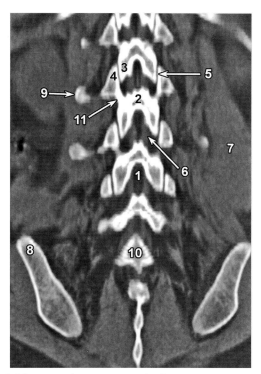

Figure 3-36 ▶ **Coronal CT Image.** Lumbar laminae. **1.** Posterior epidural fat L3-4 level **2.** Spinous process base L2 **3.** Inferior articular process L1 **4.** Superior articular process L2 **5.** L1-2 facet joint **6.** Ligamentum flavum **7.** Psoas muscle **8.** Iliac crest **9.** Transverse process L2 **10.** L5 spinous process base **11.** Pars interarticularis.

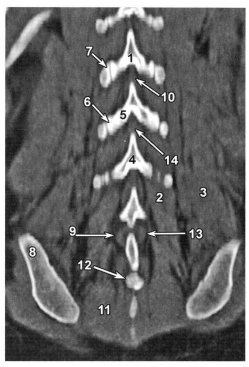

Figure 3-37 ▶ **Coronal CT Image.** Lumbosacral spinous processes. **1.** L1 spinous process **2.** Multifidus muscle **3.** Erector spinae muscle **4.** L3 spinous process **5.** L2 lamina **6.** Inferior articular facet L2 **7.** Superior articular facet L2 **8.** Iliac crest **9.** Right L4-5 interspinalis lumborum muscle **10.** L1-2 interspinous ligament **11.** Right multifidus muscle posterior to sacrum **12.** S1 spinous process **13.** Left L4-5 interspinalis lumborum muscle **14.** L2-3 interspinous ligament.

SACRAL ANATOMY

Douglas S. Fenton, M.D.

COMPUTED TOMOGRAPHY (CT) AXIAL OBLIQUE SACRUM

SUPERIOR TO INFERIOR

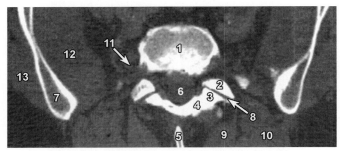

Figure 4-1 ▶ CT Axial Oblique. L5-S1 disc level. **1.** L5-S1 intervertebral disc **2.** S1 superior articular facet **3.** L5 inferior articular facet **4.** L5 lamina **5.** Spinous process L5 **6.** Thecal sac **7.** Iliac crest **8.** L5-S1 facet joint **9.** Multifidus muscle **10.** Erector spinae muscle group **11.** L5 nerve root **12.** Iliacus muscle **13.** Gluteus medius muscle.

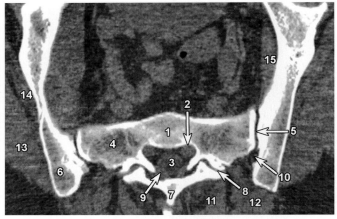

Figure 4-2 ▶ CT Axial Oblique. S1 vertebral body level. **1.** S1 vertebral body **2.** S1 nerve root **3.** Thecal sac **4.** Sacral ala **5.** Sacroiliac joint, synovial portion **6.** Iliac crest **7.** Median sacral crest **8.** Inferior L5-S1 facet joint **9.** Ligamentum flavum **10.** Sacroiliac joint, fibroligamentous portion **11.** Multifidus muscle **12.** Erector spinae muscle group **13.** Gluteus medius muscle **14.** Gluteus minimus muscle **15.** Iliacus muscle.

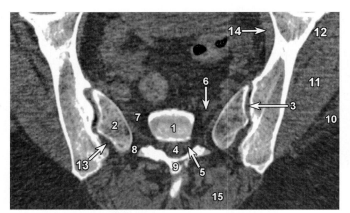

Figure 4-3 ▶ CT Axial Oblique. S1-2 disc level. **1.** S1-2 intervertebral disc, remnant **2.** Sacral ala **3.** Sacroiliac joint, synovial portion **4.** Thecal sac **5.** S2 nerve root **6.** S1 nerve root **7.** S1 ventral sacral foramen **8.** S1 dorsal sacral foramen **9.** Median sacral crest **10.** Gluteus maximus muscle **11.** Gluteus medius muscle **12.** Gluteus minimus muscle **13.** Sacroiliac joint, fibroligamentous portion **14.** Iliacus muscle **15.** Multifidus muscle.

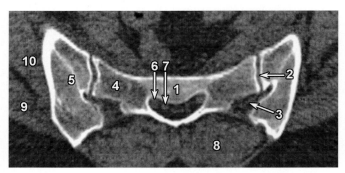

Figure 4-4 ▶ CT Axial Oblique. S2 vertebral body level. **1.** S2 vertebral body **2.** Sacroiliac joint, synovial portion **3.** Sacroiliac joint, fibroligamentous portion **4.** Sacral ala **5.** Iliac bone **6.** S2 nerve root **7.** S3 nerve root **8.** Multifidus muscle **9.** Gluteus maximus muscle **10.** Gluteus medius muscle.

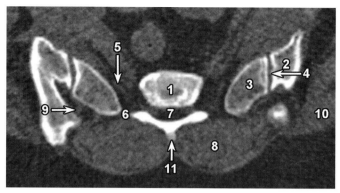

Figure 4-5 ▸ CT Axial Oblique. S2-3 disc level. **1.** S2-3 intervertebral disc, remnant **2.** Iliac bone **3.** Sacral ala **4.** Sacroiliac joint, synovial portion **5.** S2 nerve root exiting through S2 ventral sacral foramen **6.** S2 dorsal sacral foramen **7.** Sacral canal **8.** Multifidus muscle **9.** Sacroiliac joint, fibroligamentous portion **10.** Gluteus maximus muscle **11.** Median sacral crest.

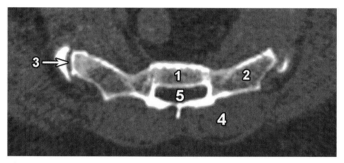

Figure 4-6 ▸ CT Axial Oblique. S3 vertebral body level. **1.** S3 vertebral body **2.** Sacral ala **3.** Sacroiliac joint, synovial portion **4.** Multifidus muscle **5.** Sacral canal.

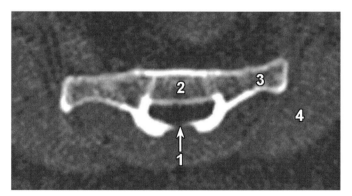

Figure 4-7 ▸ CT Axial Oblique. Lower S4 vertebral body level. **1.** Sacral hiatus **2.** S4 vertebral body **3.** Sacral ala **4.** Gluteus maximus muscle.

MAGNETIC RESONANCE IMAGING (MRI) AXIAL OBLIQUE SACRUM

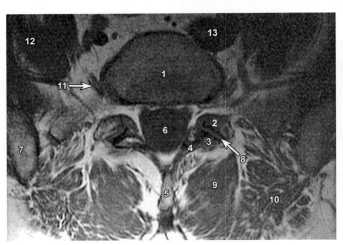

Figure 4-8 ▶ MR T1-weighted Axial Oblique. L5-S1 disc level. **1.** L5-S1 intervertebral disc **2.** S1 superior articular facet **3.** L5 inferior articular facet **4.** L5 lamina **5.** Spinous process L5 **6.** Thecal sac **7.** Iliac crest **8.** L5-S1 facet joint **9.** Multifidus muscle **10.** Erector spinae muscle group **11.** L5 nerve root **12.** Iliopsoas muscle **13.** Aorta.

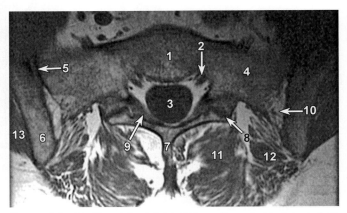

Figure 4-9 ▶ MR T1-weighted Axial Oblique. S1 vertebral body level. **1.** S1 vertebral body **2.** S1 nerve root **3.** Thecal sac **4.** Sacral ala **5.** Sacroiliac joint, synovial portion **6.** Iliac crest **7.** Median sacral crest **8.** Inferior L5-S1 facet joint **9.** Ligamentum flavum **10.** Sacroiliac joint, fibroligamentous portion **11.** Multifidus muscle **12.** Erector spinae muscle group **13.** Gluteus medius muscle.

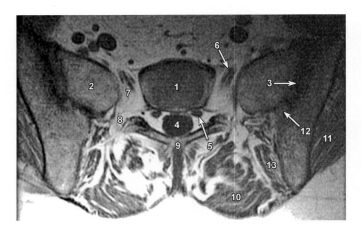

Figure 4-10 ▶ MR T1-weighted Axial Oblique. S1-2 disc level. **1.** S1-2 intervertebral disc, remnant **2.** Sacral ala **3.** Sacroiliac joint, synovial portion **4.** Thecal sac **5.** S2 nerve root **6.** S1 nerve root **7.** S1 ventral sacral foramen **8.** S1 dorsal sacral foramen **9.** Median sacral crest **10.** Multifidus muscle **11.** Gluteus maximus muscle **12.** Sacroiliac joint, fibroligamentous portion **13.** Erector spinae muscle group.

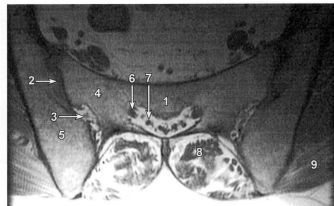

Figure 4-11 ▶ MR T1-weighted Axial Oblique. S2 vertebral body level. **1.** S2 vertebral body **2.** Sacroiliac joint, synovial portion **3.** Sacroiliac joint, fibroligamentous portion **4.** Sacral ala **5.** Iliac bone **6.** S2 nerve root **7.** S3 nerve root **8.** Multifidus muscle **9.** Gluteus maximus muscle.

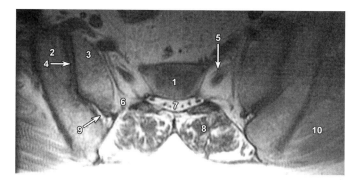

Figure 4-12 ▶ **MRI T1-weighted Axial Oblique.** S2-3 disc level. **1.** S2-3 inter-vertebral disc, remnant **2.** Iliac bone **3.** Sacral ala **4.** Sacroiliac joint, synovial portion **5.** S2 nerve root exiting through S2 ventral sacral foramen **6.** S2 dorsal sacral foramen **7.** Sacral canal **8.** Multifidus muscle **9.** Sacroiliac joint, fibroligamen-tous portion **10.** Gluteus maximus muscle.

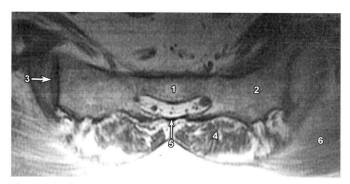

Figure 4-13 ▶ **MRI T1-weighted Axial Oblique.** S3 vertebral body level. **1.** S3 vertebral body **2.** Sacral ala **3.** Sacroiliac joint, synovial portion **4.** Multifidus muscle **5.** Sacral hiatus **6.** Gluteus maximus muscle.

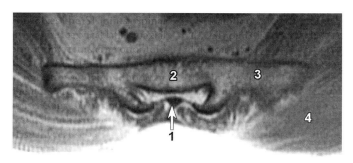

Figure 4-14 ▶ **MRI T1-weighted Axial Oblique.** S4 vertebral body level. **1.** Sacral hiatus **2.** S4 vertebral body **3.** Sacral ala **4.** Gluteus maximus muscle.

COMPUTED TOMOGRAPHY (CT)
SAGITTAL SACRUM

MIDLINE TO LATERAL

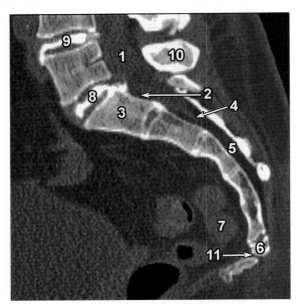

Figure 4-15 ▶ Midline Sagittal CT of the Sacrum. 1. Thecal sac **2.** Ventral epidural space **3.** S1 vertebral body **4.** Filum terminale/cauda dura **5.** Epidural fat in sacral spinal canal **6.** First coccygeal vertebral segment **7.** Rectosigmoid colon **8.** L5-S1 intervertebral disc, contrast from discogram **9.** L4-5 intervertebral disc, contrast from discogram **10.** L5 spinous process **11.** Sacrococcygeal joint.

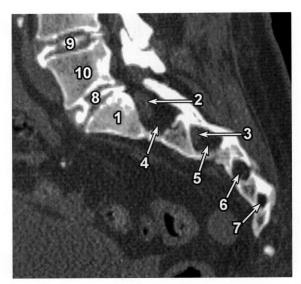

Figure 4-16 ▶ Off Midline Sagittal CT of the Sacrum. Mid foramen level. **1.** S1 vertebral body **2.** S1 nerve root **3.** S2 nerve root **4.** S1 sacral foramen **5.** S2 sacral foramen **6.** S3 sacral foramen **7.** S4 sacral foramen **8.** L5-S1 intervertebral disc, contrast from discogram **9.** L4-5 intervertebral disc, contrast from discogram **10.** L5 vertebral body.

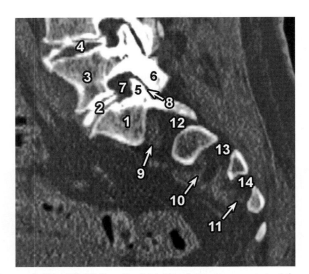

Figure 4-17 ▶ Off Midline Sagittal CT of the Sacrum. Lateral foramen level. **1.** S1 vertebral body **2.** L5-S1 intervertebral disc, contrast from discogram **3.** L5 vertebral body **4.** L4-5 intervertebral disc, contrast from discogram **5.** S1 superior articular process **6.** L5 inferior articular process **7.** L5-S1 neural foramen **8.** L5-S1 facet joint **9.** S1 nerve root **10.** S2 nerve root **11.** S3 nerve root **12.** S1 dorsal foramen **13.** S2 dorsal foramen **14.** S3 dorsal foramen.

MAGNETIC RESONANCE IMAGING (MRI) SAGITTAL SACRUM

MIDLINE TO LATERAL

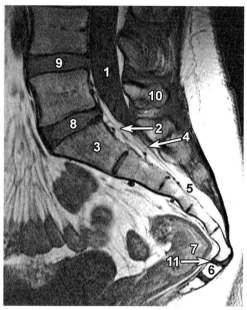

Figure 4-18 ► Midline Sagittal T1-weighted MRI of the Sacrum. **1.** Thecal sac **2.** Ventral epidural space **3.** S1 vertebral body **4.** Filum terminale/cauda dura **5.** Epidural fat in sacral spinal canal **6.** First coccygeal vertebral segment **7.** Rectosigmoid colon **8.** L5-S1 intervertebral disc **9.** L4-5 intervertebral disc **10.** L5 spinous process **11.** Sacrococcygeal joint.

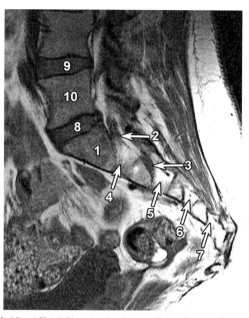

Figure 4-19 ► Off Midline Sagittal T1-weighted MRI of the Sacrum. Mid foramen level. **1.** S1 vertebral body **2.** S1 nerve root **3.** S2 nerve root **4.** S1 sacral foramen **5.** S2 sacral foramen **6.** S3 sacral foramen **7.** S4 sacral foramen **8.** L5-S1 intervertebral disc **9.** L4-5 intervertebral disc **10.** L5 vertebral body.

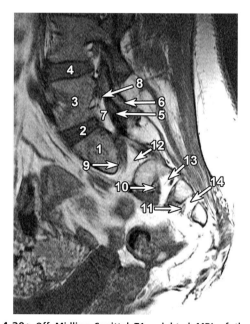

Figure 4-20 ► Off Midline Sagittal T1-weighted MRI of the Sacrum. Lateral foramen level. **1.** S1 vertebral body **2.** L5-S1 intervertebral disc **3.** L5 vertebral body **4.** L4-5 intervertebral disc **5.** S1 superior articular process **6.** L5 inferior articular process **7.** L5-S1 neural foramen **8.** L5 nerve root **9.** S1 nerve root **10.** S2 nerve root **11.** S3 nerve root **12.** S1 foramen, fat signal intensity **13.** S2 foramen, fat signal intensity **14.** S3 foramen, fat signal intensity.

COMPUTED TOMOGRAPHY (CT) CORONAL OBLIQUE SACRUM

ANTERIOR TO POSTERIOR

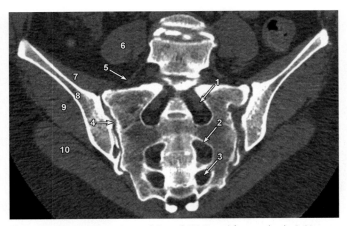

Figure 4-21 ▸ **Oblique Coronal Sacral CT.** Ventral foramen level. **1.** S1 nerve root in ventral S1 sacral foramen **2.** S2 nerve root in ventral S2 sacral foramen **3.** S3 nerve root in ventral S3 sacral foramen **4.** Sacroiliac joint, synovial portion **5.** Lumbosacral trunk **6.** Psoas muscle **7.** Iliacus muscle **8.** Iliac bone **9.** Gluteus medius muscle **10.** Gluteus maximus muscle.

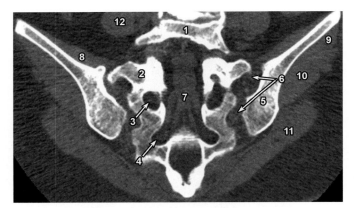

Figure 4-22 ▸ **Oblique Coronal Sacral CT.** Spinal canal level. **1.** L5 vertebral body **2.** Sacral ala **3.** S1 nerve root **4.** S2 nerve root **5.** Iliac bone **6.** Sacroiliac joint, fibroligamentous portion **7.** Thecal sac termination **8.** Iliacus muscle **9.** Gluteus minimus muscle **10.** Gluteus medius muscle **11.** Gluteus maximus muscle **12.** Psoas muscle.

ANTERIOR TO POSTERIOR

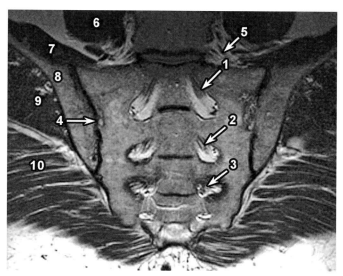

Figure 4-23 ▶ MRI T1-weighted Coronal Oblique. Ventral foramen level. **1.** S1 nerve root in ventral S1 sacral foramen **2.** S2 nerve root in ventral S2 sacral foramen **3.** S3 nerve root in ventral S3 sacral foramen **4.** Sacroiliac joint, synovial portion **5.** Lumbosacral trunk **6.** Psoas muscle **7.** Iliacus muscle **8.** Iliac bone **9.** Gluteus medius muscle **10.** Gluteus maximus muscle.

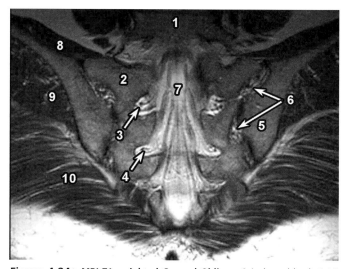

Figure 4-24 ▶ MRI T1-weighted Coronal Oblique. Spinal canal level. **1.** L5 vertebral body **2.** Sacral ala **3.** S1 nerve root **4.** S2 nerve root **5.** Iliac bone **6.** Sacroiliac joint, fibroligamentous portion **7.** Thecal sac termination **8.** Iliacus muscle **9.** Gluteus medius muscle **10.** Gluteus maximus muscle.

NOMENCLATURE FOR LUMBAR DISC DISEASE

Leo F. Czervionke, M.D.

DISCUSSION

The preferred terminology for describing disc "degeneration" and disc "displacement" has been the subject of debate and controversy for decades. Debate is still ongoing regarding the appropriate definition and usage of this terminology.

The most widely accepted recommended classification of lumbar disc pathology was formulated by a combined task force organized in the 1990s by the American Society of Spine Radiology (ASSR), the American Society of Neuroradiology (ASNR), and the North American Spine Society (NASS). The nomenclature recommendations formulated by this consensus task force were first published in 2001[1,2] and have been either endorsed, supported, or web-linked by the following organizations as of February 2003:

1. American Academy of Orthopedic Surgeons (AAOS)
2. American Academy of Physical Medicine and Rehabilitation (AAPM&R)
3. American Society of Neuroradiology (ASNR)
4. American Society of Spine Radiology (ASSR)
5. Joint Section on Disorders of the Spine and Peripheral Nerves of the American Association of Neurological Surgeons (AANS)
6. Congress of Neurological Surgeons (CNS)
7. European Society of Neuroradiology (ESNR)
8. North American Spine Society (NASS)
9. Physiatric Association of Spine, Sports, and Occupational Rehabilitation (PASSOR)

In spite of the broad support for usage of this nomenclature by the above organizations, confusion and controversy are still ongoing in regard to the proper usage of this terminology in the day-to-day clinical and imaging practice setting.[3] Presented below is a summary of this standard system of nomenclature as used to describe lumbar disc displacement with additional comments regarding the limitations and controversy concerning this nomenclature system used for describing disc displacement. This nomenclature system was established based on the morphologic appearance of the lumbar intervertebral disc as viewed on images.

It is important to bear in mind that this terminology was specifically designed for describing *lumbar* disc pathology, although this terminology is often applied to cervical and thoracic disc disease as well. Some problems do arise when this system of nomenclature is applied to disc disease in the cervical and thoracic sections of the spine. Some author comments and observations are included below to address these issues and other controversies regarding this classification system where appropriate.

A summary of the existing disc classification[1] with regard to disc displacement, along with our added commentary follows:

Disc Degeneration. The current classification of disc nomenclature includes disc degeneration, annular fissures (tears), and various types of disc herniations, with spondylosis deformans and intervertebral osteochondrosis being under the more general heading of degenerative or traumatic lesions of the intervertebral disc.

Comments: Controversy arises because there is no universal agreement as to when a *normally aging disc* becomes a *pathologically deranged disc*. Therefore no attempt is made in this section to discuss the nebulous concept of what constitutes disc degeneration as shown with imaging, from either a histologic or biomechanical perspective. This subject is dealt with in more detail in Chapter 17 concerning "internal disc derangement."

Spondylosis deformans (vertebral osteophytosis) in general is believed to be the result of the normal aging process of the disc, although its exact etiology is still poorly understood. Anterior and lateral vertebral osteophytes are usually not considered pathologic. However, osteophytes, during their development, can become inflamed and when this occurs, can be a source of intense localized back pain. Posterior or posterolateral vertebral osteophytes are also often considered pathologic because they can encroach upon the spinal canal, spinal cord, or nerve roots within the spinal canal or neural foramina. The term *intervertebral osteochondrosis* would be more accurately phrased as *discogenic vertebral osteochondrosis* because the vertebral endplate irregularities, endplate sclerosis, and reactive vertebral marrow abnormalities in this condition are induced by the degenerative disc process. Annular *tears* are more appropriately called *annular fissures* because "tear" implies a traumatic etiology, which is probably not the cause of annular fissures in most cases.

Disc Bulging. A bulging disc is not a herniated disc by definition. A "bulging" disc, as defined in this classification system, is a disc that extends beyond the outer vertebral body margins by more than 3 mm circumferentially (**Figs. 5-1 and 5-2**). The modifier "generalized" or "circumferential" may be used if the disc margin extends greater than 180 degrees (greater than 50%) of the disc circumference. The term *asymmetric disc bulge* is used if the disc bulges greater than 180 degrees but less than 360 degrees of the disc circumference (**Fig. 5-3**).

Comments: If the disc extends beyond the outer vertebral margins by 360 degrees (100%) of the disc circumference, it should be called a *bulging disc*, which is the same as a *diffuse disc bulge*, a *symmetric disc bulge*, a *generalized disc bulge*, or a *circumferential disc bulge*. We prefer to use the term *asymmetric disc bulge* to describe a broad-based extension of the disc margin that involves greater than 90 degrees but less than 360 degrees of the disc circumference. However, the current classification[1] defines an *asymmetric disc bulge* as one that involves greater than one half of the disc circumference and a *broad-based disc protrusion* as one that

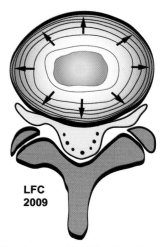

Figure 5-1 ▶ Bulging Intervertebral Disc (*arrows*). Axial plane. Other terms used to described the bulging disc include circumferential, symmetric, and generalized or diffuse disc bulge. The outer disc contour extends beyond the vertebral body margin in all directions.

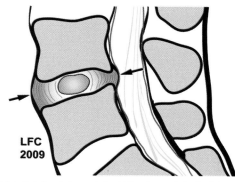

Figure 5-2 ▶ Bulging Intervertebral Disc (*arrows*). Sagittal plane. The anterior and posterior disc margins extend beyond the vertebral body margin to a similar degree.

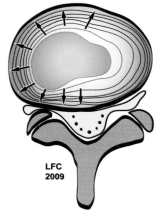

Figure 5-3 ▶ Asymmetric Disc Bulge (*arrows*). According to the present standard of nomenclature, this is a bulging disc that extends greater than 180 degrees of the disc circumference but not 360 degrees of the outer disc margin (i.e., is not symmetric or entirely circumferential).

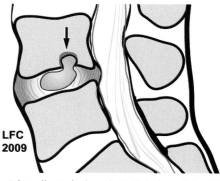

Figure 5-4 ▶ Schmorl's Node (*arrow*). Sagittal plane. A herniated disc that extends through a vertebral endplate. The classic Schmorl's node is positioned slightly posterior to the disc center in the AP (anteroposterior) dimension and most commonly involves the inferior vertebral endplate as shown here.

involves 90 to 180 degrees of the disc circumference. It is not possible with current imaging techniques to reliably differentiate a broad-based disc protrusion (which, by definition, histologically is "contained" by intact outer annular fibers) from a broad-based asymmetric bulging disc.

Disc Herniation. A disc herniation is a localized displacement of the disc margin beyond the usual confines of the disc. There are three major types of disc herniations based on the existing recommended classification, which is based on the morphologic imaging appearance of the disc as seen on computed tomography (CT) or magnetic resonance (MR): (1) disc protrusion, (2) disc extrusion, and (3) intravertebral disc herniation (Schmorl's node), which causes vertebral endplate deformity (*Fig. 5-4*). A **disc protrusion** is defined as a localized contour abnormality involving less than 180 degrees (less than 50% of the disc circumference) with a wide base where the disc projects beyond the vertebral body margin in all imaging planes. To quote the original publication, disc "protrusion is present if the greatest distance, in any plane, between the

edges of the disc material beyond the disc space is less than the distance between the edges of the base, in the same plane. The base is defined as the cross-sectional area of disc material at the outer margin of the disc space of origin, where disc material displaced beyond the disc space is continuous with disc material within the disc space."[1] Disc protrusions that involve less than 90 degrees (less than 25%) of the disc circumference are considered to be "focal" or "localized" disc protrusions (*Figs. 5-5 to 5-7*). Disc protrusions involving 90 to 180 degrees of the disc circumference are referred to as *broad-based disc protrusions* using this standard nomenclature[1,4,5] (*Fig. 5-8*).

A **disc extrusion** is a focal disc contour abnormality, less than 25% of the disc contour, that has a narrow neck in at least one imaging plane, axial or sagittal (*Figs. 5-9 and 5-10*). To quote the original publication, a disc "extrusion is present when, in at least one plane, any one distance between the edges of the disc material beyond the disc space is greater than the distance between the edges of the base, or when no continuity exists between the disc

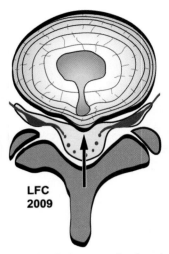

Figure 5-5 ► **Small, Localized Disc Protrusion** (*arrow*). Axial plane. This is a focal disc herniation with a wide base relative to the apex (*arrow*) that occupies less than 25% of the disc circumference. Histologically, the outermost layers of the annulus are intact, the nuclear material only extending through inner annular layers in this illustration.

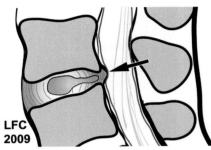

Figure 5-6 ► **Small Localized Disc Protrusion**. Sagittal plane, corresponding to the axial illustration in Figure II-1-3. The posterior disc margin indents the ventral aspect of the thecal sac (*arrow*). The posterior disc margin extends to a greater degree posteriorly than the anterior disc margin extends anteriorly. It may be difficult to differentiate a disc extrusion from protrusion based on a single sagittal image alone. Note that the nuclear material extends through inner annular lamellae, but outer annular layers remain intact.

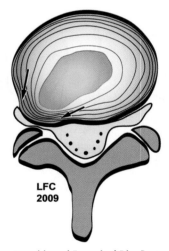

Figure 5-7 ► **Large Broad-based Foraminal Disc Protrusion.** The base of the protruding disc (*arrows*) is wider than its apex. Because this involves less than 25% of the disc circumference, this is still considered a *localized* disc protrusion based on current nomenclature. A foraminal disc extrusion with a wide base has an identical outer contour on cross-sectional imaging (see Fig. II-1-15). Because both are types of herniation, the distinction is not clinically important.

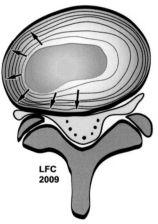

Figure 5-8 ► **Broad-based Disc Protrusion** (*arrows*). According to the currently accepted nomenclature, a *broad-based* disc protrusion is a disc herniation with a very wide *base* that involves 90 to 180 degrees of the disc circumference. I personally believe that any disc displacement that involves more than 25% of the disc circumference is not likely to represent a disc herniation histologically, that is, the outer annular fibers are likely to be intact. I, therefore, prefer to refer to any broad-based disc displacement that involves more than 90 degrees of the disc circumference as an *asymmetric disc bulge* (see Fig. II-1-3 for comparison).

material beyond the disc space and that within the disc space."[1] A disc extrusion has a relatively narrow neck relative to the apex of the disc fragment.

Disc Sequestration. A disc extrusion may be in continuity with the parent disc or separated from the parent disc, which is called *sequestered disc* or *free disc fragment*. Sequestered discs may be located at the disc level in the epidural space (*Fig. 5-11*). Often when this occurs, two distinct disc fragments are located at the disc level, which I call the "double fragment sign." Sequestered disc fragments commonly migrate above or below the parent disc level (*Fig. 5-12*). Herniated discs that migrate above or below the disc level may or may not be sequestered disc fragments, because the

migrated disc fragment above or below the intervertebral disc level may or may not be in continuity with the parent intervertebral disc. Rarely, sequestered discs may extend through the thecal sac into the subarachnoid space, a situation referred to as *intradural disc herniation* (*Fig. 5-13*).

Comments: A herniated disc fragment often contains portions of the nucleus pulposus as well as components of the inner and outer annulus, and sometimes portions of the cartilaginous end-plate.[6] Therefore the phrase *herniated nucleus pulposus* does not always completely describe the composition of the herniated disc fragment. Terms such as *prolapsed* or *ruptured discs* should be avoided in describing disc displacement.

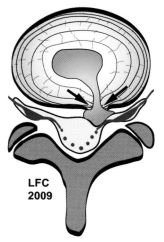

Figure 5-9 ▶ Disc Extrusion. Left paramidline, axial plane. The extruded disc has a narrow neck (*arrows*) where the nucleus extends through the outer annulus, that is, the base of disc fragment is relatively narrow compared with the apex of the fragment.

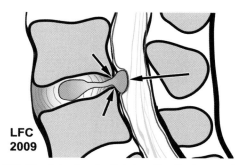

Figure 5-10 ▶ Disc Extrusion. Sagittal plane. The disc fragment (*long arrow*), composed of nuclear material and often fragments of the annulus and/or cartilaginous endplate, causes deformity of the ventral aspect of the thecal sac. The disc extrusion has a narrow neck (*small arrows*) where it penetrates the outer annulus.

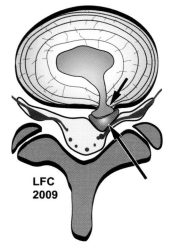

Figure 5-11 ▶ Sequestered Disc Fragment. At the intervertebral disc level. Typically, two disc fragments are present, which I refer to as a *double fragment sign*. An extruded disc (*short arrow*) is in continuity with the parent intervertebral disc. A separate *free* or *sequestered* disc fragment (*long arrow*) compresses the thecal sac and medial portion of nerve root at the intervertebral disc level.

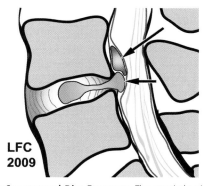

Figure 5-12 ▶ Sequestered Disc Fragment. The superiorly migrated, sequestered disc (*long arrow*) is in the ventral epidural space posterior to the vertebral body. A smaller extruded disc fragment is at the intervertebral disc level, and this fragment (*short arrow*) is in continuity with the parent intervertebral disc. Both disc fragments cause ventral thecal sac deformity.

It is unfortunate that the terms *protrusion* and *extrusion* were introduced into this classification. The term *disc herniation* may have been sufficient and is believed to be the least confusing term for describing a focal disc displacement in everyday practice.[5] The fundamental problem with subdividing disc herniations into protrusions or extrusions arises because it is not possible to discern the histologic nature of internal disc derangement precisely with current imaging techniques. The current system of nomenclature attempts to assess outer annular integrity based on the morphologic appearance of the outer disc contour. However, it is not possible to definitively differentiate a histologic disc protrusion (contained by outer annular fibers) from a histologic disc extrusion (not contained by annular fibers) based on the imaging appearance of the disc contour with existing imaging techniques (*Figs. 5-14 and 5-15*).

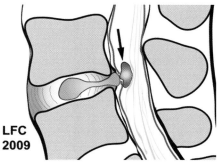

Figure 5-13 ▶ Sequestered Intradural Disc Herniation. An extruded disc fragment (*arrow*), separated from the parent disc, has ruptured through the anterior portion of the thecal sac into the subarachnoid space and is in direct contact with intrathecal nerve roots of the cauda equina.

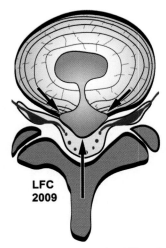

Figure 5-14 ▶ Wide-based (broad-based) Midline Disc Extrusion. There is a wide gap in the completely disrupted posterior portion of the outer annulus (*small arrows*) allowing the disc fragment to escape into the ventral epidural space where the extruded disc deforms the ventral surface of the thecal sac (*long arrow*). The base of the disc fragment is wide where it breaches the annulus (*short arrows*) relative to the smaller apex of the fragment (*long arrow*). Because one cannot determine with certainty whether outer annular fibers are completely disrupted based on the contour of the outer disc margin on cross-sectional imaging, a wide-based histologic disc extrusion cannot be differentiated from a moderate-sized or large focal disc protrusion.

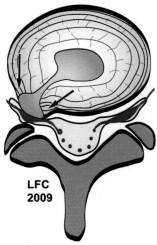

Figure 5-15 ▶ Foraminal Disc Extrusion. This is also referred to as a *lateral disc herniation* or *far lateral disc herniation*. Intraforaminal disc herniations often have a broad neck where they breach the annulus (*arrows*). Therefore, a foraminal disc protrusion is difficult or impossible to differentiate from a foraminal disc extrusion based on the imaging appearance of the outer disc contour on cross-sectional imaging (see Fig. 5-7). The foraminal disc herniation illustrated here is an extrusion histologically, because the nuclear fragment extends through all layers of the annulus posterolaterally on the right. The disc herniation compresses the nerve root within the neural foramen (intervertebral neural canal).

Histologically, a disc protrusion is a focal displacement of the disc nucleus and/or inner annulus through a defect in the annulus, with a variable number of outer annular fibers intact present. This is called a *contained disc*. In the pathologic literature, if the inner annular fibers are disrupted by protrusion of the nucleus, this is sometimes referred to as *internal mass displacement*.[7]

Regardless of the degree of circumferential focal contour abnormality, from the imaging standpoint, a disc protrusion by definition has a wide neck at the outer vertebral body margin.

Histologically, a disc extrusion is a focal extension of disc material beyond the confines of the annulus that extends through all layers of the annulus. If a focal disc contour abnormality has a narrow neck, as seen on one or more imaging planes, this is said to be consistent with a disc "extrusion", implying that all outer annular layers have been breached. However, it is not possible to say with certainty, based on imaging, whether or not all the annular layers are actually disrupted (see Fig. 5-11). Therefore we believe it is best to refer to large focal disc *protrusions* or *extrusions* simply as large *disc herniations*, so that the referring clinician reading the report of the imaging study knows beyond doubt that a significant disc abnormality is present.

Disc Size. In describing the size of the herniated disc in a report, a subjective semiquantitative size modifier should be used, such as *tiny*, *small*, *medium-sized*, or *large* to describe the size of the disc herniation.[4] Alternatively, some interpreters prefer to subjectively judge the size of a disc herniation relative to its encroachment upon the spinal canal and use the subjective terms *mild*, *moderate*, or *severe* to describe compromise of the spinal canal by the herniated disc.[4]

Disc Location. Regarding reporting of the location of the disc herniation (protrusion or extrusion), a disc herniation in the vertebral (central) canal may be located in a midline (central) position or paramidline (paracentral, left central, or right central) position.[1,4] In the intervertebral neural canal (neural foramen), the disc

fragment may be in the medial or lateral aspect of the neural canal (see Fig. 5-12). In the medial portion of the neural foramen, the disc herniation may be described as being at the disc level or infrapedicular. Extraforaminal disc herniations also occur, sometimes called *far lateral* disc herniations.[1] Migrated disc fragments in the epidural space may be at the suprapedicular, pedicular, or infrapedicular level.[8] A superiorly or inferiorly migrated herniated disc located medial to the pedicle is located in the lateral recess (also called the *subarticular zone*) and usually affects the nerve root, which lies adjacent to that pedicle.

Other Descriptive Modifiers. The use of the descriptive modifiers *focal* and *broad-based* are often not used consistently or accurately by persons reporting imaging studies according to the current system of nomenclature. In particular, the modifier *broad-based* is used loosely by some image study interpreters in describing nearly any disc contour abnormality from a small disc protrusion (which, by definition, always has a relatively *wide* base) to a circumferential disc bulge.

It is important to describe the effect of the disc displacement upon adjacent neural structures within the thecal sac, axillary root pouch, or neural foramen.[9] Any associated inflammatory mass or peridiscal hematoma occurring adjacent to a disc herniation should also be described in terms of its size and extent if present.

If possible, for optimal surgical planning purposes, it would be desirable to accurately describe the precise location of a given disc fragment in terms of its position with respect to the outer annulus, posterior longitudinal ligament, and thecal sac. However, this is often not possible within the limits of existing imaging techniques. Therefore we do not recommend using the terms *contained*, *uncontained*, *submembranous*, or *subligamentous* to describe disc herniations. Furthermore, these terms are not widely understood by image interpreters and clinicians alike. For example, from the surgeon's perspective, a *contained herniation* may include disc protrusion or subligamentous extrusion, and a *noncontained herniation* may include transligamentous extrusion or sequestration.[10]

In the routine imaging practice, for reporting disc disease and disc displacement, it is generally best to keep descriptions relatively concise and simple if possible. Those terms listed above and other terms pertaining to disc disease are described in detail in the excellent glossary at the end of the thorough disc nomenclature paper by Fardon and Milette.[1]

Cervical and Thoracic Disc Herniations. The majority of disc herniations in the cervical and thoracic spines, small or large, are disc protrusions because they have a relatively wide neck. Tiny midline or paramidline disc protrusions are extremely common in the cervical region and often asymptomatic. Disc extrusions do occur in both the cervical and thoracic spine. Cervical disc herniations are limited in their lateral extent by buttressing the effect of the uncinate processes. Although disc fragments may extend into the medial aspect of the cervical neural foramina, lateral disc herniations are rare in the cervical region. Cervical disc herniations are commonly superimposed upon generalized cervical disc bulging. Cervical and thoracic disc herniations may calcify along their outer margin and these are sometimes called *hard discs*.[1] These calcified herniated discs should not be confused with posterior vertebral osteophytes, which commonly form adjacent to a bulging or protruding cervical disc (so-called *disc-osteophyte complex*).

SUMMARY

It is important that the image study interpreter and referring clinician have a mutual understanding regarding the terminology being used in describing the imaging appearance of disc disease and disc displacement. Whether a herniated disc is a protrusion or extrusion is less important than the nature, location, and extent of the disc displacement and their effects on adjacent anatomic structures.

References

1. Fardon DF, Milette PC. Nomenclature and classification of lumbar disc pathology. Recommendations of the Combined Task Forces of the North American Spine Society, American Society of Spine Radiology, and American Society of Neuroradiology. *Spine (Phila Pa 1976)*. 2001;26(5):E93-E113.
2. Fardon DF, Milette PC. Nomenclature and Classification of Lumbar Disc Pathology: Recommendations of the Combined Task Forces of the North American Spine Society, American Society of Spine Radiology, and American Society of Neuroradiology. March 2001 [updated February 2003]; Available from: http://www.asnr.org/spine_nomenclature/.
3. Murtagh FR. The importance of being earnest—about disk nomenclature. *AJNR Am J Neuroradiol*. 2007;28(1):1-2.
4. Bailey WM. A practical guide to the application of AJNR guidelines for nomenclature and classification of lumbar disc pathology in magnetic resonance imaging (MRI). *Radiography*. 2006;12(2):175-182.
5. Milette PC. The proper terminology for reporting lumbar intervertebral disk disorders. *AJNR Am J Neuroradiol*. 1997;18(10):1859-1866.
6. Resnick D. Degenerative diseases of the vertebral column. *Radiology*. 1985;156(1):3-14.
7. Kramer J. *Intervertebral Disk Disease*. 2nd ed. New York: Thieme, 1992.
8. Wiltse LL, Berger PE, McCulloch JA. A system for reporting the size and location of lesions in the spine. *Spine*. 1997;22(13):1534-1537.
9. Khalatbari K, Azar M, Gazic FK. Reporting terminology for lumbar disk herniations: axial segmentation of the preneural foraminal portion of the lumbar nerve roots. *AJNR Am J Neuroradiol*. 2005;26(9):2430-2431; author reply 2431.
10. Ito T, Takano Y, Yuasa N. Types of lumbar herniated disc and clinical course. *Spine (Phila Pa 1976)*. 2001;26(6):648-651.

SECTION

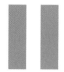

PAINFUL SPINE DISORDERS

ABDOMINAL AORTIC ANEURYSM

Leo F. Czervionke, M.D.

CLINICAL PRESENTATION

A sixty-five-year old white female with severe chronic obstructive pulmonary disease (COPD), hypertension, hyperlipidemia, and a 3-week history of mild-to-moderate intensity low back pain and abdominal pain. The patient has smoked one pack of cigarettes per day for the past 30 years. Physical examination reveals a pulsatile abdominal "mass."

IMAGING PRESENTATION

Computed tomography (CT) revealed a 7-cm diameter aneurysm of the infrarenal abdominal aorta *(Figs. 6-1 to 6-4)*. The thoracic aorta was markedly tortuous. The patient underwent arteriography, which documented the following findings: Aortic neck diameter adjacent to aneurysm—33 mm; maximal aortic aneurysm lumen diameter—58 mm; terminal aortic diameter—42 mm.

CLINICAL COURSE

The patient was not considered a surgical candidate for open aortic aneurysm repair because of her severe COPD and therefore underwent endovascular repair of the abdominal aortic aneurysm with insertion of an aortoiliac stent graft. The procedure was complicated by inadvertent rupture of the left common iliac artery, requiring interposition of an iliofemoral graft. The patient later developed an incisional hernia. She developed intermittent urinary tract infections requiring antibiotic therapy. A 2-year follow-up CT scan revealed diminished size of the aneurysm sac, measuring 5.9 × 4.4 cm in transverse diameter. Some calcium was observed in the intramural thrombus in the aneurysm sac, but no endoleak was observed.

DISCUSSION

An abdominal aortic aneurysm (AAA) is defined as an ectatic region of the aorta exceeding twice the normal diameter (approximately 3 cm). AAA should always be considered in an elderly patient with low back pain. However, abdominal aortic aneurysms are an uncommon cause of isolated low back pain but can cause severe back pain in the setting of a rupturing or dissecting aortic aneurysm. Aortic aneurysms rarely occur before age 50 but are found in 2% to 4% of the population after the age of 50.[1] For each decade beyond 65 years, the prevalence of AAA increases by 2% to 4% per decade. Average age of diagnosis of AAA is between 65 and 70 years old. Abdominal aortic aneurysms are more common in men.

The presence of coronary artery disease and peripheral vascular disease, as well as a family history of AAA, are strong risk factors.[1] Cigarette smoking is a particularly strong risk factor for the development of abdominal aortic aneurysms.[2-4] Smoking is believed to cause degradation in elastin within arterial walls.[5] Ruptured AAA and aortic dissection (AD) are significant causes of mortality in persons over age 65 years, accounting for nearly 1% of deaths. Rupture of an AAA and aortic dissection account for an estimated 15,000 deaths annually in the United States.[6] Aortic dissection and ruptured aortic aneurysm are life-threatening conditions that should always be considered in the diagnosis of back pain. The mortality for untreated aortic dissection reportedly increases at a rate of 1% to 3% per hour during the first 24 hours of illness.[3] For patients who have a rupturing AAA, the overall 30-day survival is reported to be as low as 11% despite rapid surgical intervention.[3]

Aortic Dissection

The incidence of aortic dissection (AD) is highest between ages 50 and 70 with a 5:1 male to female preponderance. The diagnosis is missed initially in up to 40% of these patients,[3] because they often lack the classic presentation, that is, a sharp, knifelike, tearing pain; 80% of aortic dissection patients are hypertensive. Other risk factors include smoking, hyperlipidemia, bicuspid aortic valve, coarctation of the aorta, decelerating trauma, cocaine usage, and inflammatory conditions of the aorta. Disorders that damage the aortic wall or are associated with an elastic deficiency in arterial walls predispose to aortic dissection; these include collagen vascular disorders, and Marfan, Ehlers-Danlos, Turner, and Noonan syndromes. Patients with aortic dissection may present with neurologic findings including cerebral and spinal cord ischemia. Quadriplegia, paraplegia, or unilateral paresthesias may also occur. Aortic dissection is caused by an intimal tear allowing luminal blood to extend into the medial layer of the aortic wall, forming a false channel or lumen within the media.

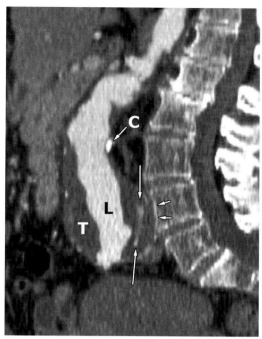

Figure 6-1 ▶ Abdominal Aortic Aneurysm, Peripheral Thrombus. Sagittal CTA image obtained following bolus IV contrast enhancement. Infrarenal abdominal aortic aneurysm causes smooth bone remodeling along anterior surface of L4 vertebral body (*short arrows*). Circumferential intra-aneurysmal thrombus located anterior (*T*) and posterior to contrast opacified aortic lumen (*L*). Curvilinear non-Calcified hyperdensity (*long arrows*) in thrombus posterior to aneurysm lumen represents opacified crescentic blood collection within posterior portion of thrombu.
C Calcified atheromatous plaque.

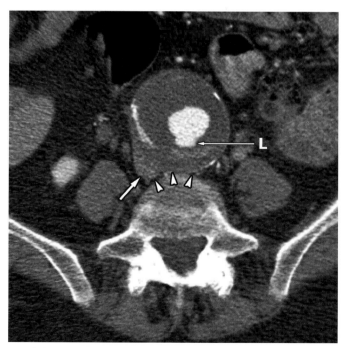

Figure 6-2 ▶ Abdominal Aortic Aneurysm, Likely Contained Rupture. Axial Contrast enhanced CTA image at L4-5 level. Focal posterior extension of contrast opacified aneurysm lumen (*L*) into posterior thrombus. The posterior aneurysm wall conforms to the anterior vertebral disc/vertebral margin (*arrowheads*), a finding that may be seen with chronic "contained" rupture. Note focal protuberance (*arrow*) of right posterolateral wall of aneurysm.

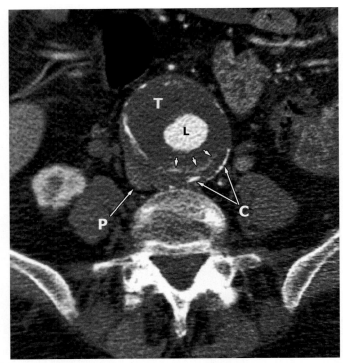

Figure 6-3 ▶ **Abdominal Aortic Aneurysm, Crescent Sign.** Axial Contrast enhanced CTA image of infrarenal abdominal aortic aneurysm. Relatively small aneurysm lumen (*L*) relative to thrombus (*T*). Outer wall of aneurysm has a discontinuous peripheral rim of calcification (*C*). Note more subtle crescentic hyperdensity (*small arrows*) with posterior thrombus representing a *crescent sign* which may indicate impending rupture. Demonstrated is focal protuberance (*P*) of the right posterolateral wall of the aneurysm.

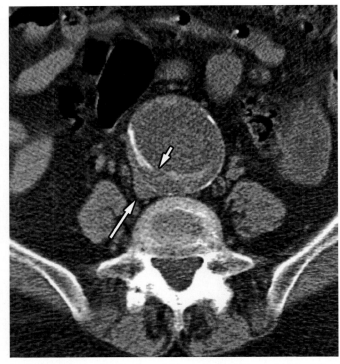

Figure 6-4 ▶ **Abdominal Aortic Aneurysm, Possible Impending Rupture.** Axial unenhanced CT image, L4-5 level. Note the focal discontinuity in the circumferential calcified plaque posterolaterally on the right (*short arrow*) and the focal protuberance of the outer aortic wall posterolaterally on the right (*long arrow*). These findings are worrisome for impending rupture.

Ruptured Aortic Aneurysm

The classic clinical triad of hypotension, abdominal pain, and a palatial mass occurs in less than 50% of patients who have a rupturing AAA.[3] Patients with rupturing AAA more commonly present with back pain, left lower-quadrant pain, flank pain, syncope, or lower-extremity paresthesias and therefore initially may be misdiagnosed as having renal colic or diverticulitis. The mortality rate in acute aortic rupture is approximately 60%,[4] whereas chronic ruptures may evolve over months with chronic low back pain. Aortic ruptures may occur at a relatively smaller diameter in females.[6] Observational evidence suggests that the presence of intraluminal thrombus may have a protective effect, because there tends to be relatively less intraluminal thrombus in ruptured aneurysms compared with nonruptured aneurysms.[1,7]

Inflammatory aneurysm is an older term used to describe a noninfectious aneurysm subtype that ruptures slowly producing an inflammatory response and adhesions in the retroperitoneal and prevertebral tissues surrounding the aorta.[8] The etiology of inflammatory aneurysms is not always known, but may be related to periaortic retroperitoneal fibrosis and possibly may be caused by autoimmune disease, such as rheumatoid arthritis, systemic lupus erythematosus, or giant cell arteritis.

Infectious (mycotic) aneurysms are uncommon, representing 1% to 2% of aortic aneurysms, but have a significantly higher incidence of rupture.[8,9] Hematogenous seeding of the aorta usually occurs because of septicemia, most commonly due to endocarditis. Most infected aortas occur in the thoracic or suprarenal abdominal aorta. Infected aortic aneurysms rarely cause infection in the adjacent spine.[9,10] Infections usually produce irregular vertebral bone destruction.[11] Discovertebral osteomyelitis or renal or psoas muscle infections may rarely cause infection of the aorta.[9] Tuberculous vertebral osteomyelitis and associated psoas muscle infections may extend to involve the aorta.[10,12]

Chronic contained ruptures of the aorta are relatively rare, occurring in approximately 2% of aortic aneurysms going to surgery.[4] Chronic contained ruptures (also called "leaking" or "sealed" ruptures) may incite a perianeurysmal inflammatory and fibrotic response, and these slowly enlarging aneurysms may erode the adjacent vertebrae, which can be responsible for the low back pain in these patients. Chronic contained ruptures of the aorta tend to cause smooth erosion of the vertebrae.[11] Support from the adjacent vertebrae may provide a tamponade effect for the chronic contained rupturing aneurysm.[13]

Penetrating atherosclerotic ulcers are found in 2% to 10% of patients examined for significant aortic abnormalities and may present with symptoms similar to aortic dissection, that is, chest pain and back pain. Penetrating aortic ulcers may result in hematoma formation in the aortic media but are not believed to be a common cause of aortic dissection. They can result in false aneurysm formation and, rarely, transmural rupture of the aorta.[14]

IMAGING FEATURES

Although abdominal aortic aneurysms (AAA) in patients who present with back pain may be overlooked based solely on clinical findings, when imaging is used to diagnose, findings that are quite characteristic of AAA will be shown. An AAA is diagnosed when the cross-sectional diameter of the abdominal aorta is 3 cm or greater (Figs. 6-1 to *6-6*). Computed tomography (CT), magnetic

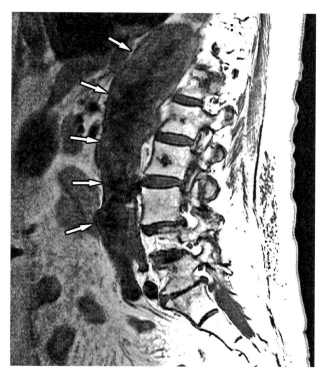

Figure 6-5 ▶ Abdominal Aortic Aneurysm. Sagittal T1-weighted MR image of the lumbar spine reveals a large tubular shaped T1 hypointense abdominal aortic aneurysm (*arrows*) located anterior to the vertebrae. The aneurysm measures 5.5 cm diameter. The aneurysm has a multilobular outer marginal contour. It is difficult to differentiate the aneurysm lumen from intra-aneurysmal thrombus based on T1-weighted images.

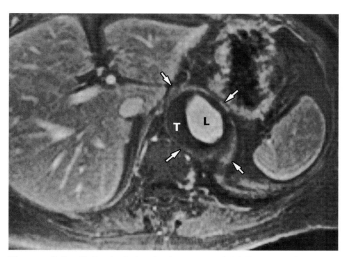

Figure 6-6 ▶ Abdominal Aortic Aneurysm. Axial fat-saturated, contrast enhanced 3D gradient echo (VIBE) MR image. Same patient as in Figure 5. The hyperintense aneurysm lumen (*L*) can be differentiated from the thrombus (*T*) on the VIBE image. Cross sectional diameter asymmetry (*arrows*) is a more worrisome finding than overall aortic tortuosity in assessing an aneurysm's tendency for rupture.

resonance (MR), computed tomographic angiography (CTA), magnetic resonance angiography (MRA), and conventional angiography are invaluable for diagnosing the features of aortic aneurysms, in establishing the prognosis, and for surgical planning prior to surgical or endovascular repair.

Aortic Ruptures

Aortic ruptures more commonly occur when the aortic diameter exceeds 5 cm and usually occur along the posterolateral wall of the abdominal aorta.[2] A retroperitoneal hematoma adjacent to an abdominal aortic aneurysm (AAA) is the most common imaging finding of AAA that has ruptured. Prior to actual rupture, it is important to recognize imaging findings that are warning signs for possible rupture of an AAA:

1. **Draped aorta sign.**[15] This is considered the most reliable sign of impending aortic rupture but can be seen with chronic contained ruptures also. This sign is considered positive if the posterior wall of the aorta is not identifiable as being distinct from adjacent structures or when the aorta closely conforms to the contour of adjacent vertebral bodies (see Fig. 6-2).
2. **Aortic cross-sectional diameter exceeding 5-cm diameter** (see Figs. 6-1 to 6-6). There is a high likelihood of rupture when the aorta exceeds 7 cm in diameter.[1] The cross-sectional lumen/thrombus ratio tends to increase with increasing aortic size.
3. **Cross-sectional diameter asymmetry.** The risk of aortic rupture is much higher when the transverse aortic diameter is greater than 5 cm.[2,5] A focal protrusion along the posterolateral aspect of the aorta may be a sign of an impending rupture (see Figs. 6-1 to 6-4). Cross-sectional aortic asymmetry is more significant than overall tortuosity of the aorta in considering the risk of aortic rupture (see Fig. 6-6).[2]
4. **An aortic diameter that enlarges at a rate of 10 mm or more per year.** This should raise concern regarding possible rupture and is an indication for surgical repair.[16]
5. **A focal discontinuity of peripheral wall calcifications.** This is more commonly observed in unstable or ruptured aneurysms (see Fig. 6-4).[1]
6. **Crescent sign.** A well-defined noncalcified, crescent-shaped region of increased attenuation within the thrombus of a large abdominal aortic aneurysm is a CT sign of acute or impending rupture.[17,18] The crescentic hyperdensity represents hematoma within the thrombus (see Fig. 6-1).
7. **Chronic contained ruptures.** These tend to cause smooth vertebral erosions, whereas infections more commonly cause irregular bone destruction when adjacent vertebrae are involved.[11,19]
8. **Ill-defined soft tissue.** Inflammatory aneurysms and infectious aneurysms characteristically have ill-defined soft tissue obscuring the para-aortic and prevertebral soft tissues on CT scanning and MR imaging.[8]

Aortic Dissection

Imaging findings include ectatic or aneurysmal dilation of the aorta and presence of an intimal flap separating the true lumen from a false lumen. The intimal flaps occur more commonly in the aortic arch and proximal descending thoracic aorta and frequently extend into the great neck vessels.

Penetrating atherosclerotic ulcers are found in 2% to 10% of patients examined for significant aortic abnormalities and may manifest with symptoms similar to aortic dissection, that is, chest pain and back pain. Ulcers are focal luminal projections into the aortic wall, typically located in the descending aorta, and are usually associated with severe atherosclerotic disease. Penetrating

aortic ulcers may result in hematoma formation in the aortic media but are not believed to be a common cause of aortic dissection. They are rarely associated with an intimal flap but may result in false aneurysm formation in the aortic wall and, rarely, transmural rupture of the aorta.[14]

DIFFERENTIAL DIAGNOSIS

The imaging appearance of aortic aneurysm is characteristic and is usually not confused with other disorders.

TREATMENT

1. **Medical therapy:** Includes drugs for controlling systemic hypertension and hyperlipidemia. Used for initial treatment of aortic aneurysms less than 5 cm in diameter and may be used for initial therapy for aortic dissections and penetrating atherosclerotic ulcers, depending on the clinical situation.
2. **Endovascular aneurysm repair (EVAR):** Current treatment of choice for uncomplicated abdominal aortic aneurysms less than 5 cm in diameter and patients with large (greater than 6 cm diameter) aneurysms who cannot undergo open surgical repair.
3. **Open surgical repair:** Usually reserved for large aortic aneurysms (greater than 6 cm diameter), complicated aortic aneurysms, infected aneurysms,[19] infected stent grafts, or aortoenteric fistulas.[1] Open surgical repair is used for treatment of complicated post-stent graft endoleaks.[20] An open surgical procedure is used for grafting the site of intimal disruption in acute aortic dissections and for treating penetrating aortic ulcers that do not respond to medical therapy if endovascular graft repair is not feasible.

References

1. Rakita D, Newatia A, Hines JJ, et al. Spectrum of CT findings in rupture and impending rupture of abdominal aortic aneurysms. *Radiographics.* 2007; 27(2):497-507.
2. Fillinger MF, Racusin J, Baker RK, et al. Anatomic characteristics of ruptured abdominal aortic aneurysm on conventional CT scans: Implications for rupture risk. *J Vasc Surg.* 2004;39(6):1243-1252.
3. Winters ME, Kluetz P, Zilberstein J. Back pain emergencies. *Med Clin North Am.* 2006;90(3):505-523.
4. Lai CC, Tan CK, Chu TW, Ding LW. Chronic contained rupture of an abdominal aortic aneurysm with vertebral erosion. *CMAJ.* 2008;178(8): 995-996.
5. Schuchmann JA. Back and thigh pain of unusual etiology complicates rehabilitation after bilateral total knee arthroplasty. *Am J Phys Med Rehabil.* 2008;87(7):585-589.
6. Broder J, Snarski JT. Back pain in the elderly. *Clin Geriatr Med.* 2007;23(2):271-289, v.
7. Siegel CL, Cohan RH, Korobkin M, et al. Abdominal aortic aneurysm morphology: CT features in patients with ruptured and nonruptured aneurysms. *AJR Am J Roentgenol.* 1994;163(5):1123-1129.
8. Arrive L, Correas JM, Leseche G, et al. Inflammatory aneurysms of the abdominal aorta: CT findings. *AJR Am J Roentgenol.* 1995;165(6): 1481-1484.
9. Macedo TA, Stanson AW, Oderich GS, et al. Infected aortic aneurysms: imaging findings. *Radiology.* 2004;231(1):250-257.
10. Chao TC, Chou WY, Teng HP, Hsu CJ. Osteomyelitis of multiple lumbar vertebrae associated with infected aortic aneurysm: a case report. *Kaohsiung J Med Sci.* 2003;19(9):481-485.
11. Choplin RH, Karstaedt N, Wolfman NT. Ruptured abdominal aortic aneurysm simulating pyogenic vertebral spondylitis. *AJR Am J Roentgenol.* 1982;138(4):748-750.

12. Falkensammer J, Behensky H, Gruber H, et al. Successful treatment of a tuberculous vertebral osteomyelitis eroding the thoracoabdominal aorta: a case report. *J Vasc Surg.* 2005;42(5):1010-1013.

13. Gandini R, Chiocchi M, Maresca L, et al. Chronic contained rupture of an abdominal aortic aneurysm: from diagnosis to endovascular resolution. *Cardiovasc Intervent Radiol.* 2008;31(Suppl 2):S62-S66.

14. Welch TJ, Stanson AW, Sheedy PF 2nd, et al. Radiologic evaluation of penetrating aortic atherosclerotic ulcer. *Radiographics.* 1990;10(4):675-685.

15. Halliday KE, al-Kutoubi A. Draped aorta: CT sign of contained leak of aortic aneurysms. *Radiology.* 1996;199(1):41-43.

16. Lederle FA, Johnson GR, Wilson SE, et al. Rupture rate of large abdominal aortic aneurysms in patients refusing or unfit for elective repair. *JAMA.* 2002;287(22):2968-2972.

17. Gonsalves CF. The hyperattenuating crescent sign. *Radiology.* 1999;211(1):37-38.

18. Mehard WB, Heiken JP, Sicard GA. High-attenuating crescent in abdominal aortic aneurysm wall at CT: A sign of acute or impending rupture. *Radiology.* 1994;192(2):359-362.

19. Diekerhof CH, Reedt Dortland RW, Oner FC, Verbout AJ. Severe erosion of lumbar vertebral body because of abdominal aortic false aneurysm: Report of two cases. *Spine.* 2002;27(16):E382-E384.

20. Baum RA, Stavropoulos SW, Fairman RM, Carpenter JP. Endoleaks after endovascular repair of abdominal aortic aneurysms. *J Vasc Interv Radiol.* 2003;14(9 Pt 1):1111-1117.

ANEURYSMAL BONE CYST

Leo F. Czervionke, M.D.

CLINICAL PRESENTATION

The patient is a 10-year-old female with a 7-month history of upper back pain, scapular pain, and rib pain. The patient developed bilateral lower extremity weakness 3 weeks prior to presentation.

IMAGING PRESENTATION

Magnetic resonance (MR) imaging reveals a solid and cystic mass containing heterogeneous regions of high, low, and intermediate signal intensity *(Fig. 7-1)*. The mass predominantly involves the posterior vertebral arch of T3 on the left, with some involvement of the T3 vertebral body on the left. Computed tomography (CT) shows a large soft tissue mass that has destroyed the T3 spinous process, left lamina, and left pedicle, and extends into the vertebral body *(Fig. 7-2)*.

DISCUSSION

The lesion that has become known as "aneurysmal bone cyst" was originally described by Van Arsdale in 1893, who referred to this lesion as a "ossifying hamartoma."[1] The term *aneurysmal bone cyst* was first used for describing these lesions in 1942 by Jaffe and Lichtenstein.[2] Aneurysmal bone cysts are rare, benign, yet locally destructive; they are expansile, highly vascular bone lesions.[3] They represent approximately 1% to 2% of primary bone "tumors,"[4] although they are not true neoplasms. The majority of aneurysmal bone cysts arise in the metaphysis of the long bones. Approximately 10% to 20% of aneurysmal bone cysts occur in the axial skeleton.[5] Spinal aneurysmal bone cysts occur most frequently in the thoracic spine, followed by the lumbar spine, cervical spine, and least commonly in the sacrum.[4,6,7] Aneurysmal bone cysts in the sacrum or pelvis tend to be more aggressive lesions that cause extensive bone destruction *(Figs. 7-2 to 7-8)*.[3,8] Spinal aneurysmal bone cysts nearly always arise in the posterior vertebral arch but frequently extend into the ipsilateral pedicle and vertebral body, epidural space, or adjacent neural foramen (see Figs. 7-1 and 7-2). They rarely extend into the nearby ribs or adjacent vertebrae.

The majority of patients who present with aneurysmal bone cyst are younger than age 20, and there is a slight female predilection;[4,7] 95% of patients with spine lesions present with back pain, usually slow in onset.[3] These patients may have scoliosis. Myelopathy or radiculopathy may be present if the spinal cord or nerve roots are compressed. Paresthesias, loss of anal sphincter tone, leg weakness, and urinary retention may occur with spinal or sacral aneurysmal bone cysts depending on their location and extent.[3]

Secondary aneurysmal bone cysts may arise in or adjacent to other primary bone tumors in a small percentage of cases, especially in giant cell tumors and osteoblastomas, but they also occasionally occur in osteosarcomas, chondroblastomas, fibrous histiocytomas, and less commonly in other bone tumors.[4,9,10] The etiology of aneurysmal bone cysts is unknown. It is possible that some of these tumors arise secondary to vascular anomalies such as arteriovenous (AV) fistula formation in bone secondary to trauma or neoplasm. Hereditary influences are believed to play a role in a significant number of *primary* aneurysmal bone cysts. Translocations or deletions in chromosomes 16 and 17 have been demonstrated in some patients.[11,12]

Histologically, the typical aneurysmal bone cyst is composed of blood-filled cavities with surrounding trabecular and solid elements comprised of vascularized stromal tissues containing multinucleated osteoclastic giant cells, spindle cells, fibroblasts, myofibroblasts, hemosiderin deposits, and a variable amount of cartilage and osteoid that may be mineralized.[4]

IMAGING FEATURES

Aneurysmal bone cysts are expansile, osteolytic lesions that arise in the posterior vertebral arch.[9] They can cause localized cortical thinning, bone erosion, or destruction, which may be visible on radiographs and CT and MR images. Because lesions commonly extend into the vertebral body, the pedicle on the side of the tumor is often eroded or destroyed (see Fig. 7-2). Cortical thinning and bone destruction are best demonstrated by CT. There is often a thin rim of cortical bone along the expanded remodeled margin of the tumor and a sharp zone of transition between the tumor and adjacent normal bone (see Fig. 7-4). There may be mineralized osteoid or cartilaginous elements in the septated or solid portions of the lesion histologically.[4] Occasionally, a sufficient quantity of this calcification is present in the lesion, which is then visible on CT images or radiographs. Patients with aneurysmal bone cysts may present with vertebral collapse visible as vertebral planum on radiographs or CT.[13]

These tumors typically are comprised of multiloculated cavities containing cystic bloody liquid and debris, with adjacent septations and some solid elements (see Fig. 7-1). The cysts appear hypodense and of mixed density on CT and are heterogeneous in intensity on

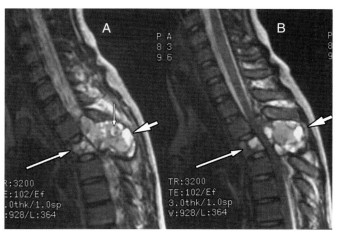

Figure 7-1 ▶ T3 Vertebral Aneurysmal Bone Cyst. T2-weighted left parasagittal MR image **A** and mid sagittal image **B**. The aneurysmal bone cyst predominantly involves the posterior vertebral arch of T3 (*short arrow*). The lesion contains multiple ovoid areas of heterogeneous signal intensity that has replaced the left posterior vertebral arch and left posterolateral aspect of the vertebral body (*long arrow*). At least one loculation (*thin arrow in image* **A**) contains a fluid/fluid level, which is vertical on the image with the patient supine. The lesion extends into the epidural space causing cord compression. The lesion was largely cystic in nature at surgery, containing multiple loculated cystic collections of bloody liquid.

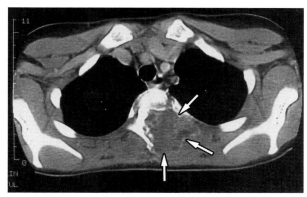

Figure 7-2 ▶ T3 Vertebral Aneurysmal Bone Cyst. Contrast enhance axial CT image. Minimal contrast enhancement is seen along the margin of the lesion (*arrows*). The lesion was almost entirely cystic in nature at surgery containing multiloculated bloody liquid at different stages of metabolic degradation. Ovoid hypodense areas with the lesion represent lower density liquid-filled cystic cavities. More dense areas within the lesion represent cystic cavities containing more proteinaceous bloody liquid.

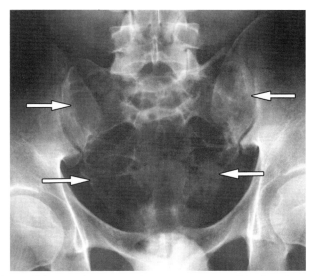

Figure 7-3 ▶ Sacral Aneurysmal Bone Cyst. 25-year-old male patient with 2-month history of low-back pain and hamstring distribution pain. AP radiograph of sacrum shows a subtle low a density "bubbly lesion" throughout the sacrum (*arrows*), which is slightly less dense compared to the normal density of the iliac bones. This lesion could easily be overlooked on this radiograph, possible mistaken for overlying bowel.

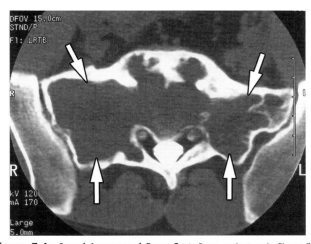

Figure 7-4 ▶ Sacral Aneurysmal Bone Cyst. Same patient as in Figure 7-3. Axial CT Image reveals a homogeneous hypodense lesion (*arrows*) that occupies almost the entire sacral contents, sparing the cortical margins of the sacrum. The sacroiliac joints and adjacent cortex remains intact.

MR. Fluid and fluid levels may be visible on CT or MR with the denser T2 hypointense liquid and sediment visible posteriorly and T2 hyperintense liquid visible anteriorly.[4,5,7,8] In some cases, the aneurysmal bone cyst contains a mixture of both cystic and solid components; 3% to 7% of aneurysmal bone cysts lack cystic elements, and those appear as solid "tumors" on CT and MR images.[6] Some aneurysmal bone cysts appear entirely homogeneous in density on CT and homogeneous in signal intensity on MR, containing homogeneous liquid (see Figs. 7-4 to 7-8).

Aneurysmal bone cysts tend to be enhanced heterogeneously after IV contrast administration. Solid or septated portions of the tumor are enhanced after IV contrast. The cystic cavities show no significant contrast after iodinated contrast enhancement, but the margins of the cyst often enhance (see Figs. 7-2 and 7-7). The liquid within the cyst may accumulate the paramagnetic contrast agent, so the cystic contents may enhance faintly and homogeneously after paramagnetic contrast administration (see Fig. 7-7). Solid portions of the "cyst" enhance more intensely. Aneurysmal bone cysts commonly extend into the epidural space or adjacent neural foramen where they can compress the spinal cord or nerve roots (see Fig. 7-1, *B*).[14] The extraosseous extent is best shown with MR imaging.

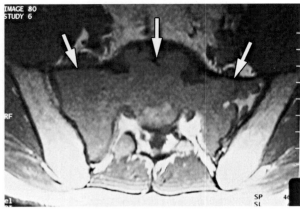

Figure 7-5 ▶ Sacral Aneurysmal Bone Cyst. Axial T1 weighted MR image corresponding to same slice location as CT image in Figure 7-4. The sacrum (*arrows*) is uniformly hypointense relative to the iliac bones.

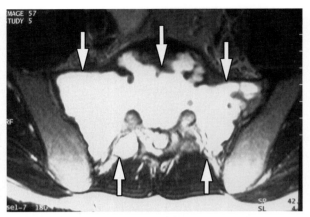

Figure 7-6 ▶ Sacral Aneurysmal Bone Cyst. Same patient as in Figure 7-5. Corresponding T2 weighted MR axial image. The sacral contents are almost entirely filled by homogeneously T2 hyperintense liquid (*arrows*).

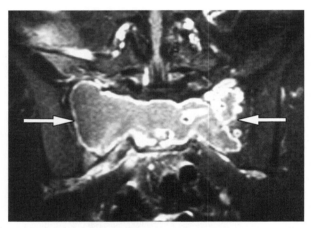

Figure 7-7 ▶ Sacral Aneurysmal Bone Cyst. Same patient as Figures 7-4 to 7-6. Contrast enhanced fat saturated coronal T1-weighted MR image. There is faint enhancement of the cystic contents within the sacrum. The margins of the cyst (*arrows*) enhance more intensely than the central portion of the cyst.

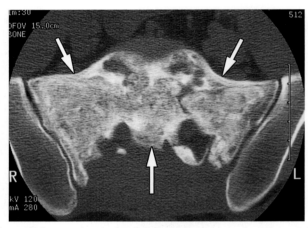

Figure 7-8 ▶ Sacral Aneurysmal Bone Cyst. Same patient as in Figures 7-3 to 7-7. Following sacral curettage, the sacral cavity was packed with morsellized bone allograft resulting in heterogeneous hyperdense appearance of the sacrum (*arrows*) on this axial postoperative CT scan. Compare with preoperative CT scan, Figure 7-4.

Angiography demonstrates hypervascularity along the margins of the aneurysmal bone cysts[8] or throughout the lesion in the case of predominantly solid lesions. Cervical aneurysmal bone cysts may encase the vertebral artery.[15]

Radionuclide bone scanning typically shows increased blood flow to the lesion and increased uptake in the solid portions of the tumors. Predominantly cystic lesions show increased uptake along the periphery of the aneurysmal bone cyst where vascularity is usually greatest. Predominantly cystic aneurysmal bone cysts have a "doughnut" appearance on bone scans, the cystic center of the lesion being photopenic.[4] A photopenic doughnut appearance may also be seen with giant cell tumors.[7]

DIFFERENTIAL DIAGNOSIS

1. **Giant cell tumor:** Tends to occur in young to middle-aged adults. These tumors are expansile lesions that may arise in the posterior vertebral arch, vertebral body, or sacrum. Smaller lesions are confined to the bone and have a thin shell of expanded bone. Larger lesions tend to break through the cortex and may involve the paravertebral soft tissues (***Figs. 7-9 and 7-10***). Aneurysmal bone cysts may arise within or adjacent to giant cell tumors.

2. **Lymphoma:** May be confused with aneurysmal bone cyst on radiographs or CT. Lymphoma can cause an osteolytic, expansile lesion in bone and may be confused with the solid form of aneurysmal bone cyst on radiographs, CT, and MR. Lymphoma is typically a solid tumor, lacking cystic components. Lymphoma may remain confined to the marrow cavity of the involved vertebra or sacrum. Large lymphomas may break through the cortex into the adjacent soft tissues. Lymphoma is often very radiosensitive and may respond dramatically to radiation therapy (***Fig. 7-11***).

3. **Metastasis:** May manifest as an osteolytic expansile mass in the posterior vertebral elements, vertebral bodies, or sacrum. Look for other metastases elsewhere in the spine and skeleton.

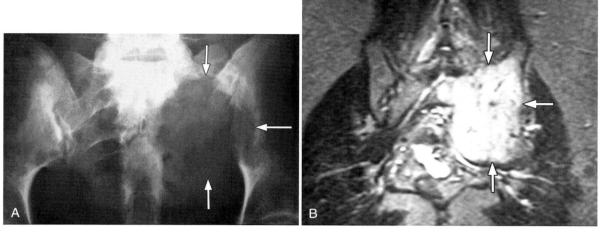

Figure 7-9 ▶ Sacral Giant Cell Tumor. 25-year-old female patient with vague pelvic and lumbosacral pain. AP radiographic image **A** reveals a large ovoid radiolucent region (*arrows*) in the left sacral wing representing an osteolytic lesion. In coronal T2-weighted MR image **B**, the left sacral wing and portion of the left iliac wing are replaced by a heterogeneous T2 hyperintense soft-tissue mass (*arrows*), which obliterates the left sacroiliac joint.

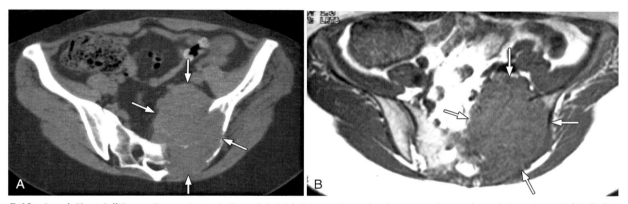

Figure 7-10 ▶ Sacral Giant Cell Tumor. Same patient as in Figure 7-9. Axial CT image **A** reveals a large expansile mass (*arrows*) destroying the left half of the sacrum and medial portion of the left iliac bone. The mass is nearly homogeneous in density, similar that of muscle. A large anterior exophytic component of the mass (*anterior arrows*) extends into the pelvic soft tissues. In corresponding axial T1-weighted MR image **B**, the mass (*arrows*) is nearly homogeneous, hypointense relative to bone marrow and slightly hyperintense relative to muscle. The mass obliterates the left sacroiliac joint.

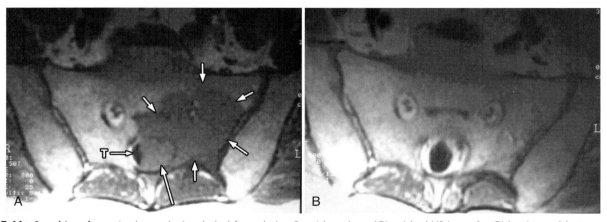

Figure 7-11 ▶ Sacral Lymphoma. Involves predominantly the left sacral wing. On axial unenhanced T1-weighted MR image **A**, a T1 hypointense (*short arrows*) is seen in the left sacral wing. A component of the mass extends into the left S1 neural foramen and into the sacral spinal canal (*long arrow*) where it displaces the thecal sac (*T*) to the right. On unenhanced T1-weighted MR image **B** obtained 6 months later following radiation therapy, the sacrum appears normal and the tumor in the left S1 neural foramen and sacral spinal canal has resolved completely.

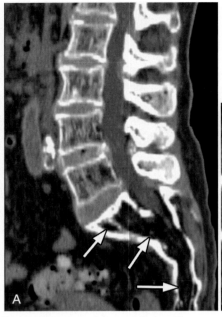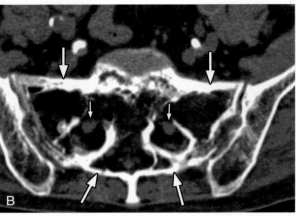

Figure 7-12 ▶ **Diffuse Replacement of the Sacral Cancellous Bone by Fat.** Sagittal CT image **A** and axial CT image **B**. The cortical margins of the sacrum (*arrows in image* **A**, *long arrows in image* **B**) are thickened and sclerotic but not expanded. Hypodense fatty tissue replace's the sacral cancellous bone and also fills the sacral spinal canal and neural foramina adjacent to the S1 nerve roots (*short arrows in image* **B**).

Metastases are usually heterogeneous lesions that infiltrate the marrow cavities of bone but also produce cortical bone destruction and commonly invade the epidural space or paraspinal soft tissues.

4. **Plasmacytoma:** Fairly homogeneous solid masses that frequently occur in the setting of multiple myeloma. Plasmacytomas may arise in the paraspinal soft tissues, vertebrae, or sacrum. Bone lesions may remain confined to the marrow cavity but can remodel and erode the cortex.

5. **Osteoblastoma:** Can mimic aneurysmal bone cyst except that usually disorganized bone formation is present in the tumor. Osteoblastomas usually arise in the posterior vertebral arch in young persons. Occasionally, osteoblastomas may contain aneurysmal bone cysts.

6. **Telangiectatic osteosarcoma:** An aggressive appearing and behaving malignant bone tumor that may involve the vertebral body, posterior arch, or both. These tumors usually have poorly defined margins with a permeative or moth-eaten appearance in the adjacent bone. Telangiectatic osteosarcomas may contain blood-filled cavities displaying fluid/fluid levels, which resemble aneurysmal bone cyst formation in the tumor.

7. **Fatty replacement of the sacrum:** Rarely, the sacrum is completely replaced by fatty marrow, which may be confused with an aneurysmal bone cyst as shown by CT. However, MR imaging reveals the fatty nature of this tissue within the sacrum (*Fig. 7-12*).

PROGNOSIS AND TREATMENT

Aneurysmal bone cysts are histologically benign lesions and usually have good prognosis but can recur after therapy. Post adolescence, the tumor size may stabilize. Many methods have been used to treat aneurysmal bone cysts. Some aneurysmal bone cysts will recur after treatment, especially if they are not excised completely.

Treatment includes the following:

1. **Therapeutic embolization:** Can be used as the initial or sole treatment of aneurysmal bone cysts if there is no neurologic impairment, vertebral fracture, or spinal instability.[9,16,17] Embolization alone may be sufficient to arrest tumor growth and alleviate the patient's back pain. If embolization fails, other treatment options outlined below are still available. Embolization is more commonly performed before surgical excision or curettage of aneurysmal bone cysts.[18]

2. **Surgical excision and curettage:** Method often used for lesions larger than 5 cm in diameter.[3] En bloc removal allows the greatest chance for a complete cure.[9,13] Preoperative embolization is useful to devascularize the tumor beforehand to minimize blood loss and allows removal of a greater portion of the lesion.[15,18] With spinal aneurysmal bone cysts, en bloc removal may not be possible because of the presence of vital nearby neural or vascular structures. The spine frequently has to be surgically fused after removal of the tumor, especially if vertebral collapse or vertebral subluxation has occurred. Fusion is often necessary in the immature spine after aneurysmal bone removal to minimize the development of kyphosis.[2,18]

3. **Intralesional curettage and bone grafting:** Method considered by many to be the procedure of choice for smaller lesions (less than 5 cm diameter) to preserve anatomic function and minimize deformity.[3] The cyst may recur after curettage alone, so adjunctive therapy is often used.[13]

4. **Radiotherapy:** Has been used alone to treat aneurysmal bone cysts.[9] Radionuclide ablation of an aneurysmal bone cyst has been described.[19] More commonly, adjunctive radiotherapy

after embolization, curettage, or excision is used, especially when the lesion cannot be completely removed. However, radiotherapy carries the risk of developing a posts radiation sarcoma years later.[3,20,21]

5. **Adjuvant cryotherapy:** Used after curettage in some patients.[20,22]

6. **Adjuvant chemical cautery:** Performed using phenol and acid alcohol after curettage. This method is not recommended with sacral lesions.[3]

7. **Sclerotherapy:** Intralesional percutaneous injection of sclerosing agents such as calcitonin and methylprednisolone has been described.[23]

8. **Repeat curettage:** Most commonly used along with intralesional bone grafting or radiotherapy to treat recurrent aneurysmal bone cysts .[3]

References

1. Van Arsdale WW. Ossifying hamartoma. *Ann Surg*. 1893;18:8-17.
2. Jaffe JL, Lichtenstein L. Solitary unicameral bone cyst with emphasis on the roentgen picture. *Arch Surg*. 1942;44:1004-1025.
3. Papagelopoulos PJ, Choudhury SN, Frassica FJ, et al. Treatment of aneurysmal bone cysts of the pelvis and sacrum. *J Bone Joint Surg Am*. 2001;83-A: 1674-1681.
4. Rodallec MH, Feydy A, Larousserie F, et al. Diagnostic imaging of solitary tumors of the spine: what to do and say. *Radiographics*. 2008;28: 1019-1041.
5. Pennekamp W, Peters S, Schinkel C, et al. Aneurysmal bone cyst of the cervical spine (2008:7b). *Eur Radiol*. 2008;18:2356-2360.
6. Suzuki M, Satoh T, Nishida J, et al. Solid variant of aneurysmal bone cyst of the cervical spine. *Spine*. 2004;29:E376-381.
7. Murphey MD, Andrews CL, Flemming DJ, et al. From the archives of the AFIP. Primary tumors of the spine: radiologic pathologic correlation. *Radiographics*. 1996;16:1131-1158.
8. Pogoda P, Linhart W, Priemel M, et al. Aneurysmal bone cysts of the sacrum: clinical report and review of the literature. *Arch Orthop Trauma Surg*. 2003;123:247-251.
9. Boriani S, De Iure F, Campanacci L, et al. Aneurysmal bone cyst of the mobile spine: report on 41 cases. *Spine*. 2001;26:27-35.
10. Kransdorf MJ, Sweet DE. Aneurysmal bone cyst: concept, controversy, clinical presentation, and imaging. *AJR Am J Roentgenol*. 1995;164:573-580.
11. Oliveira AM, Chou MM, Perez-Atayde AR, Rosenberg AE. Aneurysmal bone cyst: a neoplasm driven by upregulation of the USP6 oncogene. *J Clin Oncol*. 2006;24:e1; author reply e2.
12. Panoutsakopoulos G, Pandis N, Kyriazoglou I, et al. Recurrent t(16;17) (q22;p13) in aneurysmal bone cysts. *Genes Chromosomes Cancer*. 1999;26: 265-266.
13. Codd PJ, Riesenburger RI, Klimo P Jr, et al. Vertebra plana due to an aneurysmal bone cyst of the lumbar spine: case report and review of the literature. *J Neurosurg*. 2006;105:490-495.
14. Chan MS, Wong YC, Yuen MK, Lam D. Spinal aneurysmal bone cyst causing acute cord compression without vertebral collapse: CT and MRI findings. *Pediatr Radiol*. 2002;32:601-604.
15. Khalil IM, Alaraj AM, Otrock ZK, et al. Aneurysmal bone cyst of the cervical spine in a child: case report and review of the surgical role. *Surg Neurol*. 2006;65:298-303; discussion 303.
16. Koci TM, Mehringer CM, Yamagata N, Chiang F. Aneurysmal bone cyst of the thoracic spine: evolution after particulate embolization. *AJNR Am J Neuroradiol*. 1995;16:857-860.
17. DeRosa GP, Graziano GP, Scott J. Arterial embolization of aneurysmal bone cyst of the lumbar spine: a report of two cases. *J Bone Joint Surg Am*. 1990;72:777-780.
18. Garg S, Mehta S, Dormans JP. Modern surgical treatment of primary aneurysmal bone cyst of the spine in children and adolescents. *J Pediatr Orthop*. 2005;25:387-392.
19. Bush CH, Drane WE. Treatment of an aneurysmal bone cyst of the spine by radionuclide ablation. *AJNR Am J Neuroradiol*. 2000;21:592-594.
20. Marcove RC, Sheth DS, Takemoto S, Healey JH. The treatment of aneurysmal bone cyst. *Clin Orthop Relat Res*. 1995:157-163.
21. Frassica FJ, Frassica DA, Wold LE, et al. Postradiation sarcoma of bone. *Orthopedics*. 1993;16:105-106, 109.
22. Schreuder HW, Veth RP, Pruszczynski M, et al. Aneurysmal bone cysts treated by curettage, cryotherapy and bone grafting. *J Bone Joint Surg Br*. 1997;79:20-25.
23. Rai AT, Collins JJ. Percutaneous treatment of pediatric aneurysmal bone cyst at C1: a minimally invasive alternative: a case report. *AJNR Am J Neuroradiol*. 2005;26:30-33.

ANKYLOSING SPONDYLITIS

Leo F. Czervionke, M.D.

CLINICAL PRESENTATION

The patient is a 65-year-old female with a history of chronic low back and neck pain and markedly reduced mobility in the cervical and lumbar region. Her records have noted the diagnosis of ankylosing spondylitis for 20 years. She has always been and remains HLA-B27 negative; 15 years ago she developed Crohn's disease, which has been controlled with sulfasalazine (Azulfidine). Bilateral total hip replacement procedures were performed 13 years ago. She has recently become weak in both lower extremities and has developed peripheral neuropathy and bladder dysfunction. Physical examination reveals absent lower extremity reflexes and loss of position sense in both feet. Presumptive diagnosis of cauda equina syndrome was made.

IMAGING PRESENTATION

Anteroposterior (AP) and lumbar spine radiographs (*Figs. 8-1 and 8-2*) reveal symmetric fusion of both sacroiliac (SI) joints and a bamboo configuration of the spine. The vertebral bodies have a squared off configuration and vertebral body syndesmophytes are visible at all lumbar and visualized lower thoracic levels. There is calcification of the intervertebral discs and posterior interspinous and supraspinatus ligaments. Syndesmophytosis and bilateral SI joint fusion are demonstrated on the radiographs and magnetic resonance (MR) images (*Figs. 8-1 to 8-5*). There is diffuse lumbar dural ectasia and multiple arachnoid diverticula eroding the lamina at several lumbar levels (see Figs. 8-4, 8-5; *Fig. 8-6*). The nerve rootlets are adherent to the posterolateral aspect of the thecal sac in and adjacent to the arachnoid diverticula giving a "vacant" thecal sac appearance consistent with chronic arachnoiditis. The intervertebral discs are heterogeneous on MR secondary to intradiscal calcification or ossification (see Figs. 8-2, 8-4, and 8-5).

DISCUSSION

Ankylosing spondylitis (AS), also called *Marie-Strümpell disease*, is a seronegative (rheumatoid factor-negative) disorder causing sacroiliitis, enthesopathy, and spondyloarthropathy, with variable peripheral joint involvement. This is a complex, often debilitating condition with insidious onset and a variable degree of involvement in the spine. The socioeconomic impact of AS on the patient, her family, and on the healthcare system in general cannot be understated.[1] Of all patients with ankylosing spondylitis, 95% are HLA-B27 positive compared with 8% of control white populations;[2] 5% of patients with clinical and imaging manifestations of AS are HLA-B27 negative, as in the patient described earlier. HLA-B27 is a genetically encoded antigenic protein found on the surface of leukocytes in some persons. Approximately 1% of patients who are HLA-B27 positive will develop a rheumatoid factor–negative spondyloarthropathy (ankylosing spondylitis, psoriatic arthropathy, Reiter's disease, and arthritis of inflammatory bowel disease). HLA-B27 is believed to play an important role in initiating and perpetuating the T-cell–mediated immune process, which leads to the manifestations of AS[2] in most patients with this disorder. It has been postulated that some external antigenic agent, possibly a microbial agent, may trigger an abnormal response by T-cells to the HLA-B27/peptide complexes that form in these patients.[2] Cytokines, such as interleukin-10, as well as genetic and environmental factors, are also believed to play a role.[1] The resulting inflammatory cellular infiltrates target cortical bone, cartilage, and ligaments adjacent to fibrocartilaginous and synovial joints. Many of the manifestations of AS are the result of an exaggerated reparative response to this inflammatory process.[2]

The prevalence of AS is between 0.2% and 0.8% in whites.[3,4] AS occurs five times more commonly in men than in women. Juvenile ankylosing spondylitis can occur as well. AS disease progression tends to spread cephalad from the SI joints to the lumbar spine and eventually may involve the thoracic and cervical spine, although spinal involvement is variable and may not be contiguous.[5] Women tend to have a milder course of disease progression, and spinal involvement has a tendency to be more discontiguous in women.[5] Patients with AS usually present between the ages of 15 and 35 with severe low back or sacroiliac pain and stiffness of the spine and joints.[6] The patient presents with low back pain or sacroiliac pain, back stiffness, and sometimes sciatic pain. Constitutional symptoms such as anorexia, weight loss, and low-grade fever may also be present.[6] Patients who present later in life tend to have a better prognosis. Early onset of disease or involvement of the hip joints is usually associated with poor prognosis.[6] With time, severe osteoporosis develops, and the paraspinal muscles tend to become atrophic because of disuse.[7] The inadequately supported, brittle spine becomes very susceptible to spinal fractures, which can contribute significantly to the morbidity of these patients.[2] It is important to be aware that cauda equina syndrome may occur in patients with AS.[8,9] The etiology of cauda equina syndrome in patients with ankylosing spondylitis is controversial. Cauda equina syndrome may develop in AS patients in the absence of

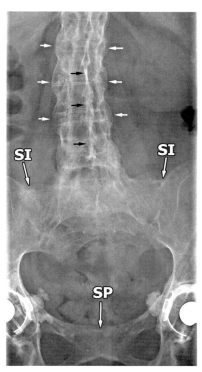

Figure 8-1 ▶ **Ankylosing Spondylitis.** AP lumbar spine radiograph. Sacroiliac joints (*SI*) are fused. Bamboo shaped spine due to syndesmophyte formation laterally (*small white arrows*). Interspinous/supraspinous ligamentous calcification or ossification (*black arrows*). Symphysis pubis (*SP*) is sclerotic and fused. Note bilateral hip prostheses.

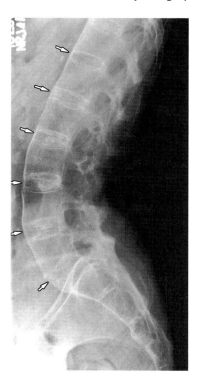

Figure 8-2 ▶ **Ankylosing Spondylitis.** Lateral lumbar spine radiograph. Squared-off configuration of vertebral bodies due to paraspinous ligamentous ossification along anterior vertebral body margins and syndesmophyte formation (*arrows*) along anterior disc margins. Note calcification and/or ossification of the lumbar intervertebral discs. Generalized osteopenia of visualized spine.

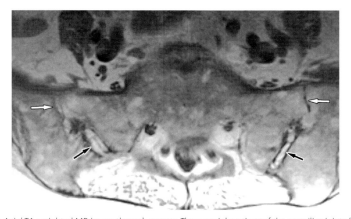

Figure 8-3 ▶ **Ankylosing Spondylitis.** Axial T1-weighted MR image through sacrum. The synovial portions of the sacroiliac joints (*white arrows*) are fused. Fibro-ligamentous portions of the SI joints (*black arrows*) are not fused.

mass effect upon the cauda equina in AS patients. It has been postulated that in AS patients, arachnoid adhesions secondary to arachnoiditis, tether the cauda equina nerve rootlets to arachnoid diverticula.[8,10] Inflammation of the arachnoid within these diverticula in AS patients has been described.[11] Indeed, this could be the cause of the cauda equina syndrome in the patient presented above.

A discussion of the detailed clinical and radiographic criteria for diagnosis of AS is beyond the scope of this discussion but can be found elsewhere.[1,6] Sacroiliitis is the hallmark of AS and usually

occurs early in the disease. Initially, one SI joint may be more affected than the other, but as the disease progresses, the sacroiliac involvement characteristically becomes bilaterally symmetric. Ankylosing spondylitis begins as an erosive arthropathy affecting the synovial portions of the SI joints bilaterally and usually symmetrically. Erosions begin first on the iliac side of the SI joints and then involve both cortical surfaces of the synovial portion of the SI joints. The SI joint spaces widen, the adjacent cortical margins later become sclerotic, and eventually the SI joints fuse in a bilaterally symmetric fashion (see Fig. 8-3, *Fig. 8-7*). The fibrous portions

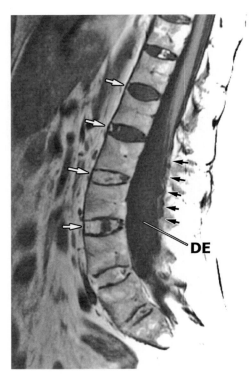

Figure 8-4 ▶ Ankylosing Spondylitis. Sagittal T1-weighted MR image lumbar spine. Vertebral bodies have a squared off appearance. T1 hypointense thin anterior longitudinal ligament ossification in continuity with syndesmophytes (*white arrows*) along the anterior disc margin. Diffuse lumbar dural sac ectasia (*DE*). Nerve rootlets of cauda equina from L2 to L4 level are adherent to the posterior thecal sac margin (*black arrows*) consistent with chronic arachnoiditis. Note heterogeneous signal intensity within the intervertebral discs due to calcification and or ossification. Also note smooth vertebral endplate depressions resulting in "ballooning" of the intervertebral discs sometimes called "fish mouth" intervertebral discs.

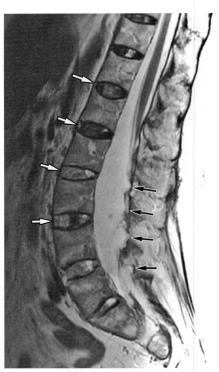

Figure 8-5 ▶ Ankylosing Spondylitis. Sagittal T2-weighted MR image lumbar spine, corresponding to Figure 4. Rootlets of the cauda equina are adherent to the posterior portion of the thecal sac where small arachnoid diverticula are located (*black arrows*). Appearance is consistent with chronic arachnoiditis. Note squared-off vertebral bodies, anterior ligamentous ossification (*white arrows*), and heterogeneous intradiscal signal intensity.

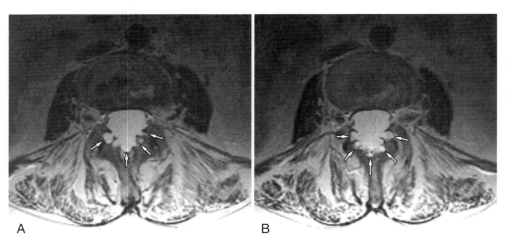

Figure 8-6 ▶ Ankylosing Spondylitis. Same patient as in Figures 8-1 to 8-5. Axial T2-weighted MR images **A** and **B** reveal a largely "vacant" thecal sac with arachnoid diverticula (*arrows*) eroding the lamina bilaterally. The nerve rootlets of the cauda equina are difficult to visualize, since they are adherent to the posterior thecal sac within or adjacent to the diverticula. Appearance is consistent with chronic arachnoiditis.

of the SI joints may also be involved but usually do not fuse to the same degree as the synovial portions of the SI joints. Ankylosing spondylitis may be limited to the SI joints, but AS has a predilection for the axial skeleton, affecting fibrocartilaginous and synovial joints and adjacent vertebrae. The lumbar spine is often affected, but the thoracic and cervical spine may also be involved to a variable degree. Some portions of the spine may not be significantly involved. Sometimes AS affects the lumbar and cervical spine with relative sparing of the thoracic spine.

In AS, in the acute inflammatory phase, cortical bone damage occurs, and this phase is relatively short compared with the reparative and bone deposition phase.[2] In the spine, this is manifested

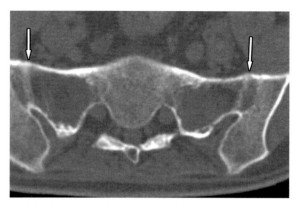

Figure 8-7 ▸ Ankylosing Spondylitis. Axial CT image reveals ankylosis of the synovial portion (*arrows*) of both sacroiliac joints.

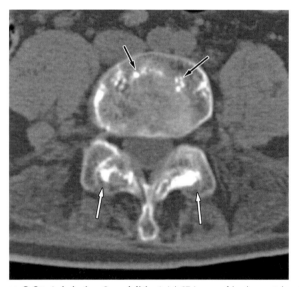

Figure 8-9 ▸ Ankylosing Spondylitis. Axial CT image of lumbar vertebra. The facet joints (*white arrows*) are fused and areas of dense sclerosis are located in the adjacent articular facets and laminae. Several focal calcifications (*black arrows*) are located in the intervertebral disc anteriorly.

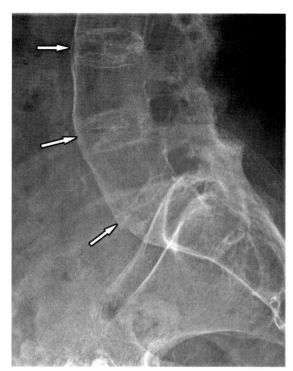

Figure 8-8 ▸ Ankylosing Spondylitis. Same patient as Figures 8-1 to 8-6. Lateral radiograph of lumbosacral junction. Syndesmophytes (*arrows*) are seen as thin vertical ossifications along the anterior disc margin continuous with the ossified anterior longitudinal ligament. Note intradiscal calcification and/or ossification. Diffuse osteopenia in visualized vertebrae.

early on as an erosive arthropathy, which may involve synovial and fibrocartilaginous joints. The cortical erosions begin along the corners of the vertebral bodies at the discovertebral junction (Romanus lesions), most often beginning at the thoracolumbar junction, but can eventually progress to involve the entire spine. Sclerotic lesions often develop at the corner of vertebral bodies (*shiny corner* sign).[6] The erosions undergo a reparative process leading to adjacent sclerosis. The bone reparative response is not confined to the damaged cortex. The bone deposition continues to involve adjacent ligaments and the outer annulus of the disc, resulting in thin vertically oriented syndesmophytes *(Fig. 8-8)*. The involved vertebral bodies typically develop a *squared-off* appearance, in part due to post erosive cortical sclerosis and also due to paraspinous ligamentous calcification and eventual ossification (see Figs. 8-2, 8-4, 8-5, and 8-8).

AS is an inflammatory enthesopathy (enthesitis), that is, an inflammatory condition that affects ligamentous and tendinous attachments in the spine, hips, and shoulders and sometimes affects the more peripheral appendicular joints. Paraspinous

ligamentous abnormalities are very common, beginning early in the disease, and can represent a prominent manifestation of this disease.

In ankylosing spondylitis, early inflammation occurs where the outer fibers of the annulus fibrosus (*Sharpey's fibers*) insert into the corners of the vertebral bodies. These outer annular fibers ossify along with thin ossifications of the paraspinal ligaments to form syndesmophytes, which are seen as thin vertically oriented ossifications of the anterior longitudinal ligament and lateral paraspinal ligaments that extend along the anterior and lateral vertebral body margins from mid-vertebral level to adjacent mid-vertebral level, in continuity with the ossified outer annular fibers of adjacent intervertebral discs (see Figs. 8-4, 8-5, and 8-8). This results in the so-called *bamboo spine* appearance (see Fig. 8-1). The syndesmophytes that develop in psoriatic and Reiter's spondyloarthropathies tend to be larger, more exuberant, asymmetric bony excrescences arising along the discovertebral margins.

In ankylosing spondylitis, the zygapophyseal (facet) joints undergo an erosive arthropathy initially, but later become sclerotic and eventually fuse *(Fig. 8-9)*. The vertebrae in AS are very brittle because of osteoporosis and are prone to fracture. The fractures are frequently transverse in orientation and may form pseudoarthroses. These pseudoarthroses may extend transversely through the vertebrae or through the intervertebral disc.

Severe kyphosis of the thoracolumbar spine and early onset degenerative disc disease often develop in patients with AS. The intervertebral disc is a fibrocartilaginous joint and intradiscal calcifications, and ossifications frequently develop in the intervertebral disc that have a unique heterogeneous signal intensity

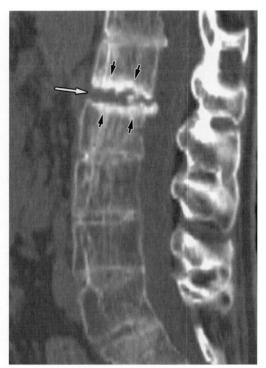

Figure 8-10 ▶ Chronic Noninfectious Spondylodiscitis, Longstanding Ankylosing Spondylitis. The L1-2 intervertebral disc space is widened (*white arrow*). The adjacent cortical vertebral endplates are irregular and sclerotic (*black arrows*). Note squared-off configuration of the lumbar vertebral bodies and generalized osteopenia.

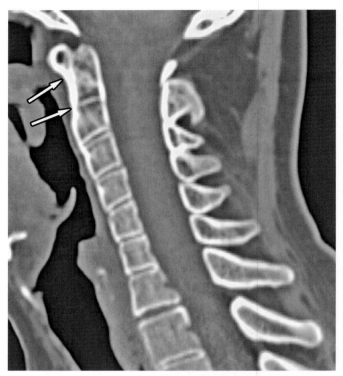

Figure 8-11 ▶ Ankylosing Spondylitis. Sagittal cervical spine CT reformatted image reveals ankylosis of the atlanto-axial joint and ossification of the anterior longitudinal ligament (*arrow*) anteriorly at the C1-3 levels. Mid- and lower-cervical vertebral bodies have a squared-off or trapezoidal configuration. No syndesmophytes in lower cervical spine.

appearance on MR imaging (see Figs. 8-4 and 8-5). Some of this intradiscal signal may be due to formation of fatty intradiscal bone marrow.[12] AS may manifest as a spondylodiscopathy, which can be mistaken for infectious spondylodiscitis. The vertebral endplates often become irregular secondary to cortical erosions and adjacent endplate sclerosis develops (**Fig. 8-10**). Frank dissolution of the endplates, commonly seen in discovertebral infection, however, does not usually occur.

Other spinal joints can also be involved in ankylosing spondylitis, including the zygapophyseal (facet) joints (see Fig. 8-9), costotransverse joints, costovertebral joints, and the atlantoaxial joint. Cartilage in these joints and adjacent cortical bone go through a phase of erosive arthropathy, followed by marginal cortical bone sclerosis and eventually fusion of the affected joints. The atlantoaxial joint is more commonly involved in rheumatoid arthritis, but if involved, adjacent ligaments can become thickened and the odontoid may become eroded, similar to that seen in rheumatoid arthritis. The atlantoaxial joint in AS usually becomes fused (**Fig. 8-11**). In rheumatoid arthritis, the atlantoaxial joint widens secondary to erosion and subluxation. The sternoclavicular, acromioclavicular joints, and pubic symphysis may be affected in both men and women.[5]

Peripheral joints can be involved as well but are less commonly involved than in rheumatoid arthritis. The hip and shoulder joints are more commonly involved than the more peripheral joints of the hands and feet, especially in women and children with this disorder. Periarticular demineralization is not a feature of AS when peripheral joints are involved, as it is with rheumatoid arthritis.[6] Instead, after the erosive phase, sclerosis of the adjacent cortical

bone usually ensues, sometimes followed by peripheral joint fusion.

Extracelluar manifestations of AS may occur. Iritis occurs in up to 20% of patients. Possible cardiac manifestations include chamber enlargement, conduction abnormalities, pericarditis, and aortic insufficiency. Pulmonary fibrosis and upper pulmonary lobe cavitation may occur. Patients with AS may have concomitant inflammatory bowel disease or amyloidosis, which may result in renal failure.[6]

IMAGING FEATURES

Radiographs or computed tomography (CT) are used to detect and assess the extent of the erosive arthropathy, cortical bone sclerosis, paraspinal ligamentous ossifications, discovertebral abnormalities, disc calcification/ossification, spinal joint arthroses, and peripheral joint involvement in all stages of the disease, as described above in the discussion. CT is best for detection of subtle cortical erosions of the SI joints, vertebral bodies, costotransverse joints, and costovertebral joints. CT is the procedure of choice for evaluating for fractures that may develop. With MRI, one is able to detect the above abnormalities as well. MRI is particularly valuable for detecting the presence of active inflammation within bone, joints, and ligaments when fat-saturated imaging techniques are used, with and without IV contrast enhancement with paramagnetic contrast agents. The presence of spinal cord compression by displaced fracture fragments or associated epidural hematoma formation is evaluated using MRI.

Sacroiliac Joint Disease

Sacroiliac (SI) joint inflammation, marginal sclerosis, and fusion occur early in AS and are often the first imaging manifestations of the disease. Some patients with AS exhibit only SI joint involvement. Erosions first begin on the iliac side of the SI joints and areas of adjacent sclerosis develop. Eventually, both sides of the SI joint are involved. SI joint fusion nearly always involves the synovial portion of the SI joint but the fibroligamentous portion of the joint may also be fused.[6] Fusion of the SI joints often occurs early in the disease, and although involvement may initially be unilateral, it usually progresses rapidly so that both SI joints are symmetrically involved. These abnormalities are well shown with radiographs, CT, or MRI (see Figs. 8-1, 8-3, and 8-7).

Enthesitis/Enthesopathy

Paraspinal ligaments and ligamentous soft tissues adjacent to the large and small joints of the spine, hips, shoulders, symphysis pubis, and sternomanubrial joints may become ill-defined and calcify, giving them a fuzzy "whiskered" appearance on radiographs and CT images. The same process may occur at ligamentous and tendinous attachments to the pelvis such as the ischial tuberosities and at tendinous insertions on the long bones. The inflamed ligaments are T2 hyperintense on fat-saturated MR imaging and are enhanced after administering IV contrast. The posterior interspinous and supraspinous ligaments of the lumbar spine late in the disease are often densely calcified or ossified, visible on AP radiographs as a sclerotic vertical stripe projecting over the middle of the spine, which has been called a *dagger sign* (see Fig. 8-1).[6]

Anterolateral Vertebral Body Osteitis/Spondylitis

Osteitis causes classic anterior vertebral endplate abnormalities in AS, called *Romanus lesions*,[13] which are best demonstrated with CT or MRI. These lesions are the result of endplate cortical erosions and the inflammatory response to these erosions. These lesions are located at the anterior corners of the vertebral bodies.[13,14] On MRI, Romanus lesions are T1 hypointense and T2 hyperintense at the anterior corners of the vertebral bodies, which may be enhanced after administration of IV contrast.[14,15] On CT, the tiny erosions are initially radiolucent, but then reactive bone formation occurs and the vertebral corners become sclerotic, giving the vertebral body corners a *white, shiny* appearance.[6] This reactive bone response along with the characteristic paraspinous ligamentous ossifications (syndesmophytes) gives the vertebral body a squared-off appearance.[6] Syndesmophytes are thin vertical ossifications of the anterior and lateral paraspinal ligaments that merge imperceptibly with the outermost layers of the annulus fibrosus (see Figs. 8-2, 8-4, 8-5, and 8-8). Syndesmophytes give the spine its bamboo configuration late in the disease (see Fig. 8-1).

Spinal Joint Abnormalities

Cortical erosions, sclerosis, capsular calcifications, and eventually fusion frequently involve the margins of synovial joints of the spine including the zygapophyseal (facet) joints (see Fig. 8-9; ***Figs. 8-12, and 8-13***), costovertebral joints, and costotransverse joints and may also involve the atlantoaxial joint. Cervical spine involvement frequently results in bilaterally symmetric fusion of the cervical facet joints (see Figs. 8-12 and 8-13).

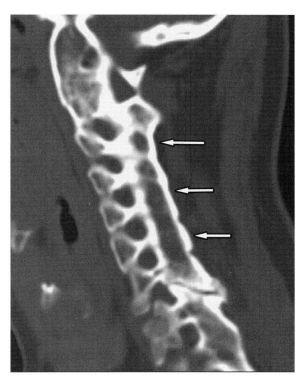

Figure 8-12 ▶ Ankylosing Spondylitis. Same patient as in Figure 8-11. Parasagittal CT reformatted image through cervical articular processes. The cervical facet joints are all fused into a single column of bone (*arrows*).

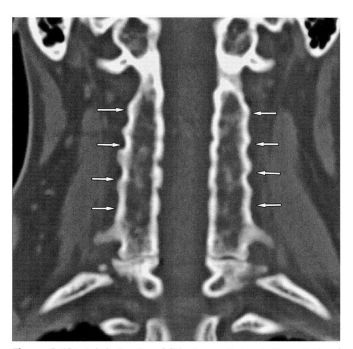

Figure 8-13 ▶ Ankylosing Spondylitis. Same patient as in Figures 8-11 and 8-12. Coronal reformatted CT image of cervical spine. Symmetric fusion of all cervical facet joints results in a solid bilateral columns of bone (*arrows*).

Noninfectious Spondylodiscitis

Localized or diffuse areas of bone erosion may occur in the vertebral endplates in AS, referred to as *Andersson lesions.*[6,16] These occur radiographically in 8% of patients with AS.[17] On CT, there is focal or diffuse vertebral endplate irregularity, which may be confused for infectious discitis (see Fig. 8-10). Late in the healing phase, the adjacent bone becomes sclerotic. Interestingly, these lesions have the same MR imaging features and evolution as the advanced degenerative discogenic vertebral endplate abnormalities described by Modic.[18] The vertebral endplates are irregular, and early on there is T1 hypointense, T2 hyperintense reactive signal disturbance in the marrow adjacent to the endplate as in Modic type 1 discogenic endplate disease. Usually, the adjacent disc is T2 hypointense, similar to a degenerating disc rather than the T2 hyperintense disc seen in infectious discitis. Later, as healing occurs, the marrow adjacent to the endplate becomes T1 hyperintense and eventually T1 and T2 hypointense as sclerosis develops adjacent to the endplate.[14]

Osteoporosis and Fish Vertebrae

In patients with AS, the vertebral endplates are usually thin, sclerotic structures lacking significant irregularity. In the later stages of the disease, osteoporosis is often a dominant feature. As in any patient with severe osteoporosis, smooth concave endplate depressions may develop, giving the vertebral body a *fish vertebra* appearance.[6] When this happens, the corresponding intervertebral disc space has been described as having a *ballooned* appearance, which some refer to as a *fish mouth* intervertebral disc (see Fig. 8-4).

Intradiscal Abnormalities

Calcifications, ossifications, and even bone marrow may form in the intervertebral discs late in the later stages of the disease and are demonstrated well on radiographs (see Figs. 8-2 and 8-8) and on CT images. On MR images, these intradiscal calcifications/ossifications have a characteristic appearance, appearing as heterogeneous areas of high and low T1 signal intensity within the intervertebral discs (see Figs. 8-4 and 8-5).

Dural ectasia may develop, which results in an overall large size of the spinal canal, particularly in the lumbar region (see Figs. 8-4, 8-5, and 8-6). Dural ectasia may be seen in other conditions such as neurofibromatosis type 1, Marfan syndrome, and Ehlers-Danlos disease.[9]

Arachnoid diverticula may develop, which cause lobular laminar erosions that erode into the lumbar lamina, visible on CT and MR images (see Figs. 8-5 and 8-6). The presence of arachnoid diverticula are highly suggestive (and possibly pathognomonic) of AS. Cauda equina nerve rootlets may prolapse into these diverticula, or the cauda equina rootlets may be tethered to the margins of these diverticula by adhesions (see Figs. 8-5 and 8-6), which likely form secondary to chronic arachnoiditis.[8,9]

Spinal Fractures

In patients with ankylosing spondylitis, spinal fractures are usually highly unstable injuries that most commonly occur in

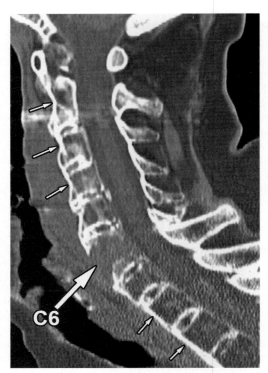

Figure 8-14 ► Ankylosing Spondylitis, Acute Transverse "Banana" Fracture through C6 Vertebra. Sagittal CT image. The upper and lower halves of the C6 vertebral body are widely separated (*large arrow*). Small arrows point to ossification of the anterior longitudinal ligament. Note intradiscal calcifications at multiple levels, commonly seen in ankylosing spondylitis.

the cervical region and next most commonly occur at the thoracolumbar junction.[19] Although nondisplaced fractures may occur, these fractures are typically highly unstable and may be associated with cord injury (*Figs. 8-14 to 8-16*). The fractures in AS tend to be transversely oriented and may extend through the vertebral body or intervertebral disc and usually extend through the posterior vertebral elements. The fractures are best demonstrated with CT or MRI. The adjacent anterior and posterior paraspinal ligaments are usually disrupted, which is best shown with MRI. Cord compression and contusion are best evaluated with MRI. The patient may develop a pseudoarthrosis at the site of the fracture. Avascular necrosis may also occur in these patients.[19]

DIFFERENTIAL DIAGNOSIS

1. **Reiter's syndrome** (uveitis, urethritis and reactive spondyloarthropathy) **and psoriatic arthritis** (spondyloarthropathy and psoriasis skin condition): Also referred to as *seronegative* (rheumatoid factor-negative) *spondyloarthropathies.* SI joint involvement tends to be asymmetric in both conditions. Syndesmophytes and paraspinous ligamentous ossifications tend to be more bulky in configuration and asymmetric compared with the very thin vertically oriented syndesmophytes and paraspinous ligamentous ossifications seen in AS. Peripheral joint involvement tends to be a more dominant

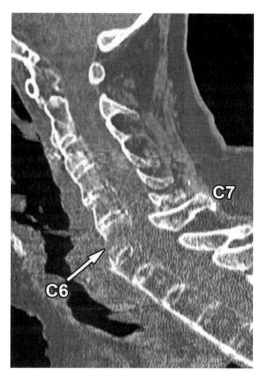

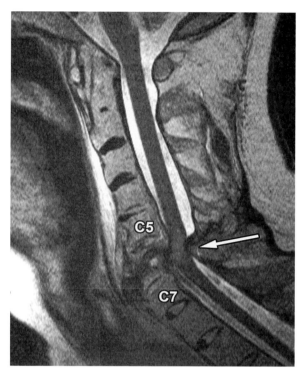

Figure 8-15 ▶ **Ankylosing Spondylitis.** Same patient as in Figure 8-14. Sagittal CT image obtained 3 days after patient was placed in halo traction device and subsequently became acutely paraplegic. The spine above the mid-C6 fracture (*arrow*) is subluxed posteriorly, and the spinal canal is now markedly narrowed by posteriorly subluxed C6 vertebral body fragment and base of C7 spinous process. The C6 spinous process is subluxed posteriorly relative to the C7 spinous process, indicating disruption of the C6-7 interspinous ligaments.

Figure 8-16 ▶ **Ankylosing Spondylitis.** Same patient as in Figures 8-14 and 8-15. Sagittal T2 weighted MR image obtained while patient was in a halo traction device. Marked cord compression occurred at C6-7 level, secondary to posterior subluxation of the spine above the mid-C6 vertebral fracture. The cord is compressed anteriorly by the posteriorly displaced upper portion of the C6 vertebral body and posteriorly by the base of the C7 spinous process (*arrows*) and ligamentum flavum. Note T2 hyperintense edema in the cord at C6 level due to cord compression.

feature in these two conditions. Psoriatic arthritis affects hands more commonly, whereas Reiter's syndrome affects the feet more than the hands. Psoriatic arthritis may precede or occur after development of the characteristic psoriatic skin rash; 80% of Reiter's syndrome patients are HLA-B27 positive; 50% of psoriatic arthritis patients are HLA-B27 positive.

2. **Arthritis of inflammatory bowel disease:** Also known as a *seronegative spondyloarthropathy*. Patients with AS may have inflammatory bowel disease, as in the patient presented in this case.

3. **Infectious sacroiliitis:** Usually unilateral SI joint disease with rapid onset of clinical symptoms and rapid osteolytic bone destruction.

4. **Rheumatoid arthritis:** Rarely involves the SI joints. Spinal involvement is most commonly in the cervical atlantoaxial joint, where joint laxity and subluxation occurs. The odontoid process is usually eroded.

5. **Juvenile rheumatoid arthritis**: Age at onset in childhood or adolescence. Vertebral growth centers are affected. SI joints may be involved and eventually fuse. Causes a peripheral joint enthesopathy, but usually not a spinal enthesopathy.

6. **Infectious spondylodiscitis**: Usually causes dissolution of the cortical endplates and little endplate sclerosis early in the process. Later, with healing, the endplates may look irregular and sclerotic. The intradiscal contents are typically T2 hyperintense in active discitis because of the presence of inflammatory tissue and increased water content in the infected. The disc in tuberculous spondylodiscitis may not be T2 hyperintense, and the endplate irregularity and sclerosis could mimic that seen in patients with ankylosing spondylitis, depending on the stage of the process.

7. **Alkaptonuria (ochronosis):** Rare inherited autosomal recessive disorder of phenylalanine and tyrosine metabolism, resulting in accumulation of homogentisic acid in the tissues. This disorder causes extensive degeneration and calcification of cartilaginous joints throughout the body including multilevel disc calcification that could be confused with intradiscal calcifications of AS (*Figs. 8-17 and 8-18*). Multilevel vertebral osteophytosis in this disorder somewhat resembles the bamboo spine of AS (see Figs. 8-1 and 8-2). Cartilage in the SI joints is densely calcified, which may be confused with SI joint fusion (see Fig. 8-14). Patients with ochronosis may have aortic valvular disease similar to that which may occur in AS.

TREATMENT

There is no known treatment available that targets the underlying mechanism that produces the inflammation in AS. Treatment is directed at controlling the inflammation with the goal of producing a long-term remission of symptoms, but this is often not attained.[20]

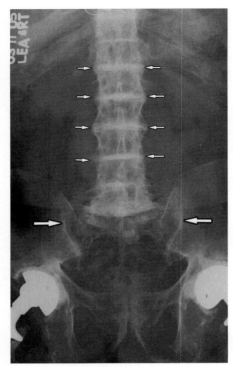

Figure 8-17 ▸ **Alcaptonuria (Ochronosis).** AP lumbar spine radiograph. The spine has a bamboo appearance due to presence of bilaterally symmetric vertebral osteophyte formations and paraspinous ligamentous ossifications at every disc level (*small arrows*). The intervertebral discs are all diffusely calcified. The sacroiliac joint spaces (*large arrows*) are diffusely calcified as well simulating SI joint fusion. Bilateral total hip prostheses.

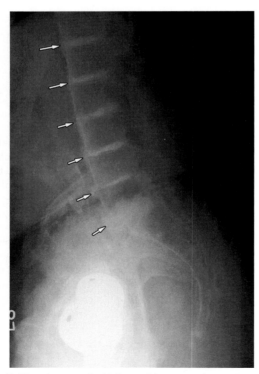

Figure 8-18 ▸ **Alcaptonuria (Ochronosis).** Same patient as in Figure 8-13. Lateral lumbar spine radiograph reveals ill-defined continuous ossification of anterior longitudinal ligament and squared-off appearance of vertebral bodies, which may be confused with that seen in ankylosing spondylitis. Note diffuse dense calcification of the intervertebral discs.

1. **Nonsteroidal anti-inflammatory drugs (NSAIDs):** Given first, but the symptoms of AS may not be controlled over time with these drugs.[1,20]
2. **Antirheumatic drugs** (e.g., sulfasalazine): Given as the second line of treatment, but their efficacy has not been proved.[20]
3. **Intra-articular anesthetic/steroid injections:** May be useful to control pain in cases where there is localized inflammation in one or a few joints.
4. **Intravenous bisphosphonate** (pamidronate): Has been shown to be effective in some AS patients.
5. **Intravenous corticosteroid therapy** (e.g., IV methylprednisolone): May be necessary in NSAID-refractory active AS.[20]
6. **Gold salts, antimalarial drugs, and azathioprine** (Azasan, Imuran): Have been used in some cases with varying success.[20]
7. **Adjunct physical therapy and a long-term exercise program:** Necessary and beneficial in many AS patients.
8. **Surgery:** May be necessary to stabilize the spine or when joint integrity becomes compromised.[20] Patients who develop cervical spine fractures often are treated with traction reduction followed by halo-vest immobilization. Extreme caution must be used when using halo-vest immobilization in these patients, because this device can accentuate or cause cord disruption in some patients with unstable cervical spine fracture dislocations (see Figs. 8-14 to 8-16). If fracture reduction does not occur or if there is fracture nonunion, surgical stabilization is required.[21] If the fracture is accompanied by an epidural hematoma, this usually requires surgical decompression. If vertebral subluxations, spinal stenosis, or severe kyphoscoliosis occur, this often requires surgical intervention.

References

1. Sieper J, Braun J, Rudwaleit M, et al. Ankylosing spondylitis: an overview. *Ann Rheum Dis.* 2002;61(Suppl 3):iii8-iii18.
2. Roberts S, Butler RC. Inflammatory mediators as potential therapeutic targets in the spine. *Curr Drug Targets Inflamm Allergy.* 2005;4:257-266.
3. Braun J, Bollow M, Remlinger G, et al. Prevalence of spondylarthropathies in HLA-B27 positive and negative blood donors. *Arthritis Rheum.* 1998;41:58-67.
4. van der Linden SM, Khan MA. The risk of ankylosing spondylitis in HLA-B27 positive individuals: a reappraisal. *J Rheumatol.* 1984;11:727-728.
5. Braunstein E, Martel W, Moidel R. Ankylosing spondylitis in men and women: a clinical and radiographic comparison. *Radiology.* 1982;144:91-94.
6. Resnick D. Ankylosing spondylitis. In: Resnick D, ed. *Diagnosis of Bone and Joint Disorders.* 4th ed. Philadelphia: Saunders; 2002;2:1023-1081.
7. Sage M, Gordon T. Muscle atrophy in ankylosing spondylitis: CT demonstration. *Radiology.* 1983;149:780.
8. Arslanoglu A, Aygun N. Magnetic resonance imaging of cauda equina syndrome in long-standing ankylosing spondylitis. *Australas Radiol.* 2007;51:375-377.
9. Tyrrell PN, Davies AM, Evans N. Neurological disturbances in ankylosing spondylitis. *Ann Rheum Dis.* 1994;53:714-717.
10. Mitchell M, Sartoris D, Moody D, Resnick D. Cauda equina syndrome complicating ankylosing spondylitis. *Radiology.* 1990;175:521-525.
11. Byrne E, McNeill P, Gilford E, Wright C. Intradural cyst with compression of the cauda equina in ankylosing spondylitis. *Surg Neurol.* 1985;23:162-164.
12. Malghem J, Lecouvet FE, Francois R, et al. High signal intensity of intervertebral calcified disks on T1-weighted MR images resulting from fat content. *Skeletal Radiol.* 2005;34:80-86.
13. Romanus R, Yden S. Destructive and ossifying spondylitis changes in rheumatoid ankylosing spondylitis. *Acta Orthop Scand.* 1952;22:88-99.

14. Hermann KG, Althoff CE, Schneider U, et al. Spinal changes in patients with spondyloarthritis: comparison of MR imaging and radiographic appearances. *Radiographics.* 2005;25:559-569; discussion 569-570.

15. Jevtic V, Kos-Golja M, Rozman B, McCall I. Marginal erosive discovertebral "Romanus" lesions in ankylosing spondylitis demonstrated by contrast enhanced Gd-DTPA magnetic resonance imaging. *Skeletal Radiol.* 2000;29: 27-33.

16. Andersson O. Roentgenbilden vid spondylarthris ankylopoetica. *Nord Med Tidskr.* 1937;14:2000-2003.

17. Kabasakal Y, Garrett SL, Calin A. The epidemiology of spondylodiscitis in ankylosing spondylitis: a controlled study. *Br J Rheumatol.* 1996;35: 660-663.

18. Modic MT, Steinberg PM, Ross JS, et al. Degenerative disk disease: assessment of changes in vertebral body marrow with MR imaging. *Radiology.* 1988;166:193-199.

19. Wang Y-F, Teng MM-H, Chang C-Y, et al. Imaging manifestations of spinal fractures in ankylosing spondylitis. *AJNR Am J Neuroradiol.* 2005;26: 2067-2076.

20. Dougados M, Dijkmans B, Khan M, et al. Conventional treatments for ankylosing spondylitis. *Annals of the Rheumatic Diseases.* 2002;61(Suppl 3): iii40-50.

21. Reiter MF, Boden SD. Inflammatory disorders of the cervical spine. *Spine.* 1998;23:2755-2766.

ARACHNOID CYST

Leo F. Czervionke, M.D.

CLINICAL PRESENTATION

The patient is a 72-year-old female with longstanding gait disturbance, spasticity, back pain, right hip pain, and lower extremity hyperreflexia. No bowel or bladder dysfunction. No thoracic sensory level. Based on clinical findings, obtained lumbar magnetic resonance (MR) study to rule out lumbar disc herniation, which was negative. Obtained additional thoracic and cervical MR studies because of hyperreflexia.

IMAGING PRESENTATION

Thoracic MR study revealed a fusiform T1 hypointense, T2 hyperintense fluid collection within the thecal sac displacing the spinal cord anteriorly from the C3 level to approximately the C6 level consistent with a posterior arachnoid cyst (*Figs. 9-1 and 9-2*).

DISCUSSION

Spinal arachnoid cysts are uncommon. They are intradural-extramedullary or extradural collections of cerebrospinal fluid (CSF)–like fluid, most commonly occurring in the thoracic spinal canal dorsal to the thoracic spinal cord. Intradural arachnoid cysts are less common than extradural arachnoid cysts (*Figs. 9-3 and 9-4*).[1] Patients with arachnoid cysts usually present between the ages of 20 and 50, but these cysts can occur at any age and any spinal level[2]; 85% are located in the thoracic spinal canal, 15% in the cervical spinal canal (*Figs. 9-5 and 9-6*), and 5% in the lumbar spinal canal.[3] The majority of spinal arachnoid cysts are located dorsal to the spinal cord (see Fig. 9-1).

Primary (congenital) arachnoid cysts are almost always intradural and represent meningeal duplication cysts where the arachnoid layer, comprised of two layers of cuboidal epithelium, is split into two layers by the fluid collection, so the wall of the arachnoid cyst is lined by a single layer of cuboidal epithelium. Primary arachnoid cysts are almost always located dorsal to the cord. A hydrodynamic theory has been postulated regarding the formation of arachnoid cysts in which CSF pulsation is said to expand congenitally weakened areas in the arachnoid. Posterior intradural arachnoid cysts are believed to arise in the region of the septum posticum of Schwalbe.[4] Secondary (acquired) arachnoid cysts (also called *subarachnoid cysts*) may occur after trauma, hemorrhage, surgery, or infection (arachnoiditis), and are believed to be secondary to developing adhesions, which can result in loculation of a CSF collection. Secondary arachnoid cysts may be intradural or extradural.

Spinal arachnoid cysts are a type of meningeal cyst, which have been classified by Naybors and colleagues.[5] Type 1 cysts are spinal extradural meningeal cysts without spinal nerve root fibers (see Fig. 9-2). Type 2 meningeal cysts are spinal extradural meningeal cysts with spinal nerve root fibers. Type 3 cysts are spinal intradural meningeal cysts (see Fig. 9-1). Type 2 meningeal cysts include the common Tarlov-type perineural cysts (spinal nerve root diverticula) that frequently occur within the spinal or sacral neural foramina.

Patients with arachnoid cysts can present with back pain or be myelopathic with hyperreflexia, paraparesis, paresthesias, or bladder/bowel incontinence. Radiculopathy can also occur. Ventral cysts are more likely to cause weakness and myelopathic signs.[6] Some patients with arachnoid cysts are asymptomatic; the cysts are discovered incidentally on thoracic MR studies performed for other reasons. Back pain is the most common manifesting complaint, followed by sensory changes, urinary incontinence, and weakness.[5] An intermittent waxing and waning clinical course is typical, which clinically may simulate multiple sclerosis.[2] Postural changes can accentuate or alleviate the symptoms.[5] Cyst enlargement is attributed to the presence of a ball-valve–type obstruction allowing CSF to flow into but not out of the cyst.[2,7] Pain associated with arachnoid cysts may be accentuated during the Valsalva maneuver.[2] If the arachnoid cyst is not removed, the adjacent spinal cord may become atrophic. Arachnoid cysts may be associated with scoliosis, syringohydromyelia and rarely spinal dysraphism (meningomyelocele or diastematomyelia).[3,8] If an associated syringohydromyelia occurs, the syrinx typically extends above the level of the cyst.[9] Arachnoid cysts have no malignant potential.

IMAGING FEATURES

Arachnoid cysts are ellipsoid-shaped fluid collections usually located dorsal to the spinal cord, typically extending over a length of two to four vertebral segments or greater (see Figs. 9-1 to 9-3) or less commonly are more localized (see Figs. 9-5 and 9-6). Extradural arachnoid cysts may extend into adjacent neural foramina, sometimes resembling a dumbbell configuration. Plain radiographs are of no value in the diagnosis of arachnoid cysts. In the past they were diagnosed with computed tomography (CT)

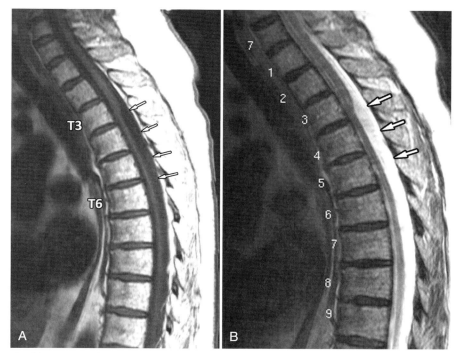

Figure 9-1 ▶ Thoracic Arachnoid Cyst. Sagittal T1-weighted MR image, **A**, and sagittal T2-weighted MR image, **B**, reveal widening of the CSF space posterior to the spinal cord from the mid T3 level to approximately the T6 level, representing an intradural arachnoid cyst (*arrows*). Note deformity of the posterior cord surface from T3 to T6 due to compression or cord atrophy. The upper margin of the cyst is probably at the mid-T3 level. The lower extent of the cyst is not defined.

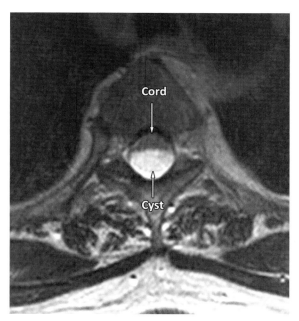

Figure 9-2 ▶ Thoracic Arachnoid Cyst. Same patient as in Figure 9-1. Axial T2-weighted MR image shows flattening of the spinal cord posteriorly, likely by compression from the posterior intradural arachnoid cyst.

myelography (see Fig. 9-4). The cyst may fill immediately on injection of intrathecal contrast, fill not at all, or there may be a delayed filling of the cyst if a small communication exists between the cyst and the intradural CSF. These cysts are usually detected today with MRI.

Because the cyst wall of primary (congenital) arachnoid cysts is only one cell layer thick, it cannot be seen with MRI. Secondary (acquired) arachnoid cyst walls may be visible if the wall is composed of adhesions, which of course may be many cell layers thick. Extradural arachnoid cysts may compress the thecal sac, and the

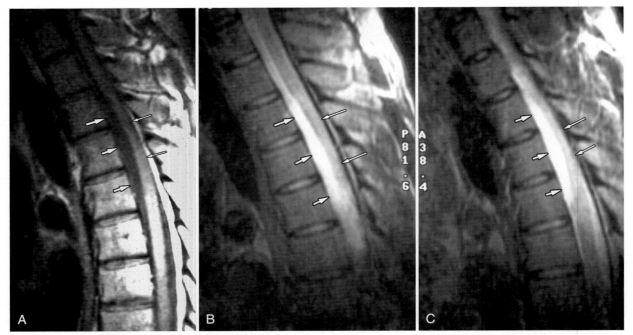

Figure 9-3 ▶ Thoracic Arachnoid Cyst. Sagittal T1-weighted MR image, **A** and contiguous sagittal T2-weighted images, **B** and **C**. Fusiform TI hypointense and T2 hyperintense cyst (*short, thick arrows*) causes smooth indentation of the ventral cord surface and posterior displacement of the spinal cord (*long, thin arrows*) extending over three vertebral levels. It is difficult to determine whether or not this cyst is intradural or extradural in location based on these images.

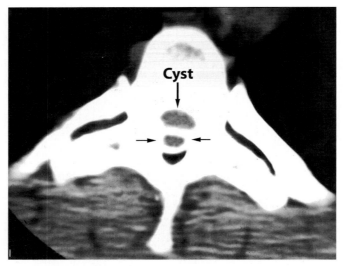

Figure 9-4 ▶ Thoracic Arachnoid Cyst. Same patient as in Figure 8-3. Axial Post myelogram CT Image. Intrathecal contrast (*small arrows*) surrounds the relatively hypodense spinal cord. The cyst does not opacify with intrathecal contrast and is extradural in location, ventral to the thecal sac.

thecal sac wall may be mistaken for the cyst wall (***Fig. 9-7***). The liquid in the cyst usually has signal intensity identical to CSF and is T1 hypointense and T2 hypointense. Therefore the only finding on MR may be widening of the CSF space dorsal to the spinal cord and smooth extrinsic indentation of the dorsal surface of the spinal cord, which may simulate cord thinning and atrophy.[9] Sometimes there is a focal indentation of the cord surface at the superior extent of the arachnoid cyst (see Fig. 9-1). Pulsatile or nonpulsatile CSF

may be seen in the arachnoid cyst. If nonpulsatile, the cyst liquid is slightly more T2 hyperintense than the pulsatile CSF in the adjacent thecal sac (see Figs. 9-5 and 9-6).

Because the MRI appearance of an intradural arachnoid cyst may simulate cord atrophy, a myelogram-CT may be necessary to confirm presence of an arachnoid cyst. The arachnoid cyst on initial myelographic CT images has an intradural-extramedullary mass configuration with a classic intradural *cap sign*. The

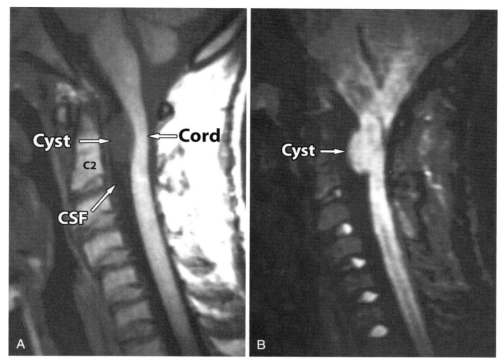

Figure 9-5 ▶ Cervical Arachnoid Cyst. At C2 level cyst deforms and displaces the spinal cord posteriorly. The cyst is hypointense relative to the cord, but is slightly hyperintense relative to CSF on sagittal T1-weighted image, **A**. The cyst is slightly more intense than CSF on the T1-weighted image, **A**, and isointense relative to the cord on the sagittal proton density-weighted conventional spin echo image, **B**, obtained with echo time (TE) = 25 msec and recovery time (TR) = 2500 msec.

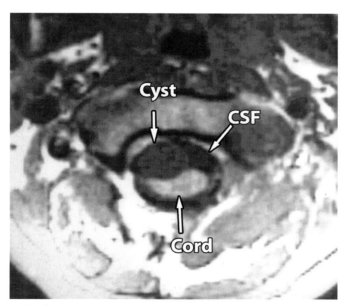

Figure 9-6 ▶ Cervical Arachnoid Cyst, C2 level. Same patient as in Figure 8-5. Axial T1-weighted MR image. The cyst is centered to the right of midline and indents the right anterior cord surface. The cyst is hypointense relative to the cord but slightly more intense than cerebrospinal fluid.

intrathecal myelographic contrast may eventually leak into the cyst from minutes to hours after intrathecal contrast instillation, so if post-myelographic CT imaging is delayed, it may not be possible to differentiate the opacified intrathecal contrast from opacified liquid in the cyst. Hence, it is important to perform the post-CT imaging immediately after the myelogram (see Fig. 9-4). Arachnoid cysts do not show enhancement after IV contrast is administered, but normally enhancing epidural veins adjacent to the cyst may be mistaken for enhancement of the outer cyst margin (Fig. 9-7).

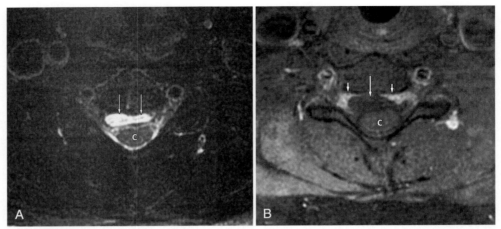

Figure 9-7 ▶ Cervical Ventral Epidural Cyst. The cyst (*arrows*) is hyperintense on fat-satirated T2-weighted MR image, **A**, relative to the spinal cord (C) and displaces the thecal sac posteriorly. On gadolinium-enhanced axial fat-saturated T1-weighted MR image, **B**, the cyst (*long arrow*) does not enhance after IV contrast administration. Adjacent anterior epidural venous plexus (*short arrows*) does enhance with contrast.

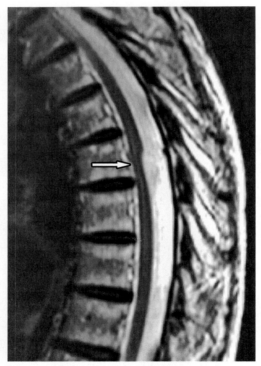

Figure 9-8 ▶ Small Posterior Intradural Arachnoid Cyst Versus Transdural Spinal Cord Herniation. No surgical confirmation. Sagittal T2-weighted MR image of thoracic spine. Both conditions may have a similar appearance on MR imaging with focal concavity along posterior surface of the spinal cord (*arrow*).

DIFFERENTIAL DIAGNOSIS

1. **Transdural herniation of the spinal cord:** An uncommon condition that has likely been underdiagnosed or misdiagnosed in the past. Transdural spinal cord herniation causes a focal cord deformity that may be confused with an intradural arachnoid cyst both clinically and on images *(Fig. 9-8)*; 40% of these patients present with back pain.[10] Patients with this condition may also present with Brown-Séquard syndrome. In transdural cord herniation, the spinal cord protrudes or herniates through a dural defect. The cord is usually tethered to the anterior (most common) or anterolateral dural surface in this condition.[11] Rarely, the dural defect is posteriorly located.[10] The cord can have a very bizarre appearance on MR imaging *(Figs. 9-9 and 9-10)*. Dorsal transdural cord herniations are almost all associated with previous surgery.[10]

   The most common MR imaging appearance of transdural cord herniation is a focal indentation in the dorsal cord surface,

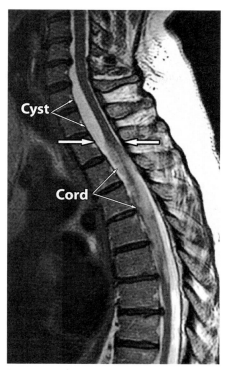

Figure 9-9 ▶ Multilevel Idiopathic Transdural Spinal Cord Herniation. No history of trauma. Sagittal T2-weighted MR image, thoracic spine. Note the cyst anterior to the spinal cord from C7 to the T2 level. Abrupt change in spinal cord shape (*between large arrows*) at mid T2 level. The spinal cord is elongated and has a "smudgy" appearance in part because of volume averaging with CSF space laterally on either side. The thoracic cord resumes a normal shape and configuration at the T7 level. Posterior disc protrusion shown at T7-8 level.

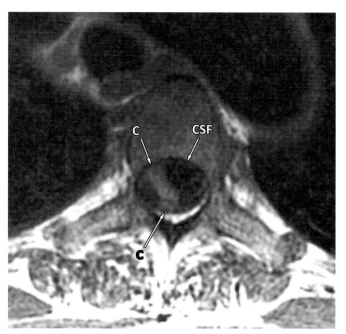

Figure 9-10 ▶ Transdural Spinal Cord Herniation. Same patient as in Figure 8-9. T1-weighted axial MR image through mid-horacic spine. Note the bizarre, arcuate-shaped spinal cord (*C*) hat appears to be attached to the dura along right anterolateral and posterior surfaces of the thesal sac. Prominent CSF space or cyst located to left of the cord and smaller CSF spaqe to the right of the cord.

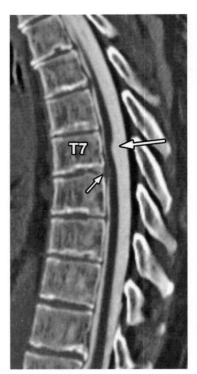

Figure 9-11 ▶ Transdural Cord Herniation Versus Anterior Dural-Cord Adhesions Associated with T7-8 Disc Herniation. Sagittal post myelogram CT image. A focal indentation (*long arrow*) is seen in the dorsal cord surface resembling a dorsal arachnoid cyst. The anterior cord surface is in close proximity with the thecal sac anteriorly. No evidence of arachnoid cyst at CT-myelography. Note small disc protrusion-herniation at T7-8 level (*short arrow*) causes mild anterior thecal sac deformity.

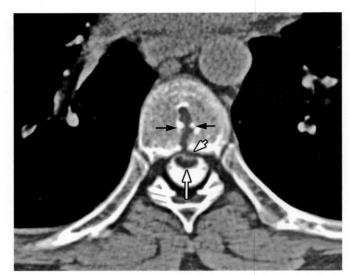

Figure 9-12 ▶ Nuclear Trail Sign. Same patient as in Figure 8-11. Axial post myelogram CT image through inferior T7 vertebral endplate level. *Nuclear trail sign* seen as a defect with sclerotic margins (*black arrows*) in inferior endplate of T7, related to T7-8 disc herniation. The spinal cord (*long white arrow*) is in close proximity to the thecal sac anteriorly. Small herniated disc (*short white arrow*) causes indentation of left ventral aspect of thecal sac and spinal cord.

and the cord typically is in contact with the anterior or anterolateral dural surface (see Fig. 9-8). This is believed to be secondary to the cord protruding through a defect in the thecal sac. However, dural adhesions tethering the cord to the anterior thecal sac can have an identical appearance *(Fig. 9-11)*. The etiology of the dural defect is not known. Many believe a congenital dural defect predisposes one to this condition. In some cases, an intradural arachnoid cyst is present dorsal to the cord, which may predispose formation of the dural defect .[11] However, in some cases, there is no associated arachnoid cyst present. Dural cysts and pseudomeningoceles may form adjacent to the dural defect,[10] and the cord may herniate into these dural pouches.

In some cases, thoracic disc herniation may predispose one to this condition.[11] The herniated disc may cause a defect in the anterior portion of the thecal sac, predisposing it to cord herniation. Alternatively, inflammation associated with the disc herniation could result in dural adhesions that form between the thecal sac and the spinal cord. One should always look for a so called *nuclear trail sign* on MR or CT adjacent to a thoracic spinal cord when thoracic arachnoid cyst or transdural thoracic spinal cord herniation is suspected (Figs. 9-11 and *9-12*).[12]

2. **Spinal cord atrophy:** May occur after cord injury secondary to trauma or ischemia. Post-traumatic atrophy of the spinal cord may be difficult in some cases to differentiate from an arachnoid cyst. A myelogram followed by CT scanning

may be necessary in this situation to exclude an intradural or extradural cystic mass causing cord compression.

TREATMENT

1. No treatment is necessary if the arachnoid cyst is small, stable in size, and asymptomatic.[2]
2. Surgical removal is the procedure of choice for symptomatic or enlarging arachnoid cysts. The entire cyst wall should be removed or the cyst may recur. If the cyst is very large and complete excision is not possible, the cyst is widely fenestrated or marsupialized and a shunt tube is placed within the cyst, which drains into the pleural or peritoneal cavity.[2,3]

References

1. Galzio RJ, Zenobii M, Lucantoni D, Cristuib-Grizzi L. Spinal intradural arachnoid cyst. *Surg Neurol.* 1982;17(5):388-391.
2. Hughes G, Ugokwe K, Benzel EC. A review of spinal arachnoid cysts. *Cleve Clin J Med.* 2008;75(4):311-315.
3. Abou-Fakhr FS, Kanaan SV, Youness FM, et al. Thoracic spinal intradural arachnoid cyst: report of two cases and review of literature. *Eur Radiol.* 2002;12(4):877-882.
4. Lake PA, Minckler J, Scanlan RL. Spinal epidural cyst: theories of pathogenesis. Case report. *J Neurosurg.* 1974;40(6):774-778.
5. Nabors MW, Pait TG, Byrd EB, et al. Updated assessment and current classification of spinal meningeal cysts. *J Neurosurg.* 1988;68(3):366-377.
6. Wang MY, Levi AD, Green BA. Intradural spinal arachnoid cysts in adults. *Surg Neurol.* 2003;60(1):49-55; discussion, 56.

7. Sklar E, Quencer RM, Green BA, et al. Acquired spinal subarachnoid cysts: evaluation with MR, CT myelography, and intraoperative sonography. *AJR Am J Roentgenol.* 1989;153(5):1057-1064.

8. Rabb CH, McComb JG, Raffel C, Kennedy JG. Spinal arachnoid cysts in the pediatric age group: an association with neural tube defects. *J Neurosurg.* 1992;77(3):369-372.

9. Silbergleit R, Brunberg JA, Patel SC, et al. Imaging of spinal intradural arachnoid cysts: MRI, myelography and CT. *Neuroradiology.* 1998;40(10): 664-668.

10. Watters MR, Stears JC, Osborn AG, et al. Transdural spinal cord herniation: imaging and clinical spectra. *AJNR Am J Neuroradiol.* 1998;19(7): 1337-1344.

11. Wada E, Yonenobu K, Kang J. Idiopathic spinal cord herniation: report of three cases and review of the literature. *Spine.* 2000;25(15):1984-1988.

12. Spissu A, Peltz MT, Matta G, Cannas A. Traumatic transdural spinal cord herniation and the nuclear trail sign: case report. *Neurol Sci.* 2004;25(3): 151-153.

ARACHNOIDITIS

Douglas S. Fenton, M.D.

CLINICAL PRESENTATION

The patient is a 67-year-old woman who presented in early 2005 with mild, low back pain and severe pain and numbness from the knees down. The patient gave a history of back surgery 40 years previously and has had some problems with her back ever since. She had an epidural steroid injection in February 2004 but began to feel numbness in her left leg, beginning in July 2004 that progressed to bilateral leg pain and tingling in the feet. The pain from her knees down was rated at 8/10 and was characterized as deep, achy, and burning. Her pain occurred with activity and at rest. The patient denied any bowel or bladder symptoms.

IMAGING PRESENTATION

Sagittal and axial T2-weighted magnetic resonance (MR) images reveal a single thickened cord of soft tissue extending from a normal-appearing and normal-positioned conus medullaris to the lumbosacral junction. The thecal sac has a featureless appearance, and one does not see the normal intrathecal nerve roots that would be expected. This thickened cord represents adhesion of the intrathecal nerve roots into a solitary cord *(Fig. 10-1)*.

DISCUSSION

Lumbar arachnoiditis is an inflammatory condition of the arachnoid membrane that surrounds the spinal cord and its roots that eventually results in adhesions and clumping of nerve roots, thus the synonym *chronic adhesive arachnoiditis*. Quincke, in 1893, is credited with the initial description of arachnoiditis and with linking it to syphilis, gonorrhea, tuberculosis, and extension of infections from the middle ear.[1] Currently, arachnoiditis is usually associated with substances that are injected into the subarachnoid space (myelographic contrast media, anesthetics, and steroids), infection, trauma, surgery (both intradural and extradural), and intrathecal hemorrhage.[2] The oily contrast media iodophendylate (Pantopaque) has been estimated to cause radiographic arachnoiditis in approximately 70% of cases, whereas the early water-soluble agents caused arachnoiditis much less.[3] The residua of Pantopaque myelography can still be seen today in routine imaging of elderly patients. Pantopaque has a high density and therefore is radiopaque on plain films *(Fig. 10-2)* and computed tomography (CT) *(Fig. 10-3)*. Pantopaque's oily characteristics make it readily apparent

on MR *(Fig. 10-4)*. The clinical symptoms of arachnoiditis were seen in only about 1% of the total cases.[3] Today's water-based contrast agents have further decreased the incidence of both radiologic arachnoiditis (imaging findings of arachnoiditis without symptoms) and clinical arachnoiditis (imaging findings and symptoms of arachnoiditis).

Three membranes, the arachnoid, dura, and pia, cover and protect the spinal cord and nerve roots. The arachnoid membrane is very thin and fragile. It does not have innervation or vascularization and therefore it heals poorly.[4] The pathogenesis of arachnoiditis is similar to the repair process of serous membranes in that there is a negligible inflammatory cellular exudate and a prominent fibrinous exudate. The fibrinous exudate covers the nerve roots and causes them to stick to each other and the thecal sac. During the repair phase, as arachnoiditis progresses, dense collagenous adhesions are formed by proliferating fibrocytes.[5] Burton[6] reviewed 100 patients with arachnoiditis and described the process beginning with a radiculitis or inflammation of the pia-arachnoid with associated hyperemia and swelling of the nerve roots. This was followed by fibroblast proliferation and collagen deposition that caused adherence of the nerve roots to each other and to the thecal sac. As arachnoiditis proceeded to its end stage, there was complete encapsulation of the nerve roots, which were atrophic and hypoxemic.

The patient with clinical arachnoiditis can demonstrate a myriad of symptoms, each of which taken alone could point to a different etiology. Back pain is one of the most frequent manifesting symptoms, which often begins unilaterally and may become bilateral later.[7] However, certain bizarre symptoms can serve as clues to the proper diagnosis. The patient may describe a "burning sensation in the sacral region, gripping or clawing pain down the back of one or both legs not of sciatic distribution, tingling pain in the insteps, burning at the inner aspects of the knees, or tingling and pain in the feet. The symptoms often persist at rest and at night."[8] The patient may also have urinary urgency, frequency, and incontinence. There may be unexplained skin rashes and itching, loss of sensation below the affected area, or partial/complete paralysis of the lower extremities.[9]

Potential complications of arachnoiditis are cauda equina syndrome and arachnoiditis ossificans. The cauda equina syndrome is often a late complication of arachnoiditis with symptoms of paresthesias, bowel and bladder abnormalities, and potentially paralysis. Arachnoiditis ossificans is calcification and/or ossification of the spinal meninges. A bony metaplasia of the arachnoid membrane occurs, which can compress the spinal nerves, resulting

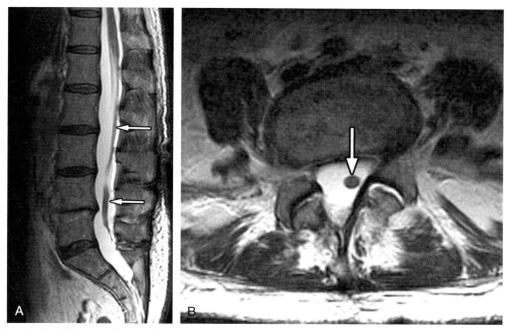

Figure 10-1 ▸ Lumbar Arachnoiditis. Sagittal T2-weighted MR image of the lumbar spine, **A**, and axial T2-weighted MR image, **B**, at the level of L4-5 demonstrates a single intrathecal thickened neural element *(arrows)* from the conus medullaris to the sacrum compatible with nerve root adhesions.

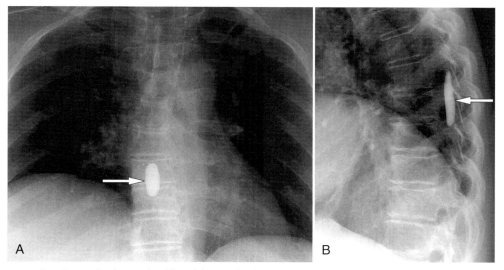

Figure 10-2 ▸ Pantopaque. Posterior-anterior *(image A)* and lateral *(image B)* radiographs. There is an ovoid region of increased density within the spinal canal in the midthoracic region compatible with Pantopaque *(arrow)*. Prior to the advent of water-based myelographic contrast media, the oil-based Pantopaque contrast was instilled during myelography and then removed after imaging. In many patients, a small residual of contrast remained and stays with the patient indefinitely.

in severe, intractable pain, paraparesis, and bowel/bladder abnormalities.[10]

IMAGING FEATURES

The original radiographic description of arachnoiditis was demonstrated by myelography. Jorgensen[11] and Delamarter[4] have classified cases of arachnoiditis based on their radiographic appearance. Mild arachnoiditis (Jorgensen type I, Delamarter group I) may show only lack of filling of one or more nerve root sleeves or focal adhesion of nerve roots. As arachnoiditis progresses to a moderate degree, there is greater nerve root adhesion with peripheral adherence of the nerve roots to the thecal sac giving the "featureless" or "empty sac" appearance *(Fig. 10-5)* (Jorgensen type I, Delamarter group II). These myelographic findings are better visualized on the postmyelogram CT *(Fig. 10-6)* including intrathecal "cysts," which are actually regions of cerebrospinal fluid (CSF) that have been walled off by the adhesions. As arachnoiditis becomes more severe, there is greater nerve root clumping *(Fig. 10-7)* and leptomeningeal adhesions, where one can see angular defects in the contrast column and a mass of fibrotic nerves (Jorgensen type II, Delamarter group III), which can cause a myelographic block.[12]

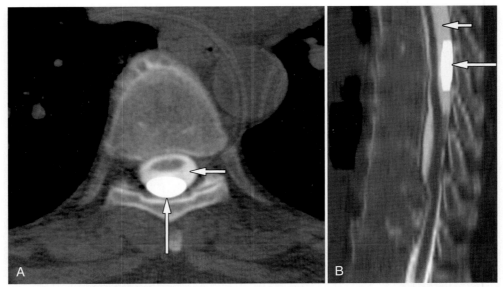

Figure 10-3 ▶ Pantopaque on CT myelography. Same patient as in Figure 10-2. Axial water-based contrast myelogram, **A**, *(mid thoracic region)* and sagittal reformatted image, **B.** Note the ovoid region of increased density within the dependent *(posterior)* aspect of the thecal sac *(long arrow)* that is compatible with Pantopaque. This density is greater than that of the water-based contrast *(short arrow)* within the thecal sac used for recent myelography.

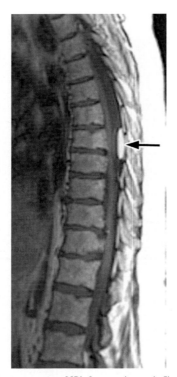

Figure 10-4 ▶ Pantopaque on MRI. Same patient as in Figures 10-1 and 10-2. Sagittal T1-weighted MR image shows the same ovoid region of homogeneously increased signal intensity *(arrow)*. Oil, like fat, demonstrates increased T1 signal intensity.

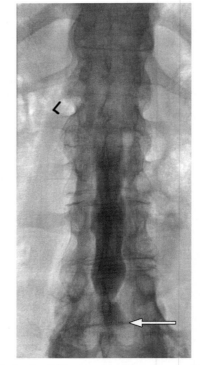

Figure 10-5 ▶ Arachnoiditis. Anteroposterior radiograph of the lumbar spine obtained post-myelogram demonstrates a smooth appearance of the thecal sac contour. There is also complete absence of filling of the thecal sac caudal to L4-5 (*arrow*). A normal myelogram shows outpouchings at or just inferior to the level of each pedicle where the segmental nerve root exits.

MR imaging is now the preferred method for evaluating arachnoiditis because it can achieve the diagnosis without the potential for further irritation of the arachnoid membrane by lumbar puncture or the introduction of contrast media. T2-weighted MR images can best demonstrate the clumped nerve roots (see Fig. 10-1), peripherally adhered nerve roots *(Fig. 10-8)*, and adhesions *(Fig. 10-9)*. Although arachnoid adhesions can be enhanced, the addition of intravenous contrast to the MR examination does not appear to be of much assistance in the diagnosis of arachnoiditis.[13]

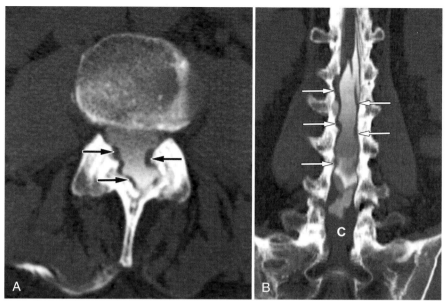

Figure 10-6 ▶ Arachnoiditis with Peripherally Adhesed Nerve Roots. Same patient as in Figure 10-5. Axial Image, **A,** and coronal reformatted image, **B.** Lumbar spine post-myelogram shows adherence of the nerve roots to the periphery of the thecal sac *(arrows)*. On the coronal image, contrast does not fill the thecal sac caudal to L4-5 because of extreme clumping of nerve roots. *C,* Clumped nerve roots.

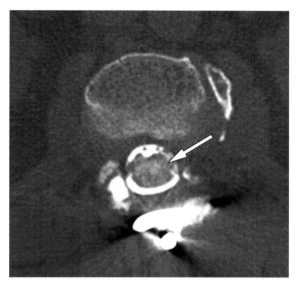

Figure 10-7 ▶ Central Nerve Root Clumping with Fibrous Adhesions. Axial CT image from a lumbar myelogram. There is a mass-like density in the central thecal sac *(arrow)* without evidence of discrete nerve roots, which is compatible with severe arachnoiditis.

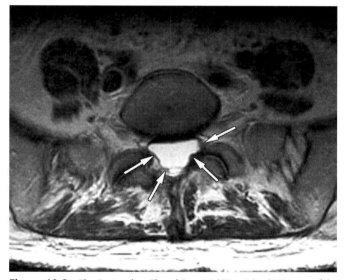

Figure 10-8 ▶ The Featureless Thecal Sac. Axial T2-weighted MR image of the lumbar spine. The individual nerve roots are adhered to the walls of the thecal sac *(arrow).*

DIFFERENTIAL DIAGNOSIS

1. **Spinal stenosis**: Nerve roots are clumped but not adhesed. There is often tortuosity of the nerve roots cephalad to the region of stenosis *(Fig. 10-10)*.
2. **Neoplasm of the cauda equina:** Usually demonstrates very significant contrast enhancement, unlike arachnoiditis. There may be associated cysts and/or evidence of hemorrhage.
3. **Intradural metastases:** Demonstrate significant enhancement.

4. **Carcinomatous meningitis:** Often appears as nerve root enhancement without clumping *(Fig. 10-11)*.

TREATMENT

The prognosis for patients with arachnoiditis is poor. Complete pain relief is impossible in most cases.

1. **Conservative management:** The preferred method, including pain management with narcotics, steroids, and spinal cord stimulation. Direct spinal cord stimulation is an alternative to

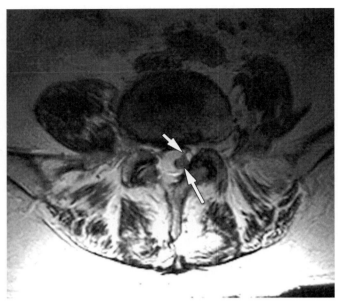

Figure 10-9 ▶ Focal Adhesions. Axial T2-weighted Image of the lumbar spine demonstrates a focal mass of adhesed nerve roots in the left side of the thecal sac *(long arrow)* with a curvilinear adhesion extending from the focal mass to the left ventral thecal sac wall *(short arrow)*.

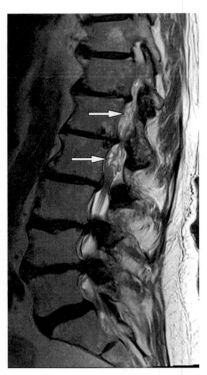

Figure 10-10 ▶ Spinal Stenosis. A narrowed spinal canal can lead to an appearance of adhesions; however, with spinal stenosis, the nerves are not thickened or adhesed to each other. Sagittal T2 MR image demonstrates very tortuous nerves, particularly cephalad to the spinal stenosis *(arrows)*.

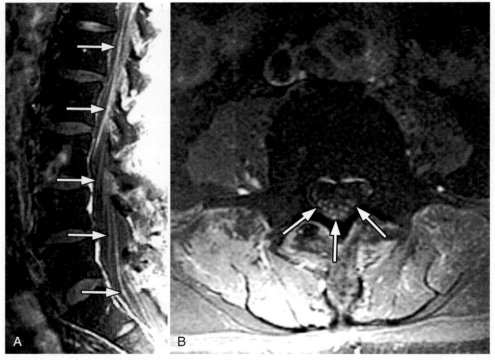

Figure 10-11 ▶ Carcinomatous Meningitis. Sagittal post-contrast T1-weighted MR image, **A,** and axial post-contrast T1-weighted MR image, **B** show the nerve root enhancement of carcinomatous meningitis *(arrows)*. The individual nerve roots can be thickened but are not typically clumped.

narcotics; however, it provides an average reduction of the patient's pain by 50% in studies up to 7 years after insertion of the device. Because this is a limited success rate, a spinal cord stimulator trial is often attempted for 5 to 7 days to discover which patients may have success.[9]

2. **Surgical treatment:** Removal of scar tissue by microsurgical lysis, laminectomy, dural decompressive grafting, and posterolateral fusion with instrumentation[14] may provide temporary relief. However, the scarring often returns after a short time.

References

1. Horrax G. Generalized cisternal arachnoiditis simulating cerebellar tumor: its surgical treatment and end results. *Arch Surg.* 1924;9:95.
2. Quiles M, Marchisello PJ, Tsairis P. Lumbar adhesive arachnoiditis: etiologic and pathologic aspects. *Spine.* 1978;3:45-50.
3. Hansen EB, Fahrenkrug A, Praestholm J. Late meningeal effects of myelographic contrast media with special reference to Metrizamide. *Br J Radiol.* 1978;51:321.
4. Delamarter R, Ross J, Masaryk T, et al. Diagnosis of lumbar arachnoiditis by magnetic resonance imaging. *Spine.* 1990;15:4304-4310.
5. Smolik E, Nash F. Lumbar spinal arachnoiditis: a complication of the intervertebral disc operation. *Ann Surg.* 1951;133:490-495.
6. Burton CV. Lumbosacral arachnoiditis. *Spine.* 1978;3:24-30.
7. Hoffman GS. Spinal arachnoiditis: what is the clinical spectrum? *Spine.* 1983;8:538-540.
8. Bourne IH. Lumbo-sacral adhesive arachnoiditis: a review. *J R Soc Med.* 1990;83:262-265.
9. Wright MH, Denney LC. A comprehensive review of spinal arachnoiditis. *Orthop Nurs.* 2003;22:215-219.
10. Tetsworth K, Ferguson L. Arachnoiditis ossificans of the cauda equina. *Spine.* 1986;11:765-766.
11. Jorgensen J, Hansen PH, Steenskrow V, Ovesen N. A clinical and radiological study of chronic lower spinal arachnoiditis. *Neuroradiology.* 1975;9:139-144.
12. Lumbardi G, Passerini A, Migliavacca F. Spinal arachnoiditis. *Br J Radiol.* 1962;35:314-320.
13. Johnson CE, Sze G. Benign lumbar arachnoiditis: MR imaging with gadopentetate dimeglumine. *AJR Am J Roentgenol.* 1990;155:873-880.
14. Brammah T, Jayson M. Syringomyelia as a complication of spinal arachnoiditis. *Spine.* 1994;29:2603-2605.

ARTERIOVENOUS FISTULA

Douglas S. Fenton, M.D.

CLINICAL PRESENTATION

The patient is an 82-year-old man who has noted progressive walking difficulty and weakness in the legs over the last 6 months. Patient had an L3-L5 lumbar decompression 2 years earlier for spinal stenosis and noticed only partial improvement in his symptoms. Patient feels he is weak from the hips inferiorly. He can stand for only 5 minutes and walk for just 200 yards before his legs become weak. He has collapsed several times when he was unable to sit down. The patient now walks with the aid of a cane in his right hand and has developed a scoliosis. Patient denies radicular pain. Patient has occasional incontinence. Electromyogram (EMG) demonstrates severe chronic multilevel lumbar radiculopathies on the left with diffuse sensory and motor peripheral neuropathy.

IMAGING PRESENTATION

Sagittal and axial T2-weighted magnetic resonance (MR) images demonstrate a long segment region of abnormal increased signal intensity involving much of the central spinal cord from the mid thoracic region to the conus medullaris. There are multiple small ovoid regions of intermediate signal intensity along the dorsal aspect of the spinal cord. The findings represent arteriolized venous structures secondary to an extradural arteriovenous fistula with spinal cord ischemia that is likely secondary to venous hypertension and the high flow of shunted arterial blood from the fistula leading to deprivation of blood or "steal" from the spinal cord (*Fig. 11-1*).

DISCUSSION

Spinal arteriovenous malformations (AVMs) and arteriovenous fistulas (AVFs) are a group of various disorders. By definition, an AVM is an abnormal communication between the arterial and venous systems. This connection may be a simple fistula or a more complex communication. It is important to recognize the signs and symptoms of a spinal AVM because it can, in its early stages, resemble various causes of low back pain and weakness. Many patients have undergone surgical procedures for symptoms presumably related to spinal stenosis and/or foraminal narrowing only to discover later that the problem was a spinal AVM.

Traditionally, spinal AVMs have been classified as types I to IV, but more recently, Spetzler and colleagues[1,2] have offered a new classification system based on specific anatomic and pathophysiologic factors. These factors include whether the AVM is extradural or intradural, ventral or dorsal, or intramedullary in location and whether there are single or multiple feeding branches.

Initial symptoms related to venous congestion include paresthesias and/or radicular pain.[3,4] Low back pain is frequently seen. There may be weakness and gait abnormalities. Symptoms are progressive and often ascending.[5] Later in the disease process, bowel and bladder incontinence, erectile dysfunction, and urinary retention can be seen.[4]

Type I (Intradural Dorsal AVF)

Intradural dorsal arteriovenous fistulas (AVFs) are the most common type of spinal AVF, representing 60% to 80% of spinal AVMs. They are most common in males (5:1) and are more commonly found in the thoracic region.[6] Patients with AVFs usually present in the fifth to seventh decade of life. Type I fistulas are composed of a single radicular feeding artery (type I-A) or multiple radicular feeding arteries (type I-B) that communicate(s) with the venous system of the spinal cord at the dural sleeve of the nerve root.[2] Whether there are single or multiple radicular feeding arteries, there remains only a single intradural fistula. This then leads to compromise of spinal cord venous outflow with arteriolization of the coronal venous plexus, venous hypertension, and progressive myelopathy.[1,2]

Type II (Intramedullary AVM)

Intramedullary arteriovenous malformations (AVMs) have a nidus (Latin for "nest") similar to intracranial AVMs.[1] They have been referred to as classic AVMs or glomus-type lesions. Intramedullary AVMs are the second most common type of spinal AVM, representing 19% to 45% of cases.[7,8] Type II lesions are found equally in men and women and manifest in the third or fourth decade of life.[9] These AVMs are associated with aneurysms in up to 44% of cases and typically manifest with hemorrhage, either parenchymal or subarachnoid, or compression-induced acute myelopathy.[1,9] Intramedullary AVMs are further subdivided into compact or diffuse depending on the vascular architecture of the nidus.[2] These lesions can have single or multiple feeding arteries from branches of the anterior spinal artery (ASA) and posterior spinal artery (PSA). They are characterized by high pressure, relatively low resistance, and high blood flow.[1]

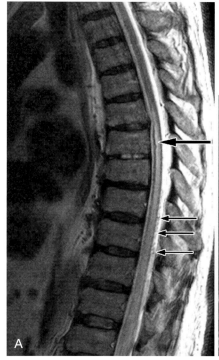
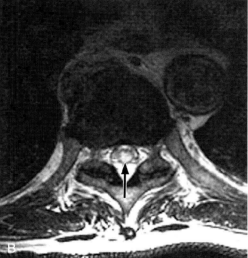

Figure 11-1 ► **Arteriovenous Fistula with Spinal Cord Ischemia.** Long segment region of abnormal increased T2 signal intensity involving the mid- and lower-thoracic spinal cord on sagittal image **A** *(large arrow)*. Note the multiple small regions of intermediate signal intensity on the dorsal aspect of the spinal cord *(small arrows)*. Axial T2-weighted MR image **B** reveals the central location of the T2 abnormality *(arrow)*.

Type III (Extradural-Intradural AVM)

Type III lesions, extradural-intradural arteriovenous malformations, are also known as *juvenile* or *metameric AVMs*. These lesions respect no tissue boundary and can involve bone, muscle, skin, spinal canal, spinal cord, and nerve roots.[1,2] These lesions are invested along a particular somite level. When the lesion involves the entire somite level, it has been called *Cobb's syndrome*.[2] Type III AVMs are extremely rare and have a poor prognosis. They usually manifest early in life with bruits and myelopathy.[10]

Type IV (Intradural Ventral AVF)

Type IV, or perimedullary-type arteriovenous malformations (AVMs), are located in the ventral midline subarachnoid space.[1,2] These lesions arise directly from the ASA and are true fistulas without an intervening capillary network.[1] Blood flow is rapid through these fistulas and can produce flow-related aneurysms and venous hypertension.[1] Over time, the size and flow of the fistula increase, and the signs and symptoms related to progressive vascular steal and spinal cord compression become more pronounced.[1,2] These patients can present with progressive venous hypertension myelopathy or hemorrhage.[10] These fistulas have been subdivided into three subtypes based on the size and flow through them.[11] Type IV-A lesions are small and have a single feeder. Blood flow is slow through Type IV-A lesions and venous hypertension is moderate.[1] Type IV-B lesions are intermediate with a major feeder from the ASA and minor feeders at the level of the fistula.[2] Type IV-C

lesions are giant fistulas with large shunt volumes and large tortuous draining veins.[10] The high flow through Type IV-C lesions leads to vascular steal from the spinal cord arterial supply and spinal cord ischemia.[2]

Extradural Arteriovenous Fistulae

Extradural arteriovenous fistulae arise from a direct connection between an extradural artery, usually arising from a branch of a radicular artery, and an extradural vein of the epidural venous plexus.[1,2] This leads to engorgement of the epidural venous system, compression of the spinal cord and nerve roots, and progressive myelopathy.[1] High venous pressure in the epidural venous system can lead to intradural venous hypertension.[1,2] The high flow of shunted arterial blood from these fistula can also lead to steal from the spinal cord and ischemia.[1,2]

Conus Medullaris AVM

The conus medullaris AVM consists of multiple feeding arteries, multiple niduses, and a complex venous drainage.[1] There are multiple arteriovenous shunts that arise from the ASA and PSA with glomus-type niduses. These AVMs are always located in the conus medullaris and cauda equina but can also extend along the entire filum terminale.[1] Clinically, they can manifest with venous hypertension, ischemia, compression, or hemorrhage, but unlike other spinal AVMs, they frequently produce symptoms of radiculopathy and myelopathy at the same time.[1]

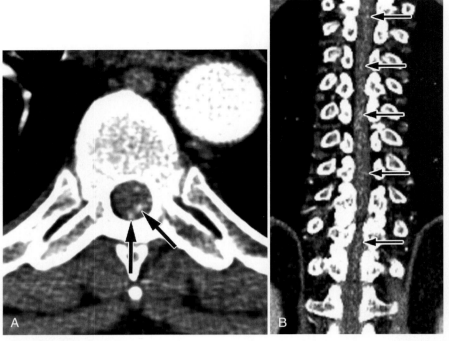

Figure 11-2 ▶ Abnormal Serpentine Enhancing Vessels (*arrows*). Shown along the posterior aspect of the spinal cord on post-contrast axial CT image **A** and coronal reformatted image **B**.

IMAGING FEATURES

Myelography demonstrates multiple curvilinear filling defects in the contrast column along the surface of the negative defect of the spinal cord. Computerized tomography (CT) may demonstrate an enlarged spinal cord and also enhance vessels along the surface of the spinal cord (*Fig. 11-2*). Magnetic resonance (MR) imaging has a distinct advantage in that it will demonstrate whether or not there are signal changes intrinsic to the spinal cord compatible with edema and/or ischemia. When the spinal cord is affected, T1-weighted MR images demonstrate an enlarged hypointense spinal cord. The spinal cord may demonstrate increased T2 signal centrally as well as flow voids along the cord surface (*Fig. 11-3*). Heterogeneous signal can occasionally be seen if there is associated hemorrhage. T1-weighted post-contrast imaging will show multiple enhancing vessels (*Fig. 11-4*).

The gold standard imaging modality for spinal vascular malformation is catheter angiography. Although there have been advances with CT angiography and MR angiography in identifying the level of the fistula and normal arterial anatomy,[12-15] catheter angiography is the only definitive method for diagnosing the type of vascular malformation, the feeding vessels, nidus architecture, and venous outflow and therefore also gives a roadmap as to the treatment plan (*Fig. 11-5*).

One of the most important parts in evaluating a spinal vascular malformation, aside from the malformation itself, is the identification of the artery of Adamkiewicz (AA). The AA is the largest anterior radiculomedullary artery with a diameter of 0.8 to 1.3 mm.[15] The AA is the main arterial supply to the lower one-third of the spinal cord and therefore must not be interrupted during endovascular or surgical treatment. The AA originates from a left intercostal or lumbar artery in 68% to 73% of patients and at the

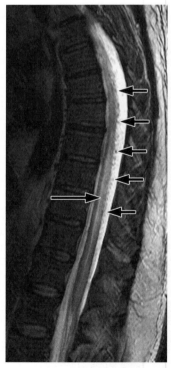

Figure 11-3 ▶ Abnormal Dorsal Flow Voids and Spinal Cord Ischemia. Sagittal T2-weighted MR image with abnormal long segment spinal cord T2 signal abnormality (*long arrow*) with multiple regions of intermediate signal on the dorsal cord surface compatible with dilated vessels (*short arrows*).

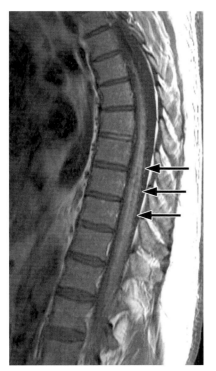

Figure 11-4 ▶ Abnormal Vasculature. (Same patient as in Figure 11-3.) Sagittal post contrast T1-weighted MR image reveals mild enhancement of the abnormal vasculature on the dorsal spinal cord surface (*arrows*).

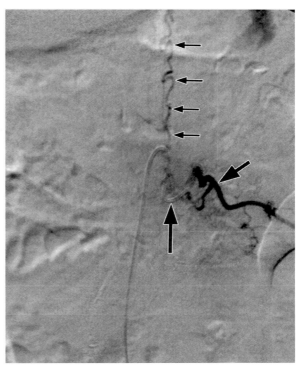

Figure 11-5 ▶ Arteriovenous Fistula. Conventional catheter angiogram subtracted view. The faint outline of a catheter (*long arrow*) is identified. A left-sided segmental artery is opacified with contrast (*short arrow*) as well as a serpentine arteriolized vein (*small arrows*).

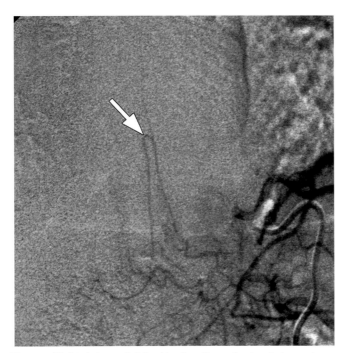

Figure 11-6 ▶ Artery of Adamkiewicz. Conventional catheter angiogram shows the classic appearance of the hairpin turn (*arrow*) seen with opacification of the artery of Adamkiewicz. One can see this angiographic appearance with any radiculomedullary artery.

level of the ninth to twelfth intercostal artery in 62% to 75% of patients.[15] The AA and ASA classically form a hairpin turn (***Fig. 11-6***). The spinal cord, embryonically, occupies the full length of the spinal canal including the 8 to 10 coccygeal sclerotomes. At full term, the ascent of the "extra" coccygeal sclerotomes causes the redundancy of the vessels cephalad forming the hairpin turn.

DIFFERENTIAL DIAGNOSIS

1. **Normal cerebrospinal fluid (CSF) pulsations on MRI:** This type of signal "abnormality" is usually posterior to the spinal cord (***Fig. 11-7***). It can have a variable appearance and can be extinguished using specific pulse sequences.
2. **Tortuous intradural nerve roots from lumbar spinal canal stenosis (*Fig. 11-8*):** With severe spinal canal stenosis, the intradural nerve roots can be prolapsed cephalad or caudal and have a similar appearance to tortuous vessels; however, the nerve roots do not enhance, or occasionally enhance only minimally.
3. **Spinal cord neoplasm** (astrocytoma, ependymoma, cavernous angioma) (***Fig. 11-9***): Post-contrast imaging should readily demonstrate an enhancing mass lesion. There can be increased vascularity associated with these neoplasms; however, they are typically not enlarged.
4. **Intradural extramedullary neoplasms** (paraganglioma): Paragangliomas can have a prominent surrounding vascular supply, but there is also an enhancing mass.
5. **Collateral venous flow:** Occlusion of the inferior vena cava (IVC) may result in shunting of venous outflow into epidural

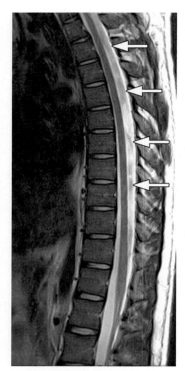

Figure 11-7 ▸ **CSF Pulsation Artifact.** Artifacts can be seen within the CSF posterior to the spinal cord (*arrows*). These should not be confused with the punctate vascular abnormalities seen with arteriovenous fistula (AVF). The spinal cord has normal signal intensity as opposed to those with spinal AVF.

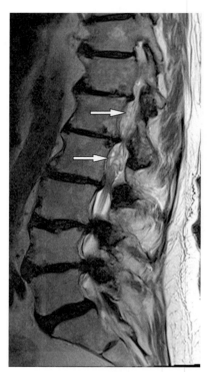

Figure 11-8 ▸ **Nerve Root Tortuosity.** The intrathecal nerve roots cranial, and sometimes caudal, to a region of severe spinal stenosis can become tortuous *(arrows)* and have the appearance of abnormal vessels.

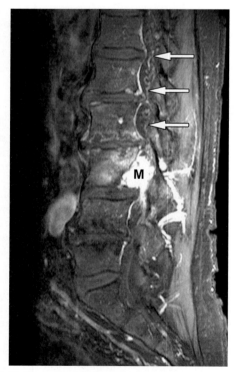

Figure 11-9 ▸ **Tumor Vascularity.** Sagittal post-contrast T1 MR image demonstrates serpentine vasculature on the dorsum to the spinal cord *(arrows)*; however, one can readily identify the mass *(M)* that these vessels are supplying.

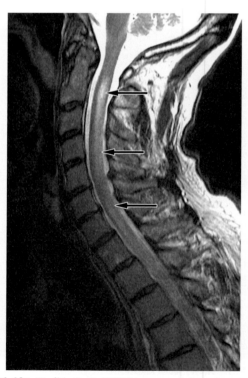

Figure 11-10 ▸ **Myelitis.** Sagittal T2 MR image reveals long segment spinal cord T2 abnormality *(arrows)* but no abnormal vessels.

and/or intradural veins. One should evaluate the IVC for its size and patency.

6. **Myelitis:** This can have an appearance similar to venous hypertension caused by AVF on T2-weighted acquisitions. Both myelitis and AVF can demonstrate long segment T2 abnormality involving the spinal cord (*Fig. 11-10*). AVF demonstrates increased vascularity, whereas myelitis does not.

TREATMENT

1. **Type I** (intradural dorsal) **AVFs:** Can be successfully treated surgically using a posterior approach. The intradural arterialized vein is identified along the nerve root and traced to its exit point at the margin of the dural root sleeve. The vein is then surgically interrupted with cauterization and microscissors.[2]

2. **Type II** (intramedullary) **AVMs:** Have been successfully treated with endovascular embolization;[16] however, the typical treatment remains surgical extirpation.[1] Through a combination of embolization and open surgery, Spetzler and colleagues have achieved gross total resections of intramedullary AVMs in 92% of patients.[1]

3. **Type III** (extradural-intradural) **AVMs:** Are primarily treated with embolization because of their diffuse involvement of neural structures, bone, and soft tissue. Surgery is reserved to decompress the mass along the nerve roots and spinal cord.[1] A complete cure is not a realistic goal. Treatment should be performed to reduce mass effect, venous hypertension, and vascular steal to reduce the patient's symptoms.[2]

4. **Types IV-A and IV-B** (intradural ventral) **AVFs:** Are treated surgically from an anterior or anterolateral approach. The key to surgical success is preservation of the ASA and its branches during obliteration of the fistula.[2] Type IV-C AVFs, because of their complex architecture and multipedicled feeders, are best treated with embolization.[1,2,11]

5. **Conus medullaris AVMs:** Are treated with combined endovascular embolization and surgery.[2] Care must be taken to separate the ASA and PSA branches from the lesion. Surgical decompression of the spinal cord and nerve roots can give significant relief to the patients.[1,2]

6. **Extradural AVFs:** Are treated with endovascular embolization.[17] Surgery is limited to patients requiring local decompression.[2]

References

1. Spetzler RF, Detwiler PW, Riina HA, Porter RW. Modified classification of spinal cord vascular lesions. *J Neurosurg.* 2002;96:145-156.
2. Kim LJ, Spetzler RF. Classification and surgical management of spinal arteriovenous lesions: arteriovenous fistulae and arteriovenous malformations. *Neurosurgery.* 2006;59(Suppl 3):S195-S201.
3. Jellema K, Canta LR, Tijssen CC, et al. Spinal dural arteriovenous fistulas: clinical features in 80 patients. *J Neurol Neurosurg Psychiatry.* 2003;74:1438–1440.
4. Krings T, Geibprasert S. Spinal dural arteriovenous fistulas. *AJNR Am J Neuroradiol.* 2009;30:639-648.
5. Koenig E, Thron A, Schrader V, et al. Spinal arteriovenous malformations and fistulae: clinical, neuroradiological and neurophysiological findings. *J Neurol.* 1989;236:260–266.
6. Berenstein A, Lasjaunias P. In: *Surgical Neuroangiography: Endovascular Treatment of Spine and Spinal Cord Lesions.* Berlin: Springer-Verlag; 1992:1-109.
7. Bao Y-H, Ling F. Classicization and therapeutic modalities of spinal vascular malformations in 80 patients. *Neurosurgery.* 1997;40:75-81.
8. Mourier KL, Gobin YP, George B, et al. Intradural perimedullary arteriovenous fistulae results of surgical and endovascular treatment in a series of 35 cases. *Neurosurgery.* 1993;32:885-891.
9. Niimi Y, Berenstein A, Setton A, Neophytides A. Embolization of spinal dural arteriovenous fistulae: results and follow up. *Neurosurgery.* 1997;40:675-682.
10. Ferch RD, Morgan MK, Sears WR. Spinal arteriovenous malformations: a review with case illustrations. *J Clin Neurosci.* 2001;8:299-304.
11. Anson JA, Spetzler RF. Classification of spinal arteriovenous malformations and implications for treatment. *BNI Quarterly.* 1992;8:2-8.
12. Saraf-Lavi E, Bowen BC, Quencer RM, Sklar EM, et al. Detection of spinal dural arteriovenous fistulae with MR imaging and contrast-enhanced MR angiography: sensitivity, specificity, and prediction of vertebral level. *AJNR Am J Neuroradiol.* 2002;23:858-867.
13. Pattany PM, Saraf-Lavi E, Bowen BC. MR angiography of the spine and spinal cord. *Top Magn Reson Imaging.* 2003;14:444-460.
14. Nakayama Y, Awai K, Yanaga Y, et al. Optimal contrast medium injection protocols for the depiction of the Adamkiewicz artery using 64-detector CT angiography. *Clin Radiol.* 2008;63:880-887.
15. Yoshioka K, Niinuma H, Ehara S, et al. MR angiography and CT angiography of the artery of Adamkiewicz: state of the art. *Radiographics.* 2006;26:S63-S73.
16. Ausman JI, Gold LH, Tadavarthy SM, et al. Intraparenchymal embolization for obliteration of an intramedullary AVM or the spinal cord: technical note. *J Neurosurg.* 1977;47:119-125.
17. Niimi Y, Berenstein A. Endovascular treatment of spinal vascular malformations. *Neurosurg Clin N Am.* 1999;10:47-71.

ATLANTOAXIAL ROTATORY FIXATION

Leo F. Czervionke, M.D.

CLINICAL PRESENTATION

The patient is a 59-year-old disabled man with longstanding left hemiparesis after intracerebral hemorrhage secondary to right basal ganglia atrioventricular (AV) malformation. Patient now presents with chronic headaches and torticollis. The patient's head and neck are rigid on physical examination.

IMAGING PRESENTATION

Stable appearance of the brain is compared with multiple previous magnetic resonance (MR) studies. On cervical spine radiographs, the head is tilted down and rotated to the left (*Fig. 12-1*) consistent with torticollis. On computed tomography (CT) scan of the cervical spine, there is clockwise rotatory subluxation of the C1 vertebra relative to C2 (*Figs. 12-2 to 12-5*).

DISCUSSION

Atlantoaxial rotatory fixation (AARF) is also called *atlantoaxial rotatory subluxation* or *fixed atlantoaxial rotatory subluxation*. In AARF, the atlas (C1) is either rotated about the odontoid process or the C1 lateral mass on one side is anteriorly subluxed and *rotated* relative to the relatively *fixed* C1-2 facets on the opposite side. The degree of atlantoaxial "rotation" in most cases occurs within the normal range of rotation of the atlantoaxial joint.

AARF is one cause of acquired torticollis and is more commonly encountered in children than in adults)[1]. Although considered by some to be rare in adults, the radiographic appearance of AARF is not uncommonly seen in adults in routine practice. AARF may occur spontaneously, secondary to spasmodic torticollis, often after an upper respiratory infection,[2,3] after major or minor cervical trauma,[2,4] secondary to C1-2 arthritis (osteoarthritis, rheumatoid arthritis, and ankylosing spondylitis),[5,6] or congenital anomalies, or is associated with infection (Grisel's syndrome). Atlanto-occipital subluxation commonly occurs in patients with Down syndrome. Mongolism may also be associated with atlanto-occipital subluxation (AOS) and AARF.[7,8] Atlantoaxial rotary fixation has been reported after disabling cerebral infarction, caused by constant head posturing to the same side (see Figs. 12-1 to 12-5).[9]

AARF may be mistakenly diagnosed on radiographic images in normal children. Relatively minor degrees of apparent AARF or nonfixated C1-2 rotary subluxation in children may be considered within normal limits.[10] In the absence of trauma or torticollis, this diagnosis should always be questioned in children. Fluoroscopic evaluation may be required to determine whether actual rotatory *fixation* exists.

Anatomically, the C1-2 articulations are unique in the spine. The capsules surrounding the lateral C1-2 (facet) joints are relatively lax compared with other facet joints, whereas the ligaments surrounding the odontoid process such as the transverse, apical, and alar ligaments are relatively less compliant. Normally, the head can be rotated 90 degrees to the left and right, and one half of this rotation is made possible by the atlantoaxial articulations,[1] the other one half allowed for by rotation of other cervical facet joints and the atlanto-occipital joints. The transverse ligament of the dens keeps the dens in close proximity to the anterior arch of C1, and the alar ligaments limit the extent of rotation of C1 relative to C2 from approximately 25 to 56 degrees.[1,11-13] When hyper-rotational stress is placed on the C1-2 joints, rotatory subluxation can occur without disruption of the alar or other periodontoid ligaments.[14] The alar ligaments are most resistant to dynamic loads placed on the C1-2 articulations.[14]

The cause of the rotatory fixation is not always known but is believed to be related initially to swollen, redundant capsular and synovial tissues surrounding the lateral and anterior atlantoaxial articulations, secondary to inflammation or trauma. In many cases, there is no known etiology for AARF. In adults, this condition is often associated with severe degenerative disease of the upper cervical facets and may or may not be associated with torticollis (*Figs. 12-6 to 12-8*). Atlantoaxial rotatory fixation may be associated with anomalies of the atlanto-occipital or atlantoaxial articulations such as atlanto-occipital fusion (*Figs. 12-9 and 12-10*). In some cases, AARF occurs secondary to congenital maldevelopment of the ligaments adjacent to these articulations. In these cases, the involved ligaments become edematous, hyperemic, and lax, which predisposes them to AARF.

Concomitant muscle spasm may occur, especially in the acute post-traumatic setting. The muscle spasm usually involves the sternocleidomastoid muscle resulting in torticollis. Later on, capsular adhesions or contractures develop.[15] The torn or thickened capsule may also invaginate into the lateral C1-2 (facet) joints, or meniscal-like synovial folds may form and extend into the lateral atlantoaxial (C1-2 facet) joints, thereby preventing or impairing rotational movement.[5]

Atlantoaxial rotatory fixation has been classified into four types by Fielding[15]:

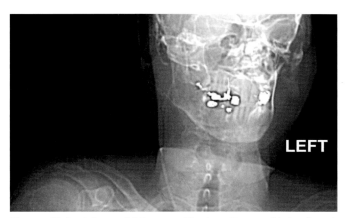

Figure 12-1 ▶ Atlantoaxial Rotatory Fixation. AP scout digital radiograph obtained prior to CT scan. The head and mandible are turned to the left in this patient with torticollis.

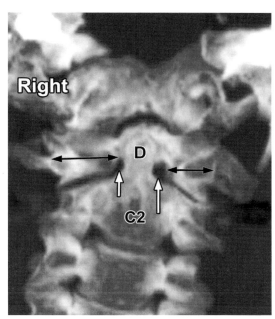

Figure 12-2 ▶ Atlantoaxial Rotatory Fixation. Same patient as in Figure 12-1. 3D surface rendered coronal CT image is equivalent to an anteroposterior (AP) *open mouth* radiograph. There is asymmetry of the lateral masses of C1. The right lateral mass of C1, which is anteriorly subluxed relative to C2, appears relatively wide *(long horizontal black arrow)* and the left lateral mass of C1, which is posteriorly subluxed relative to C2, appears relatively narrow *(short horizontal black arrow)*. The spaces between the dens *(D)* and the lateral masses of C1 are asymmetric. Because this is a 3D projection equivalent to a radiographic projection, the right lateral mass of C1 paradoxically appears closer to the dens *(short white arrow)*, whereas the left lateral mass appears further from the dens *(long white arrow)*. In reality, the opposite is actually true *(see Figure 12-3)*.

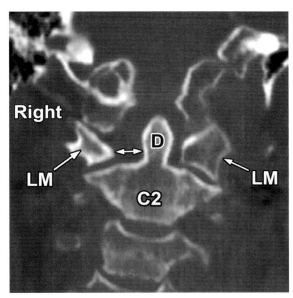

Figure 12-3 ▶ Atlantoaxial Rotatory Fixation. Coronal thin section reformatted CT image obtained through the odontoid process *(dens)*, corresponding to Figure 12-2. In reality, the space *(two headed arrow)* between the anteriorly subluxed right lateral mass of C1 and the dens *(D)* is actually widened *(compare with radiograph in Figure 12-2)*. The space between the left lateral mass of C1 and the dens is actually narrowed *(long arrow)*.

Rarely, a fifth type occurs in which both AARF and atlanto-occipital rotary subluxation are present.[1] AARF may also occur in Grisel's syndrome, which is nontraumatic atlantoaxial subluxation occurring after infection or surgery in the head and neck region, resulting in ligamentous laxity surrounding the atlantoaxial joints.[16] Occasionally, the infected ligaments will rupture.[1]

Patients with AARF present clinically with varying degrees of neck pain, diminished range-of-neck rotation, and the head is characteristically tilted, slightly flexed, and rotated to the side opposite the torticollis. Usually the patient has no neurologic deficit unless concomitant atlantoaxial subluxation is present. If there is hyper-rotation of the neck, the vertebral artery may be compromised.[1]

Torticollis may occur with or without atlantoaxial rotatory fixation. Congenital anomalies of the sternocleidomastoid muscle (e.g., congenital fibrosis), painful neck conditions such as myositis, lymphadenitis, and tumors of the cervical spine may cause contraction of the sternocleidomastoid muscle, resulting in torticollis in the absence of AARF.[1] These patients will have contraction of the sternocleidomastoid (SCM) muscle on the side opposite to the side the head is facing. In patients with both torticollis and AARF, the SCM muscle contraction occurs on the same side the head is facing.[1] If torticollis does not resolve in 1 to 2 weeks, the diagnosis of AARF should be entertained. When atlantoaxial subluxation or AARF develops after prolonged involuntary neck posturing, an underlying diagnosis of dystonia should be considered.[3]

Type 1. AARF without anterior displacement of the atlas. The odontoid acts as the pivot point (center of rotation). The transverse and alar ligaments of the dens are intact. (Most common type) (see Figs. 12-1 to 12-8).

Type 2. AARF with anterior displacement of the atlas by 3±5 mm. One articular mass acts as the pivot point. The transverse ligament is abnormal or deficient (second most common type) (see Figs. 12-9 and 12-10).

Type 3. AARF with anterior displacement of the atlas by greater than 5 mm. The transverse and alar ligaments are abnormal or deficient.

Type 4. AARF with posterior displacement of the atlas. (Rarest type associated with hypoplasia of the dens).

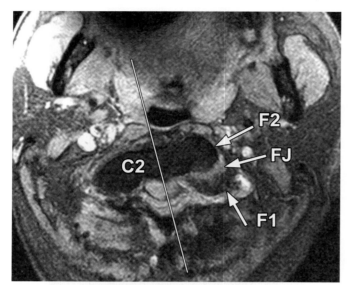

Figure 12-10 ▶ Occipital-Atlantal Assimilation (OA Fusion) Associated with Atlantoaxial Rotatory Fixation. Same patient as in Figure 12-9. On axial gradient echo MR image, the inferior C1 facet *(F1)* is rotated posteriorly relative to the left superior C2 facet *(F2)*. The left C1-2 facet joint *(FJ)* is widened. The line represents AP axis of C2 vertebra.

In cases of upper cervical trauma, fat-saturated T2-weighted MR images or STIR images should be obtained in all cases. If concomitant atlantoaxial rotatory fixation and cord compression is present, this is best demonstrated on sagittal CT reformatted images or on sagittal MR images (see Fig. 12-9). Severe trauma can also result in atlantoaxial rotatory subluxation or rarely dislocation, which is best demonstrated with CT.[23] In these cases, there is usually significant damage or rupture of the alar and transverse ligaments of the dens.

Atlanto-occipital dislocation (AOD) is rarely associated with AARF. However, in cases of severe upper cervical trauma, atlanto-occipital dislocation can occur, which is a life-threatening, often fatal condition.[24] In patients who survive this injury, severe respiratory distress is often present because of brainstem injury or retropharyngeal hematoma compressing the airway.[25] Anterior AOD is commonly evaluated on radiographs or sagittal CT images using the Power's ratio,[26] which is defined as the ratio of the distance between the basion (B) and the posterior arch of C1 (C), divided by the distance between the opisthion (O) and anterior arch of C1 (A). If the BC/OA ratio is greater than 1, this indicates anterior atlanto-occipital dislocation. However, this ratio can be less than 1 (within normal limits) and therefore misleading in posterior AOD or longitudinal AOD. Furthermore, this ratio is unreliable in patients with congenital anomalies of the foramen magnum or in fracture of the posterior arch of C1.[24,27] (For additional discussion of the Power's ratio and other measurements for assessing upper cervical instability, refer to Chapter 32, "Hangman's Fracture").

mass and the dens is actually greater than the distance between the dens and posteriorly subluxed C1 articular pillar, as demonstrated on thin section coronal and axial CT images (see Figs. 12-3 and 12-4). Rotatory subluxation is well demonstrated with multiplanar CT (see Figs. 12-3 to 12-8).[19] Three-dimensional (3D) surface-rendered CT imaging may be helpful for presurgical evaluation of these patients,[19,21] but 3D surface-rendered images are not required for the diagnosis of this condition.

The radiographic appearance of C1-2 rotary fixation may be indistinguishable from patients with torticollis without true rotatory "fixation."[2] Cinefluoroscopy, or a *functional* CT study, may be needed to confirm that the rotational anomaly is actually *fixed*, which can be confirmed by having the patient rotate the head in various positions during fluoroscopy or CT, respectively.[2,12]

Active inflammation involving the C1-2 articulations is well demonstrated on fat-saturated T2-weighted MR images or short tau inversion recovery (STIR) images, but fat-saturated contrast-enhanced T1-weighted images are most sensitive to the presence of inflammation in and adjacent to the joints or in the vertebrae, intervertebral disc, and paraspinal ligaments in general. Radionuclide bone scanning will be positive if active bone turnover is taking place, as in the case of a healing fracture or active inflammation in the C1-2 vertebrae.

In the setting of trauma, AARF may be associated with fractures of the atlas, odontoid process, or lateral masses of C2.[22] Cervical fractures are best evaluated with multiplanar CT scanning, but associated soft tissue injury to the spinal cord or paraspinous ligaments is best demonstrated with MR imaging.

MRI should be obtained in every patient with suspected trauma to the atlanto-occipital or atlantoaxial region, because it allows direct evaluation of the spinal cord for possible cord compression, evaluation of possible cord or brainstem edema, and for assessment of the paraspinal ligaments and retropharyngeal soft tissues.

DIFFERENTIAL DIAGNOSIS

The clinical and radiographic appearance of AARF is characteristic and usually no differential diagnosis is considered. Difficulties in diagnosis may arise when associated fractures, atlantoaxial subluxation, or atlanto-occipital subluxation are also present. Because an infectious process involving the C1-2 region is one cause of AARF, neck infection must be ruled out in all cases.

TREATMENT

There is controversy as to how this condition should be treated. Treatment varies and depends on severity and duration of the abnormality. Treatment of AARF can be difficult, especially in chronic cases, where the rotational anomaly is truly fixed. An attempt at correcting the rotational deformity by forcibly turning the head usually causes significant neck pain, and this should not be performed.

1. **Soft cervical collar, rest, and analgesics:** Minor degrees of early AARF after acute trauma, for example, can be treated conservatively, and the rotational anomaly often resolves spontaneously.[4] For minor and acute cases, a soft cervical collar, rest, and analgesics may be sufficient.[28]

2. **Injections:** Anesthetic or steroid injections into the C1-2 joints can relieve pain associated with AARF but do not correct the head tilt or rotational deformities because intra-articular injections do not relieve muscle spasm or dissolve ligamentous adhesions.[1] Steroidal agents should not be given if infection is suspected.

3. **Skull traction:** Treatment by skull traction has been used in some patients in the post-traumatic setting, but its use is

controversial and potentially dangerous; traction may cause additional injury to the spinal cord.[15,27]

4. **Arthrodesis and/or posterior cervical fusion:** C1-2 lateral mass arthrodesis and/or posterior cervical fusion has been performed in some patients for treatment of AARF.[29]

5. **Antibiotics:** The primary treatment of Grisel's syndrome is medical. The microbial organism should be isolated and treated with the appropriate antibiotic.[16] If a neck abscess is present, it may require surgical drainage.

References

1. Roche CJ, O'Malley M, Dorgan JC, Carty HM. A pictorial review of atlantoaxial rotatory fixation: key points for the radiologist. *Clin Radiol.* 2001;56(12):947-958.
2. Kowalski HM, Cohen WA, Cooper P, Wisoff JH. Pitfalls in the CT diagnosis of atlantoaxial rotary subluxation. *AJR Am J Roentgenol.* 1987;149(3):595-600.
3. Dalvie S, Moore AP, Findlay GF. C1/C2 rotary subluxation due to spasmodic torticollis. *J Neurol Neurosurg Psychiatry.* 2000;69(1):135-136.
4. Sobolewski BA, Mittiga MR, Reed JL. Atlantoaxial rotary subluxation after minor trauma. *Pediatr Emerg Care.* 2008;24(12):852-856.
5. Chang H, Found EM, Clark CR, et al. Meniscus-like synovial fold in the atlantoaxial (C1-C2) joint. *J Spinal Disord.* 1992;5(2):227-231.
6. Leventhal MR, Maguire JK, Jr., Christian CA. Atlantoaxial rotary subluxation in ankylosing spondylitis: a case report. *Spine (Phila Pa 1976).* 1990;15(12):1374-1376.
7. Menezes AH, Ryken TC. Craniovertebral abnormalities in Down's syndrome. *Pediatr Neurosurg.* 1992;18(1):24-33.
8. Stein SM, Kirchner SG, Horev G, Hernanz-Schulman M. Atlanto-occipital subluxation in Down syndrome. *Pediatr Radiol.* 1991;21(2):121-124.
9. Mori K, Hukuda S, Katsuura A, et al. Spontaneous atlantoaxial rotatory fixation in old age after cerebral infarction: case report. *Spine.* 2000;25(16):2137-2140.
10. Villas C, Arriagada C, Zubieta JL. Preliminary CT study of C1-C2 rotational mobility in normal subjects. *Eur Spine J.* 1999;8(3):223-228.
11. Penning L, Wilmink JT. Rotation of the cervical spine: a CT study in normal subjects. *Spine (Phila Pa 1976).* 1987;12(8):732-738.
12. Dvorak J, Hayek J, Zehnder R. CT-functional diagnostics of the rotatory instability of the upper cervical spine. Part 2. An evaluation on healthy adults and patients with suspected instability. *Spine (Phila Pa 1976).* 1987;12(8):726-731.
13. Dvorak J, Panjabi M, Gerber M, Wichmann W. CT-functional diagnostics of the rotatory instability of upper cervical spine. 1. An experimental study on cadavers. *Spine (Phila Pa 1976).* 1987;12(3):197-205.
14. Goel VK, Winterbottom JM, Schulte KR, et al. Ligamentous laxity across C0-C1-C2 complex: axial torque-rotation characteristics until failure. *Spine (Phila Pa 1976).* 1990;15(10):990-996.
15. Fielding JW, Hawkins RJ. Atlantoaxial rotatory fixation. (Fixed rotatory subluxation of the atlantoaxial joint). *J Bone Joint Surg Am.* 1977;59(1):37-44.
16. Wetzel FT, La Rocca H. Grisel's syndrome. *Clin Orthop Relat Res.* 1989;(240):141-152.
17. Wortzman G, Dewar FP. Rotary fixation of the atlantoaxial joint: rotational atlantoaxial subluxation. *Radiology.* 1968;90(3):479-487.
18. Hopla DM, Mazur JM, Bass RM. Cervical vertebrae subluxation. *Laryngoscope.* 1983;93(9):1155-1159.
19. Cowan IA, Inglis GS. Atlantoaxial rotatory fixation: improved demonstration using spiral CT. *Australas Radiol.* 1996;40(2):119-124.
20. Ajmal M, O'Rourke SK. Odontoid Lateral Mass Interval (OLMI) asymmetry and rotary subluxation: a retrospective study in cervical spine injury. *J Surg Orthop Adv.* 2005;14(1):23-26.
21. Duan S, Huang X, Lin Q, Chen G. Clinical significance of articulating facet displacement of lateral atlantoaxial joint on 3D CT in diagnosing atlantoaxial subluxation. *J Formos Med Assoc.* 2007;106(10):840-846.
22. Fuentes S, Bouillot P, Palombi O, et al. Traumatic atlantoaxial rotatory dislocation with odontoid fracture: case report and review. *Spine (Phila Pa 1976).* 2001;26(7):830-834.
23. Amirjamshidi A, Abbassioun K, Khazenifar M, Esmailijah A. Traumatic rotary posterior dislocation of the atlas on the axis without fracture: report of a case and review of literature. *Surg Neurol.* 2009;71(1):92-97; discussion 8.
24. Ahuja A, Glasauer FE, Alker GJ Jr, Klein DM. Radiology in survivors of traumatic atlanto-occipital dislocation. *Surg Neurol.* 1994;41(2):112-118.
25. Cohen A, Hirsch M, Katz M, Sofer S. Traumatic atlanto-occipital dislocation in children: review and report of five cases. *Pediatr Emerg Care.* 1991;7(1):24-27.
26. Powers B, Miller MD, Kramer RS, et al. Traumatic anterior atlanto-occipital dislocation. *Neurosurgery.* 1979;4(1):12-17.
27. Labbe JL, Leclair O, Duparc B. Traumatic atlanto-occipital dislocation with survival in children. *J Pediatr Orthop B.* 2001;10(4):319-327.
28. Muniz AE, Belfer RA. Atlantoaxial rotary subluxation in children. *Pediatr Emerg Care.* 1999;15(1):25-29.
29. El Masry MA, El Assuity WI, Sadek FZ, Salah H. Two methods of atlantoaxial stabilisation for atlantoaxial instability. *Acta Orthop Belg.* 2007;73(6):741-746.

CHAPTER 13

BURST FRACTURE

Douglas S. Fenton, M.D.

CLINICAL PRESENTATION

The patient is a 24-year-old female who states that at approximately 2:30 P.M. today, she jumped off a second-floor balcony for fun. The patient states that she landed on her feet on a grassy surface. The patient states that she had immediate onset of low back pain. The patient, at this time, rates that pain at 9 out of 10. She states it is constant and aching in nature and made worse with any movements. The patient denies leg pain, neck pain, paresthesias, or alteration in motor function. The patient states that she has a numb feeling in both hips and has been incontinent of urine.

IMAGING PRESENTATION

Frontal and lateral radiographs reveal compression of the superior and inferior L2 endplates with bone fragments and anterior and posterior extension of bone compatible with a burst fracture. There is evidence of spinal stenosis at the fracture level from the retropulsed fragment *(Fig. 13-1)*.

DISCUSSION

Thoracolumbar fractures can be divided into several different types including wedge-compression deformities, flexion-distraction injuries (including Chance [seat belt] fractures) and burst fractures.[1,2] Approximately 90% of all spinal fractures occur in the thoracolumbar spine with burst fractures comprising 10% to 20% of them).[3,4]

Burst fractures result from an axial compressive load applied to the spinal column with varying degrees of flexion and/or rotation. There is centripetally oriented disruption of the vertebral body. There is typically a comminuted vertical fracture of the vertebrae originating near the region of the basivertebral vein (88% of cases) with unilateral (38.7%) or bilateral (46.6%) posterior element fractures, anterior wedge deformity (average height loss of 35.4%), increased interpediculate distance (81%), and a retropulsed fragment into the spinal canal, usually from the posterosuperior corner of the vertebral body causing significant narrowing of the spinal canal (average anterosposterior canal compromise of 57.3%).[5] The comminuted fracture of the superior endplate may extend through the vertebral body to connect with a comminuted fracture of the inferior endplate (type A fracture). The more common classic burst fracture (type B) has retropulsion of bone into the spinal canal from a fracture of the posterosuperior endplate with an intact inferior endplate. Type B fractures can lead to acute or late kyphosis. A type C fracture is a rare, isolated fracture of the inferior endplate.[3] Type D fractures are burst fractures with lateral translation, and type E is a unilateral burst fracture.[3]

The T12-L2 vertebrae are the most vulnerable to burst fractures. Above T12, the facet joints limit extension and the costotransverse and costovertebral joints add stability.[6] Below L2, stability is added by the psoas muscle and strong intraspinous and supraspinous ligaments.[7] At the thoracolumbar junction, the facet joints change from coronal to sagittal orientation, and the spine changes from kyphosis to lordosis allowing for greater flexion, extension, and sliding motion during trauma.[6]

The stability of a thoracolumbar burst fracture is a topic of much debate because stability is the most important determinant for the choice of treatment.[8] Instability can be defined as the loss of the spine's ability to maintain relationship between the vertebrae under normal physiologic loads. The two-column concept of spinal stability was described by Holdsworth.[9] The spine is divided into anterior and posterior columns. The anterior column consists of the vertebral body, intervertebral disc, and anterior and posterior longitudinal ligaments. The posterior column consists of the pedicles, articular facets, ligamentum flavum, and the interspinous and supraspinous ligaments. A three-column concept was introduced by Denis.[3,10] In the three-column concept, the posterior column remains the same; however, the Holdsworth's anterior column is divided into anterior and middle columns. The middle column is in essence the posterior half of Holdworth's anterior column. The middle column contains the posterior half of the vertebral body, the posterior annulus fibrosis, and the posterior longitudinal ligament *(Fig. 13-2)*.[8-10] Holdsworth considered burst fractures to be stable, because although the anterior column (Denis' anterior and middle columns) was compressed, the posterior column was sufficiently intact. Denis believed that involvement of the middle column was sufficient evidence to consider the fracture to be unstable. Denis' three-column theory is the more widely used concept today; however, since the advent of magnetic resonance imaging (MRI), evaluation of the posterior ligamentous complex (supraspinous ligament, interspinous ligament, ligamentum flavum, and facet joint capsules) has been used to assess stability of a thoracolumbar burst fracture. If the posterior ligamentous complex demonstrates abnormal increased T2-weighted signal intensity, then this would suggest relative instability.[11,12] Radiographic signs of instability also include widening of the interspinous distance, translation of greater than 2 mm, kyphosis of greater than 20 degrees, loss of 50% or more, and fractures of the articular processes.[13]

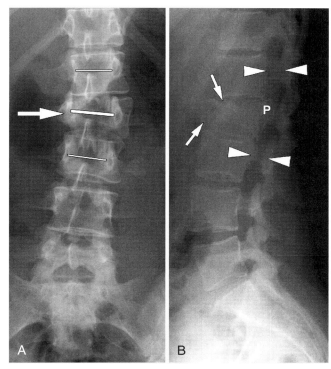

Figure 13-1 ▶ Burst Fracture. Frontal radiograph demonstrates decreased height of the L2 vertebral body *(arrow)* and widening of the interpediculate distance *(white line in comparison with levels above and below)*. The lateral radiograph shows the L2 vertebral fracture to be comminuted *(arrows)* along with compression of both the superior and inferior endplates. There is retropulsion of a fragment of bone *(P)* from the posterosuperior aspect of L2, which causes spinal canal narrowing. The normal anteroposterior dimension of the spinal canal is depicted between the arrowheads at L1 and L3.

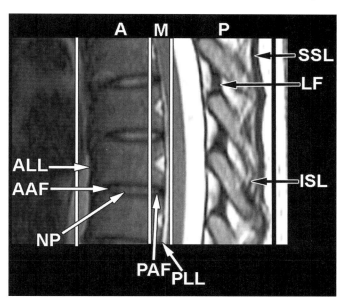

Figure 13-2 ▶ Three-column Concept of Spine Stability. On sagittal imaging, the spine is divided into anterior *(A)*, middle *(M)* and posterior *(P)* columns. The anterior column consists of the anterior longitudinal ligament *(ALL)*, the anterior anulus fibrosis *(AAF)*, and the nucleus pulposus *(NP)*. The middle column consists of the posterior annulus fibrosis *(PAF)* and posterior longitudinal ligament *(PLL)*. The posterior column consists of all structures posterior to the posterior longitudinal ligament including the ligamentum flavum *(LF)*, interspinous ligament *(ISL)*, and supraspinous ligament *(SSL)* and facet joint capsules *(not pictured)*.

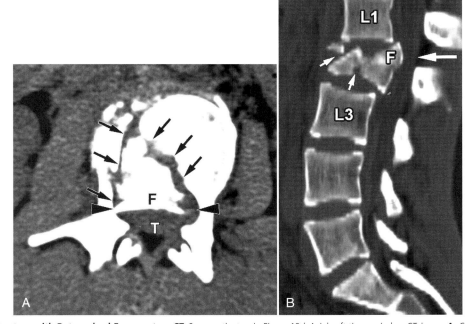

Figure 13-3 ▶ Burst Fracture with Retropulsed Fragment on CT. Same patient as in Figure 13-I. Axial soft tissue window CT, image **A.** Comminuted vertebral fracture *(arrows)* with retropulsion of a fracture fragment *(F)* causing moderate to severe compression of the thecal sac *(T)* and regions of the lateral recesses *(arrowheads)*. Sagittal bone window CT, image **B,** reveals the comminution of the vertebral body *(small arrows)* and the retropulsed fragment *(F)* causing narrowing of the central spinal canal *(large arrow)*.

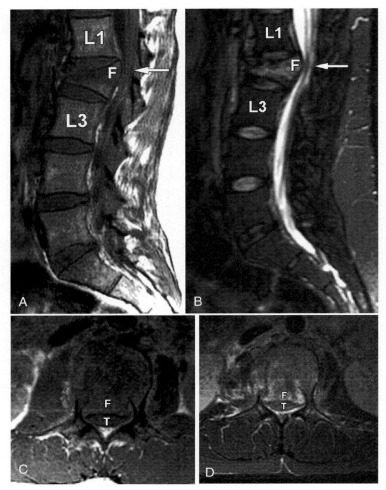

Figure 13-4 ▶ Burst Fracture with Retropulsed Fragment on MRI. Same patient as in Figures 13-1 and 13-3. Sagittal T1-weighted MR image **A,** and fat-saturated T2-weighted MR image **B.** Superior and inferior endplate compression deformity of L2 with kyphotic angulation. The L2 vertebral body displays decreased T1/increased T2 signal intensity compatible with marrow edema. There is retropulsion of bone *(F)* from the posterosuperior L2 vertebral body causing central canal stenosis *(arrow).* Axial T1-weighted MR image **C** and fat-saturated T2-weighted MR image **D** better demonstrate the degree of spinal canal narrowing and the relationship of the fracture fragment *(F)* to the thecal sac *(T).*

Patients with thoracolumbar burst fractures present with back pain and/or back tenderness on palpation. Neurologic injury from burst fractures is common, seen in nearly two thirds of patients.[5] Because the spinal cord terminates at the same level of typical thoracolumbar fractures, patients can present with bowel and bladder signs and decreased movement/sensation in the lower extremities.

IMAGING FEATURES

Many of the typical burst fracture findings can be seen with plain film radiographs. On the lateral view, one can see the wedge-shaped fracture deformity, the degree of kyphosis, widening of the interspinous distance if there is ligamentous disruption, and any translation of the vertebral body (see Fig. 13-1, *B*). On the anteroposterior view, one can see widening of the interpediculate distance (see Fig. 13-1, *A*) and/or widening of the interspinous distance. Computed tomography (CT), with sagittal and coronal reformatted images, is

superior to plain film radiographs in that one can directly visualize the posteriorly directed bone fragment and assess the degree of spinal canal and/or neural foraminal narrowing. Aside from the vertebral compression fracture, one is able to discern fractures of the neural arch. One can also see indirect signs of ligamentous disruption (interspinous widening, facet articulation separation, and vertebral body translation). CT using bone algorithm best defines the fractures, and soft tissue algorithm is best to evaluate central canal and foraminal compromise *(Fig. 13-3).* On MRI, abnormal decreased T1 and increased T2 signal intensities are seen in the affected vertebrae. Kyphotic angulation can be measured. Spinal canal narrowing from the retropulsed fragment can be assessed *(Fig. 13-4).* MRI is being used more often in thoracolumbar fractures because of its ability to demonstrate soft tissue injury. Ligamentous injury is suggested by abnormal increased T2 or short tau inversion recovery (STIR) signal intensity in the regions of the various ligaments. MRI will also demonstrate abnormal signal intensity in the spinal cord if it has been injured or demonstrate the presence or absence of a hematoma in the spinal canal.

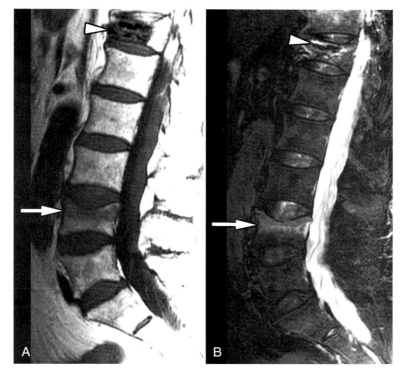

Figure 13-5 ▶ Osteoporotic Compression Deformity. Sagittal T1-weighted MR image, **A**, and fat-saturated T2-weighted MR image, **B**. Compression of the superior endplate of L4 with a band of decreased T1 signal intensity (*arrow*, image **A**) and increased T2 signal intensity (*arrow*, image **B**) paralleling the superior endplate. There is no evidence of a retropulsed fragment. Note the chronic compression deformity of the T12 vertebral body, which has been percutaneously treated with vertebral augmentation (*arrowhead*).

DIFFERENTIAL DIAGNOSIS

1. **Osteoporotic compression (wedge compression) fractures:** These can appear similar to a burst fracture; however, the retropulsion of bone, if it occurs, is minimal, although it is typically from the posterosuperior portion of the vertebral body. There is also no widening of the interpediculate distance. T1 signal changes are often limited to an endplate and parallel that endplate (*Fig. 13-5*).

2. **Flexion distraction injuries:** Such fractures at the thoracolumbar region are commonly called *Chance fractures*. These unstable fractures disrupt both the posterior and middle columns and often extend into the anterior column. One may see a horizontal fracture through the spinous process (*Fig. 13-6*) and posterior elements or, less commonly, separation of the spinous processes caused by ligamentous disruption. The tensile strength of the ligaments is greater than that of the bone, and therefore the bone will fracture before the ligaments fail.[14] Abnormal low T1 signal intensity can be seen in the compressed vertebral body, often with a cleft representing a fracture line.

3. **Pathologic compression fractures:** These typically demonstrate complete replacement of the vertebral body marrow with decreased T1/increased T2 signal intensity and enhancement and may have an associated soft tissue mass (*Fig. 13-7*).

TREATMENT

1. **Conservative treatment** is considered appropriate for thoracolumbar burst fractures without neurologic deficit. A review of the literature demonstrated no statistically significant difference in functional outcome 2 years after conservative or operative treatment for thoracolumbar fractures without neurologic deficit.[15] Conservative treatment typically consists of a combination of bed rest, functional rehabilitation, a body cast/orthosis, and postural reduction.

2. **Operative treatment** is considered appropriate in patients with an unstable burst fracture and a neurologic deficit. Surgical goals include decompression of the spinal canal, restoration of vertebral height, and alignment and prevention of further spinal deformity.[8]

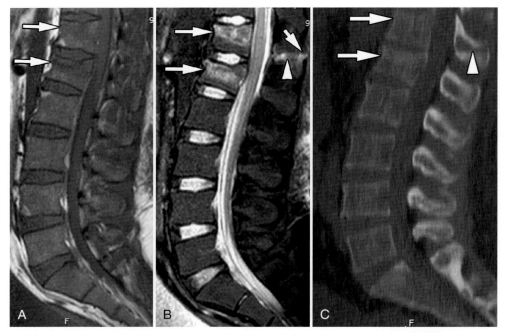

Figure 13-6 ► **Flexion-distraction Injury.** Linear band of decreased T1 signal intensity and increased T2 signal intensity paralleling the compressed superior endplates of the T12 and L1 vertebral bodies (*long arrows*) on sagittal T1-weighted MR image **A** and fat-saturated T2-weighted MR image **B**. One can also appreciate abnormal increased T2 signal intensity through the middle of the T12 spinous process (*arrowhead*) secondary to traumatic disruption of the supraspinous ligament (*short arrow*). Midline sagittal CT image **C** in the same patient demonstrates mild compression of the superior endplates of T12 and L1 (*arrows*) and a linear fracture through the T12 spinous process (*arrowhead*).

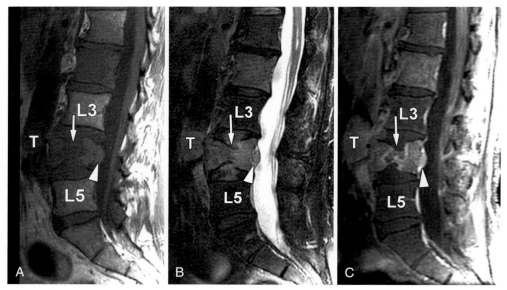

Figure 13-7 ► **Pathologic Fracture.** Sagittal T1-weighted MR image **A,** fat-saturated T2-weighted MR image **B,** and fat-saturated post-contrast T1-weighted MR image **C**. There is abnormal decreased T1 signal intensity, increased T2 signal intensity and enhancement throughout the L4 and L2 vertebral bodies compatible with metastatic disease. The L4 vertebral body is compressed with a central cleft (*arrow*) as well as retropulsion of pathologic bone into the ventral epidural space (*arrowhead*). Also noted is a tumor (*T*) within the inferior vena cava ventral to the L4 vertebral body from contiguous spread.

References

1. Shuman WP, Rogers JV, Sickler ME, et al. Thoracolumbar burst fractures: CT dimensions of the spinal canal relative to postsurgical improvement. *AJR Am J Roentgenol.* 1985;145:337-341.
2. McAfee PC, Yuan HA, Fredrickson BE, Lubicky JP. The value of computed tomography in thoracolumbar fractures. *J Bone Joint Surg Am.* 1983;65:461-473.
3. Denis F. The three-column spine and its significance in the classification of acute thoracolumbar spinal injuries. *Spine.* 1983;8:817-831.
4. Kraemer WJ, Schemitsch EH, Lever J, et al. Functional outcome of thoracolumbar burst fractures without neurological deficit. *J Orthop Trauma.* 1996;10:541-544.
5. Atlas SW, Regenbogen V, Rogers LF, Kim KS. The radiographic characterization of burst fractures of the spine. *AJR Am J Roentgenol.* 1986;147:575-582.
6. Brant-Zawadzki M, Jeffrey RB, Minagi H, Pitts LH. High resolution CT of thoracolumbar fractures. *AJNR Am J Neuroradiol.* 1982;3:69-74.
7. Gui L, Savini R, Sgattoni M. Surgical stabilization of fractures of the thoracic and lumbar spine by Harrington's technique. *Ital J Orthop Traumatol.* 1980;6:157-173.
8. Dai LY, Jiang SD, Wang XY, Jiang LS. A review of the management of thoracolumbar burst fractures. *Surg Neurol.* 2007;67:221-231.
9. Holdsworth FW. Fractures, dislocations and fracture-dislocations of the spine. *J Bone Joint Surg Am.* 1970;52:1534-1551.
10. Denis F. Spinal instability as defined by the three-column spine concept in acute spinal trauma. *Clin Orthop.* 1984;189:65-76.
11. Oner FC, van Gils AP, Dhert WJ, Verbout AJ. MRI findings of thoracolumbar spine fractures: a categorisation based on MRI examination of 100 fractures. *Skeletal Radiol.* 1999;28:433-443.
12. Dai LY, Ding WG, Wang XY, et al. Assessment of ligamentous injury in patients with thoracolumbar burst fractures using MRI. *J Trauma.* 2009;66:1610-1615.
13. Petersilge CA, Emery SE. Thoracolumbar burst fracture: evaluating stability. *Semin Ultrasound CT MR.* 1996;17:105-113.
14. Davis JM, Beall DP, Lastine C, et al. Chance fracture of the upper thoracic spine. *AJR Am J Roentgenol.* 2004;183:1475-1478.
15. Yi L, Jingping B, Gele J, et al. Operative versus non-operative treatment for thoracolumbar burst fractures without neurological deficit. Cochrane Database of Systematic Reviews 2006, Issue 4. Art. No.: CD005079. DOI: 10.1002/14651858.CD005079.pub2.

CAUDA EQUINA SYNDROME

Douglas S. Fenton, M.D.

CLINICAL PRESENTATION

The patient is a 24-year-old female who presents acutely with low back pain and urinary incontinence. She has seen several physicians and has had several emergency room visits in the last 6 months for escalating back and leg pain. She had an imaging study that demonstrated a small focal disc herniation at L3-4. She has been taking over-the-counter pain medications ever since. This afternoon she took a nap and when she woke up she felt that her feet were swollen. She cannot move her toes. When she went to the bathroom, she lost control of her bladder. She feels numb from the waist down. Her legs show a sensory deficit at the lower outer mid leg in approximately the L5 distribution. She has intact hip flexion and knee extension. She is unable to flex or extend her ankles. She has intact distal pulses. She has brisk symmetric patellar reflexes. She has no Achilles reflex and a Babinski reflex cannot be obtained on either side.

IMAGING PRESENTATION

Sagittal and axial T2-weighted magnetic resonance (MR) images reveal a very large soft tissue mass extending posteriorly to occupy the entire spinal canal at the level of the L3-4 disc. This mass appears to be connected to the L3-4 disc and has similar signal intensity to disc material. The findings are compatible with a large disc herniation. On the axial T2-weighted MR image, there is obliteration of the normal cerebrospinal fluid (CSF)–containing thecal sac from the disc herniation, which incorrectly makes this image look T1-weighted (*Fig. 14-1*).

DISCUSSION

Cauda equina syndrome (CES) has been defined as low back pain, unilateral or usually bilateral sciatica, saddle sensory disturbances, bladder and bowel dysfunction, and variable lower extremity motor and sensory loss including paraplegia.[1-3] The clinical diagnosis of CES should not be made unless there is bladder, bowel, or sexual function abnormality.[1-3]

The cauda equina is formed by the nerve roots caudal to the level of the conus medullaris. The cauda equina syndrome can result from any lesion that compresses the cauda equina and causes a dysfunction of multiple lumbar and sacral nerve roots. The most common etiology of CES is a large central lumbar disc herniation

at the L4-5 or L5-S1 level. Patients may be predisposed to CES if they have a congenitally narrow spinal canal or an acquired spinal stenosis. Some other etiologies of cauda equina syndrome include a traumatic injury, neoplasm, spinal anesthesia, spinal epidural hematoma, abscess, late stage ankylosing spondylitis, inferior vena cava thrombosis, and iatrogenic causes such as chiropractic manipulation or postoperative complications.[4-8] There is no gender or race predilection for CES; however, atraumatic CES is most often seen in adults secondary to surgical morbidity, disc degeneration, neoplasm, and abscess. If a young adult presents with CES, a large midline disc herniation should be suspected.[9]

Patients with CES often present with bilateral leg symptoms that include sciatica, weakness, sensory changes, and gait disturbances. The symptoms can vary greatly: from mild paresis to complete paralysis, paresthesia to complete anesthesia, difficulty walking to inability to ambulate. There can be minimal to no back pain. Bowel or bladder incontinence can present alone or in combination. The urinary incontinence of CES is due to overflow from an asensate bladder with high volumes.[9,10] Most clinicians divide CES into two categories: CES with established urinary retention or incomplete CES in which there is reduced urinary sensation, loss of desire to void, or a poor stream, but no established retention or overflow.[11,12] It is important to know whether the patient is incontinent to urine at the time of presentation because this has a very poor prognosis.[13]

The diagnosis of CES begins with a good history and the finding of any of the classic symptoms of CES. A physical examination can narrow the differential. With CES, the patient's reflexes may be diminished or absent. Hyperactive reflexes may signify a lesion above the cauda. Likewise, a positive Babinski sign should lead one away from the diagnosis of CES and toward an upper motor neuron lesion. The urinary bladder can be catheterized to evaluate for a significant urine volume with little to no urge to void.[10]

IMAGING FEATURES

Plain radiographs have limited value in the evaluation of CES. One may occasionally find a traumatic fracture or destructive changes that could point toward a potential source of a patient's CES. Computed tomography (CT) is a better choice than plain radiography because it can better demonstrate spinal canal narrowing and its potential causes, be it a fracture, large disc herniation, metastatic lesion, hematoma, or other compressive lesion. A myelogram with a postmyelogram CT is more sensitive than a plain CT; however,

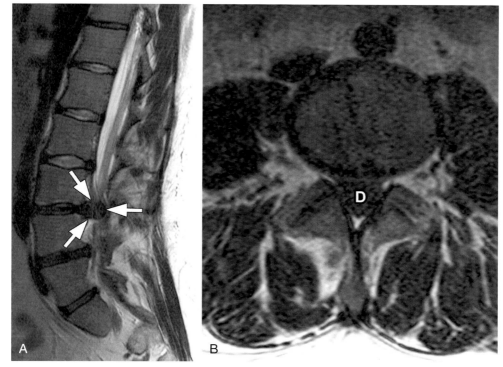

Figure 14-1 ▶ Large Lumbar Disc Herniation. Sagittal T2-weighted MR image **A** and axial T2-weighted MR image **B** at the L3-4 disc level. Large disc herniation (*arrows*, image **A**) completely obliterates the thecal sac at L3-4. Axial image, **B**, demonstrates absence of the normal increased T2-weighted signal intensity of the thecal sac because the disc herniation (*D*) occupies all the available space.

it is a more invasive test and will occasionally need more than one puncture of the dura, (lumbar and cervical) if there is a complete myelographic block to assess the full extent of the abnormality *(Fig. 14-2)*. Magnetic resonance imaging (MRI), given its greater soft tissue discrimination, can readily discern the relationship between the offending lesion and the cauda equina and often obviate the need for CT with or without myelography *(Fig. 14-3)*.[14] T2-weighted MR images are valuable because they render CSF bright and the intrathecal nerve roots of decreased signal intensity. It is difficult to see the relationship of an offending lesion and the cauda equina by T1-weighted MR imaging because both the intrathecal CSF and nerve roots are of decreased signal intensity *(Fig. 14-4)*.

DIFFERENTIAL DIAGNOSIS

The cauda equina syndrome does not have a differential diagnosis because it is not a single entity. It is a clinical syndrome that can be caused by any compressive lesion of the lumbar and sacral nerve roots. What is important is differentiating the causes of CES, which include the following:

1. Large midline lumbar disc herniations (see Fig. 14-1)
2. Traumatic injury *(Fig. 14-5)*
3. Neoplasm
4. Spinal epidural hematoma (see Fig. 14-3)
5. Spinal anesthesia

6. Epidural abscess/phlegmon *(Fig. 14-6)*
7. Late stage ankylosing spondylitis
8. Inferior vena cava thrombosis
9. Iatrogenic causes (chiropractic manipulation or postoperative complications such as hematoma)

TREATMENT

Surgical management. If a patient is discovered to have a potentially reversible cause of CES, then surgery is recommended. Management would depend on what the cause of the patient's CES is; however, because most cases of CES are secondary to a large midline lumbar disc herniation, surgical decompression with discectomy should be performed. The debate lies in the urgency of the surgical decompression. When a person presents with CES, it is understandable to think that the quicker to decompression, the better chance for recovery; however, ethical considerations would not allow this hypothesis to be tested.[11] One review suggests that only patients with CES without urinary retention should have urgent surgical decompression because outcomes of surgery in those with urinary retention have no bearing on the timing of the surgery.[15] A large review of cases of CES suggests that surgical intervention within 48 hours of the onset of symptoms will produce better outcomes than if surgery is delayed.[4] A reanalysis of these same data suggests that intervention within 24 hours of onset of symptoms demonstrates a better prognosis in patients with CES, whether or not there is urinary retention.[16]

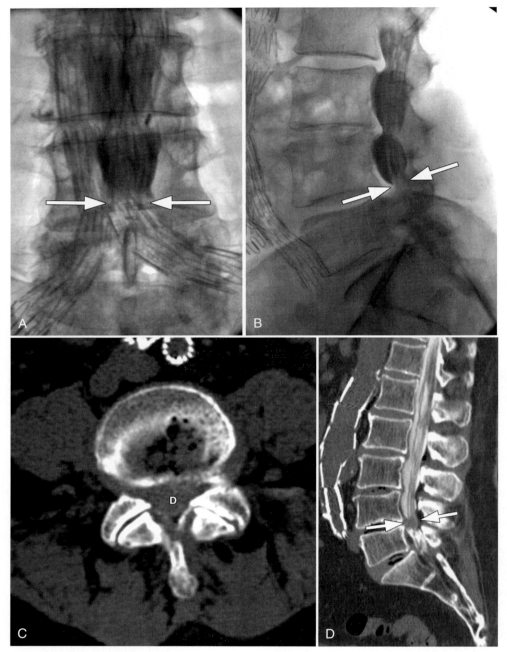

Figure 14-2 ▶ Myelographic Block from Large Disc Herniation. Frontal, **A,** and lateral, **B,** lumbar myelogram images. Axial, **C,** and reformatted sagittal, **D,** CT images after myelography. Nearly complete obliteration of the contrast-filled spinal canal at the L4-5 disc level *(arrows). D* = Disc material.

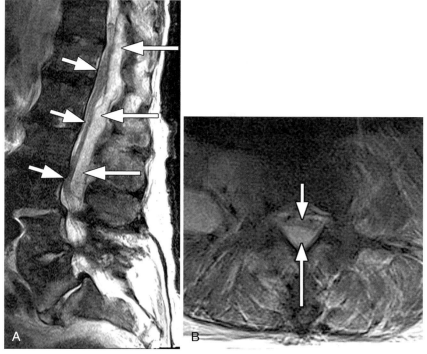

Figure 14-3 ▶ Spinal Epidural Hematoma. Long-segment region of intraspinal increased T2 signal intensity on sagittal image **A** (*long arrows*). The spinal cord and cauda equina (*short arrows*) are displaced anteriorly. Axial T2-weighted MR image **B** shows the hematoma posteriorly (*long arrow*) and the spinal cord ventrally (*short arrow*).

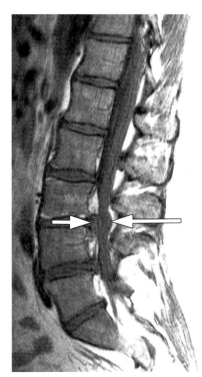

Figure 14-4 ▶ Disc Herniation on TI-Weighted MRI. Same patient as in Figure 14-1. One can readily identify the ventral portion of the disc herniation (*short arrow*); however, the extruded portion posteriorly has similar signal intensity to normal CSF and is therefore easily overlooked (*long arrow*).

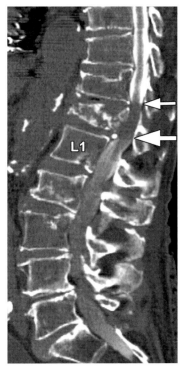

Figure 14-5 ▶ Traumatic Vertebral Injury. Sagittal reformatted CT image post-myelogram. Traumatic burst fracture of T12 with retropulsion of bone. There is complete obstruction to the flow of contrast both caudal and cranial to T12. Contrast injection was initially performed at L3, evaluating only the lower level of the obstruction (*large arrow*). A cervical puncture with additional contrast administration was necessary to evaluate the upper level of the obstruction (*small arrow*).

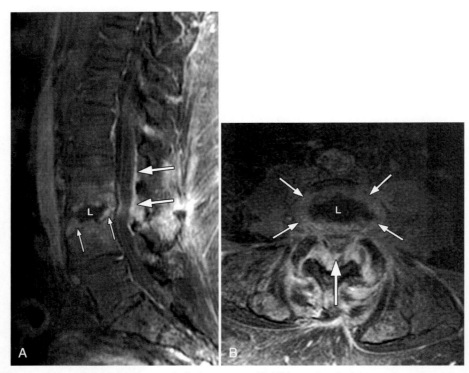

Figure 14-6 ▶ Discitis/Osteomyelitis with Epidural Abscess. Sagittal post-contrast T1 MR image **A** and axial post-contrast T1-weighted MR image **B**. Enhancement of the L4-5 intervertebral disc (*small arrows*), liquefaction of the central disc (*L*), and enhancement in the epidural space (*large arrows*).

References

1. Aho AJ, Auranen A, Pesonen K. Analysis of cauda equina symptoms in patients with lumbar disc prolapse. *Acta Chir Scand*. 1969;135:413-420.
2. Choudhury AR, Taylor JC. Cauda equina syndrome in lumbar disc disease. *Acta Orthop Scand*. 1980;51:493-499.
3. Kostuik JP, Harrington I, Alexander D, et al. Cauda equina syndrome and lumbar disc herniation. *J Bone Joint Surg Am*. 1986;68:386-391.
4. Ahn UM, Ahn NU, Buchowski JM, et al. Cauda equina syndrome secondary to lumbar disc herniation: a meta-analysis of surgical outcomes. *Spine*. 2000;25:1515-1522.
5. Boukobza M, Guichard JP, Boissonet M, et al. Spinal epidural hematoma: report of 11 cases and review of the literature. *Neuroradiolgy*. 1994;36:456-459.
6. Busse JW, Hsu WS. Rapid progression of acute sciatica to cauda equina syndrome. *J Manipulative Physiol Ther*. 2001;24:350-355.
7. Mohit AA, Fisher DJ, Matthews DC, et al. Inferior vena cava thrombosis causing acute cauda equina syndrome: case report. *J Neurosurg*. 2006;104:46-49.
8. Rigler ML, Drasner K, Krejcie TC, et al. Cauda equina syndrome after continuous spinal anesthesia. *Anesth Analg*. 1991;72:275-281.
9. Della-Giustina DA. Emergency department evaluation and treatment of back pain. *Emerg Med Clin North Am*. 1999;17:877-893.
10. Anderson JT, Bradley WE. Neurogenic bladder dysfunction in protruded lumbar disk and after laminectomy. *Urology*. 1976;8:94-96.
11. Lavy C, James A, Wilson-MacDonald J, Fairbank J. Cauda equina syndrome. *BMJ*. 2009;338:881-884.
12. DeLong WB, Polissar N, Neradilek B. Timing of surgery in cauda equina syndrome with urinary retention: meta-analysis of observational studies. *J Neurosurg Spine*. 2008;8:305-320.
13. Qureshi A, Sepp P. Cauda equina syndrome treated by surgical decompression: the influence of timing on surgical outcome. *Eur Spine J*. 2007;16:2143-2151.
14. Coscia M, Leipzig, T, Cooper D. Acute cauda equina syndrome. *Spine*. 1994;19:475-478.
15. Gleave JR, MacFarlane R. Prognosis for recovery of bladder function following lumbar central disc prolapse. *Br J Neurosurg*. 1990;4:205-209.
16. Todd NV. Cauda equina syndrome: the timing of surgery probably does influence outcome. *Br J Neurosurg*. 2005;19:301-306.

CHIARI TYPE I MALFORMATION

Douglas S. Fenton, M.D.

CLINICAL PRESENTATION

The patient is a 62-year-old man who has been under a physician's care for fainting spells for the last 6 months. He has also had symptoms of numbness in his shoulders, arms, and hands, which has become worse over the last few years. He also has paresthesias and numbness on the right side of his neck and face. The patient describes problems with balance and urinary urgency. On neurologic examination, the patient has some difficulty with tandem gait. His strength is normal. He has numbness on the right side from C2 through C4 and has an absent right biceps reflex.

IMAGING PRESENTATION

Sagittal T1- and T2-weighted magnetic resonance (MR) imaging obtained demonstrates a long-segment region of cerebrospinal fluid (CSF)–signal intensity within the cervical spinal cord from C2-T2. There is also pointing of the cerebellar tonsil, which extends through the foramen magnum consistent with Chiari type I malformation with syringomyelia (*Fig. 15-1*).

DISCUSSION

The Chiari malformation is characterized by inferior herniation of the cerebellar tonsils through the foramen magnum. The various types of Chiari malformation, I to III, are a continuum of posterior fossa hindbrain development. The general consensus is that the main abnormality in Chiari I is underdevelopment of the occipital bone with an otherwise normal posterior fossa brain volume.[1]

The Chiari I malformation is usually congenital but can, on occasion, be acquired.[2] Symptoms of Chiari malformation do not often arise until the patient is in the late thirties. Depending on the degree of cerebellar tonsillar herniation, the size of the foramen magnum, and which structures may be compressed, the presentation of a Chiari malformation can vary from no symptoms to very severe. The clinical presentation of Chiari I can be related to direct compression of the brainstem or spinal cord or to cerebrospinal fluid disturbances such as hydrocephalus.[3] Headache, the most frequent symptom, might be the only manifestation of Chiari I or it can be absent altogether. The Chiari I headache is often occipito-suboccipital and may worsen with Valsalva maneuver/cough, change in posture, or physical exertion.[4] Other symptoms include neck pain, balance problems, muscle weakness, numbness, or other abnormal feelings in the arms or legs, dizziness, vision problems, difficulty swallowing, ringing or buzzing in the ears, hearing loss, vomiting, insomnia, or depression.[5]

The incidence of Chiari I malformation, with tonsillar herniation greater than 5 mm through the foramen magnum, is approximately 0.5% to 0.75%.[6,7] However, if one includes tonsillar herniation of 2 mm below the foramen magnum, then the sensitivity of predicting symptomatic patients is 100% with a specificity of 98.5%. If the lowest extent of the tonsils is 3 mm, then the sensitivity is 96% with a specificity of 99.5%.[8] Therefore, borderline Chiari I is diagnosed radiographically with 3 to 5 mm of caudal descent of the cerebellar tonsils. One can be more definite in the diagnosis if there is 5 mm or more descent, pointed tonsils, and/or crowding at the craniocervical junction. Most series report a slight female preponderance for Chiari I.[9,10]

A syringomyelia, an abnormal collection of fluid within the spinal cord, occurs in approximately 14% to 75% of patients with Chiari I.[11] Cavitation may occur in the spinal cord in 20% to 40%, and 60% to 90% of symptomatic patients have an associated syrinx.[3] There have been many hypotheses regarding why a syrinx cavity develops in Chiari patients. Some have proposed that CSF is unable to pass through the fourth ventricle because of the crowding of the posterior fossa. The systolic pulsations of CSF are then redirected from the fourth ventricle to the central canal of the spinal cord ("water-hammer" effect) with the creation of a syrinx and progressive cavitation.[12] Another theory suggests a ball-valve obstruction at the foramen magnum with a pressure difference created between the intracranial contents and spinal canal during patient coughing or Valsalva maneuver.[13] During coughing or Valsalva maneuver, fluid that would normally be forced into the head may be directed into the spinal cord through extracellular pathways because of obstruction at the foramen magnum.[14] There are also reported cases of spontaneous regression of Chiari-associated syrinx.[15]

Skeletal anomalies are often seen in conjunction with Chiari I malformation, including scoliosis in 40% to 60%, basilar invagination in 25% to 50%, and Klippel-Feil in 5% to 10%. The posterior fossa is small and there may be a short clivus.

Chiari II malformations have displacement of the cerebellar vermis and tonsils into the spinal canal with caudal displacement of the brainstem and elongation of the fourth ventricle.[6] Type III malformations are rare and are characterized by herniation of the medulla and cerebellum into a high cervical meningocele.[6] Chiari II and III malformations are readily recognized early in life due to their associated meningoceles.[6] Chiari I malformations are frequently undetected until later in childhood or adulthood.

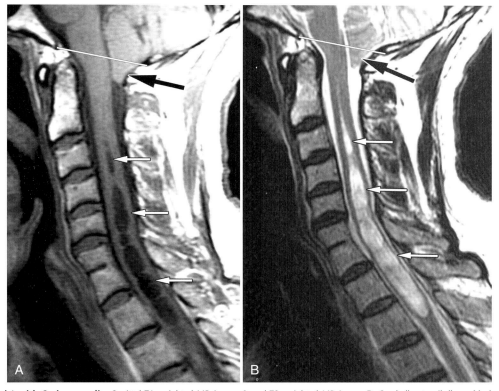

Figure 15-1 ▶ Chiari I with Syringomyelia. Sagittal T1-weighted MR image **A** and T2-weighted MR image **B.** Cerebellar tonsil *(large black arrow)* is approximately 10 mm inferior to the foramen magnum *(white line between basion anteriorly and opisthion posteriorly)*. The tonsil has a pegged appearance. Long-segment region of CSF signal intensity within the spinal cord from C2-T2 *(small white arrows)*. Findings compatible with Chiari type I malformation with associated syringomyelia.

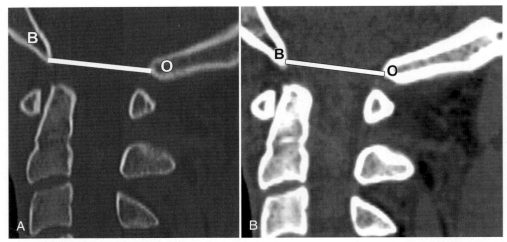

Figure 15-2 ▸ **Floor of the Foramen Magnum.** Cerebellar tonsillar measurement is made in relationship to the floor of the foramen magnum. Sagittal reconstructed CT images using bone algorithm (image **A**) and standard soft tissue algorithm (image **B**) demonstrate the floor of the foramen magnum as a line drawn between the midpoint of the basion (*B*) and the midpoint of the opisthion (*O*).

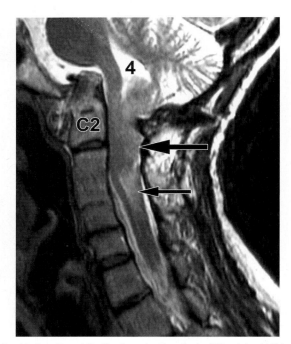

Figure 15-3 ▸ **Chiari I Malformation with Cord Ischemia and Basilar Invagination.** Sagittal T2-weighted MR image reveals 15 mm ectopia of the cerebellar tonsil (*large arrow*), elongation of the fourth ventricle (*4*) and increased T2 signal intensity within the cervical cord more inferiorly (*small arrow*), compatible with cord ischemia. Note the presence of basilar invagination with the dens of C2 projecting through the foramen magnum, almost in contact with the undersurface of the pons. There is also significant spinal canal narrowing at the craniocervical junction.

IMAGING FEATURES

On computerized tomography (CT) or magnetic resonance imaging (MRI), the cerebellar tonsils should be at least 5 mm below the foramen magnum for the radiographic criterion of Chiari I to be fulfilled. The foramen magnum is delineated by a line drawn between the midpoint of the anterior border of the foramen magnum/tip of the clivus (basion) and midpoint of the posterior border of the foramen magnum (opisthion) *(Fig. 15-2)*. The shape of the inferior tonsils is pointed or pegged (see Fig. 15-1). The fourth ventricle is normal in position but may be elongated *(Fig. 15-3)*. A syringohydromyelia is identified in many patients. The syrinx cavity is best imaged with MRI. The syrinx has the imaging characteristic of CSF and therefore demonstrates decreased T1 signal, increased T2 signal, and no enhancement *(Fig. 15-4)*. MR cinematic phase-contrast (Cine PC) imaging can be performed to

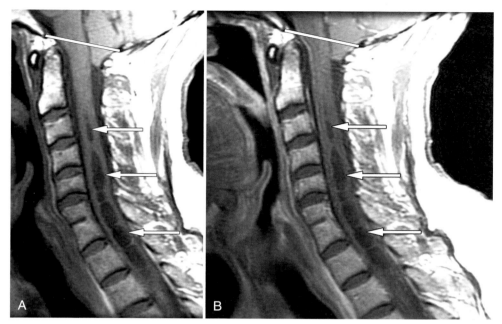

Figure 15-4 ▶ Syrinx. Same patient as in Figure 15-1 with 10-mm cerebellar tonsillar ectopia. No evidence is apparent of enhancement of the syringomyelia *(arrows)* between the sagittal pre-contrast T1 MR image **A** and sagittal post-contrast MR image **B.**

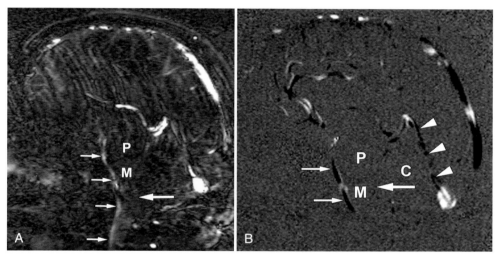

Figure 15-5 ▶ CSF Flow Study. Midline sagittal phase contrast image **A** and reverse image **B** performed to evaluate the presence or absence of CSF pulsation in patient with Chiari type I malformation. Pulsation *(small arrows)* can be seen ventral to the pons (P) and medulla (M) but not in between the brainstem and cerebellum *(large arrow)*. Note flow-related signal in the straight sinus *(arrowheads)*.

evaluate whether there is normal CSF pulsation ventral and dorsal to the cervicomedullary junction either before or after surgery *(Fig. 15-5)*.

DIFFERENTIAL DIAGNOSIS

1. **Low-lying cerebellar tonsils**: Cerebellar tonsillar tissue can normally extend 2 to 3 mm through the foramen magnum.
2. **CSF leak or lumbar drain overshunting**: These etiologies cause a differential in pressures with higher CSF pressure in the brain and lower CSF pressure inferior to the brain. This CSF hypotension "pulls" brain tissue downward *(Fig. 15-6)*.
3. **Increased intracranial pressure**: Increased intracranial pressure from an intracranial mass or from chronic ventriculoperitoneal shunting can "push" brain tissue downward *(Fig. 15-7)*.

TREATMENT

The treatment of symptomatic Chiari I malformation is surgical. The controversy lies in the asymptomatic patient. Many believe

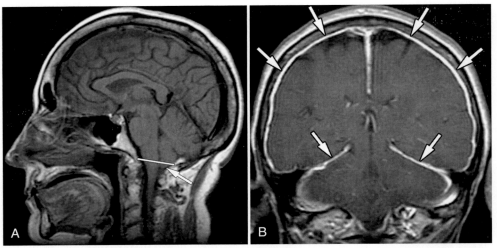

Figure 15-6 ▸ **Cerebellar Tonsillar Herniation Secondary to Inferior Pull.** Sagittal T1-weighted MR image **A** and coronal post-contrast T1-weighted MR image **B** in patient with a lumbar drain. Sagittal image demonstrates mild cerebellar tonsillar ectopia *(arrow)*. Note the diffuse, thick enhancement of the cerebral and cerebellar meninges *(arrows)* secondary to overaggressive lumbar drainage.

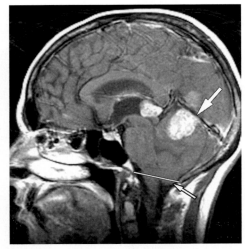

Figure 15-7 ▸ **Cerebellar Tonsillar Herniation Secondary to Superior Push.** Metastatic disease. Midline sagittal T1-weighted post-contrast MR image reveals several enhancing lesions with the more prominent cerebellar metastasis *(large arrow)* and its associated edema, causing mild inferior cerebellar tonsillar displacement *(small arrow)*.

that if the patient is asymptomatic and does not have a syrinx, then conservative management of symptoms can be performed. If the asymptomatic patient has a syrinx, then surgical decompression is considered. There have been many different surgical approaches for the symptomatic patient without or with syrinx, including plugging of the obex, placement of a stent in the fourth ventricle, extensive posterior fossa craniectomy, and multiple cervical laminectomies.[16] During the pediatric section of the 2000 meeting of the American Association of Neurological Surgeons, surgeons were surveyed regarding the surgical approach they took for Chiari I malformation; 9% recommended surgery in asymptomatic patients.[17] In symptomatic patients, 20% recommended osseous decompression, 30% recommended osseous decompression with dural grafting, 25% performed osseous decompression with dural grafting and intradural dissection of adhesion, and 30%

recommended osseous decompression with dural grafting, intradural dissection, and tonsillar manipulation and resection.[16,17]

References

1. Stovner LJ, Bergan U, Nilsen G, Sjaastad O. Posterior cranial fossa dimensions in the Chiari I malformation: relation to pathogenesis and clinical presentation. *Neuroradiolgy.* 1993;35:113-118.
2. Huang PP, Constantini S. "Acquired" Chiari I malformation. *J Neurosurg.* 1994;80:1099-1102.
3. Milhorat TH, Chou MW, Trinidad EM, et al. Chiari I malformation redefined: clinical and radiographic findings for 364 symptomatic patients. *Neurosurgery.* 1999;44:1005-1017.
4. Pascual J, Oterino A, Berciano J. Headache in type I Chiari malformation. *Neurology.* 1992;42:1519-1521.
5. Chiari malformation fact sheet. National Institute of Neurological Disorders and Stroke. Available at http://www.ninds.nih.gov/disorders/chiari/detail_chiari.htm. (accessed May 26, 2009).

6. Elster AD, Chen MY. Chiari I malformations: clinical and radiologic reappraisal. *Radiology*. 1992;183:347-353.
7. Meadows J, Kraut M, Guarnieri M, et al. Asymptomatic Chiari type I malformations identified on magnetic resonance imaging. *J Neurosurg*. 2000;92:920-926.
8. Barkovikch AJ, Wippold FJ, Sherman JL, Citrin CM. Significance of cerebellar tonsillar position on MR. *AJNR Am J Neuroradiol*. 1986;7:795-799.
9. Levy WJ, Mason L, Hahn JF. Chiari malformation presenting in adults: a surgical experience in 127 cases. *Neurosurgery*. 1983;12:377-390.
10. Pillay PK, Awad IA, Little JR, Hahn JF. Symptomatic Chiari malformation in adults: a new classification based on magnetic resonance imaging with clinical and prognostic significance. *Neurosurgery*. 1991;28:639-645.
11. Oakes WJ. Chiari malformations, hydromyelia, syringomyelia. In: Wilkins RH, Rengachary SS, eds. Neurosurgery. Vol 3. New York: McGraw-Hilll; 1996:3593-3616.
12. Gardner WJ, Angel J. The mechanisms of syringomyelia and its surgical correction. *Clin Neurosurg*. 1959;6:131-140.
13. Williams B. On the pathogenesis of syringomyelia: a review. *J R Soc Med*. 1980;73:798-806.
14. Ball MJ, Dayan AD. Pathogenesis of syringomyelia. *Lancet*. 1972;2:799-801.
15. Sung WS, Chen YY, Dubey A, Hunn A. Spontaneous regression of syringomyelia: review of the current aetiological theories and implications for surgery. *J Clin Neurosci*. 2008;15:1185-1188.
16. Alden TD, Ojemann JG, Park TS. Surgical treatment of Chiari I malformation: indications and approaches. *Neurosurg Focus*. 2001;11:E2.
17. Haroun RI, Guarnieri M, Meadow JJ, et al. Current opinions for the treatment of syringomyelia and Chiari malformations: survey of the Pediatric Section of the American Association of Neurological Surgeons. *Pediatr Neurosurg*. 2000;33:311-317.

CHORDOMA

Leo F. Czervionke, M.D.

CLINICAL PRESENTATION

The patient is a 49-year-old male who presented with drainage from a painful area of soft tissue swelling in the posterior perianal region. The drainage ceased but the pain and swelling persisted, so a computed tomography (CT) scan of the sacrum was obtained.

IMAGING PRESENTATION

Large, lobulated heterogeneously enhancing mass was shown centered at the sacrococcygeal junction. On CT the mass involves the lower sacrum and coccyx causing bone destruction (*Figs. 16-1 and 16-2*). Portions of the remaining sacral vertebrae adjacent to the mass are sclerotic. The mass contained focal calcifications or islands of remnant vertebral bone. The mass is T1 hypointense and T2 hyperintense relative to the normal sacral vertebrae (*Figs. 16-3 to 16-5*).

DISCUSSION

Chordomas are bone tumors that arise from embryologic remnants of the notochord. They represent approximately 3% of malignant bone tumors; 50% of them arise from the sacrococcygeal region, 35% in the clival region, and 15% from the vertebral bodies.[1,2] Vertebral body chordomas most commonly occur in the cervical region, next most commonly in the lumbar region, and least commonly in the thoracic spine.

Chordomas usually manifest as slowly growing tumors in middle-aged patients, usually presenting between the ages of 30 and 70. Manifesting symptoms depend on the tumor location. Sacrococcygeal chordomas are twice as common in males as in females, but there is an equal male-female incidence in clival chordomas.[3] Sacrococcygeal chordomas extend far more commonly anterior to the sacrum than posteriorly.[3] Sacrococcygeal tumors manifest as painful swellings in the sacrococcygeal region. Vertebral chordomas may be associated with pain, numbness, weakness, and bowel or bladder dysfunction, secondary to cord compression. Thoracic chordomas may present with pain, swallowing difficulty, and hoarseness if they extend into the posterior mediastinum.[4] Posterior mediastinal chordomas can be highly malignant tumors.[5]

Chordomas are malignant tumors that commonly recur locally and less commonly metastasize to the lymph nodes, lungs, or other

bones. The 5-year survival rate is approximately 75% and 10-year survival is 35%.[6]

Chordomas are usually soft, bulky lobulated masses when they manifest. They arise from the bone but almost always have an extraosseous soft tissue component.[2] There are three histologic subtypes: (1) Clear cell tumors (most common type) contain intracytoplasmic vacuoles within "physaliphorous" cells. They typically have a mucoid matrix divided by multiple fibrous septations. (2) Chondroid tumors contain cartilaginous tissue, usually type II collagen, and often have immunohistochemical markers including cytokeratin (CK), epithelial membrane antigen (EMA), and sometimes carcinoembryonic antigen (CEA).[7] Chondroid chordomas arise most commonly at the spheno-occipital synchondrosis, where they involve the adjacent clivus. (3) Sarcomatous chordoma is a highly malignant, poorly differentiated tumor.

IMAGING FEATURES

Chordoma is a heterogeneous bone-destroying tumor involving the sacrococcygeal region, clivus, or vertebral body. Vertebral body lesions often are associated with a bulky anterior epidural mass that may compress the spinal cord. On CT, amorphous clumps of calcification or islands of residual bone are often contained in the tumor, more common in sacrococcygeal tumors (see Figs. 16-1 and 16-2). A combination of bone destruction and adjacent bone sclerosis is typical (see Figs. 16-1 and 16-2).[8] The tumor is usually heterogeneous on CT and magnetic resonance (MR) imaging. With MR, the tumor contains heterogeneous tissue that is predominantly T1 hypointense and T2 hyperintense (see Figs. 16-3 and 16-4). The tumor contains prominent T2 hypointense septations in up to 70% of cases (see Fig. 16-3).[1,4] Areas of hemorrhagic necrosis are common within the tumor.[4] The foci of T2 hypointensity in chordomas usually represent hemosiderin.[9] Calcifications occur in only 15% of chordomas,[1] but remnants of native bone within the tumor secondary to bone destruction are common in clival and sacrococcygeal chordomas. Intense heterogeneous enhancement is typical after IV contrast administration,[4] but some tumors enhance to a far lesser degree (see Figs. 16-4 and 16-5). The tumor may cause neural foraminal marginal expansion and erosion. Foraminal tumors can have a dumbbell configuration.

With vertebral chordomas, the anterior portion of the vertebral body is usually spared.[1] The epidural or paraspinal component of vertebral chordomas is often greater than the bony portion of the

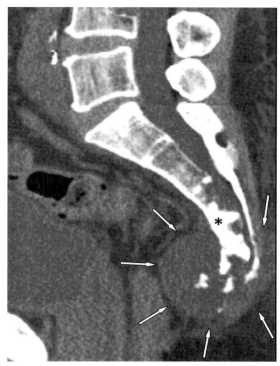

Figure 16-1 ▶ **Sacrococcygeal Chordoma.** Sagittal reformatted CT image of the sacrum reveals a soft tissue mass *(arrows)* causing bone destruction in the lower sacrum and coccyx. The soft tissue component of the mass is centered anterior to the sacrococcygeal junction and contains islands of vertebral remnants. There are regions of sclerosis (*) in the adjacent sacrum.

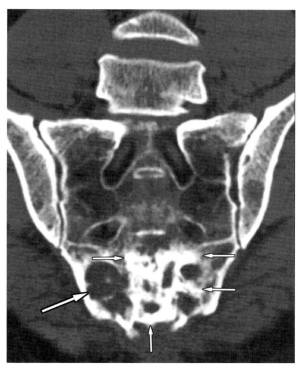

Figure 16-2 ▶ **Sacrococcygeal Chordoma.** Same patient as in Figure 16-1. Coronal reformatted CT posterior to the soft tissue mass. Note areas of sclerosis *(small arrows)* in the lower sacrum and an osteolytic area *(large arrow)* in the right lower sacrum.

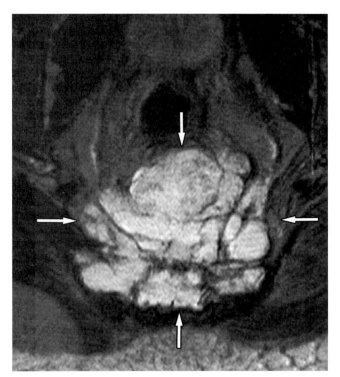

Figure 16-3 ▶ **Sacrococcygeal Chordoma.** Same patient as in Figures 16-1 and 16-2. Coronal T2-weighted MR image anterior to the sacrum. Multilobulated predominantly T2 hyperintense mass *(arrows)* contains multiple T2 hypointense septations.

vertebral tumor *(Figs. 16-6 and 16-7)*. The epidural tissue characteristically extends along the posterior or lateral annular margins of adjacent vertebral bodies and drapes across the posterior or lateral margin of the adjacent disc (see Figs. 16-6 and 16-7).[1] This pattern of spread is highly suggestive of vertebral chordoma. The epidural component of the tumor classically has been described as having a "mushroom" shape or "collar button" configuration that spans one to three vertebrae, contacting the posterior margin of adjacent intervertebral discs.[1,2]

Cervical chordomas may span multiple contiguous vertebral levels.[2] The tumor may involve the posterior portion of the intervertebral disc, which is not surprising because the posterior portion of the nucleus pulposus is the last developing structure to undergo notochordal regression.

Chordomas most commonly occur at the skull base involving the clivus. Clival chordomas usually manifest as lobulated, prepontine masses that invade and destroy the clivus. They may contain clumps of calcification and typically enhance heterogeneously *(Fig. 16-8)*.

DIFFERENTIAL DIAGNOSIS OF SACROCOCCYGEAL AND SACRAL CHORDOMA

1. **Sacral metastases:** These can occur anywhere in the sacrum but more commonly involve the upper or mid portion of the sacrum. Sacral metastases typically are heterogeneous marrow-infiltrating lesions associated with bone destruction and usually enhance heterogeneously *(Fig. 16-9)*.

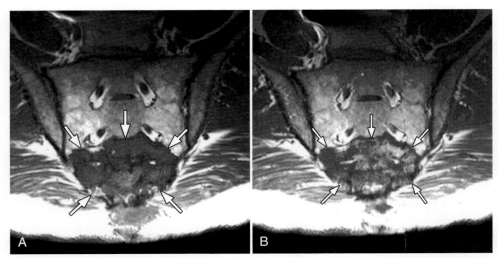

Figure 16-4 ▶ Sacrococcygeal Chordoma. Same patient as in Figures 16-1 to 16-3. Coronal pre- and postcontrast MR imaging. The mass *(arrows)* involves the lower sacrum and is relatively T1 hypointense relative to the upper sacral segments on unenhanced T1-weighted MR image **A.** Portions of the mass enhance heterogeneously *(arrows)* as shown on contrast enhanced image **B.**

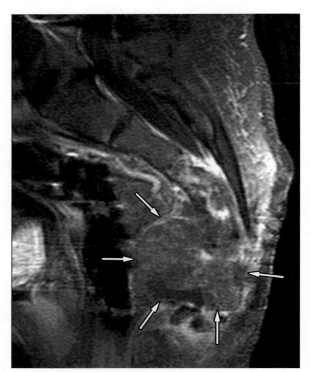

Figure 16-5 ▶ Sacrococcygeal Chordoma. Same patient as in Figures 16-1 to 16-4. The mass *(arrows)* is relatively hypointense on contrast enhanced fat saturated mid-sagittal MR image through the sacrococcygeal region. A few small heterogeneous regions of contrast enhancement are located within the mass but the majority of the mass does not enhance appreciably following IV contrast.

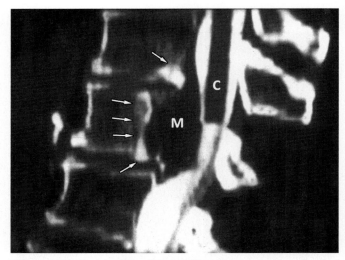

Figure 16-6 ▶ Vertebral Chordoma at T12 Level. On post myelogram sagittal CT image, tumor erodes into the posterior portion of the T12 vertebral body causing osteolysis and adjacent bone sclerosis *(arrows)* in the T11 and T12 vertebral bodies. The epidural component of the mass *(M)* extends into spinal canal causing ventral thecal sac deformity and posterior displacement of the conus medullaris *(C)*. Note that the mass is closely applied to the posterior margin of the T11-T12 and T12-L1 discs.

2. **Lymphoma:** When lymphoma involves the sacrum, a solid mass that typically is a T1 hypointense, T2 hyperintense marrow-infiltrating bone lesion is found. Lymphoma of the sacrum may be confined to the sacrum or extend through the cortex with a soft tissue component. Lymphoma can occur anywhere in the sacrum but favors the sacral wing region

(Figs. 16-10 and 16-11). Sacral lymphomas are often highly radiosensitive tumors that may resolve completely after a course of radiotherapy (Fig. 16-11).

3. **Plasmacytoma:** A plasma cell tumor is a distinct mass usually occurring in a patient with multiple myeloma. Plasmacytomas may or may not expand the bone. They are usually fairly

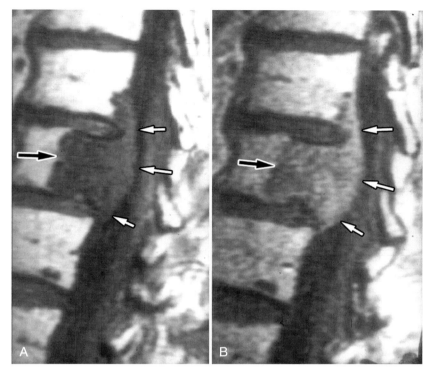

Figure 16-7 ▶ **Vertebral Chordoma at T12 Level.** Same patient as in Figure 16-6. Sagittal precontrast T1-weighted MR image **A** and postcontrast MR image **B.** Note the enhancement of the mass *(white arrows)* in the epidural space and posterior portion of the T12 vertebral body *(black arrow).* The mass *(white arrows)* contacts the posterior annulus of the T11-12 and T12-L1 discs and protrudes into the spinal canal.

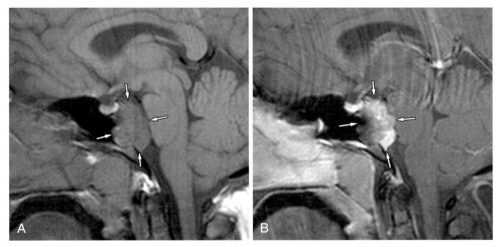

Figure 16-8 ▶ **Clival Chordoma (Chondroid Type).** Sagittal pre- and postcontrast T1-weighted MR images **A** and **B.** Heterogeneously enhancing mass *(arrows)* in the prepontine cistern causes flattening of the anterior belly of the pons. The anterior portion of the mass involves the clivus and protrudes into the posterior portion of the sphenoid sinus *(anterior arrow in images **A** and **B**).*

homogeneous on T1-weighted and T2-weighted MR images and usually enhance intensely with contrast. The adjacent marrow may be heterogeneous due to diffuse infiltration of the marrow by multiple myeloma. Sacral plasmacytomas favor the upper portion of the sacrum or thoracic vertebrae *(Fig. 16-12).*

4. **Giant cell tumor:** A heterogeneous, expansile lesion within the vertebra or sacrum. This may expand the cortex or break through the cortex into the adjacent soft tissues. On MR imaging, this is a T1 hypointense and T2 hyperintense expansile lesion that may contain cystic areas with loculated fluid/fluid levels. Predominantly solid giant cell tumors are difficult to differentiate from lymphoma by imaging *(Fig. 16-13).*

5. **Meningioma:** May occur along the clivus but usually does usually not invade the clivus. Meningioma rarely originates in

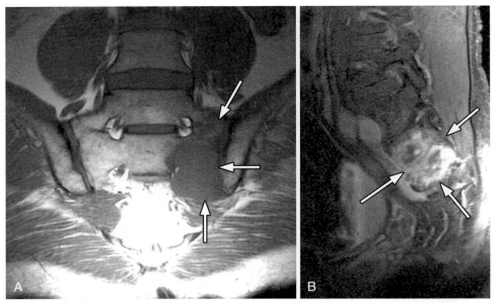

Figure 16-9 ► **Sacral Metastasis Originating from Myoepithelial Carcinoma of the Right Parotid Gland.** On T1-weighted MR image **A,** the mass *(arrows)* is T1 hypointense relative to the normal vertebral marrow. The tumor predominantly involves the left sacral wing. On sagittal contrast-enhanced fat-saturated T1-weighted MR image **B,** obtained through the left sacral wing, the mass *(arrows)* enhances heterogeneously.

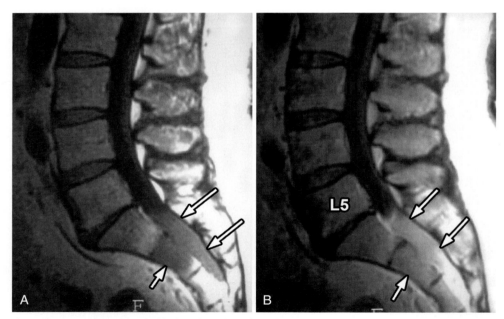

Figure 16-10 ► **Sacral Lymphoma.** Involves S2 vertebral body and sacral spinal canal. Unenhanced sagittal T1-weighted MR image **A** and sagittal contrast-enhanced T1-weighted MR image **B.** The tumor in the S2 vertebral body *(short arrow)* and spinal canal *(long arrows)* is T1 hypointense relative to the normal sacral marrow and enhances moderately following IV contrast administration. *L5* = L5 vertebral body.

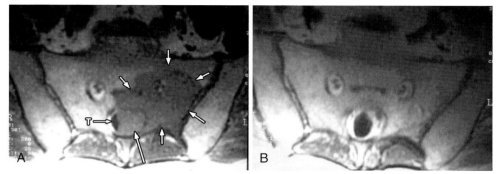

Figure 16-11 ▶ Sacral Lymphoma. Involves the S2 vertebral body, left sacral wing, and sacral spinal canal. Same patient as in Figure 16-10. On axial unenhanced T1-weighted MR image **A,** the T1 hypointense lesion *(short arrows)* is seen in the left sacral wing. A component of the mass extends into the left S1 neural foramen and into the sacral spinal canal *(long arrow)* where it displaces the thecal sac *(T)* to the right. On unenhanced T1-weighted MR image **B** obtained 6 months later following a course of radiotherapy, the sacrum appears normal and the tumor in the left S1 neural foramen, and sacral spinal canal has resolved.

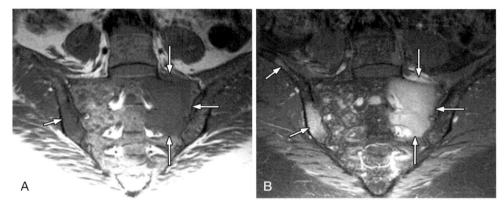

Figure 16-12 ▶ Sacral Plasmacytoma in Patient with Multiple Myeloma. A plasmacytoma *(long arrows)* replaces the left sacral wing. The lesion is nonexpansile and homogeneous on T1-weighted MR image **A** and enhances intensely with contrast as shown on contrast-enhanced fat-saturated T1-weighted MR image **B**. Smaller plasmacytomas *(short arrows)* are located in the right iliac wing. The bone marrow in other portions of the iliac wings, sacrum, and L5 vertebral body is heterogeneous in image **A** and enhances heterogeneously in image **B** secondary to diffuse infiltration of the bone marrow by multiple myeloma.

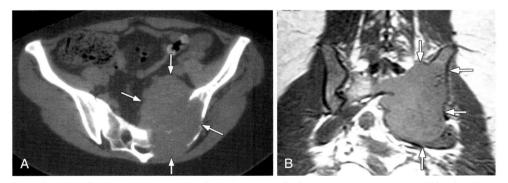

Figure 16-13 ▶ Large Sacral Giant Cell Tumor. Large intrasacral and exophytic presacral soft tissue component in 25-year-old female with vague lumbosacral pain and pelvic discomfort. Axial CT image **A** shows a large mass *(arrows)* destroying the left half of the sacrum, crossing the left sacroiliac joint, and extending into the left iliac bone. A large component of the mass *(anterior arrows)* extends into the prevertebral soft tissues. On axial T1-weighted MR image **B,** a large bulky mass *(arrows)*, displaying nearly homogeneous signal intensity, is replacing the left half of the sacrum, obliterates the left sacroiliac joint, and involves the left iliac wing. Sacral lymphoma can have a similar appearance.

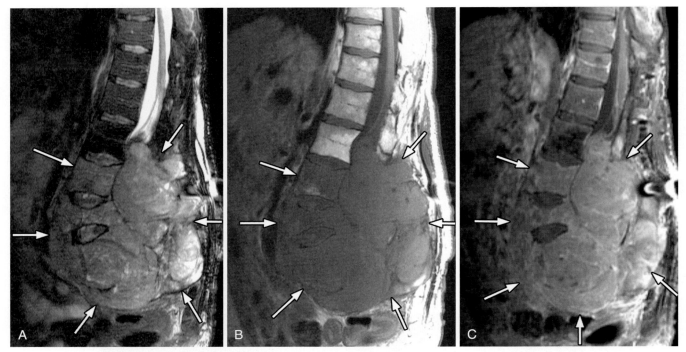

Figure 16-14 ► **Rare Malignant Lumbosacral Meningioma.** The patient is paraplegic and has lost bowel and bladder control due to involvement of the cauda equina. A very large multilobulated mass *(arrows in images* **A, B,** *and* **C***)* replaces the sacrum and lower lumbar vertebrae and has expanded into the lumbosacral spinal canal and paraspinal soft tissues. The mass is heterogeneous and T2 hyperintense relative to the normal vertebrae on T2-weighted sagittal MR image **A.** The mass is more homogeneous in appearance on corresponding sagittal T1-weighted MR image **B.** On contrast-enhanced fat-saturated T1-weighted MR image **C,** the tumor enhances diffusely and contains enhancing curvilinear septations as shown. Note relative sparing of the lower lumbar intervertebral discs.

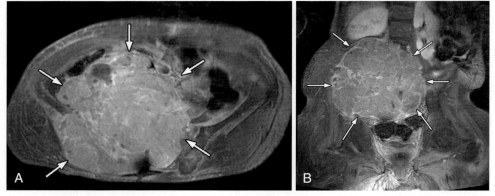

Figure 16-15 ► **Malignant Lumbosacral Meningioma.** Same patient as in Figure 16-14. In contrast-enhanced fat-saturated T1-weighted MR image **A,** a bulky mass *(arrows)* has replaced the entire sacrum and a large portion of the right iliac wing. The mass extends into the right gluteus muscles and into the pelvic soft tissues. In coronal contrast-enhanced fat-saturated T1-weighted MR image **B,** obtained through the pelvic soft tissues, the pelvic component of the mass *(arrows)* contains whorls of lobulated enhancing soft tissue separated by enhancing curvilinear septations.

the sacrococcygeal region where it can manifest as a large bulky enhancing expansile mass simulating a chordoma *(Figs. 16-14 and 16-15)*.

6. **Sacrococcygeal teratoma:** A heterogeneous mass arising in the sacrococcygeal region in a young child, containing areas of fat.

7. **Chondrosarcoma**: More commonly arises in vertebral arch or at the clivus. Look for chondroid calcification, "popcorn" or "arcuate" pattern of calcification. Calcifications are far more

common within a chondroma or chondrosarcoma than in a chordoma. Chondrosarcoma typically has S-100 protein and Vimentin immunohistochemical markers.

8. **Schwannomas or neurofibromas:** Common intradural and intraforaminal tumors. The extradural tumors usually extend into adjacent neural foramina giving them a dumbbell configuration.

9. **Benign notochordal tumor** (BNCT): A benign condition in which persistent notochordal tissue remnants are confined to

the vertebral bodies. There is no associated paraspinal or epidural soft tissue component and no destruction of adjacent vertebral endplates. It is possible that chordomas can arise from preexisting BNCT.[11] BNCT is associated with a patchy region of bone sclerosis in the affected vertebral body on CT or radiographs that may involve a large portion of the vertebral body. The abnormal region is T1 hypointense/T2 hyperintense on MR imaging.[11] BNCT may be far more common than reported because it is likely mistaken for common vertebral hemangiomas, which have similar imaging features. However, BNCT lacks the vertical bone struts and speckled MR signal intensity characteristics of vertebral hemangiomas. The cells in this condition contain glycogen granules. Immunohistochemical stains of the tissue within affected vertebral bodies show presence of Vimentin, S-100 protein, EMA, CAM5.2, AE1/AE3, and CK18.[11]

10. **Ecchordosis physaliphora:** Gelatinous soft tissue that also arises from notochordal rests anywhere from the clivus to the sacrum. This tissue is found along the posterior margin of the clivus in 2% of autopsy specimens.[1] In the spinal canal, it most commonly arises in the anterior epidural space and may simulate an epidural mass. It is usually asymptomatic. On MR imaging, it has a variable T1 signal intensity but is usually T2 hypointense relative to the spinal cord. It usually does not enhance after administration of IV contrast.[10] It may be associated with a nearby bone defect in the clivus or vertebra. There are no known cases of metastases from this condition.[10]

TREATMENT

1. **En bloc surgical excision** obtaining a wide margin of resection is performed to minimize the chance of recurrence, which is quite common in these tumors.[12-15] Vertebral tumors require partial corpectomy and usually instrumentation stabilization.

2. **Radiotherapy** alone is not sufficient for treatment of chordomas and is usually reserved for recurrent tumor or as adjuvant therapy when a wide resection of the tumor cannot be achieved.[16,17]

References

1. Smolders D, Wang X, Drevelengas A, et al. Value of MRI in the diagnosis of non-clival, non-sacral chordoma. *Skeletal Radiol.* 2003;32:343-350.
2. Wippold FJ, 2nd, Koeller KK, Smirniotopoulos JG. Clinical and imaging features of cervical chordoma. *AJR Am J Roentgenol.* 1999;172:1423-1426.
3. Walsh TM, Mayer PJ. Chordoma of the thoracic spine presenting as a second primary malignant lesion: a case report. *Spine.* 1992;17:1524-1528.
4. Murphy JM, Wallis F, Toland J, et al. CT and MRI appearances of a thoracic chordoma. *Eur Radiol.* 1998;8:1677-1679.
5. Cotler HB, Cotler JM, Cohn HE, et al. Intrathoracic chordoma presenting as a posterior superior mediastinal tumor. *Spine.* 1983;8:781-786.
6. Berven S, Zurakowski D, Mankin HJ, et al. Clinical outcome in chordoma: utility of flow cytometry in DNA determination. *Spine.* 2002;27:374-379.
7. Wojno KJ, Hruban RH, Garin-Chesa P, Huvos AG. Chondroid chordomas and low-grade chondrosarcomas of the craniospinal axis: an immunohistochemical analysis of 17 cases. *Am J Surg Pathol.* 1992;16:1144-1152.
8. Ducou le Pointe H, Brugieres P, Chevalier X, et al. Imaging of chordomas of the mobile spine. *J Neuroradiol.* 1991;18:267-276.
9. Sung MS, Lee GK, Kang HS, et al. Sacrococcygeal chordoma: MR imaging in 30 patients. *Skeletal Radiol.* 2005;34:87-94.
10. Ng SH, Ko SF, Wan YL, et al. Cervical ecchordosis physaliphora: CT and MR features. *Br J Radiol.* 1998;71:329-331.
11. Yamaguchi T, Iwata J, Sugihara S, et al. Distinguishing benign notochordal cell tumors from vertebral chordoma. *Skeletal Radiol.* 2008;37:291-299.
12. Bailey CS, Fisher CG, Boyd MC, Dvorak MF. En bloc marginal excision of a multilevel cervical chordoma: case report. *J Neurosurg Spine.* 2006;4:409-414.
13. Biagini R, Casadei R, Boriani S, et al. En bloc vertebrectomy and dural resection for chordoma: a case report. *Spine.* 2003;28:E368-372.
14. Boriani S, Chevalley F, Weinstein JN, et al. Chordoma of the spine above the sacrum: treatment and outcome in 21 cases. *Spine.* 1996;21:1569-1577.
15. Currier BL, Papagelopoulos PJ, Krauss WE, et al. Total en bloc spondylectomy of C5 vertebra for chordoma. *Spine.* 2007;32:E294-299.
16. Cheng EY, Ozerdemoglu RA, Transfeldt EE, Thompson RC, Jr. Lumbosacral chordoma: prognostic factors and treatment. *Spine.* 1999;24:1639-1645.
17. York JE, Kaczaraj A, Abi-Said D, et al. Sacral chordoma: 40-year experience at a major cancer center. *Neurosurgery.* 1999;44:74-79; discussion 79-80.

DEGENERATIVE DISC DISEASE

Leo F. Czervionke, M.D.

CLINICAL PRESENTATION

The patient is a 63-year-old female patient with a history of two back surgeries in the distant past to remove herniated discs on the left at L5-S1. Patient has had chronic intermittent left lower extremity pain and numbness for many years since the surgery, attributed to known chronic recurrent L5-S1 disc herniation. She now presents with recent development of severe low back pain when bending forward and bilateral hip pain.

IMAGING PRESENTATION

Radiograph obtained reveals intervertebral disc space narrowing at L5-S1 associated with vertebral endplate sclerosis and marginal vertebral osteophyte formation (*Fig. 17-1*). Magnetic resonance (MR) imaging reveals an enhancing full-thickness posterior annular fissure (tear) at L4-5 and a right paramidline focal posterior annular fissure at L5-S1 (*Figs. 17-2 to 17-6*). A left paramidline L5-S1 herniated disc causes left anterolateral thecal sac deformity (see Fig. 17-6).

DISCUSSION

Normal Intervertebral Disc

The intervertebral disc is a fibrocartilaginous structure comprised anatomically of a nucleus pulposus centrally, annulus fibrosus peripherally, and cartilaginous endplates superiorly and inferiorly (*Fig. 17-7*). The intervertebral disc is a fibrocartilaginous joint (it is not a synovial joint and therefore does not develop osteoarthritis). The intervertebral disc is composed of a mucopolysaccharide-rich ground substance, collagen bundles, chondrocytes, and water. The majority of the ground substance and water in the disc is located in the nucleus and inner portion of the annulus (*Fig. 17-8*); 80% of the disc collagen is either type I or type II collagen, but small amounts of types III, V, IX, and XI collagen are also present in the disc.[1]

The nucleus pulposus is centrally located in the intervertebral disc and is gelatinous in nature, composed of approximately 85% water, 15% mucopolysaccharide material, and a tiny amount of type I collagen located at the nuclear equator called the *reticular stratum*.[2] The mucopolysaccharides in the intervertebral disc are high-molecular-weight protein proteoglycans (also called *glycosaminoglycans*). These proteoglycans include chondroitin sulfate, keratin sulfate, and small amounts of hyaluronic acid. The proteoglycans are negatively charged molecules that have an affinity to bind with water.[1,3] The proteoglycans and water are concentrated in the nucleus and inner annulus. The amount of water in the disc at any given time is the result of a balance between hydrostatic forces from axial loading and intrinsic osmotic forces.[1,4,5] The proteoglycans bind water in the disc, predominantly in the nucleus and inner annulus, and are responsible for the high intrinsic hydrostatic pressure of the normal intervertebral disc, which allows the disc to resist and distribute compressive (axial loading) forces.[1] The disc height and intradiscal T2 MR signal intensity normally changes depending on the time of the day (diurnal variation).[6] This diurnal variation in intradiscal MR signal intensity is less in degenerated discs.[7] When a compressive load is placed upon the disc, water leaves the disc (predominantly through the endplates), and when the compressive load is removed, water returns to the disc.[1,6] As much as 40% to 60% of the intradiscal water can be removed by mechanical compression of the disc in vitro.[8]

The annulus fibrosus anatomically is divided into inner and outer regions (*Fig. 17-9*). The inner portion of the annulus contains less concentrated collagen, proteoglycans, and water and more closely resembles the nucleus pulposus histologically and on MR images; 80% of the collagen in the disc is type I or type II collagen.[1] The outer annular collagen is predominantly type I collagen and is arranged in 15 to 25 concentric rings.[9] These lamellae are not completely separate from adjacent lamellar rings, often splitting and obliquely joining adjacent lamella.[1,9,10] Approximately 3% of the collagen in the annulus is type V collagen, which may play a role in regulating the spatial orientation and dimensions of the lamellae.[1] Tiny, obliquely oriented or perpendicular interlamellar collagen bridges, visible on high-detail cryomicrotome images, also join the concentric lamellar rings (*Fig. 17-10*).[11,12] The outermost portion of the annulus is mainly dense fibrocartilage, concentrically arranged into lamellar bundles of mainly type I collagen, similar to the fibrocartilage found in the meniscus of the knee. These fibers are T2 hypointense on MR images (*Fig. 17-11*). These outermost annular collagen bundles, often referred to as *Sharpey's fibers*, are normally attached to the periosteum of the vertebral body corners, bone that was formed from the ring apophyes (see Fig. 17-9).[13,14] The anterior and posterior longitudinal ligaments merge imperceptibly with the outermost fibers of the annulus (*Fig. 17-12*).

The collagen bundles in the outer annulus give the disc its tensile strength, offering resistance to radially oriented (shear)

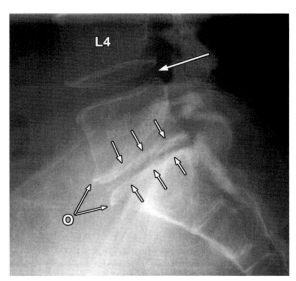

Figure 17-1 ▶ L5-S1 Intervertebral Osteochondrosis and Spondylosis Deformans. Lateral radiograph of lumbosacral junction. Marked narrowing of L5-S1 intervertebral disc with sclerosis at the adjacent vertebral endplates *(short arrows)*. Small vertebral osteophytes *(O)* arise from anterior vertebral body margins at L5-S1. Relatively normal height of L4-5 disc except for minimal narrowing of intervertebral disc space posteriorly *(long arrow)*. *L4* = L4 vertebral body.

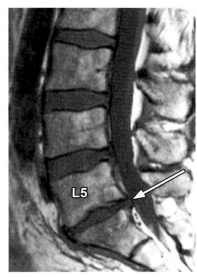

Figure 17-2 ▶ L5-S1 Posterior Disc Protrusion. Sagittal T1-weighted MR image in same patient as in Figure 17-1. The stature of the L5-S1 intervertebral disc is markedly diminished relative to normal stature of intervertebral discs above. The posterior margin of the L5-S1 disc *(arrow)* protrudes into the ventral epidural space. *L5* = L5 vertebral body.

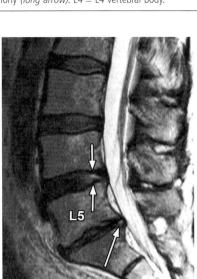

Figure 17-3 ▶ Posterior Annular Fissures. Sagittal T2-weighted MR image in same patient as in Figures 17-1 and 17-2. T2 hyperintensity zone *(short arrows)* in posterior annulus of L4-5 intervertebral disc consistent with full thickness (discographic grade 3) posterior annular fissure. Anterior portion of the L4-5 intervertebral disc is diminished in intensity relative to normal intensity L2-3 and L3-4 intervertebral discs above. The L5-S1 intervertebral disc is narrowed and diminished in intensity secondary to disc degeneration. Focal T2 hyperintense region *(long arrow)* in posterior annulus of L5-S1 disc represents a small localized annular fissure. The posterior L5-S1 disc margin protrudes into the ventral epidural space.

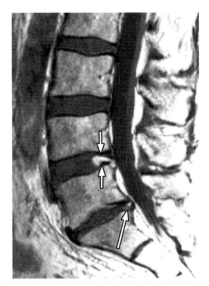

Figure 17-4 ▶ Enhancing Posterior Annular Fissures. Contrast-enhanced sagittal T1-weighted MR image corresponding to Figures 17-2 and 17-3. The full thickness L4-5 posterior annular fissure *(short arrows)* and localized posterior L5-S1 annular fissure *(long arrow)* both enhance intensely following IV contrast.

forces, which are produced when a compressive load is placed upon the nucleus and inner annulus.[15] The outermost portion of the annulus is normally innervated by both somatic and autonomic (sympathetic) sensory fibers, many of which are unmyelinated.[14] In degenerated discs, nerves may penetrate into the nucleus.[16] As the disc *degenerates*, annular fissures develop and connective tissue containing blood vessels and nerve endings infiltrate these fissures.[15]

The nerves in this connective tissue have nociceptors that detect and transmit pain sensation responsible for discogenic pain.

The cartilaginous disc endplate is made up of a fine, loosely arranged fibrillar network of predominantly type II collagen, similar to articular hyaline cartilage (see Figs. 17-7 and 17-12). The vertebral cortical bone endplate and the cartilaginous disc endplate form a unit that serves to provide structural and nutritional

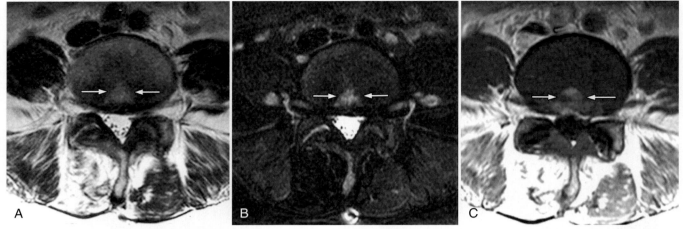

Figure 17-5 ▶ Full Thickness Posterior Annular Fissure. Axial MR images obtained through L4-5 intervertebral disc in same patient as in Figures 17-1 to 17-4. Wedge-shaped posterior annular fissure *(arrows in images* **A** *and* **B***)* is hyperintense on axial T2-weighted MR image **A** and is even more conspicuous on fat-saturated T2-weighted MR image **B.** The annular fissure *(arrows in image* **C***)* enhances on contrast-enhanced axial T1-weighted image **C.**

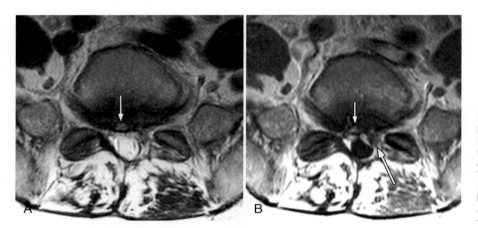

Figure 17-6 ▶ Posterior Annular Fissure. Same patient as in Figures 17-1 to 17-5. On axial T2-weighted MR image **A,** the focal T2 hyperintense zone *(arrow)* represents small, localized right paramidline posterior annular fissure. On corresponding contrast-enhanced T1-weighted MR image **B,** this localized fissure enhances *(short arrow).* A moderated-sized left paramidline disc herniation with surrounding enhancing tissue *(long arrow)* causes left anterolateral thecal sac deformity.

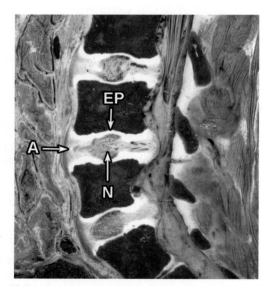

Figure 17-7 ▶ Normal Lumbar Intervertebral Discs in Adolescent Cadaver. Sagittal Cryomicrotome Image. Sagittal cryomicrotome image, cadaver. Normal intervertebral discs in adolescent. Nucleus *(N)* is distinct from outer annulus *(A)* but inner annulus has features of both nucleus and outer annulus. Well defined "white" cartilaginous endplate *(EP)* is similar to hyaline cartilage.

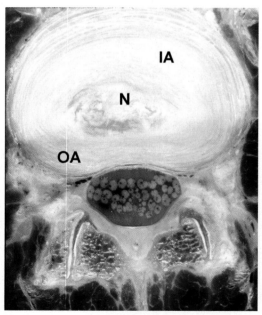

Figure 17-8 ▶ Normal Lumbar Intervertebral Disc. Axial Cryomicrotome Image in Adult Cadaver. Nucleus *(N)* and inner annulus *(IA)* are similar in appearance. Distinct concentric lamellar rings become more compact in the periphery of the outer annulus *(OA).*

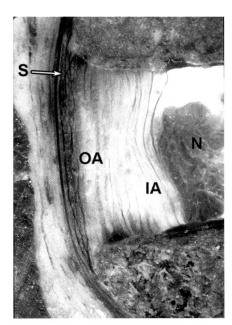

Figure 17-9 ► Sagittal Cryomicrotome Image of Anterior Annulus of Lumbar Intervertebral Disc in Adult Cadaver. The nucleus *(N)* is gelatinous material. Lamellae are more loosely arranged in inner annulus *(IA)* and more ground substance is located between lamellae in the inner annulus. The outer annulus *(OA)* contains more tightly packed lamellae. Sharpey's fibers *(S)* are densely compacted outermost annular lamellae which merge with the posterior longitudinal ligament and attach to the corners of the vertebral bodies.

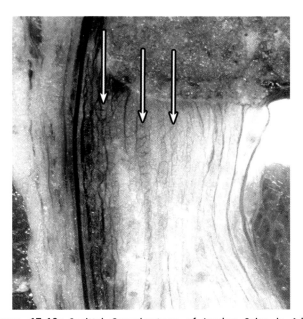

Figure 17-10 ► Sagittal Cryomicrotome of Lumbar Spine in Adult Cadaver Specimen. Fine transverse and obliquely oriented fibers *(arrows)* join the larger concentric, vertically-oriented lamellae. These tiny bridging fibers are not visible between the inner lamellae.

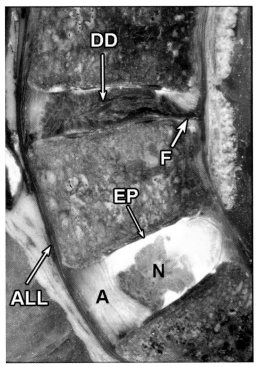

Figure 17-12 ► Sagittal Cryomicrotome of Lumbar Spine in Adult Cadaver Specimen. End stage L4-5 disc degeneration *(DD)*. The L4-5 disc, devoid of nuclear material, has become replaced almost entirely by collagenous tissue. A fissure *(F)* extends through the posterior annulus. L4-5 disc height is reduced compared with relatively normal L5-S1 intervertebral disc, which has a distinct gelatinous nucleus *(N)*, annulus *(A)* and cartilaginous endplate *(N)*. The posterior longitudinal ligament and anterior longitudinal ligament *(ALL)* are in contact with the vertebral body margin and outermost portion of the annulus. Note the anterior annulus is thicker than posterior annulus.

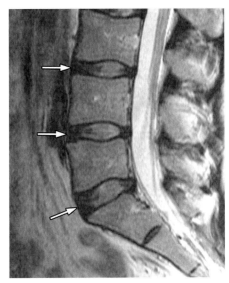

Figure 17-11 ► Sagittal T2-Weighted MR Image, Normal Spine. The outer annulus is T2 hypointense. The anterior annulus is thicker than the posterior annulus. The inner annulus and nucleus have similar intensity, being relatively T2 hyperintense compared with dark outer annulus.

support to the intervertebral disc.[17] The cartilaginous endplate is in close proximity to a rich vascular network in and adjacent to the vertebral body endplates, which facilitates the exchange of intradiscal water, nutrients, and metabolic waste. The cartilaginous endplates also provide intradiscal support and resistance to compressive (axial loading) forces.

All portions of the adult intervertebral disc are normally devoid of blood vessels. Nutrients and metabolites, for disc nourishment, pass mainly by diffusion, but some pass by active transport from blood vessels that reside in small perforations located in the vertebral cortical endplates, and these substances pass across the cartilaginous endplates into the disc.[18,19] Some water and nutrient exchange also occurs along the peripheral margin of the disc.[19] It is believed that this nutrient exchange mechanism is facilitated by compression and decompression of the disc during normal daily activity. Interference with this nutrient exchange system by discovertebral infection, for example, causes damage to the vertebral endplates and results in destruction of the intervertebral disc.

Aging Disc

There is no general agreement as to what actually constitutes a normal aging disc versus a degenerated disc or when the transition from normal to aging to degenerated disc occurs. In persons of all ages, the collagen concentration is greater in the outer annulus. With increasing age, the relative collagen content increases in the disc from cephalad to caudad, and from peripheral to central.[3,15]

The most striking changes in the intervertebral disc with advancing age occur in the disc nucleus and inner annulus. With age, the water content of the disc diminishes, but only by a relatively small amount. In children, 85% of the disc nucleus contains water, and 78% of the disc annulus contains water.[18] Intervertebral discs in patients of advanced age still contain approximately 70% water.[18] Therefore, it is estimated that the disc water content is reduced by only 15% to 20% from approximately age 10 to 70 in the "normally aging" disc. Therefore, the amount of disc *desiccation* that occurs in the normally aging disc is actually not that great on a percentage basis. In degenerating discs, a greater degree of disc dehydration is expected to occur.

The total proteoglycan content in the disc does decrease with age.[1,17,20] However, the ratio of keratin sulfate to chondroitin sulfate in the disc actually increases with age.[15,21] The collagen content in the disc increases dramatically with age[3] and may be the primary reason discs appear "dark" on T2-weighted MR images. By age 80, the "normal" disc nucleus is almost completely replaced by dense fibrocartilage, but the disc height remains preserved.

It is possible that some small annular fissures can occur as a result of the normal aging process. Small annular fissures are sometimes observed in anatomic specimens of the disc in persons 15 to 20 years of age. By age 30, annular fissures are found in nearly all anatomic disc specimens.[14]

Degeneration of the Intervertebral Disc (Disc Derangement)

There is no general consensus or unifying theory as to what actually causes or constitutes intervertebral *disc degeneration* or *disc derangement*.[22] Disc degeneration is likely caused by multiple interactive factors.[23,24] Many believe that the degenerated, internally deranged disc is the result of acceleration of the normal

aging process. It is likely that genetic factors or some metabolic dysfunction renders the disc susceptible to chronic derangement or acute disruption. In degenerating discs, the water content is definitely reduced, but it is uncertain whether water reduction occurs primarily or is secondary to reduction in proteoglycan concentration, because proteoglycan synthesis and water binding in the disc are interrelated. In the aging and degenerating disc, it is also known that collagen, which predominates normally in the disc periphery, infiltrates the inner annulus and nucleus replacing portions of the disc previously occupied by proteoglycans and water.[25] Dehydration of the disc likely predisposes it to annular fissure formation, but the exact mechanism by which annular fissure formation occurs is not known. In the end stages of disc degeneration, the disc is replaced almost entirely by amorphous fibrocartilage with no distinction between nucleus and annulus (see Fig. 17-12).[24]

An acute traumatic episode can disrupt the disc but is not likely the major factor that produces disc degeneration, as was once believed. A history of trauma is obtained in only a minority of patients who have herniated intervertebral discs. Biomechanical studies have shown that the disc is less likely than the vertebral body to fail as a result of trauma. However, repetitive microtrauma may cause damage to the osteocartilaginous endplate or intervertebral disc, which may eventually weaken the disc and make it unable to withstand daily biomechanical stress.

Because the intervertebral disc normally lacks a blood supply, nutrients and water are exchanged between capillaries and the extravascular spaces in the vertebral bodies and epidural space via the osteocartilaginous endplates and outermost annular disc margins, which function similarly to semipermeable membranes.[1,26] Metabolic disorders or inflammatory processes that damage or interfere with the exchange of water and nutrients across the endplates or at the peripheral disc margins may therefore play a role in the pathogenesis of disc degeneration.[26]

There is mounting evidence that genetic factors predispose the disc to degeneration and hence disc herniation.[23,27] Inherited genetic traits likely render the disc more susceptible to degeneration, disc herniation, or weakening of the vertebral bone.[28-31] Cytokines, such as interleukin-1, may contribute to disc degeneration by causing release of enzymes that degrade proteoglycans. Inflammatory cytokines are believed to be one of several mediators of back pain.[30] Enzymes capable of disc degradation, such as metalloproteinases and aggrecanase, occur in high concentrations in degenerating discs and in even higher concentrations in herniated discs.[32]

Regardless of the pathogenesis of disc degeneration, the result of the biomechanical stress placed upon the disc either acutely or chronically is the development of annular fissures (annular tears). Radially oriented fissures, in particular, are believed to be associated with primary biomechanical failure of the annulus, and these annular tears are consistently found in degenerated symptomatic and asymptomatic intervertebral discs viewed with discography. Radially oriented *partial* or *full-thickness* annular tears extend across and disrupt the lamellar rings (*Fig. 17-13*). Fissures that disrupt the lamellar rings should always be considered pathologic, and their presence always indicates internal disc derangement. These radially oriented fissures often involve the inner annulus initially and later extend to involve the outer annulus.[14] Annular fissures most often occur with concomitant reduction in disc height and are often associated with discogenic pain because they contain vascularized granulation tissue with nerves that have nociceptors that transmit pain sensation.

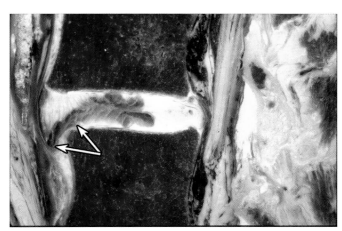

Figure 17-13 ▶ Sagittal Cryomicrotome Image of Cadaver Specimen, Lumbar Spine. A full thickness annular fissure *(arrows)* extends through the anterior annulus inferiorly.

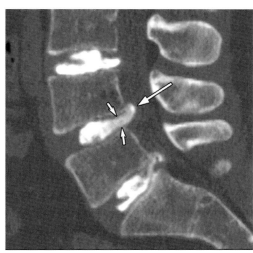

Figure 17-14 ▶ Full Thickness Posterior Annular Fissure Shown by Discography. Sagittal post-discogram CT image in patient having severe low back pain and bilateral thigh pain. Highly concordant pain response upon injection of L4-5 intervertebral disc. Shown is a large discographic grade III full thickness posterior annular fissure *(small arrows)* with contrast agent extending into a posterior herniated disc *(arrow)*.

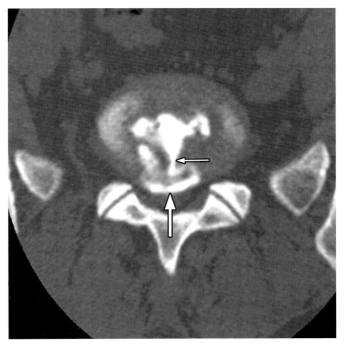

Figure 17-15 ▶ Contained Disc Extrusion. Post discography axial CT image at L4-5 level in same patient as in Figure 17-14. Injected intradiscal contrast agent fills a large grade III annular fissure *(small arrow)* that extends into a midline disc herniation *(long arrow)*. The contrast extends through all layers of the annulus, so this is a disc extrusion even though it has a relatively wide neck. The herniation is limited (contained) posteriorly by the posterior longitudinal ligament.

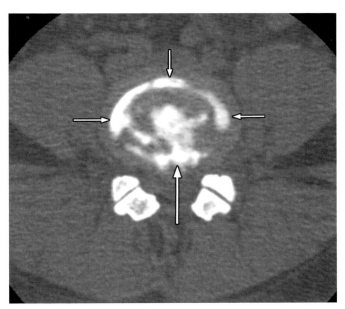

Figure 17-16 ▶ Diffusely Bulging Disc. Post discography axial CT image at L4-5 level in another patient with highly concordant pain response upon injection of this disc. A broad midline posterior annular fissure *(long arrow)* is present that does not extend to the posterior disc margin (partial thickness annular fissure). There is a large crescent-shaped annular fissure *(small arrows)* anteriorly and bilaterally.

Although some small annular fissures may form in normally aging discs, large crescent-shaped annular fissures and all radially oriented annular fissures are likely pathologic in nature *(Figs. 17-14 to 17-16)*. Crescentic annular fissures of all sizes likely contribute to the circumferential disc bulging frequently observed in degenerated discs (see Fig. 17-16). These crescent-shaped fissures cause disruption of the tiny interlamellar bridges and also the proteoglycan-rich ground substance, which results in lamellar separation.

Internal Disc Derangement Classification

Three types of annular tears (fissures) have been described and classified by Yu and colleagues[38] *(Fig. 17-17)*. This classification of annular fissures discussed here should not be confused with the grading system currently used for discography (see "Grading System for Discography" below). **Type I annular tears** are crescentic fissures that disrupt the interlamellar collagen fibers and are usually located between concentric annular lamellae (see Fig. 17-17; *Fig. 17-18*). These may be seen on MR images as crescent-shaped fissures that characteristically have high T2 signal intensity *(Fig. 17-19)*. The large concentric lamellae may remain intact adjacent to small, isolated type I fissures. This type of annular fissure may occur in the normal aging process and internal disc derangement and likely contributes to the generalized lamellar separation and annular laxity observed in the diffusely bulging disc. Large crescentic annular tears are seen in pathologic internal disc derangement (see Fig. 17-16). The small or large crescent-shaped type I annular fissures visible on routine T2-weighted MR images, usually near the periphery of the annulus, are likely pathologic (see Fig. 17-19; *Fig. 17-20*).

The **type II annular tears** are annular fissures that most people are familiar with and are the type frequently referred to in MR reporting. These are also called *radial tears*, because they extend radially from the inner annulus outward, disrupting concentric

lamellae (see Figs. 17-3 to 17-5, 17-13 to 17-15, and 17-17). The radial tear likely represents a pathologic entity rather than the result of the normal aging process. The presence of radial annular tears, along with progressive loss of cartilage in the nucleus pulposus, is the feature associated most often with disc degeneration.[12] The radial tear is the most frequent type of annular fissure visible on routine MR images, seen on T2-weighted MR images as a linear or oblong region of high–signal intensity tissue within the otherwise low-intensity outer annulus. The "bright" signal in the outer annulus, signifying the radial tear, is sometimes referred to as a T2 *high intensity zone* (see Figs. 17-3 to 17-5). Radial annular tears are frequently associated with the presence of discogenic pain as elicited by discography based on personal experience, although not all radial tears are symptomatic. Radial tears are more commonly observed in the midline posteriorly or posterolaterally in the annulus.

Type III annular tears are tiny triangular-shaped tears at the periphery of the disc, near the insertion of Sharpey's fibers into the

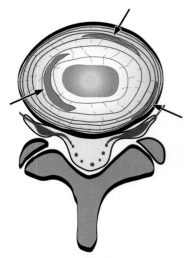

Figure 17-17 ▶ Three Types of Annular Fissures. Illustration of lumbar spine in sagittal plane demonstrating the three types of annular fissures described by Yu and colleagues (1988). Type 1 is a concentric, crescent-shaped fissure. Type 2 is a radial annular fissure. Type 3 is a tiny triangular-shaped defect in the annulus peripherally near apophyseal corner of vertebral body.

Figure 17-18 ▶ Bulging Lumbar Intervertebral Disc, Axial Plane. Illustration showing diffusely bulging lumbar intervertebral disc containing concentric (crescentic) Type 1 annular fissures *(arrows)* located in ground substance between concentric lamellar rings. These fissures are equivalent to discographic Grade 4 fissures.

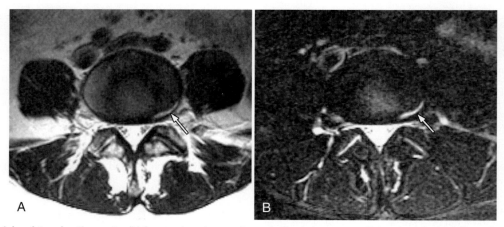

Figure 17-19 ▶ Peripheral Annular Fissure. Small left posterolateral crescentic annular fissure is an arcuate T2 hyperintensity *(arrow)* near the disc periphery on axial T2-weighted MR image **A.** The annular fissure *(arrow)* is more conspicuous on fat-saturated T2-weighted MR image **B.**

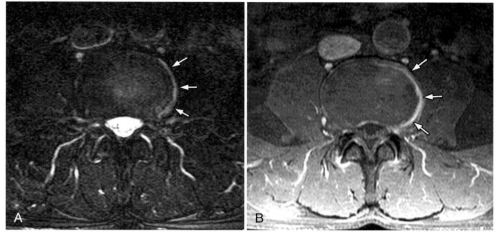

Figure 17-20 ▶ Peripheral Annular Fissures. Large left lateral crescentic annular fissure *(arrow)* is T2 hyperintense on fat-saturated T2-weighted MR image **A** and enhances *(arrow)* following IV contrast on axial fat-saturated contrast-enhanced MR image **B.**

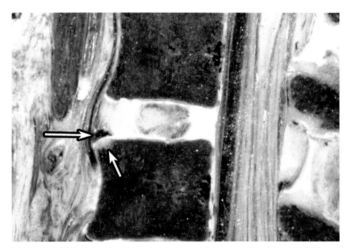

Figure 17-21 ▶ Sagittal Cryomicrotome Image of Cadaver Specimen. Photograph shows a tiny triangular shaped Type 3 annular fissure *(long arrow)* in L1-2 intervertebral disc anteriorly. Note cortical bone buildup *(short arrow)* at adjacent corner of vertebral body where a small osteophyte has formed.

vertebral endplate (see Fig. 17-17; *Fig. 17-21*). Type III tears may be quite common but are not frequently recognized on MR images because of their small size. They may be associated with Sharpey's fiber detachments from the vertebral body corners (apophysis) and therefore may occur in the process of vertebral osteophyte formation.

IMAGING FEATURES

The normal disc is fairly homogeneous in signal intensity on T1-weighted MR images and relatively hypointense relative to the vertebral marrow. The normal intervertebral disc is "dark" peripherally and "bright" centrally on T2-weighted MR images (see Fig. 17-11). The bright portion of the intervertebral disc corresponds to the nucleus pulposus and inner annulus.[25,33] The dark portion of the disc on T2-weighted MR images corresponds to the outer annulus (see Fig. 17-11).[11,25] A thin horizontal linear band of

hypointensity may be visible in the disc on MR images, which may represent the intranuclear cleft, a thin band of compacted collagenous, reticular, and elastic fibers.[2,34] A truncation artifact on MR images may simulate the intranuclear cleft.[35]

Despite the lack of agreement regarding the etiology of disc degeneration, the MR imaging features that characterize the degenerating disc are well known. With MR imaging, in aging and degenerating discs, the initial finding is reduction in intradiscal signal intensity on T2-weighted MR images.[25,36] Some use the phrase *T2 dark disc* to describe the MR appearance of aging or degenerative intervertebral discs (*Fig. 17-22*). The term *dessicated* disc is often used synonymously with T2 dark disc, but disc dehydration (desiccation) alone does not account for the reduction in intradiscal T2 signal intensity observed. The T2 hypointensity of the intervertebral disc seen on T2-weighted MR images with disc degeneration is more likely due to collagen replacement of the disc and reduction in proteoglycan content rather than reduction in overall water content of the disc. However, all of these factors contribute to the reduction in intradiscal T2 signal intensity. Rarely, internally deranged discs are largely T2 hyperintense, which may be due to diffuse infiltration of the disc by granulation tissue (*Fig. 17-23*).

As the disc continues to degenerate further and can no longer withstand biomechanical stress, the disc height diminishes. Loss of disc stature is a reliable sign of pathologic internal disc derangement. This is well demonstrated on MRI, computed tomography (CT), and plain radiographs (see Figs. 17-1 to 17-3, 17-23; *Fig. 17-24*). In advanced disc degeneration, intradiscal calcification[6] or gas formation frequently occur, which are also definite signs of severe disc degeneration, best demonstrated on CT or radiographs (see Fig. 17-24).

Many other degenerative spinal conditions may coexist with intervertebral disc degeneration including spondylosis deformans (vertebral osteophytosis), facet osteoarthritis, paraspinous ligamentous thickening, spinal stenosis, and spondylolisthesis. Whether these conditions are causally related to intervertebral disc degeneration or merely occur concomitantly with disc degeneration has not been clearly established. Potentially pain-producing active inflammation secondary to degenerative disorders involving the intervertebral disc, vertebral bodies, vertebral osteophytes, and zygoapophyseal (facet) joints is best demonstrated on MR imaging using fat-saturation techniques.[37]

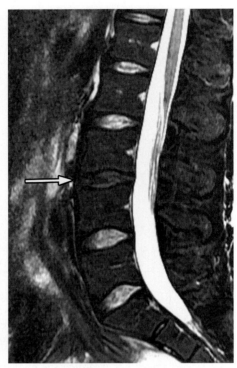

Figure 17-22 ► T2 "Dark" Disc. Sagittal fat-saturated T2-weighted MR image. The signal intensity of the L3-4 intervertebral disc *(arrow)* is diminished and the disc height is reduced slightly, relative to adjacent normal intervertebral discs.

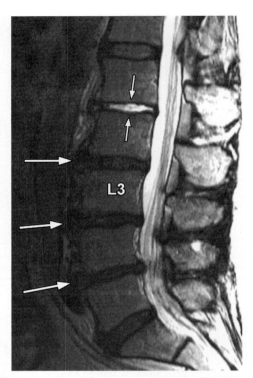

Figure 17-23 ► Multilevel Disc Degeneration (Internal Disc Derangement). Sagittal T2-weighted MR image in a patient with vague low back pain. The lower four intervertebral discs have diminished intradiscal T2 signal intensity. The L2-3, L3-4, and L4-5 discs are reduced in height relative to normal and bulge diffusely. Dark osteophytes arise from anterior vertebral body margins *(long arrows)*. The L1-2 intervertebral disc *(between small arrows)* is very T2 hyperintense probably due to infiltration of intervertebral disc by granulation tissue, mucoid material or fluid. The L1-2 vertebral cortical endplates *(small arrows)* are completely intact, so this should not be mistaken for discitis.

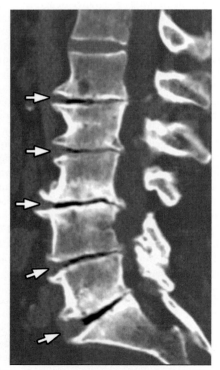

Figure 17-24 ► Multilevel Lumbar Disc Degeneration. Sagittal CT reformatted image in a patient with generalized low back pain. All lumber intervertebral discs *(arrows)* are narrowed and contain gas ("vacuum discs"). Degenerative discogenic reactive bony sclerosis involves the vertebral endplates and adjacent vertebral bodies. Prominent vertebral marginal osteophytes at all lumbar levels anteriorly and posteriorly.

Annular tears or fissures are seen on T2-weighted MR images as focal, linear, or arcuate regions of T2 hyperintensity in the disc,[39] sometime referred to as *high intensity zones* in the disc (see Figs. 17-3, 17-5, 17-19, 17-20; *Fig. 17-25*). These T2 hyperintense regions in the disc correspond anatomically to areas of mucoid degeneration in the disc.[38,40] Annular fissures are visible on MR images even in the early stages of disc degeneration.[41] Annular fissures enhance after intravenous paramagnetic contrast administration on T1-weighted MR images (see Figs. 17-4, 17-20, and 17-25). The enhancement is likely due to the presence of vascularized granulation tissue within these fissures.[39,40] It is important to stress that the presence of demonstrable annular fissures within the disc on MR images does not indicate that these fissures are necessarily the source of the patient's pain. Discography is more sensitive than MR imaging for the detection of radial annular tears.[42]

The vast majority of so called *degenerating discs* seen on radiographs, CT, or MR imaging are not symptomatic. In general, it is not possible to reliably predict based on imaging features which discs are symptomatic. Discography is the procedure of choice for diagnosing morphologic and symptomatic intervertebral disc derangement. Discography is a provocative procedure, performed by injecting a small quantity of fluid into the disc, to determine whether a given intervertebral disc is responsible for the patient's pain. The injected fluid causes a temporary increase in intradiscal pressure. This fluid is a mixture of an iodinated contrast agent and

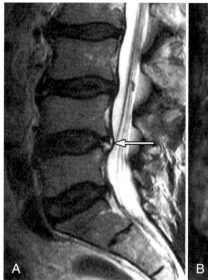 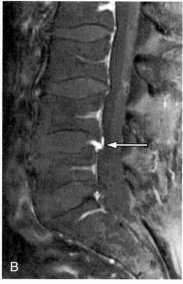

Figure 17-25 ▶ Posterior Annular Fissure, L4-5 Level. Patient with severe low back pain. Multiple T2 dark discs and a posterior annular fissure focal T2 hyperintensity zone *(arrow)* are demonstrated on T2-weighted MR image **A** at L4-5 level. The posterior annular fissure *(arrow)* enhances intensely as shown on corresponding sagittal contrast-enhanced fat-saturated T1-weighted MR image **B.**

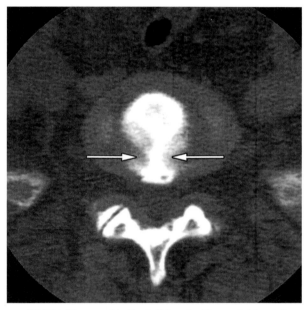

Figure 17-26 ▶ Discographic Grade 3 Annular Fissure. Axial post discogram CT image. A large midline annular fissure *(arrows)* fills with contrast and extends to the posterior disc margin following injection of contrast agent into the nucleus.

a small volume of antibiotic agent. The primary goal of performing provocative discography is to answer the following question: Is the pain generated at a given injected disc level concordant with the patient's back pain in distribution and intensity? The secondary question to answer is: How many discs injected generate concordant or partially concordant pain? Therefore, assessment of the patient's response to pain during injection of fluid into the disc is the primary reason for performing discography.

Discography is more sensitive than MR imaging for diagnosing and defining the extent of annular tears.[42] However, the morphologic appearance of the disc on discographic radiographs and on post-discogram CT scans is of secondary importance to the

patient's pain response elicited at the time of discography. Discography can provide anatomic information regarding the position of annular fissures, information that may be useful for planning the approach for certain percutaneous annular ablation procedures.

The techniques for performing discography, and discussion of the criteria used to determine whether a disc is symptomatic are beyond the scope of this chapter, but a detailed discussion of discographic technique can be found elsewhere.[43,44] The grading system currently used for discography for reporting the morphologic appearance and extent of annular fissures is a modified version of the Dallas grading system[45] as follows:

Grading System for Discography
   Grade 0. Contrast agent confined to nucleus.
   Grade 1. Radial annular tear involving inner one third of annulus.
   Grade 2. Radial annular involving middle one third of annulus.
   Grade 3. Radial annular tear involving outer one third of annulus *(Fig. 17-26)*.
   Grade 4. Complex annular tear with grade 3 radial tear plus a crescentic annular tear involving greater than 30 degrees of the disc circumference *(Fig. 17-27)*.
   Grade 5. Any full-thickness annular tear with extra-annular leakage of contrast agent.

The **diffusely degenerated disc**, which is a diffusely deranged intervertebral disc that allows the discographic contrast to infiltrate throughout the disc substance, should be added to the grading system. This pattern is commonly seen during discography *(Figs. 17-28 and 17-29)*.

Vertebral Osteochondrosis

With more advanced disc degeneration, reactive bone abnormalities often develop in the vertebral endplates and adjacent trabecular bone. This condition is referred to as *intervertebral osteochondrosis*, but the manifestations of this degenerative process in the intervertebral disc are seen in the vertebral endplates and adjacent bone marrow. On radiographs and CT images, endplate irregularities and cortical thickening occur adjacent to the

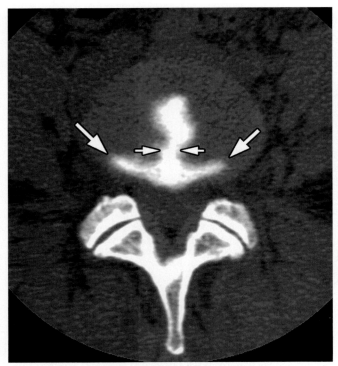

Figure 17-27 ► Discographic Grades 3 and 4 Annular Fissures. Axial post discogram CT image. A Grade 3 midline annular fissure *(small arrows)*, and peripheral crescentic Grade 4 *(large arrows)* fill with contrast following injection of contrast agent into the nucleus.

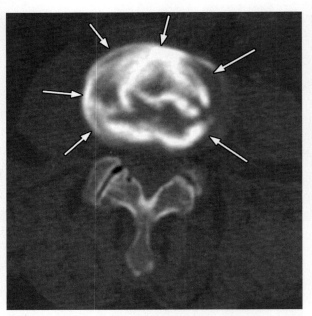

Figure 17-28 ► Diffuse Intervertebral Disc Degeneration. Axial post discogram CT image. The injected contrast agent infiltrates throughout the L3-4 intervertebral disc.

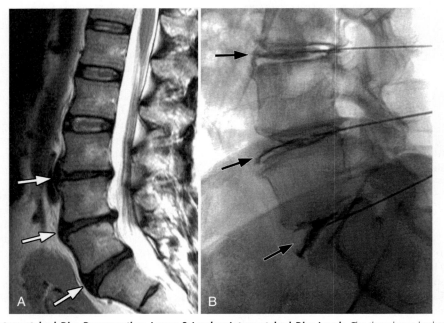

Figure 17-29 ► Diffuse Intervertebral Disc Degeneration, Lower 3 Lumbar Intervertebral Disc Levels. The three lower lumbar intervertebral discs *(arrows)*, shown on sagittal T2-weighted MR image **A,** are T2 hypointense, bulge diffusely, and have lost height relative to the normal discs more superiorly. Corresponding lateral radiograph (image **B**), in the same patient obtained during discography, shows discography needles in the lower three lumbar intervertebral discs. Injected contrast agent extends throughout these intervertebral discs *(arrows)* indicating diffuse disc degeneration.

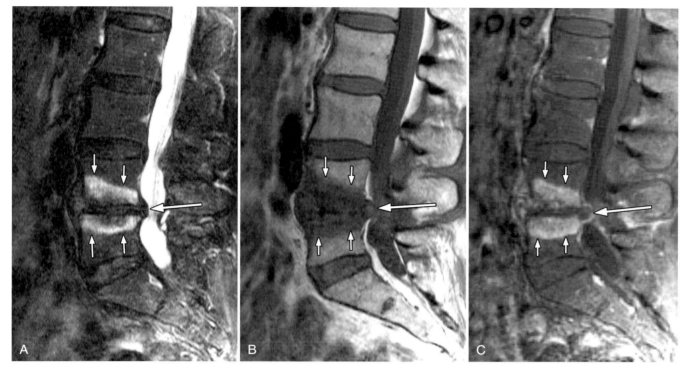

Figure 17-30 ▶ Reactive Degenerative Discogenic Intervertebral Osteochondrosis (Modic Type I) Simulating Disc Infection. On sagittal fat-saturated T2-weighted MR image **A,** the L4-5 intervertebral disc is T2 hypointense. The adjacent cortical endplates are intact but hyperintense signal *(small arrows)* is located in the vertebral body marrow adjacent to the L4-5 vertebral endplates. On sagittal T1-weighted MR image **B,** the reactive marrow is T1 hypointense *(small arrows)* and the vertebral cortical endplates are not clearly defined. On sagittal contrast-enhanced fat-saturated T1-weighted MR image **C,** intense enhancement of the reactive marrow *(small arrows)* is located adjacent to well defined cortical endplates. Note posterior disc herniation *(long arrow)* in images **A, B,** and **C.** Repeated disc aspiration biopsies failed to culture any organism; the patient had normal erythrocyte sedimentation rate (ESR) and normal serum C-reactive protein levels.

degenerated disc. Sclerosis develops in the trabecular bone adjacent to the vertebral endplates and is well demonstrated on CT and radiographs.[46]

The MR appearance of the reactive endplate signal abnormalities, which accompany intervertebral osteochondrosis, was reported independently by Sobel[46] and de Roos[47] in 1987, and was classified by Modic and colleagues[48] in 1988. Reactive vertebral body and endplate changes are visible on MR imaging and are secondary to intervertebral disc degeneration. In the majority of cases, the reactive vertebral body signal disturbance is not associated with symptoms.[49,50] **Type I** vertebral body/endplate changes represent vascularized marrow and have low signal intensity on T1-weighted MR images and high signal intensity on T2-weighted MR images *(Fig. 17-30 A-B)*. These areas adjacent to the vertebral endplates may enhance intensely after IV contrast administration, and this appearance can simulate that seen with spondylodiscitis *(Fig. 17-30 C)*. Type I reactive vertebral body/endplate changes have the greatest likelihood of being symptomatic, and when symptomatic, usually are associated with localized back pain.[49] Discography is the procedure of choice to confirm the presence of discogenic pain associated with type I endplate changes.[51] **Type II** vertebral body/endplate changes represent a more chronic phase of discogenic disease with proliferation of fatty marrow in the vertebral body adjacent to the degenerating disc and are characterized by high signal intensity on T1-weighted MR images and isointense or slightly hyperintense on T2-weighted MR images. Intervertebral discs associated with type II endplate changes occasionally may be

symptomatic with discography.[51] **Type III** vertebral body/endplate changes are usually not associated with symptoms and represent dense bone, devoid of marrow, and are dark on T1-weighted and T2-weighted MR images.

DIFFERENTIAL DIAGNOSIS

1. **Discovertebral infection** (discitis/osteomyelitis) can be confused with disc degeneration, especially when type I Modic changes are present. Although most infected discs are T2 hyperintense, occasionally infected discs are not hyperintense, such as in patients with mycobacterial injections. A needle aspiration biopsy of the disc should be performed if there is doubt based on imaging studies or clinical findings.
2. **Vertebral metastases** adjacent to the vertebral endplate are occasionally mistaken for degenerative discogenic endplate disease.

TREATMENT

1. **No treatment:** The vast majority of degenerative intervertebral discs are asymptomatic and require no treatment.
2. **Conservative therapy:** Treatment with nonsteroidal anti-inflammatory agents (NSAIDs) and physical therapy is often

prescribed for mild to moderate discogenic back pain with mixed results.

3. **Percutaneous intradiscal thermal or radiofrequency annular ablation:** Procedures such as intradiscal electrothermal therapy (IDET™) or radiofrequency annuloplasty (discTRODE™) can be effective in treating some patients experiencing discogenic pain.

4. **Surgical fusion:** The procedure of choice if less invasive procedures fail to relieve discogenic pain, especially if the discogenic pain is associated with vertebral instability.

5. **Artificial intervertebral disc replacement:** Has been used with varying success. This procedure, more commonly used in Europe, is still not widely accepted in the United States as a treatment for disc degeneration and refractory discogenic pain.[52-54]

6. **Intervertebral disc transplantation:** This an investigational surgical procedure that has been performed in the cervical spine.[55]

References

1. Gumina S, Postacchini F. Biochemistry, nutrition, and metabolism. In: Postacchini F, ed. *Lumbar Disc Herniation*. Wien, New York: Springer-Verlag; 1999:59-79.
2. Yu SW, Haughton VM, Lynch KL, et al. Fibrous structure in the intervertebral disk: correlation of MR appearance with anatomic sections. *AJNR Am J Neuroradiol*. 1989;10(5):1105-1110.
3. Sylven B. On the biology of nucleus pulposus. *Acta Orthop Scand*. 1951;20(4):275-279.
4. Urban JP, Maroudas A. Swelling of the intervertebral disc in vitro. *Connect Tissue Res*. 1981;9(1):1-10.
5. Nachemson A. Towards a better understanding of low-back pain: a review of the mechanics of the lumbar disc. *Rheumatol Rehabil*. 1975;14(3):129-143.
6. Pritzker KP. Aging and degeneration in the lumbar intervertebral disc. *Orthop Clin North Am*. 1977;8(1):66-77.
7. Boos N, Wallin A, Gbedegbegnon T, et al. Quantitative MR imaging of lumbar intervertebral disks and vertebral bodies: influence of diurnal water content variations. *Radiology*. 1993;188(2):351-354.
8. Urban JP, McMullin JF. Swelling pressure of the lumbar intervertebral discs: influence of age, spinal level, composition, and degeneration. *Spine (Phila Pa 1976)*. 1988;13(2):179-187.
9. Marchand F, Ahmed AM. Investigation of the laminate structure of lumbar disc anulus fibrosus. *Spine (Phila Pa 1976)*. 1990;15(5):402-410.
10. Inoue H, Takeda T. Three-dimensional observation of collagen framework of lumbar intervertebral discs. *Acta Orthop Scand*. 1975;46(6):949-956.
11. Czervionke LF, Haughton VM. Degenerative disease of the spine. In: Atlas SW, ed. *Magnetic Resonance Imaging of the Brain and Spine*. 3rd ed. Philadelphia: Lippincott Williams & Wilkins; 2002.
12. Yu S, Haughton VM, Sether LA, et al. Criteria for classifying normal and degenerated lumbar intervertebral disks. *Radiology*. 1989;170(2):523-526.
13. Ho PS, Yu SW, Sether LA, et al. Progressive and regressive changes in the nucleus pulposus. *Part I. The neonate. Radiology*. 1988;169(1):87-91.
14. Hirsch C, Schajowicz F. Studies on the structural changes in the lumbar annulus fibrosus. *Acta Orthop Scand*. 1952;22:185-231.
15. Adams P, Eyre DR, Muir H. Biochemical aspects of development and ageing of human lumbar intervertebral discs. *Rheumatol Rehabil*. 1977;16(1):22-29.
16. Modic MT, Ross JS. Lumbar degenerative disk disease. *Radiology*. 2007;245(1):43-61.
17. Nachemson AL. The lumbar spine: an orthopaedic challenge. *Spine*. 1976;1(1):59-71.
18. Lipson SJ. Ageing versus degeneration of the intervertebral disc. In: Weinstein JN, Wiesel SW, eds. *The Lumbar Spine*. Philadelphia: W.B. Saunders Co.; 1990;xxii, 1035.
19. Maroudas A, Stockwell RA, Nachemson A, Urban J. Factors involved in the nutrition of the human lumbar intervertebral disc: cellularity and diffusion of glucose in vitro. *J Anat*. 1975;120(Pt 1):113-130.
20. Gower WE, Pedrini V. Age-related variations in proteinpolysaccharides from human nucleus pulposus, annulus fibrosus, and costal cartilage. *J Bone Joint Surg Am*. 1969;51(6):1154-1162.
21. Nachemson A. Intradiscal measurements of pH in patients with lumbar rhizopathies. *Acta Orthop Scand*. 1969;40(1):23-42.
22. Modic MT, Herfkens RJ. Intervertebral disk: normal age-related changes in MR signal intensity. *Radiology*. 1990;177(2):332-333; discussion 3-4.
23. Modic MT. Degenerative disc disease: genotyping, MR imaging, and phenotyping. *Skeletal Radiol*. 2007;36(2):91-93.
24. Modic MT, Masaryk TJ, Ross JS, Carter JR. Imaging of degenerative disk disease. *Radiology*. 1988;168(1):177-186.
25. Sether LA, Yu S, Haughton VM, Fischer ME. Intervertebral disk: normal age-related changes in MR signal intensity. *Radiology*. 1990;177(2):385-388.
26. Ogata K, Whiteside LA. Nutritional pathways of the intervertebral disc: an experimental study using hydrogen washout technique. *Spine*. 1980;6:211-216.
27. Matsui H, Kanamori M, Ishihara H, et al. Familial predisposition for lumbar degenerative disc disease: a case-control study. *Spine (Phila Pa 1976)*. 1998;23(9):1029-1034.
28. Kawaguchi Y, Osada R, Kanamori M, et al. Association between an aggrecan gene polymorphism and lumbar disc degeneration. *Spine (Phila Pa 1976)*. 1999;24(23):2456-2460.
29. Videman T, Leppavuori J, Kaprio J, et al. Intragenic polymorphisms of the vitamin D receptor gene associated with intervertebral disc degeneration. *Spine (Phila Pa 1976)*. 1998;23(23):2477-2485.
30. Zhang Y, Sun Z, Liu J, Guo X. Advances in susceptibility genetics of intervertebral degenerative disc disease. *Int J Biol Sci*. 2008;4(5):283-290.
31. Zortea M, Vettori A, Trevisan CP, et al. Genetic mapping of a susceptibility locus for disc herniation and spastic paraplegia on 6q23.3-q24.1. *J Med Genet*. 2002;39(6):387-390.
32. Roberts S, Caterson B, Menage J, et al. Matrix metalloproteinases and aggrecanase: their role in disorders of the human intervertebral disc. *Spine (Phila Pa 1976)*. 2000;25(23):3005-3013.
33. Pech P, Haughton VM. Lumbar intervertebral disk: correlative MR and anatomic study. *Radiology*. 1985;156(3):699-701.
34. Aguila LA, Piraino DW, Modic MT, et al. The intranuclear cleft of the intervertebral disk: magnetic resonance imaging. *Radiology*. 1985;155(1):155-158.
35. Breger RK, Czervionke LF, Kass EG, et al. Truncation artifact in MR images of the intervertebral disk. *AJNR Am J Neuroradiol*. 1988;9(5):825-828.
36. Rasekhi A, Babaahmadi A, Assadsangabi R, Nabavizadeh SA. Clinical manifestations and MRI findings of patients with hydrated and dehydrated lumbar disc herniation. *Acad Radiol*. 2006;13(12):1485-1489.
37. D'Aprile P, Tarantino A, Jinkins JR, Brindicci D. The value of fat saturation sequences and contrast medium administration in MRI of degenerative disease of the posterior/perispinal elements of the lumbosacral spine. *Eur Radiol*. 2007;17(2):523-531.
38. Yu SW, Sether LA, Ho PS, et al. Tears of the anulus fibrosus: correlation between MR and pathologic findings in cadavers. *AJNR Am J Neuroradiol*. 1988;9(2):367-370.
39. Ross JS, Modic MT, Masaryk TJ. Tears of the anulus fibrosus: assessment with Gd-DTPA-enhanced MR imaging. *AJR Am J Roentgenol*. 1990;154(1):159-162.
40. Haughton V. Imaging intervertebral disc degeneration. *J Bone Joint Surg Am*. 2006;88 Suppl 2:15-20.
41. Sharma A, Pilgram T, Wippold FJ, 2nd. Association between annular tears and disk degeneration: a longitudinal study. *AJNR Am J Neuroradiol*. 2009;30(3):500-506.
42. Yu SW, Haughton VM, Sether LA, Wagner M. Comparison of MR and diskography in detecting radial tears of the anulus: a postmortem study. *AJNR Am J Neuroradiol*. 1989;10(5):1077-1081.
43. Fenton DS, Czervionke LF. *Image-Guided Spine Intervention*. Philadelphia: WB Saunders; 2002.
44. International Spine Intervention Society (ISIS). *Practice Guidelines for Spinal Diagnostic Treatment Procedures*. San Francisco, CA: ISIS; 2004.
45. Sachs BL, Vanharanta H, Spivey MA, et al. Dallas discogram description: a new classification of CT/discography in low-back disorders. *Spine (Phila Pa 1976)*. 1987;12(3):287-294.
46. Sobel DF, Zyroff J, Thorne RP. Diskogenic vertebral sclerosis: MR imaging. *J Comput Assist Tomogr*. 1987;11(5):855-858.
47. de Roos A, Kressel H, Spritzer C, Dalinka M. MR imaging of marrow changes adjacent to end plates in degenerative lumbar disk disease. *AJR Am J Roentgenol*. 1987;149(3):531-534.
48. Modic MT, Steinberg PM, Ross JS, et al. Degenerative disk disease: assessment of changes in vertebral body marrow with MR imaging. *Radiology*. 1988;166(1 Pt 1):193-199.
49. Rahme R, Moussa R. The modic vertebral endplate and marrow changes: pathologic significance and relation to low back pain and segmental instability of the lumbar spine. *AJNR Am J Neuroradiol*. 2008;29(5):838-842.

50. Chung CB, Vande Berg BC, Tavernier T, et al. End plate marrow changes in the asymptomatic lumbosacral spine: frequency, distribution and correlation with age and degenerative changes. *Skeletal Radiol.* 2004;33(7):399-404.

51. Thompson KJ, Dagher AP, Eckel TS, et al. Modic changes on MR images as studied with provocative diskography: clinical relevance—a retrospective study of 2457 disks. *Radiology.* 2009;250(3):849-855.

52. Herkowitz HN. Total disc replacement with the CHARITE artificial disc was as effective as lumbar interbody fusion. *J Bone Joint Surg Am.* 2006; 88(5):1168.

53. Shuff C, An HS. Artificial disc replacement: the new solution for discogenic low back pain? *Am J Orthop Belle:* 2005;34(1):8-12.

54. Hochschuler SH, Ohnmeiss DD, Guyer RD, Blumenthal SL. Artificial disc: preliminary results of a prospective study in the United States. *Eur Spine J.* 2002;11 (Suppl 2):S106-S110.

55. Ruan D, He Q, Ding Y, et al. Intervertebral disc transplantation in the treatment of degenerative spine disease: a preliminary study. *Lancet.* 2007; 369(9566):993-999.

DEGENERATIVE DISCOGENIC VERTEBRAL ENDPLATE DISEASE

Douglas S. Fenton, M.D.

CLINICAL PRESENTATION

The patient is a 72-year-old male whose chief complaint is left mid back pain. He states it has been going on for approximately 2 weeks. He says it is a sharp pain in the middle of his back that is elicited by certain types of movements, sneezing, coughing, or getting up from a chair. There is no clear history of trauma. He is afebrile. Recent laboratory evaluations including white blood cell count, C-reactive protein, and sedimentation rate are normal.

IMAGING PRESENTATION

Sagittal T1 and fat-saturated T2-weighted magnetic resonance (MR) images of the thoracic spine reveal decreased T1 and increased T2 signal intensity symmetrically involving the anterior endplates of a mid thoracic level with mild anterior disc height loss compatible with type 1 vertebral endplate disease (VED) *(Fig. 18-1)*.

DISCUSSION

Signal changes in the vertebral endplates and marrow are commonly seen on MR imaging of the spine. Three patterns/types were originally described by DeRoos[1] in 1987 and later became known to the general radiology population as Modic changes.[2,3] VED, particularly type 1, has been demonstrated to be strongly associated with back pain.[4-6]

VED type 1 has been described as disruption and fissuring of the endplate with regions of degeneration, regeneration, and vascular granulation tissue.[2] VED type 2 has been described as disruption of the endplates with increased reactive bone and granulation tissue, and the hematopoetic elements in the vertebrae are replaced by abundant fat (yellow marrow).[2] VED type 3 is presumed to be related to bone sclerosis.

The prevalence of VED in patients with degenerative disc disease of the lumbar spine ranges between 19% and 59%, with types 1 and 2 being the most common and type 3 being more rare.[1,3,6] VED is most commonly seen at the L4-5 and L5-S1 levels[6] and appears to increase with advancing age.[4] VED is uncommon in asymptomatic individuals. Weishaupt and colleagues [7] demonstrated a presence of VED in less than 10% of asymptomatic volunteers ages 20 to 50 and only one case of type 1 VED in 300 patients.

Several theories have been proposed as to the pathogenesis of VED. One theory suggests that VED is caused by a bacterial infection of the disc and another that microtraumas/fractures occur in the endplate.[8] Each of these can predispose the endplate and marrow to inflammatory change. Type 1 changes have a similar appearance to inflammation on MR imaging (MRI). Histologic and biochemical analyses support type I changes being an inflammatory condition. During surgery, Ohtori[9] removed the endplates of 14 patients with low back pain and VED types 1 and 2, and 4 patients without VED. Markers of inflammation, specifically tumor necrosis factor (TNF) and protein gene product (PGP) 9.5 were significantly higher in the endplates of those with VED as opposed to those without; 86% of the VED patients had PGP 9.5 as opposed to none of the controls. TNF was found in both the study group and the control group, but was significantly higher in the VED group and significantly higher in type 1 patients when compared with type 2 patients. Whether or not the patient has VED, very few PGP 9.5 fibers were present in the vertebral marrow and no TNF was observed in the marrow. The presence of these proinflammatory substances could explain why VED causes pain and why patients with type 1 VED are more strongly associated with pain. Rannou and colleagues[10] studied highly sensitive C-reactive protein (hsCRP) in groups of patients without VED, with VED type 1, and with VED type 2 and found the levels of this highly sensitive marker of low grade inflammation to be significantly higher in the type 1 group than in those in the type 2 group or in those without VED. This would further suggest that type 1 changes may reflect inflammation.

Many studies portend that type 1 VED is unstable[2,11,12] and that type 1 changes may increase in size, convert to type 2 changes, or go back to normal in a short time. Mitra and colleagues[11] showed an improvement in low back pain symptoms on conversion from type 1 to type 2 or to normal. Type 2 changes tend to remain stable for much longer.

IMAGING FEATURES

Plain radiographs and computed tomography (CT) images are very insensitive to the early changes of VED (types 1 and 2). These imaging modalities can detect the endplate sclerosis of type 3 VED. Nuclear medicine bone scan will demonstrate nonspecific increased radiotracer uptake in an area of active bone turnover and thus will be most intense with type 1 VED *(Fig. 18-2)* and less so with type 2 or type 3. Fluorodeoxyglucose positron emission

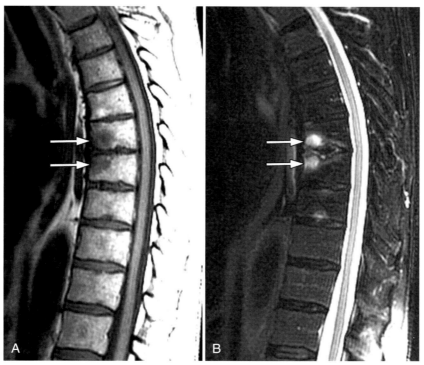

Figure 18-1 ▶ **Type 1 Vertebral Endplate Disease.** Sagittal imaging demonstrates symmetric decreased T1 signal intensity (*arrows*, image **A**) and increased T2 signal intensity (*arrows*, image **B**) along the ventral endplates of a mid-thoracic disc, mainly anteriorly. There is moderate loss of ventral disc height.

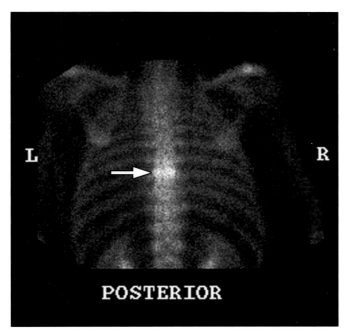

Figure 18-2 ▶ **Nuclear Medicine Bone Scan.** Posterior view. Intense region of radiotracer uptake involving a midthoracic vertebra (*arrow*).

tomography (FDG-PET) imaging does not demonstrate increased activity in areas of VED; however, this modality can be used to distinguish between severe discogenic vertebral endplate degenerative changes from vertebral osteomyelitis.[13] MRI is the imaging modality of choice for detecting and diagnosing VED; however, because VED is not a fast-acting process, it would be inappropriate to follow patients with VED with short-term MRI examinations. VED appears as bands of signal intensity that are parallel to the vertebral endplates.

1. MR imaging of type 1 VED demonstrates signal intensity that reflects its inflammatory nature: decreased T1 signal intensity, increased T2 signal intensity, and usually pronounced enhancement. There may also be linear enhancement of the intervertebral disc (*Fig. 18-3*).
2. MR imaging of type 2 VED demonstrates signal intensity that reflects its fatty nature: increased T1 signal intensity, increased T2 signal intensity, and usually without evidence of enhancement (*Fig. 18-4*).
3. MR imaging of type 3 VED demonstrates signal intensity that reflects its sclerotic nature: decreased T1 signal intensity, decreased T2 signal intensity, and usually without evidence of enhancement (*Fig. 18-5*). Plain radiographs (*Fig. 18-6*) and CT imaging of type 3 VED (*Fig. 18-7*) demonstrates high density (sclerotic) endplates.

DIFFERENTIAL DIAGNOSIS

1. **Disc infection**: Type 1 VED can appear the same as infection, however, with infection there is increased T2 signal intensity in the disc and destruction of the endplates as well as a possible soft tissue mass and epidural extension (*Fig. 18-8*).
2. **Osteoporotic compression deformity**: This can appear to be similar to type 1 VED; however, the signal changes typically involve only one vertebral body endplate, and there is an associated compression (*Fig. 18-9*).

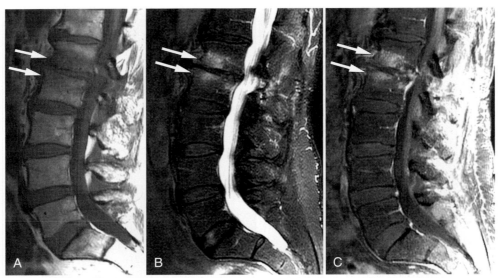

Figure 18-3 ▶ Type 1 Vertebral Endplate Disease (VED), MR Image. Sagittal T1 (**A**), fat-saturated T2 (**B**) and post-contrast, fat-saturated T1 (**C**) images. L1-2 vertebral endplates are of decreased T1 signal intensity, increased T2 signal intensity, and enhanced consistent with its inflammatory nature. The T2 abnormality can be obscured by normal fatty marrow if a fat-saturated pulse sequence is not used.

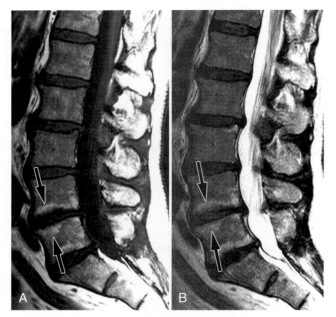

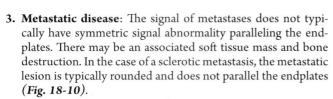

Figure 18-4 ▶ Type 2 Vertebral Endplate Disease (VED), MRI. Sagittal T1- (**A**) and T2- (**B**) weighted MR images. L4-5 vertebral endplates are of increased T1 and T2 signal intensity consistent with its fatty nature.

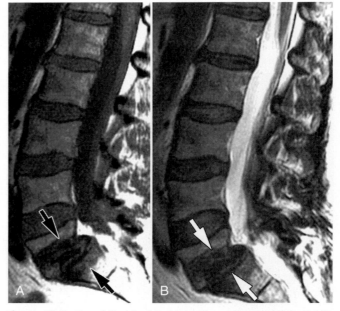

Figure 18-5 ▶ Type 3 Vertebral Endplate Disease (VED), MRI. Sagittal T1- (**A**) and T2- (**B**) weighted MR images. L5-S1 vertebral endplates are of decreased T1 and T2 signal intensity consistent with its sclerotic nature.

3. **Metastatic disease**: The signal of metastases does not typically have symmetric signal abnormality paralleling the endplates. There may be an associated soft tissue mass and bone destruction. In the case of a sclerotic metastasis, the metastatic lesion is typically rounded and does not parallel the endplates (**Fig. 18-10**).

4. **Hemodialysis spondyloarthropathy**: Has an appearance similar to disc space infection.

5. **Ankylosing spondylitis**: Endplate changes may look like type 1 VED, but there is often squaring of the vertebral body with ankylosing spondylitis.

6. **Vertebral hemangioma**: Can have a fatty appearance like type 2 VED but is usually round or patchy, not parallel to the endplates.

7. **Marrow heterogeneity**: Can appear like type 2 VED although it is usually patchy and not paralleling the endplates (**Fig. 18-11**).

8. **Radiation therapy effect**: Can appear like type 2 VED but is usually sharply marginated from radiation collimation (**Fig. 18-12**).

Text continued on page 141

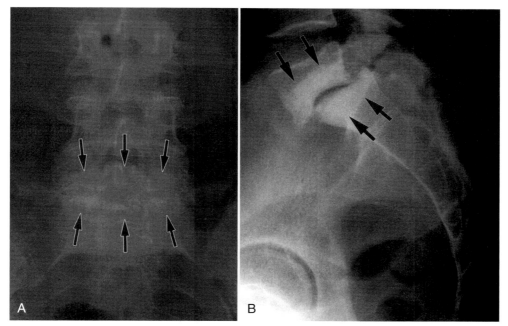

Figure 18-6 ▶ Type 3 Vertebral Endplate Disease (VED). (Same patient as in Figure 18-4.) Frontal and lateral plain radiographs. Symmetric sclerosis of the endplates at the L5-S1 level (*arrows*).

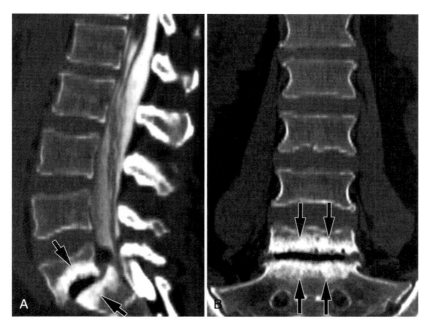

Figure 18-7 ▶ Type 3 Vertebral Endplate Disease (VED), CT. (Same patient as in Figures 18-4 and 18-5.) Reformatted sagittal (**A**) and coronal (**B**) images demonstrate high density sclerosis of the endplates at L5-S1 (*arrows*).

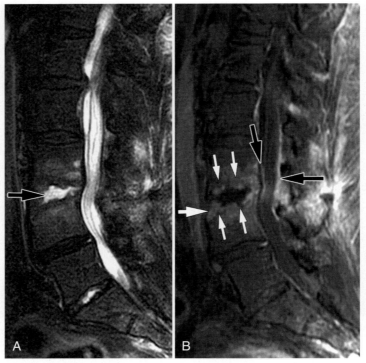

Figure 18-8 ▶ Disc Infection. Increased T2 signal intensity in the L3-4 disc (*arrow*, image **A**). Enhancement of the disc (*black arrow*) and irregularity and enhancement of the vertebral endplates (*white arrows*) on sagittal post-contrast T1 image **B**. Note enhancing phlegmon in the epidural space (*black arrows*, image **B**).

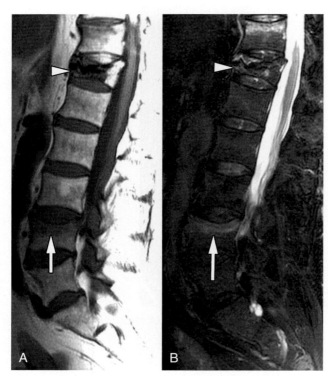

Figure 18-9 ▶ Recent Benign Compression Deformity. Signal abnormality of a compression deformity is identical to type 1 VED due to changes from bone edema and/or inflammation *(arrow)*. Compression fractures rarely have signal changes on both sides of the disc and are typically associated with a compression deformity and a history of recent trauma. Note the chronic compression deformity of T12 that has been treated with methylmethacrylate *(arrowhead)*.

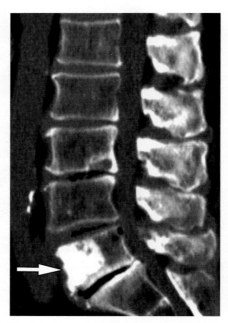

Figure 18-10 ▶ Sclerotic Metastatic Disease. Rounded sclerotic density L5 vertebral body (*arrow*). Metastatic disease is rarely linear, paralleling the endplates. Metastatic disease is often multiple. One should look for a history of a primary malignancy.

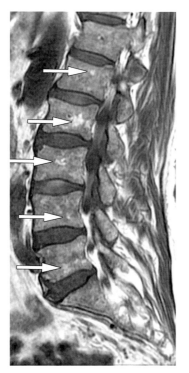

Figure 18-11 ▶ Vertebral Marrow Heterogeneity. Typically focal and patchy (*arrows*), not necessarily near the endplates with signal characteristics similar to fat; increased T1 and T2 signal intensity.

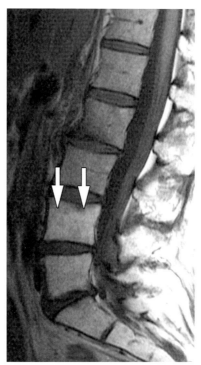

Figure 18-12 ▶ Radiation Change. Sagittal T1 demonstrates homogeneous increased signal intensity from L4 through the sacrum with a sharp linear demarcation (*arrows*) in the superior most L4, compatible with the top of the radiation field. Radiation causes change toward yellow marrow; however, it is a much more diffuse process than that adjacent to the endplates.

TREATMENT

There are no specific treatments for discogenic vertebral endplate disease. There are many instances in which VED is asymptomatic or subclinical. If one believed that a patient's pain was due to a specific VED, a short-term treatment could include injection of intradiscal steroids.[14] Spinal fusion has been considered by some as a treatment for VED; however, this is usually in conjunction with diagnosed discogenic pain.

References

1. de Roos A, Kressel H, Spritzer C, Dalinka M. MR imaging of marrow changes adjacent to end plates in degenerative lumbar disk disease. *AJR Am J Radiol.* 1987;149:531-534.
2. Modic MT, Steinberg PM, Ross JS, et al. Degenerative disk disease: assessment of changes in vertebral body marrow with MR imaging. *Radiology.* 1988;166:193-199.
3. Modic MT, Masaryk TJ, Ross JS, Carter JR. Imaging of degenerative disk disease. *Radiology.* 1988;168:177-186.
4. Kjaer P, Leboeuf-Yde C, Lorsholm L, et al. Magnetic resonance imaging and low back pain in adults: a diagnostic imaging study of 40-year-old men and women. *Spine.* 2005;30:1173-1180.
5. Albert HB, Manniche C. Modic changes following lumbar disc herniation. *Eur Spine J.* 2007;16:977-982.
6. Baithwaite I, White J, Saifuddin A, et al. Vertebral end-plate (Modic) changes on lumbar spine MRI: correlation with pain reproduction at lumbar discography. *Eur Spine J.* 1998;7:363-368.
7. Weishaupt D, Zanetti M, Hodler J, Boos N. MR imaging of the lumbar spine: prevalence of intervertebral disk extrusion and sequestration, nerve root compression, end plate abnormalities, and osteoarthritis of the facet joints in asymptomatic volunteers. *Radiology.* 1998;209:661-666.
8. Albert HB, Kjaer P, Jensen TS, et al. Modic changes, possible causes, and relation to low back pain. *Med Hypotheses.* 2008;70:361-368.
9. Ohtori S, Inoue G, Ito T, et al. Tumor necrosis factor-immunoreactive cells and PGP 9.5-immunoreactive nerve fibres in vertebral endplates of patients with discogenic low back pain and Modic type 1 or 2 changes on MRI. *Spine.* 2006;31:1026-1031.
10. Rannou F, Ouanes W, Boutron I, et al. High-sensitive C-reactive protein in chronic low back pain with vertebral endplate Modic signal changes. *Arthritis Rheum.* 2007;57:1311-1315.
11. Mitra D, Cassar-Pullicino VN, McCall IW. Longitudinal study of vertebral type 1 end-plate changes on MR of the lumbar spine. *Eur Radiol.* 2004;14:1574-1581.
12. Modic MT. Modic type 1 and type 2 changes. *J Neurosurg Spine.* 2007;6:150-151.
13. Albert HB, Petersen H, Manniche C, Hoilund-Carlsen PF. PET imaging in patients with Modic changes. *Nuklearmedizin.* 2009;48:1-3.
14. Fayad F, Lefevre-Colau MM, Rannou F, et al. Relation of inflammatory modic changes to intradiscal steroid injection outcome in chronic low back pain. *Eur Spine J.* 2007;16:925-931.

DIASTEMATOMYELIA

Douglas S. Fenton, M.D.

CLINICAL PRESENTATION

The patient is an 81-year-old female who presents with low back pain and generalized weakness in the legs. She requires a wheelchair or cane to ambulate. Her symptoms are severe and progressive. She has mild urinary incontinence.

IMAGING PRESENTATION

Midline sagittal T2-weighted magnetic resonance (MR) image reveals a low-lying spinal cord and decrease in height of the L4 vertebral body. The axial T2-weighted MR image obtained at the L4 level demonstrates that the low-lying spinal cord is split into two equal halves and separated by a cerebrospinal fluid (CSF) cleft. There is some anteroposterior-oriented low signal intensity in the L4 vertebral body. Coronal imaging (not pictured) revealed an L4 butterfly vertebra *(Fig. 19-1)*.

DISCUSSION

Diastematomyelia, also called *split cord malformation*, is a congenital malformation characterized by a division of the spinal cord and/or cauda equina in the sagittal plane, which is often associated with vertebral anomalies. The two hemicords are often separated by a bony fibrocartilaginous septum that is attached anteriorly to one or more vertebral bodies and posteriorly to the neural arches (posterior elements). The two hemicords usually (91%) rejoin into a single cord below the level of the division.[1] The cleft typically occurs between T9 and S1 in 85% of cases.[1] The cleft is exclusively in the thoracic spine in 20.6% of cases, the thoracolumbar region in 17.6%, and the lumbar in 61.8%.[1] The conus medullaris is typically low in position.[1] Diastematomyelia is the most frequent form of failed midline integration of the notochord[2] and accounts for 3.8% of all closed spinal dysraphisms.[3] Patients with diastematomyelia may be asymptomatic. When symptoms result, they can be indistinguishable from any etiology causing spinal cord tethering. Symptoms often result from tethering of the spinal cord and are secondary to associated vertebral anomalies. In children, symptoms may include foot and spinal deformities, weakness in the legs, low back pain, scoliosis, and incontinence. In adulthood, the signs and symptoms often include progressive sensory and motor problems and loss of bowel and bladder control.

The term *diastematomyelia* comes from the Greek *diastema* (cleft) and *myelos* (cord) and is irrespective of whether or not there is a bony or fibrous spur interposed between the two hemicords. Each hemicord gives rise to the ipsilateral dorsal and ventral nerve roots, although occasionally, one hemicord can give rise to three roots (ipsilateral ventral and dorsal roots and the contralateral ventral root), and the other hemicord gives rise to only the ipsilateral dorsal root.[4,5] Either way, the four normal roots (two ventral, two dorsal) arise at each level. The anterior spinal artery forms from paired primordia at the same time that diastematomyelia occurs. If there is failure of fusion of the paired primordia into a single anterior spinal artery, there may be paired anterior spinal arteries, each supplying one of the hemichords.[5] Diastematomyelia is different from diplomyelia, which is a true duplication of the spinal cord, producing two spinal cords, each of which contains one central canal, two dorsal horns, two ventral horns, and four segmental nerve roots at each level.[4]

Embryologically, diastematomyelia is a failure of midline integration resulting in two paired notochords that are separated by primitive streak cells.[6] Diastematomyelia is subcategorized into two subtypes depending on the fate of the primitive streak cells. If the streak cells develop into bone and cartilage, the two hemichords will be contained in their own dural sac separated by an osteocartilaginous spur.[6] This type of abnormality is referred to as Pang type I.[7] If the streak cells resorb or leave a thin fibrous band, the two hemichords will be contained in a single dural sac.[6] This type of abnormality is referred to as Pang type II.[7]

Diastematomyelia Type I

Type I diastematomyelia (diastematomyelia with osteocartilaginous septum) consists of two hemichords, each contained within its own dural sac and separated by a bony osteocartilaginous spur. The spur usually extends from the vertebral body to the neural arches along a midsagittal plane. Spurs can also course obliquely and may be complete or incomplete, arising from either the vertebral body or from the neural arch.[2] The two hemichords are usually the same caliber; however, the spur can occasionally split the hemichords unequally. The spur is usually located in the thoracic and/or lumbar regions and lies at the caudal end of the cord splitting.[2] The hemichords are in close proximity to the spur just cranial to the point where the hemichords will fuse into a single cord inferiorly. Vertebral anomalies are highly associated with type I and

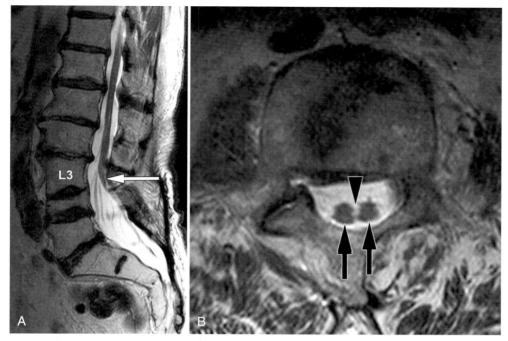

Figure 19-1 ▶ Diastematomyelia. Sagittal T2 image, **A,** and axial T2 image, **B,** of the lumbar spine. Low-lying conus at L3 level *(white arrow)*. L4 vertebral body is decreased in height secondary to it being a butterfly vertebra (not shown). Axial image reveals two hemicords *(black arrows)* with a CSF cleft between them *(arrowhead)*.

include bifid lamina, increased interpedicular distance, hemivertebrae, fused vertebrae, and disc space narrowing.[2,3,6] Scoliosis is seen in 30% to 60% of patients and is usually due to the underlying bone abnormalities.[6,8] Cutaneous hemangiomas, dyschromic patches, and hairy tufts often suggest an underlying split cord malformation. A hairy tuft high along the back is strongly associated with diastematomyelia type I or II.[3] Hydromyelia is a common finding and can involve one or both hemichords and the normal cord above and below the splitting.[2,3,6]

Diastematomyelia Type II

Type II diastematomyelia (diastematomyelia without osteocartilaginous septum) consists of two hemichords contained within a single dural sac without an intervening rigid midline septum. There are three variants of type II diastematomyelia: presence of a fibrous septum, absence of a septum, and partial cord splitting.[9] Absence of the septum is the most common type II variant.[2] Type II will demonstrate the same cutaneous stigmata and hydromyelia that are seen with type I. Vertebral anomalies are present but are usually milder than in type I. The most common vertebral anomaly in type II is the butterfly vertebrae.[2] Scoliosis is usually absent.[2] Type II is strongly associated with lipomas of the filum terminale.

IMAGING FEATURES

Plain radiographs can be an important clue as to the presence of an underlying spinal abnormality. Widening of the interpediculate distance can be identified, as can vertebral anomalies such as hemivertebra and scoliosis *(Fig. 19-2)*. A spur, if present, can be detected with plain radiography in less than 50% of cases

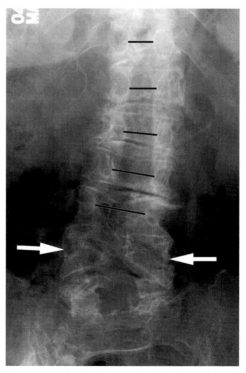

Figure 19-2 ▶ Interpedicular Distance. Frontal view of the lumbar spine. Widening of the interpedicular distance from cranial to caudal *(lines)*. Butterfly vertebra of L4 *(between white arrows)*.

(Fig. 19-3). Computerized tomography (CT) readily demonstrates an osteocartilaginous spur if present *(Fig. 19-4)* as well as vertebral anomalies *(Fig. 19-5)*. The split spinal cord can be seen with intervening CSF density *(Fig. 19-6)*. This is more evident with the administration of intrathecal contrast media. CT is also helpful for defining the anatomy of the spur for presurgical planning.

Magnetic resonance imaging (MRI), with its superior soft tissue discrimination, is the imaging modality of choice. The split cord is readily identified on axial images. Hydromyelia, if present, can be seen as increased T2-weighted signal within the normal spinal cord above or below the split and/or within each hemichord. An osteocartilaginous spur is hyperintense on T1-weighted MR images due to marrow within the spur. A fibrous septum may be isointense on T1-weighted images. The spur is often hypointense on T2-weighted imaging for either a fibrous spur *(Fig. 19-7)* of variable signal intensity or a bony spur depending on whether there is marrow within the spur *(Fig. 19-8)*. On sagittal imaging, a

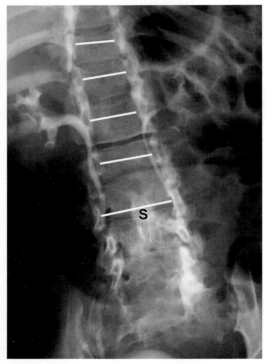

Figure 19-3 ▶ Diastematomyelia with Spur. Frontal view of the lumbar spine. Ossified spur (*S*) seen in the midline from mid L3 to inferior L4. Widening of the interpedicular distance from cranial to caudal (*lines*).

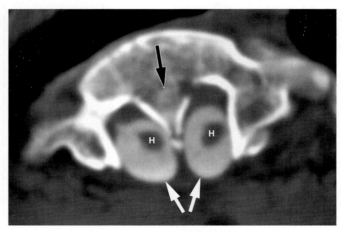

Figure 19-4 ▶ Osteocartilaginous Spur. Axial CT lumbar spine. Osteocartilaginous spur *(black arrow)* inserts between paired thecal sacs *(white arrows)* and hemicords *(H)*.

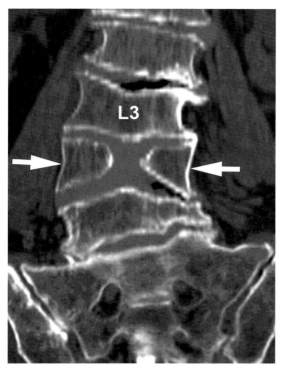

Figure 19-5 ▶ Butterfly Vertebrae. Coronal reformatted CT image demonstrates the symmetric triangular halves of the L4 butterfly vertebra *(between white arrows).*

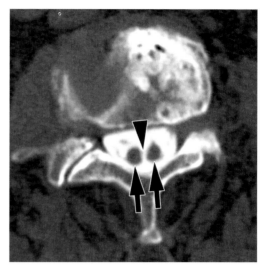

Figure 19-6 ▶ Diastematomyelia without Spur. Axial CT scan. Two hemicords are shown *(arrows)* that are contained within a single thecal sac with intervening CSF *(arrowhead).* There is no evidence of a spur in this patient; however, this imaging presentation can be seen in patients with a spur more superiorly or inferiorly.

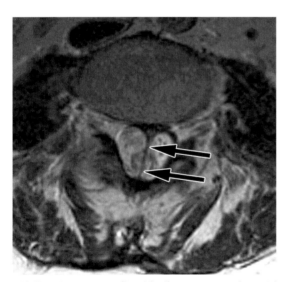

Figure 19-7 ▶ Diastematomyelia with Fibrous Spur. Axial T2-weighted MR image. Thin fibrous spur *(arrows)* separates the thecal sac and spinal cord into equal halves.

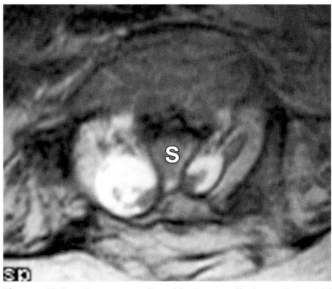

Figure 19-8 ▶ Diastematomyelia with Osteocartilaginous Spur. Axial T2-weighted image. Osseous spur *(S)* separates the thecal sac into two mildly asymmetric halves and the spinal cord into equal halves.

diastematomyelia may be underappreciated because clefting is in the midline sagittal position. The spinal cord may appear normal or slightly attenuated on sagittal imaging because of partial volume averaging with CSF between the hemichords. Vertebral anomalies are readily identified with MRI, as are cord tethering and associated fibrolipomas of the filum terminale *(Fig. 19-9).*

DIFFERENTIAL DIAGNOSIS

1. **Diplomyelia:** A true duplication of the spinal cord. There is no associated bony or fibrous septum. It may be indistinguishable radiographically from a severe, long-segment diastematomyelia.

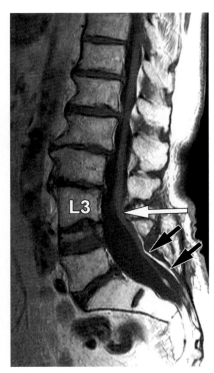

Figure 19-9 ▶ Diastematomyelia with Vertebral Anomaly, Tethered Cord and Fibrolipoma. Same patient as in Figure 19-1. Sagittal T1-weighted MR image. Low-lying spinal cord termination *(white arrow)*. Curvilinear fatty signal intensity in the posterior spinal canal *(black arrows)* compatible with fibrolipoma. Vertebral anomaly of L4 seen to be a hemivertebra on axial imaging (not shown).

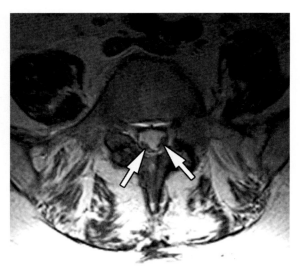

Figure 19-10 ▶ Arachnoiditis. Occasionally, arachnoiditis can have an appearance similar to diastematomyelia; however, there is no evidence of a spur and one can often see separation of individual nerve roots. Also there is no increased incidence of tethered cord or vertebral anomalies with arachnoiditis.

2. **Arachnoiditis:** Can appear as two *cords* of nerve root clumping. There is no evidence of a spur and no increased incidence of congenital vertebral anomalies *(Fig. 19-10)*.

TREATMENT

1. **Nonoperative management**: It is generally accepted that asymptomatic patients should be observed.[10]

2. **Surgical management**: Symptomatic patients need surgery that depends on the cause of the symptoms. If there is a tethered cord, then a surgical release should be performed with removal of the bony or fibrous spur and dural repair. Resection of the spur does not appear to arrest the progression of a scoliotic curve because the scoliosis is primarily due to the underlying congenital malformations of the vertebrae. Progression of a scoliotic curve should be treated surgically; however, this

treatment should be considered independent from spur resection.[10] Extreme care must be taken in overcorrecting the scoliosis in a patient with a tethered cord because the correction may cause additional stretching of the spinal cord, which could lead to significant neurologic injury.

References

1. Hilal SK, Marton D, Pollack E. Diastematomyelia in children: radiographic study of 34 cases. *Radiology.* 1974;112:609-621.
2. Rossi A, Cama A, Piatelli G, et al. Spinal dysraphism: MR imaging rationale. *J Neuroradiol.* 2004;31:3-24.
3. Tortori-Donati P, Rossi A, Cama A. Spinal dysraphism: a review of neuroradiological features with embryological correlations and proposal for a new classification. *Neuroradiology.* 2000;42:471-491.
4. Naidich TP, Harwood-Nash DC. Diastematomyelia: hemicord and meningeal sheaths; single and double arachnoid and dural tubes. *AJNR Am J Neuroradiol.* 1983;4:633-636.
5. Cohen J, Sledge CB. Diastematomyelia: an embryological interpretation with report of a case. *Am J Dis Child.* 1960;100:257-263.
6. Rossi A, Biancheri R, Cama A, et al. Imaging in spine and spinal cord malformation. *Eur J Radiol.* 2004;50:177-200.
7. Pang D, Dias MS, Ahab-Barmada M. Split cord malformation. Part I: A unified theory of embryogenesis for double spinal cord malformations. *Neurosurgery.* 1992;31:451-480.
8. Keim HA, Greene AF. Diastematomyelia and scoliosis. *J Bone Joint Surg Am.* 1973;55:1425-1435.
9. Tortori-Donati P, Rossi A, Biancheri R, Cama A. Magnetic resonance imaging of spinal dysraphism. *Top Magn Reson Imaging.* 2001;12:375-409.
10. Miller A, Guille JT, Bowen JR. Evaluation and treatment of diastematomyelia. *J Bone Joint Surg Am.* 1993;75:1308-1317.

20

DIFFUSE IDIOPATHIC SKELETAL HYPEROSTOSIS

Douglas S. Fenton, M.D.

CLINICAL PRESENTATION

The patient is a 76-year-old man who complains of neck and base of neck pain as well as debilitating headaches that awaken him at night. He also complains of shoulder pain with any overhead activity. The patient has noted some moderate swallowing difficulty over the last several years.

IMAGING PRESENTATION

Sagittal T1- and T2-weighted magnetic resonance (MR) images demonstrate flowing bone signal intensity along the ventral vertebral bodies from C3-T1. There are no degenerative changes of the intervertebral discs. The findings represent diffuse idiopathic skeletal hyperostosis (DISH). The signal intensity of this finding suggests that the regions of DISH may have gained a marrow cavity *(Fig. 20-1)*.

DISCUSSION

In 1950, Forestier and Rotes-Querol described a process that was characterized by flowing spinal osteophytes and stiffness and termed it *senile ankylosing hyperostosis.* During the next several years, many different names were given to the same condition including *Forestier disease, generalized juxtaarticular ossification of the vertebral ligaments,* and *spondylosis hyperostotica.* In 1975, Resnick further classified this process and termed it *diffuse idiopathic skeletal hyperostosis (DISH).*[1]

DISH is a common disease. It is most commonly seen in people over the age of 50. Studies have reported that 28% of people with an average age of 65 have DISH.[2] Other studies show a prevalence of DISH in 15% of women and 25% of men over the age of 50, and 26% in women and 28% in men over the age of 80.[3]

People may present with nonspecific back pain or stiffness. Dysphagia can be a complication of DISH secondary to large anterior osteophytes. Many patients are asymptomatic, with DISH being discovered incidentally.

The thoracic spine is the typical location of DISH, followed by the lumbar spine and then the cervical spine. When it occurs in the cervical spine, it often involves the lower segments. When it occurs

in the lumbar spine, it often involves the upper segments. In the thoracic region, the anterior osteophytosis is predominantly right sided. It is thought that there is a protective effect from aortic pulsation on the left side of the spine. Patients with DISH and situs inversus show ossification mainly on the left side of the thoracic spine.[4,5] The syndesmophytes of DISH project horizontally from the vertebral body and have the appearance of flowing candle wax.

DISH can have extraspinal manifestations, including enthesophytes involving the iliac wing, tendinous ossification of the knee, hyperostosis of any bone in the foot, calcaneal spurs, calcification of the Achilles tendon, osseous excrescences in the shoulder, spurs of the olecranon and hyperostosis, and spur formation in the hand and wrist.[6]

IMAGING FEATURES

DISH is predominantly a radiographic diagnosis. Forestier demonstrated the initial manifestations that were refined by Resnick and Niwayama.[4] The first of the criteria is to have flowing ossification along the anterolateral aspect of at least four contiguous vertebra. Secondly, there is preservation of disc height in the involved segment with a relative absence of degenerative changes. Lastly, there is absence of zygapophyseal ankylosis or sacroiliac degeneration. Plain radiography is the most cost-effective imaging study and may be all that is necessary to diagnose DISH. Contiguous anterior osteophytes are readily discerned with relative preservation of the disc spaces and absent/minimal facet joint degenerative changes *(Fig. 20-2)*. Computerized tomography (CT) with sagittal reformatted images can demonstrate the same findings as plain radiography *(Fig. 20-3)*. With CT, one is also able to visualize the effect the ossification has on the adjacent soft tissues. Magnetic resonance imaging (MRI) is not necessary for the diagnosis of DISH.

There are different imaging characteristics of DISH depending on whether the flowing ossification has calcified or has ossified and gained marrow elements. If it is predominantly calcified, it is hypointense on T1- and T2-weighted acquisitions. If there is a marrow cavity, DISH may appear iso- to hyperintense on T1- and T2-weighted acquisitions (see Fig. 20-1). There can be some mild enhancement of DISH when it has a marrow cavity.

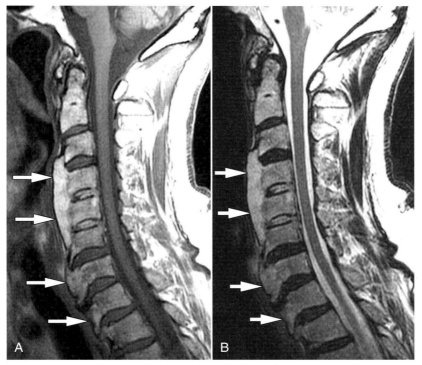

Figure 20-1 ▸ **DISH, MRI.** Sagittal T1-weighted MR image, **A,** and sagittal T2-weighted MR image, **B.** Flowing hyperintense bone along the ventral vertebral bodies *(arrows)*. Note that the disc heights are preserved.

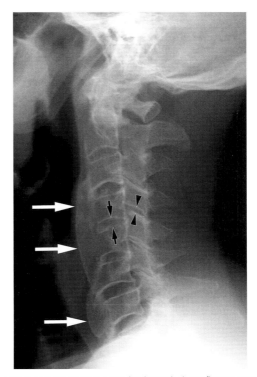

Figure 20-2 ▸ **DISH, Lateral Radiograph.** Same patient as in Figure 20-1. Lateral radiograph shows flowing ventral osteophytes *(white arrows)* with preservation of disc height *(between black arrows)* and normal facet joint articulations *(between arrowheads)*.

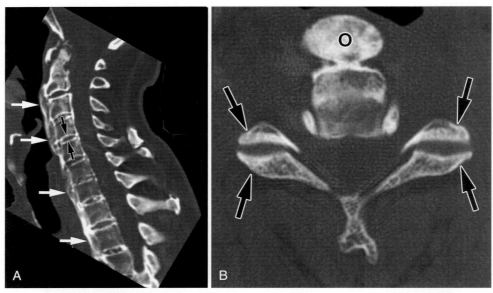

Figure 20-3 ▶ **DISH, CT.** Sagittal reformatted CT image **A,** flowing osteophytes along the ventral vertebral bodies *(white arrows)* with preservation of disc height *(black arrows).* Axial CT image **B** demonstrates normal facet joints *(arrows)* and a ventral osteophyte *(O).*

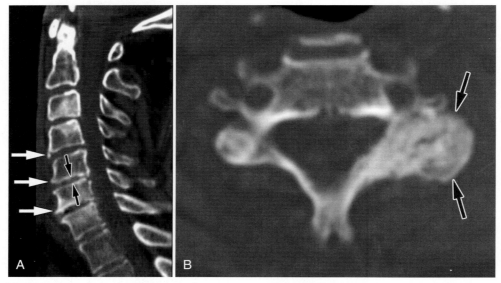

Figure 20-4 ▶ **Spondylosis.** Small ventral osteophytes *(white arrows)* are seen on sagittal reformatted CT image **A;** however, there is decrease in disc height *(black arrows).* Axial image **B** reveals facet degeneration *(arrows).*

DIFFERENTIAL DIAGNOSIS

1. **Spondylosis:** Rarely extends over four or more segments. There are often more discogenic degenerative changes and degenerative changes of the posterior elements with spondylosis *(Fig. 20-4).*
2. **Ankylosing spondylitis:** Can have syndesmophytes that appear like DISH. Ankylosing spondylitis also has a predilection for affecting the facet joints, unlike DISH *(Fig. 20-5).* One should also evaluate for associated sacroiliac joint erosions and/or ankylosis and seronegative positivity.
3. **Other spondyloarthropathies (psoriatic spondyloarthropathy, Reiter's syndrome):** As with ankylosing

spondylitis, one should evaluate for associated sacroiliac joint erosions and/or ankylosis.

TREATMENT

1. **Nonoperative therapy**: DISH is predominantly treated with nonoperative measures. For those with symptoms of back pain, physical therapy, activity modification, and nonsteroidal anti-inflammatory drugs (NSAIDs) are the main forms of treatment.
2. **Surgical therapy:** Surgery is reserved for the rare patient with DISH that causes spinal stenosis or dysphagia.

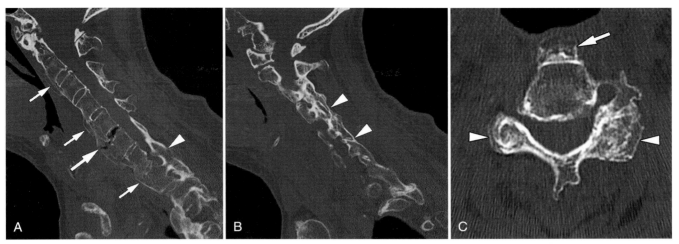

Figure 20-5 ▶ Ankylosing Spondylitis. Sagittal reformatted midline CT image **A**, sagittal off-midline reformatted image **B** and axial image **C**. Flowing anterior osteophytes appear similar to diffuse idiopathic skeletal hyperostosis (DISH) (*small white arrows*). There is also preservation of disc height. Ankylosing spondylitis has a predilection to ankylose the facet joints (*arrowheads*). Note the fracture extending through the C5-6 disc and ventral osteophyte (*large white arrow*).

References

1. Resnick D, Shaul SR, Robins JM. Diffuse idiopathic skeletal hyperostosis (DISH): Forestier's disease with extraspinal manifestations. *Radiology.* 1975;115:513-524.
2. Boachie-Adjei O, Bullough PG. Incidence of ankylosing hyperostosis of the spine (Forester's disease) at autopsy. *Spine.* 1987;12:739-743.
3. Weinfeld RM, Olson PN, Maki DD, Griffiths HJ. The prevalence of diffuse idiopathic skeletal hyperostosis (DISH) in two large American Midwest metropolitan hospital populations. *Skeletal Radiol.* 1997;26:222-225.
4. Resnick D, Niwayama G. Diffuse idiopathic skeletal hyperostosis (DISH): Ankylosing hyperostosis of Forestier and Rotes-Querol. In: Resnick D, ed. Diagnosis of Bone and Joint Disorders, vol 3. 3rd ed. Philadelphia: Saunders, 1995:1463-1495.
5. Carile L, Verdone F, Aiello A, Buongusto G. Diffuse idiopathic skeletal hyperostosis and situs viscerum inversus. *J Rheumatol.* 1989;16:1120-1122.
6. Belanger TA, Rowe DE. Diffuse idiopathic skeletal hyperostosis: Musculoskeletal manifestations. *J Am Acad Orthop Surg.* 2001;9:258-267.

DISC HERNIATION—FORAMINAL

Leo F. Czervionke, M.D.

CLINICAL PRESENTATION

The patient is a 65-year-old male with a 2-year history of progressive right thigh pain radiating down the lateral aspect of the right leg. The pain is exacerbated by walking but also present when sitting. The patient walks with a limp. Straight leg raising sign is negative. There is a diminished right knee jerk *(Figs. 21-1 and 21-2)*.

IMAGING PRESENTATION

Magnetic resonance (MR) imaging of the lumbar spine reveals a large herniated disc extending into the right L4-5 neural foramen obscuring the intraforaminal fat adjacent to the right L4 nerve root. Subtle contrast enhancement is demonstrated adjacent to the nonenhancing intraforaminal disc fragment.

DISCUSSION

Foraminal or extraforaminal disc herniations comprise approximately 10% of lumbar disc herniations. The L4 nerve root is most commonly involved.[1,2] Foraminal disc herniations tend to occur in older patients, often with little evidence of disc degeneration.[2] Posterolateral vertebral osteophytes and facet hypertrophy may contribute to the neural foraminal stenosis associated with foraminal disc herniation. The predisposing factors for lateral disc herniations are similar to other lumbar disc herniations. (Refer to discussion in Chapter 17 on lumbar disc herniation).

With foraminal or far lateral (extraforaminal) disc herniations, characteristic clinical findings are related primarily to radiculopathy in the distribution of the involved nerve root.[3-5] The radicular pain with foraminal and extraforaminal disc herniations may be extremely intense, which is believed to be due to compression of the dorsal root ganglion.[6] The pain is often located in the groin or anterior thigh, but may radiate more distally in the lower extremity. The pain may be accentuated by lateral bending. Low back pain may be present but is frequently absent or less severe than the radicular pain. The patient may experience dysesthesias or sensory loss. The knee jerk may be absent. A positive straight-leg raising sign is often present.

IMAGING FEATURES

Herniated discs that extend into the neural foramen (intervertebral foramen) usually are not detected by myelography alone, because they cause minimal or no root pouch deformity and therefore require computed tomography (CT) or MR for imaging detection *(Figs. 21-1 to 21-7)*. Foraminal and extraforaminal (far lateral) disc herniations are not uncommonly overlooked even when CT and MR imaging studies are interpreted.[8,9]

Lateral disc fragments compress the nerve roots as they course below the pedicle at a given lumbar disc level. For example, a lateral disc herniation at the L4-5 level will produce L4 radiculopathy, whereas a posterolateral disc herniation compressing the thecal sac at the same level causes L5 radiculopathy. A foraminal disc herniation may be visible on CT as an isointense or slightly hyperintense mass within the neural foramen (see Fig. 21-3). MR imaging has advantages over CT for detection of lateral disc herniation. The foraminal disc herniation is usually well demonstrated on axial T1-weighted images, which show excellent contrast between the disc material and the fat (see Figs. 21-1 to 21-6).On MR imaging, the foraminal disc herniation is usually contiguous with the parent intervertebral disc, a finding that is best demonstrated on parasagittal MR images obtained through the neural foramen (see Figs. 21-1 and 21-4). The parasagittal T1-weighted or T2-weighted Spin Echo (SE) MR images obtained through the foramen are also valuable for assessing the degree of nerve root compression (see Figs. 21-1 and 21-4). The herniated disc fragment typically does not enhance, but enhancement is nearly always demonstrated along the margin of the intraforaminal disc fragment (see Figs. 21-6 and 21-7).

Most foraminal and extraforaminal disc (far lateral) herniations tend to have a wide base where they extend beyond the vertebral body margin, and therefore the majority of foraminal disc herniations are disc protrusions by definition (see Figs. 21-5 and 21-6). However, lateral and far lateral foraminal disc extrusions also

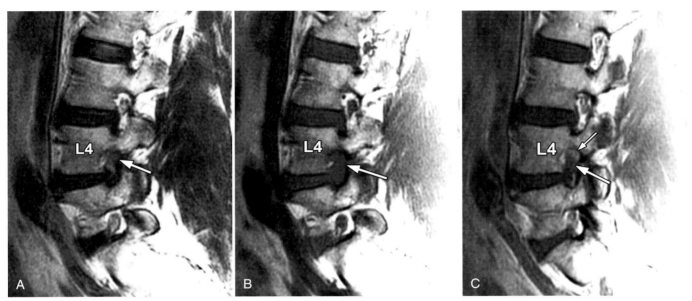

Figure 21-1 ▶ Right L4-5 Foraminal Disc Herniation. Herniated disc material *(arrows)* obscures the fat in the right L4-5 neural foramen on T2-weighted MR image **A** and T2-weighted MR image **B**. On contrast enhanced image **C**, the herniated disc *(long arrow)* does not enhance, but there is subtle contrast enhancement *(short arrow)* adjacent to the nonenhancing disc fragment.

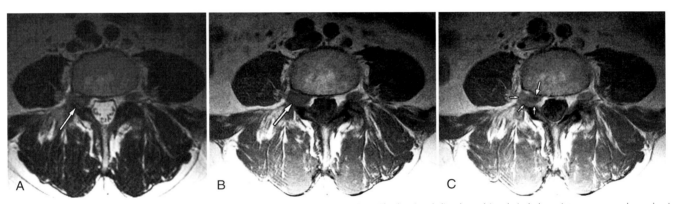

Figure 21-2 ▶ Right L4-5 Foraminal Disc Herniation. Same patient as in Figure 21-1. The herniated disc *(arrow)* is relatively hypo intense on unenhanced axial T2-weighted MR image **A** and on T1-weighted image **B**. On T1-weighted contrast enhanced MR image **C,** note the subtle contrast enhancing tissue- *(short arrows)* adjacent to the nonenhancing disc fragment *(long arrow)*.

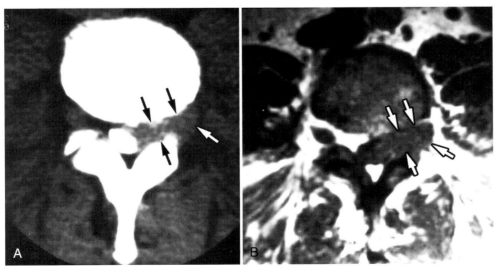

Figure 21-3 ▶ Left L3-4 Foraminal (Lateral) Disc Herniation. On axial post myelogram CT image **A,** the herniated disc *(arrows)* in the left neural foramen is less dense than the contrast in the thecal sac and adjacent vertebra but is nearly isodense relative to the paraspinal muscles. On T1-weighted axial MR image **B,** the herniated disc fragment *(arrows)* obscures fat in the left L3-4 neural foramen.

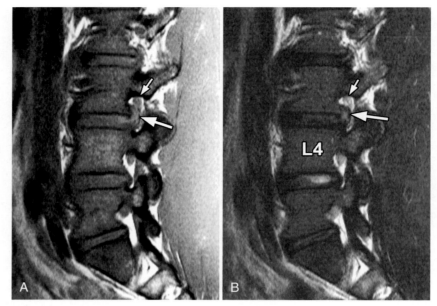

Figure 21-4 ▶ Right L3-4 Foraminal Disc Herniation. The herniated disc *(arrow)* on T1-weighted MR image **A** and T2-weighted MR image **B** is in continuity with the intervertebral portion of the disc. The foraminal disc herniation superiorly displaces the right L3 nerve root *(small arrow in image **A** and image **B**).*

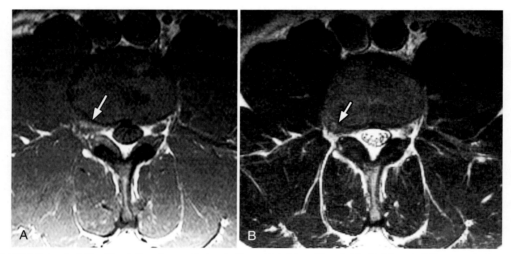

Figure 21-5 ▶ Right L3-4 Foraminal Disc Herniation. Same patient as in Figure 21-4. A broad based right L3-4 foraminal disc protrusion/herniation *(arrow)* obscures the foraminal fat adjacent to the right L3 nerve root on axial T1-weighted MR image **A** and T2-weighted MR image **B.** The herniated disc *(arrow)* is slightly T1 hyperintense relative to the intervertebral disc on image **A** and T2 isointense relative to the intervertebral disc on image **B.**

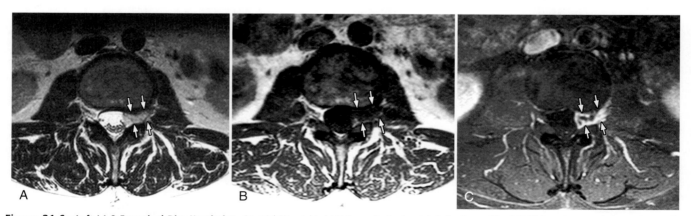

Figure 21-6 ▶ Left L1-2 Foraminal Disc Herniation. On axial T2-weighted MR image **A,** the herniated disc *(arrows)* is slight T2 hyperintense relative to the vertebra but T2 hypointense relative to intrathecal CSF. On axial T1-weighted MR image **B,** the herniated disc *(arrows)* is nearly isointense relative to CSF. Note the intense contrast enhancement *(arrows)* surrounding the nonenhancing central core of the herniated disc fragment on contrast-enhanced T1-weighted MR image **C.**

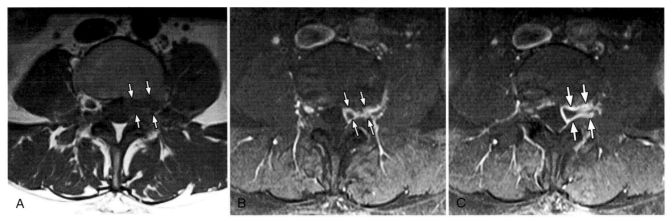

Figure 21-7 ▶ Left L3-4 Foraminal Disc Herniation. Herniated disc material *(arrows)* obscures the fat in the neural foramen on unenhanced axial T1-weighted MR image **A.** Intense contrast enhancement *(arrows)* is present along the margins, the nonenhancing central core of the herniated disc material on axial contrast enhanced T1-weighted MR images **B** and **C.**

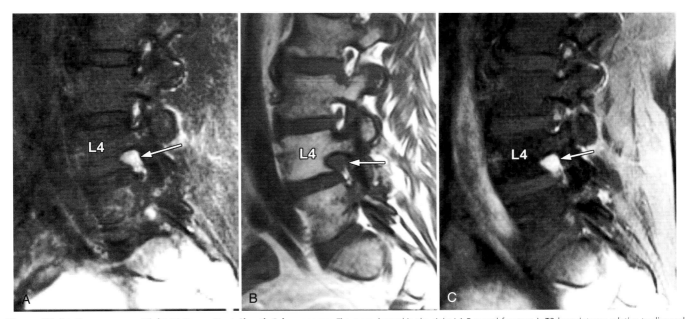

Figure 21-8 ▶ Homogeneous Right L4 Nerve Root Sheath Schwannoma. The mass *(arrow)* in the right L4-5 neural foramen is T2 hyperintense relative to disc and bone on parasagittal T2-weighted MR image **A.** The mass *(arrow)* is isointense and distinctly separate from the disc on parasagittal T1-weighted MR image **B.** The schwannoma *(arrow)* enhances intensely and homogeneously on parasagittal fat-saturated contrast-enhanced T1-weighted MR image **C.**

occur. Double disc fragments can also occur in the neural foramen or lateral to the neural foramen.[7]

DIFFERENTIAL DIAGNOSIS

1. **Schwannoma:** In the neural foramen, a schwannoma can appear similar to a foraminal disc herniation morphologically on CT or MR imaging *(Figs. 21-8 to 21-11)*.[10] On CT, schwannomas can look identical to a foraminal disc herniation (see Fig. 21-10). Most schwannomas can be differentiated from the adjacent disc by carefully examining the parasagittal MR images through the neural foramen, where the schwannoma is usually seen as a distinct mass, separate from the adjacent

intervertebral disc (see Figs. 21-8 and 21-10). Foraminal schwannomas tend to enhance homogeneously (see Fig. 21-8), whereas contrast enhancement in foraminal disc herniations nearly always occurs along the margin of the disc fragment (see Figs. 21-6 and 21-7). A minority of foraminal schwannomas have a cyst-like central component, and these tumors enhance along their margins (see Figs. 21-10 and 21-11). These schwannomas can be confused with foraminal disc herniations.

2. **Malignant nerve sheath tumor:** (These were once referred to as *neurosarcomas*.) May be indistinguishable from a schwannoma. However, contrast enhancement tends to be more heterogeneous with malignant nerve sheath tumors, and the tumor often causes destruction or deossification of the

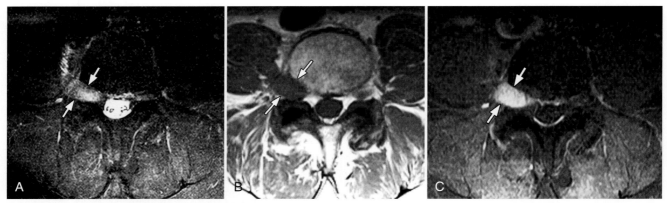

Figure 21-9 ► Homogeneous Right L4 Nerve Root Sheath Schwannoma. Same patient as in Figure 21-8. The mass *(arrows)* is relatively hyperintense relative to bone and CSF on fat-saturated T2-weighted MR image **A** and obscures the fat in the right L4-5 neural foramen on axial image **B.** The tumor *(arrows)* enhances intensely and homogeneously on contrast-enhanced fat-saturated T1-weighted MR image **C.** The tumor has enlarged the right L4-5 neural foramen by bone remodeling.

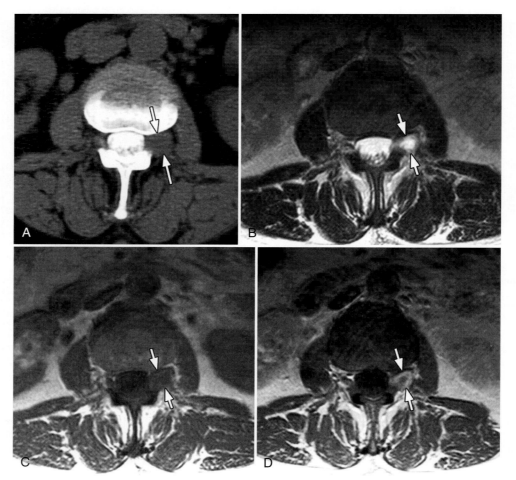

Figure 21-10 ► L2 Nerve Sheath Schwannoma. The left L2-3 intraforaminal mass *(arrows)* is nearly isointense relative to the paraspinal muscles. On T2-weighted MR image **B,** the tumor is relatively T2 hyperintense, more hyperintense centrally. The tumor *(arrows)* is slightly hyperintense relative to CSF on axial T1-weighted MR image **C.** The periphery of the tumor enhances *(arrows)* but the tumor core does not enhance, as demonstrated on axial contrast-enhanced T1-weighted MR image **D.**

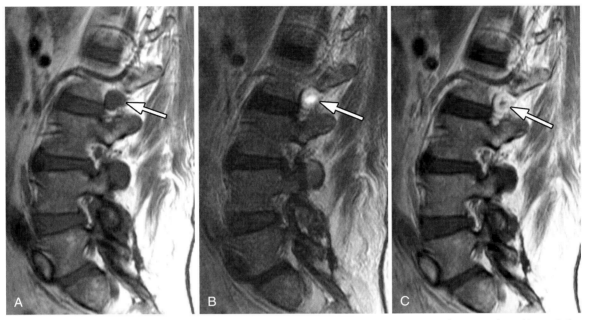

Figure 21-11 ▶ L2 Nerve Sheath Schwannoma. Parasagittal T1-weighted MR image **A**, T2-weighted MR image **B**, and contrast-enhanced image **C**. The mass *(arrow)* in the L2-3 neural foramen is T1 hypointense, T2 hyperintense (more so centrally) and displays peripheral contrast enhancement surrounding a nonenhancing central core.

adjacent bone. These tumors typically grow rapidly so early follow-up imaging is essential.

3. **Vascular tumors:** Rarely, vascular tumors can arise in the neural foramen, such as hemangioblastomas. These tumors often have aggressive imaging features and can be histologically benign or malignant. They usually cannot be differentiated from malignant nerve sheath tumors preoperatively *(Figs. 21-12 to 21-14)*.

TREATMENT

1. **Conservative therapy:** Treatment such as bed rest and administration of nonsteroidal anti-inflammatory drugs (NSAIDs) is often attempted initially, but this is often not sufficient to control the patient's radicular pain.[2]

2. **Selective nerve root injection or transforaminal epidural injection:** Such injections are extremely useful for diagnostically confirming the presence of a symptomatic lateral disc herniation and in controlling the intense radicular pain often associated with foraminal or extraforaminal disc herniation.[11] This technique should be considered the initial treatment for this condition.[2] Based on personal experience, selective nerve block or transforaminal epidural injection may obviate the need for surgery in many cases. The steroidal agent is usually mixed with a short- and/or long-acting anesthetic agent. Repeat injections may be necessary. The patient's condition should be frequently assessed. Development of leg weakness is an indication for prompt surgical intervention.

3. **Surgery:** Surgery is effective in greater than 80% of cases in reducing pain associated with lateral disc herniation.[2] Surgical excision of the foraminal herniated disc may be necessary if conservative therapy fails, if the patient cannot tolerate the pain, or if a progressive neurologic deficit occurs, or if there

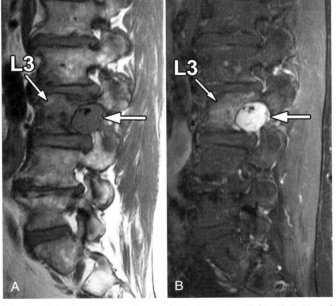

Figure 21-12 ▶ Capillary Hemangioblastoma in Right L3-4 Neural Foramen. The mass *(arrow)* on parasagittal T1-weighted MR image **A** and contrast-enhanced MR image **B** causes considerable enlargement and remodeling of the right L3-4 neural foramen and enhances heterogeneously. Signal voids in the mass represent intratumoral vessels. Note abnormal heterogeneous signal intensity in the L3 vertebral body.

are signs of lower extremity weakness. Prompt surgical intervention may be needed to prevent development of a "foot drop." Laminectomy with medial facetectomy and foraminotomy is often sufficient for removal of the foraminal disc fragment if it is accessible.[4,12] However, this approach may not be

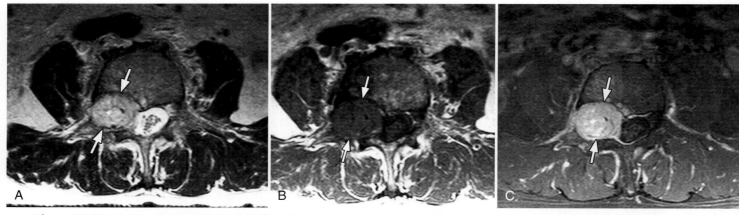

Figure 21-13 ▶ Capillary Hemangioblastoma in Right L3-4 Neural Foramen. Same patient as in Figure 21-12. On axial T2-weighted MR image **A** and axial T1-weighted MR image **B**, the mass *(arrows)* is heterogeneous in intensity and expands the right L3-4 neural foramen. The mass *(arrows)* enhances intensely contrast-enhanced fat-saturated T1-weighted MR image **C.** Vascular signal flow voids seen in the tumor.

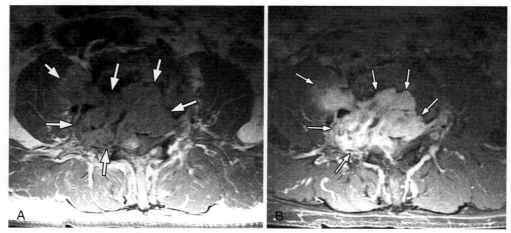

Figure 21-14 ▶ Capillary Hemangioblastoma in Right L3-4 Foramen Mimicking a Malignant Nerve Sheath Tumor. Same patient as in Figures 21-12 and 21-13, MR 17 months later. Axial unenhanced T1-weighted MR image **A** and contrast-enhanced axial T1-weighted MR image **B.** The mass *(arrows)* has increased in size considerably and is causing destruction of the adjacent L3 vertebra. The margins of the right L3-4 neural foramen are no longer well-defined. The hemangioblastoma now extends into the epidural space, where it compresses the thecal sac, and also invades the paraspinal tissues adjacent to the right psoas muscle.

sufficient to remove far lateral (extraforaminal) disc fragments.[2] A lateral fenestration procedure or a paraspinal muscle-splitting procedure may be required for removal of a far lateral disc herniation.[3,13-15] A fusion procedure is also performed if spinal instability is likely as a result of the surgical decompression procedure.[15] Disc fragments in the medial portion of the neural foramen may not be visible using a paraspinal approach.[2] Occasionally an anterolateral retroperitoneal approach is needed to remove an extraforaminal (far lateral) disc herniation.[16]

4. **Automatic percutaneous discectomy (APD):** This procedure is relatively minimally invasive and can be effective in treating some patients with lateral or far lateral disc herniations.[17]

References

1. Maroon JC, Kopitnik TA, Schulhof LA, et al. Diagnosis and microsurgical approach to far-lateral disc herniation in the lumbar spine. *J Neurosurg.* 1990;72(3):378-382.
2. Weiner BK, Fraser RD. Foraminal injection for lateral lumbar disc herniation. *J Bone Joint Surg Br.* 1997;79(5):804-807.
3. O'Hara LJ, Marshall RW. Far lateral lumbar disc herniation: The key to the intertransverse approach. *J Bone Joint Surg Br.* 1997;79(6):943-947.
4. Jackson RP, Glah JJ. Foraminal and extraforaminal lumbar disc herniation: Diagnosis and treatment. *Spine (Phila Pa 1976).* 1987;12(6):577-585.
5. Patrick BS. Extreme lateral ruptures of lumbar intervertebral discs. *Surg Neurol.* 1975;3(6):301-304.
6. Ohmori K, Kanamori M, Kawaguchi Y, et al. Clinical features of extraforaminal lumbar disc herniation based on the radiographic location of the dorsal root ganglion. *Spine (Phila Pa 1976).* 2001;26(6):662-666.
7. Abdullah AF, Wolber PG, Warfield JR, Gunadi IK. Surgical management of extreme lateral lumbar disc herniations: Review of 138 cases. *Neurosurgery.* 1988;22(4):648-653.
8. Lee IS, Kim HJ, Lee JS, et al. Extraforaminal with or without foraminal disk herniation: reliable MRI findings. *AJR Am J Roentgenol.* 2009;192(5):1392-1396.
9. Osborn AG, Hood RS, Sherry RG, Smoker WR, Harnsberger HR. CT/MR spectrum of far lateral and anterior lumbosacral disk herniations. *AJNR Am J Neuroradiol.* 1988;9(4):775-778.
10. Ashkenazi E, Pomeranz S, Floman Y. Foraminal herniation of a lumbar disc mimicking neurinoma on CT and MR imaging. *J Spinal Disord.* 1997;10(5):448-450.
11. Kurobane Y, Takahashi T, Tajima T, et al. Extraforaminal disc herniation. *Spine (Phila, 1976).* 1986;11(3):260-268.
12. Garrido E, Connaughton PN. Unilateral facetectomy approach for lateral lumbar disc herniation. *J Neurosurg.* 1991;74(5):754-756.

13. Reulen HJ, Pfaundler S, Ebeling U. The lateral microsurgical approach to the "extracanalicular" lumbar disc herniation. I: A technical note. *Acta Neurochir (Wien)*. 1987;84(1-2):64-67.

14. Wiltse L. Proceedings: Lumbar spine: Postero-lateral fusion. *J Bone Joint Surg Br*. 1975;57(2):261.

15. Kunogi J, Hasue M. Diagnosis and operative treatment of intraforaminal and extraforaminal nerve root compression. *Spine (Phila, 1976)*. 1991;16(11):1312-1320.

16. Strum PF, Armstrong GW, O'Neil DJ, Belanger JM. Far lateral lumbar disc herniation treated with an anterolateral retroperitoneal approach: Report of two cases. *Spine (Phila Pa 1976)*. 1992;17(3):363-365.

17. Onik G, Maroon J, Shang YL. Far-lateral disk herniation: Treatment by automated percutaneous diskectomy. *AJNR Am J Neuroradiol*. 1990;11(5):865-868.

DISC HERNIATION—LUMBAR

Leo F. Czervionke, M.D.

CLINICAL PRESENTATION

The patient is a 43-year-old female with an 8-day history of severe low back pain and left leg pain. Painful episode began while bending to remove clothes from a dryer. No lower extremity weakness observed. Negative straight leg raising sign. Normal lower extremity deep tendon reflexes.

IMAGING PRESENTATION

Magnetic resonance (MR) imaging was performed. A large disc herniation (extrusion) was found located on the left at the L5-S1 level. The herniated disc material compresses the left ventral aspect of the thecal sac and displaces the left S1 nerve root posteriorly (*Figs. 22-1 to 22-4*).

DISCUSSION

The levels at which 80% to 90% of herniated discs occur are the L4-5 and L5-S1 levels. However, the frequency of disc herniation at a given lumbar level tends to progress in a cephalad direction with advancing age.[1] Disc herniations may extend into the vertebral canal (central canal), lateral recess (subarticular zone), or intervertebral neural canal (neural foramen). Herniated discs may also extend vertically through the vertebral endplates (Schmorl's nodes). Most herniated discs occur in patients 40 to 60 years of age, but disc herniations may occur rarely in children, sometimes in adolescents, and not uncommonly in young adults and in the elderly.

Possibly, as many as one in three adults are believed to have asymptomatic disc herniations. The majority of patients with acute disc herniation and many patients with chronic disc herniations are symptomatic. The most common manifesting symptoms are low back and radicular pain. Symptomatic patients with radicular pain often have a positive straight leg raising sign (Lasègue sign). If the lumbar herniated disc is large, a cauda equina syndrome may be present. The low back pain associated with lumbar disc herniation is often accentuated by lumbar flexion, sitting, bending, coughing, or sneezing. The back pain often improves if the patient lies flat.

Many factors or conditions may predispose one to the development of disc herniation. Hyperflexion or hyperextension of the spine, lifting heavy objects, and exaggerated twisting movements

may all predispose one to disc herniation, particularly if the disc is already internally deranged or disrupted. Acute trauma can also predispose one to disc herniation, although often there is no acute traumatic event that can be related to the onset of symptoms.

Many patients who develop disc herniations also have coexistent internal disc derangement (*disc degeneration*) (see Fig. 22-2; *Figs. 22-5 to 22-7*). The etiology of disc degeneration is controversial, but repetitive microtrauma to the vertebra endplates is believed to interfere with the nutritional supply of the intervertebral disc, which can eventually result in internal disc derangement. Aging factors in the disc including proteoglycan replacement of the nucleus/inner annulus by predominantly type II collagen and metabolic degradation of proteoglycans with concomitant reduction in intradiscal water content (*disc desiccation*) likely play a role as well.

There is a definite familial tendency for development of disc herniation.[2] There is mounting evidence that genetic factors predispose the disc to degeneration (and hence disc herniation). Inherited genetic traits likely render the disc more susceptible to degeneration, disc herniation, or weakening of the vertebral bone. Genes that have been implicated include the following: (1) Those genes associated with the structural integrity of the disc, such as the aggrecan gene, collagen IX gene, or collagen XI gene; (2) those genes that can produce disc matrix-degrading enzymes such as the matrix metalloprotease-3 (MMP-3) gene; and (3) those genes associated with the integrity of bone structure that may be associated with osteoporosis, such as the vitamin D receptor gene and estrogen receptor genes.[3] Recently reported evidence supports a genetic basis for disc degeneration: Polymorphism of the aggrecan gene has been implicated in the development of severe multilevel disc degeneration.[4] Polymorphism of the vitamin D receptor gene may also predispose to disc degeneration.[5] A susceptibility locus for disc herniation and autosomal recessive spastic paraplegia has been found on chromosome 6.[6]

Inflammatory cytokines, such as interleukin-1, may contribute to disc degeneration by causing release of enzymes that degrade proteoglycans. Furthermore, inflammatory cytokines are involved in the mediation of back pain.[3] Enzymes capable of disc degradation, such as matrix metalloproteinases (MMPs) and aggrecanase, are present in normal discs but occur in higher concentrations in degenerating discs and even higher concentrations in herniated discs.[7] These and other enzymes are produced by cells in the disc and also by cells that invade the disc when the disc annulus or vertebral endplates becomes disrupted. It is not certain whether

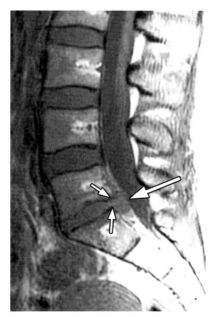

Figure 22-1 ▶ Large L5-S1 Disc Herniation (Extrusion). Sagittal T1-weighted MR image. A large herniated disc *(long arrow)* deforms the ventral margin of the thecal sac. The disc fragment is isointense relative to the intervertebral disc and hyperintense relative to CSF. The disc extrusion has a narrow "neck" or "base" at the posterior vertebral body margins *(short arrows)*.

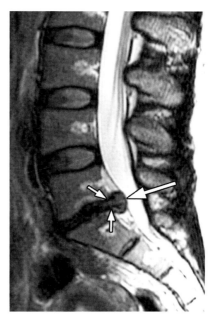

Figure 22-2 ▶ Large L5-S1 Disc Herniation. Sagittal T2-weighted MR image corresponding to Figure 22-1. A large herniated disc fragment *(long arrow)* causes ventral thecal sac indentation. The disc fragment is T2 hypointense relative to CSF but is slightly hyperintense relative to the intervertebral portion of the L5-S1 disc. The disc fragment has a narrow neck *(short arrows)* where it penetrates the outer annulus. The apex *(long arrow)* of the disc fragment is larger than the "neck" or "base" *(short arrows)* of the disc fragment. The intervertebral disc is narrowed and is dark (T2 hypointense) relative to normal discs above, consistent with L5-S1 intervertebral disc "degeneration."

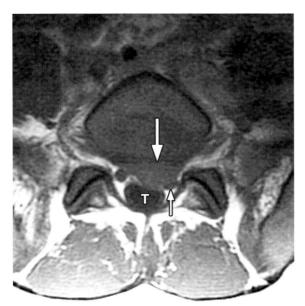

Figure 22-3 ▶ Large L5-S1 Disc Herniation. Axial T1-weighted MR image at L5-S1 intervertebral disc level in same patient as in Figures 22-1 and 22-2. The large herniated disc fragment has a broader base *(long arrow)* than apex in this plane but is still considered an extrusion because of the appearance of the disc fragment in sagittal plane. The herniated disc material is T1 hypointense relative to CSF within the thecal sac *(T)*. The herniated disc displaces the epidural fat and deforms the anterior aspect of the thecal sac on the left. The left S1 nerve root *(short arrow)* is displaced posteriorly and flattened.

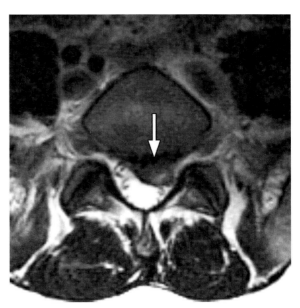

Figure 22-4 ▶ Large L5-S1 Disc Herniation. Axial T2-weighted MR image at L5-S1 intervertebral disc level in same patient as in Figures 22-1 to 22-3. The herniated disc fragment *(arrow)* is predominantly T2 hypointense relative to CSF. The thecal sac is deformed anterolaterally on the left by the herniated disc.

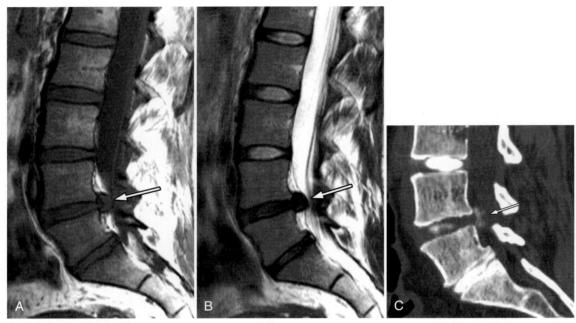

Figure 22-5 ▶ L4-5 Disc Herniation (Extrusion). On sagittal T1-weighted MR image **A,** the herniated disc fragment *(arrow)* has a narrow neck where it extends beyond the vertebral body margins. The disc fragment *(arrow)* is T1 isointense relative to the intervertebral disc and slightly more intense than intrathecal CSF. On T2-weighted MR image **B,** the herniated disc *(arrow)* is T2 hypointense relative to CSF. Intradiscal T2 intensity is much lower in L4-5 and L5-S1 intervertebral discs relative to normal intervertebral discs above, secondary to disc degeneration. On sagittal CT image, obtained following discography, the injected intradiscal contrast is seen in the L4-5 disc and within the extruded disc fragment *(arrow)* indicating presence of a full-thickness fissure (tear) in the posterior annulus.

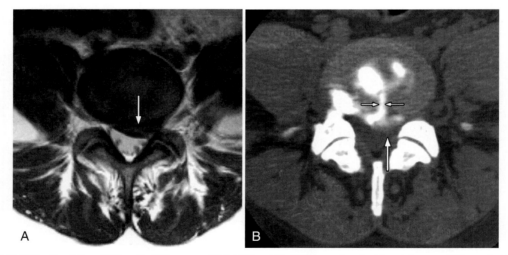

Figure 22-6 ▶ Left L4-5 Disc Herniation, MRI vs. Post Discogram CT. Axial T2-weighted MR image **A** and axial post discogram CT image **B** obtained though the L4-5 intervertebral disc level in same patient as in Figure 22-5. The disc herniation *(arrow)* has a relatively wide base and is T2 hypointense on MR image **A.** On image **B,** a full-thickness (grade 3) annular fissure *(short arrows)* fills with contrast, and the contrast extends into the herniated disc *(long arrow).*

the presence of these substances are causally related to disc degeneration or whether they are produced as a response to disc degeneration or herniation.[8]

Regardless of the underlying cause of disc degeneration, annular fissures (tears) develop in the internally deranged *degenerative* disc that may facilitate disc herniation, providing a conduit for nuclear and inner annular contents to herniate outside the confines of the disc (see Figs. 22-5 to 22-7). Grossly, the herniated disc fragment is usually composed of the disc nucleus, annular tissue, and sometimes portions of the cartilaginous endplate.[9]

A herniated disc often displaces or compresses adjacent structures such as the paraspinal ligaments, thecal sac, cauda equina, and nerve roots within the vertebral, neural foramen, or lateral recess (subarticular zone). Mechanical compression of these structures alone may not be sufficient to generate pain unless the compressed nerves or nociceptors in these tissues adjacent to the disc herniation are sensitized to pain by some other process, which is believed to be some type of inflammation.[10-13]

When an intravenous contrast agent is administered for MR evaluation of disc herniation, contrast enhancement is nearly

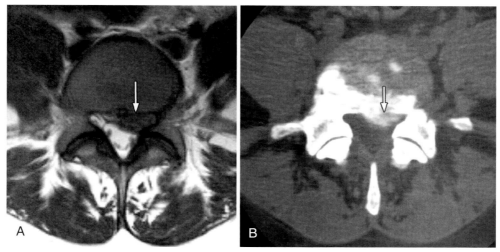

Figure 22-7 ► **Left L4-5 Disc Herniation, MRI vs. Post Discogram CT.** Axial T2-weighted MR image **A** and axial post discogram CT image **B** obtained one level below images in Figure 22-6. The herniated disc fragment *(arrow)* is T2 hypointense and is located in the left superior L5 lateral recess where it deforms the thecal sac on the left. The disc fragment *(arrow)* contains hyperdense discographic contrast agent in image **B.**

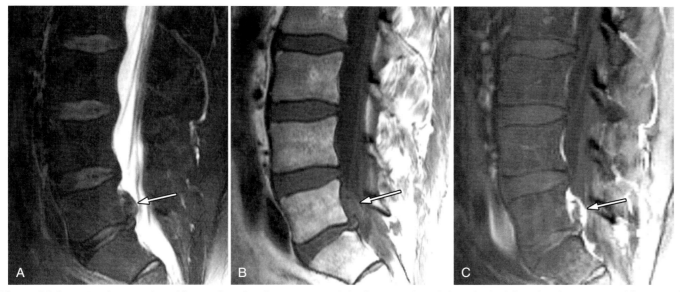

Figure 22-8 ► **L5-S1 Disc Extrusion with Superior Migration.** A sequestered disc fragment is located above disc level *(arrow)* as shown on sagittal fat-saturated T2-weighted MR image **A,** sagittal T1-weighted MR image **B,** and contrast-enhanced fat-saturated T1-weighted MR image **C.** The disc fragment centrally does not enhance, but intense peripheral contrast enhancement is demonstrated *(arrow* in **C).** On image **A,** the L5-S1 intervertebral disc is T2 hypointense and narrowed secondary to disc degeneration.

always seen in the tissue immediately adjacent to the herniated disc *(Figs. 22-8 to 22-10).* The herniated nucleus pulposus in the epidural space causes an inflammatory response in the adjacent tissues manifested by increased vascular permeability and infiltration of the inflamed tissues by leukocytes and macrophages.[13] The precise cause of this peridiscal inflammatory response is not known.[11] When a disc herniates, acidic mucopolysaccarides from the disc nucleus extend through fissures in the annulus into the epidural space, and these metabolites can incite an inflammatory reaction in the epidural space.[14] It is likely that some other biochemical mediator is also released when disc herniation occurs that hypersensitizes the compressed nerve or nearby tissue pain receptors (nociceptors) to the effects of mechanical compression.[10,14,15] Many candidates have been proposed for this biochemical

mediator of pain including nitric oxide, interleukin-1 (IL-1), interleukin-6 (IL-6), prostaglandin E_2 (PGE_2), phospholipase A2 (PLA2), tumor necrosis factor-alpha, granulocyte-macrophage colony stimulating factor, and other substances that have been found in increased amounts within herniated disc material, but their precise role is still unknown.[11,16-18] Acidic metabolites released by the herniated disc may also induce an inflammatory response adjacent to the disc fragment.[14]

An autoimmune theory has also been proposed as a cause for the peridiscal inflammation and pain associated with disc herniation. The normal intervertebral disc, lacking a blood supply, is largely sequestered from the immune system throughout most of life. When disc material herniates into the epidural space, which contains richly vascularized immunogenic tissue, the disc material

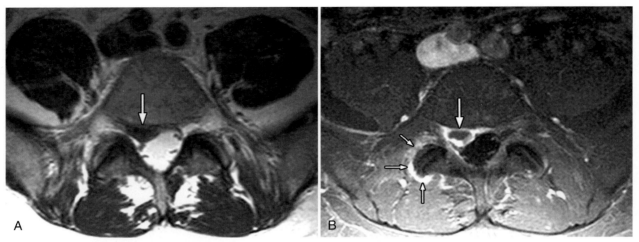

Figure 22-9 ▸ L5-S1 Disc Extrusion with Superior Migration. Same patient as in Figure 22-8. On axial T2-weighted MR image **A,** the disc fragment *(arrow)* is T2 hypointense, deforms the right anterior thecal sac margin, and encroaches upon the medial aspect of the right L5-S1 neural foramen. On corresponding axial T1-weighted MR image **B,** the disc fragment centrally does not enhance, but intense peripheral enhancement is present *(arrow)*. Note enhancement of right L4-5 facet capsule secondary to active inflammatory facet arthropathy *(small arrows)*.

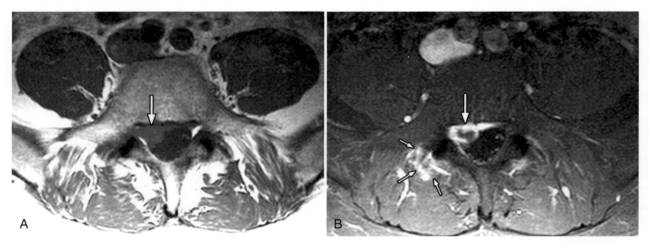

Figure 22-10 ▸ L5-S1 Disc Extrusion with Superior Migration. Shown are T1-weighted MR image **A** and contrast-enhanced fat-saturated T1-weighted MR image **B,** obtained one contiguous image level above images in Figure 22-9. In image **A,** the sequestered disc fragment *(arrow)* is T1 hyperintense relative to the CSF and obscures the epidural fat adjacent to the right L5 nerve root. In image **B,** intense enhancement *(arrow)* surrounds the nonenhancing fragment center. Note enhancement of inflamed right L4-5 parafacetal soft tissues in patient with severe low back pain and right hip and right leg pain.

acts like a foreign antigen. If this hypothesis is true, the extruded disc fragment may induce an autoimmune reaction that causes an inflammatory response. Phospholipase A2 may be involved with this process.[17,19]

IMAGING FEATURES

Herniated discs are seen with computed tomography (CT) or MR imaging as focal contour abnormalities along the disc margin. Disc herniations can be subdivided into disc protrusions or extrusions, depending on the size of the base or neck of the disc fragment where it is attached to the outer annulus. A disc protrusion has not penetrated all layers of the annulus (referred to as a *contained disc*) and by definition has a relatively wide neck or base relative to the size of the herniated disc apex in the sagittal or axial plane *(Figs. 22-11 to 22-13)*. A disc extrusion by definition penetrates all

layers of the annulus (referred to as a *noncontained disc*), and according to currently accepted nomenclature, has a relatively narrow neck (in either the sagittal or axial plane) where it extends through the annulus (see Figs. 22-1, 22-2, and 22-5).

Disc protrusions and extrusions may involute with time, which is usually associated with diminution or resolution of the patient's symptoms *(Figs. 22-14)*.[20] Disc extrusions, which are in contact with vascularized tissue in the epidural space, are far more likely to involute than protrusions.[21] Some unknown biochemical process in the epidural space likely causes the disc fragment to involute.

Radiographs do not allow direct visualization of the disc herniation, but often do demonstrate disc space narrowing, which often occurs with disc herniation. Sclerosis and marginal osteophytes may also be present along the adjacent vertebral endplates.

On myelographic radiographs or with MR myelography,[22] the herniated disc is visualized indirectly by the extrinsic deformity it produces on the thecal sac *(Fig. 22-15)*. On myelographic images,

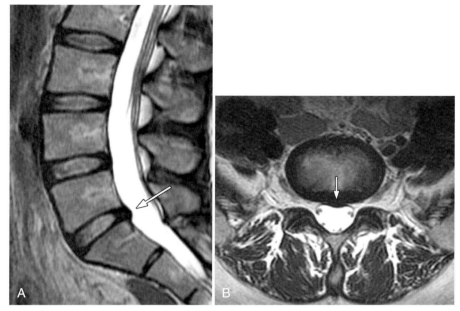

Figure 22-11 ▶ L5-S1 Disc Protrusion, No Apparent Intervertebral Disc Degeneration. The posterior annulus *(arrow)* protrudes in the midline on sagittal T2-weighted MR image **A** and axial image **B** causing mild midline ventral thecal sac indentation. Normal intensity and height of L5-S1 intervertebral disc.

the herniation may cause diminished or absent filling of the adjacent axillary root sleeve or pouch, sometimes referred to as a nerve root sleeve *defect* or *cut-off* (*Fig. 22-16*). The herniated disc fragment is seen on post-myelogram CT images as a soft tissue mass that causes extrinsic thecal sac deformity or nerve root sleeve deformity (see Figs. 22-15 and 22-16). Herniated discs are often visible on unenhanced or IV contrast-enhanced images. On plain, unenhanced CT, the herniated disc tissue is typically slightly hyperdense relative to the epidural tissues or cerebrospinal fluid (CSF) in the thecal sac (*Fig. 22-17*). Some herniated disc fragments also contain calcification, which is well demonstrated on CT. After IV contrast enhancement with CT, the vascularized epidural tissue enhances adjacent to the nonenhancing herniated disc fragment.

Occasionally, gas is visible in the epidural space on CT images of the lumbar spine. The presence of gas in the epidural space indicates that intradiscal gas (in a *vacuum disc*) has escaped through a full-thickness annular fissure into the epidural space (*Fig. 22-18*). This may or may not be associated with herniated soft tissue in the epidural space. This condition may or may not be symptomatic. If the gas collection is sufficiently large or accompanied by herniated soft tissue material, this can cause low back pain and radicular symptoms.[23]

MR imaging today is the modality of choice for evaluating disc herniation. The hallmark of a herniated disc is a focal contour abnormality along the posterior disc margin with a soft tissue mass displacing the epidural fat, nerve root, epidural veins, or thecal sac (see Figs. 22-1 to 22-10).[24] An MR scanner capable of imaging patients in an upright seated position is preferable to standard supine imaging MR scanners for detection of posterior disc herniations and anterior spondylolisthesis.[25] However, such MR scanners are not in wide clinical use at the present time.

MR not only provides morphologic information but also improves visualization of disc herniations because of the better soft tissue contrast of MR relative to CT. Midline, posterolateral, and lateral disc herniations are well seen on the T1-weighted images

because of displacement of high signal intensity fat in the lumbar epidural space or neural foramen. Fat displacement is an especially important sign in the evaluation of disc herniations, best demonstrated on T1-weighted spin-echo (SE) images (see Fig. 22-3; *Fig. 22-19*). Small disc herniations are often easier to detect on T1-weighted images (see Fig. 22-19). On T1-weighted images, the herniation appears isointense or slightly hyperintense relative to the intervertebral portion of the disc.[26]

T1 spin echo and T2 fast spin echo (FSE) or turbo spin echo (TSE) sequences are routinely used to evaluate lumbar disc disease. T1- and T2-weighted images should be obtained in sagittal and axial planes. The herniated disc is typically slightly T1 hyperintense or isointense relative to intrathecal CSF on T1-weighted images (see Figs. 22-1, 22-3, 22-5, and 22-8). The herniated disc is most often considerably T2 hypointense relative to CSF, although occasionally a disc fragment will appear relatively hyperintense on T2-weighted images, especially in chronic disc herniations or recurrent herniated discs postoperatively, which can sometimes undergo cystic degeneration.

Occasionally, extruded disc fragments are cystic or contain a cystic component, which is T1 hypointense and T2 hyperintense. These cystic disc fragments have a T2 hypointense fibrous capsule.[27,28] Cystic disc herniations are more commonly seen in disc fragments that have migrated above or below the disc level.

Nearly all herniated discs enhance along their peripheral margin after IV contrast administration, which likely is secondary to inflammatory tissue adjacent to the disc herniation (see Figs. 22-8 to 22-10 and 22-19). The disc fragment centrally usually does not enhance (see Figs. 22-9, 22-10, 22-19; *Fig. 22-20*). However, a chronic herniated disc fragment may enhance if granulation tissue invades the disc fragment. This may be seen before or after surgery. Enhancement of the intrathecal nerve root or roots being affected by the herniated disc may occur, which we refer to as *intrathecal reticulates*. This may occur preoperatively or postoperatively and may be an important cause of the patient's back pain. It is important to obtain pre- and post-contrast enhanced MR images to

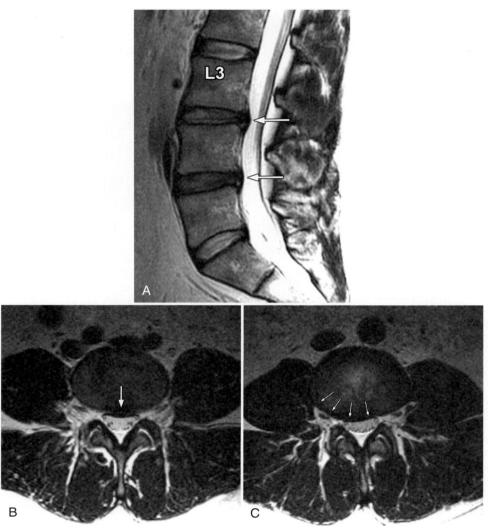

Figure 22-12 ▶ Disc Protrusions at L3-4 and L4-5 Levels Associated with Intervertebral Disc Degeneration. On sagittal T2-weighted MR image **A,** the protruding discs *(arrows)* cause mild ventral thecal sac indentation. L3-4 and L4-5 intervertebral disc height and intensity are diminished secondary to disc degeneration. Note tiny T2 high intensity focus in posterior annulus of both discs, where tiny annular fissures are located. Axial T2-weighted MR image **B,** obtained at L3-4 disc level, shows a small wide neck focal contour abnormality *(arrow)* representing a small focal disc protrusion which produces mild ventral thecal sac indentation. In sagittal T2-weighted image **C,** at the L4-5 disc level, a broad-based disc protrusion *(small arrows)* deforms right ventral aspect of thecal sac and narrows the right L4-5 neural foramen.

facilitate the diagnosis of intrathecal radiculitis associated with disc herniation. The inflamed nerve root or roots may or may not be enlarged in this condition. (See Chapter 35 for further discussion of intrathecal radiculitis.)

A small epidural hematoma may occur adjacent to a herniated disc.[29] In my experience, this rarely occurs. However, peridiscal hematomas may be underdiagnosed because they may be mistaken for peridiscal inflammatory tissue. It has been suggested that disc herniation can cause disruption of epidural veins, resulting in hematoma formation. It is not known whether epidural hematoma formation occurs at the time of disc herniation or develops later. These small hematomas are usually slightly hyperdense on CT. On T1-weighted MR images, the epidural hematoma is usually slightly more intense than the CSF and are T2 hyperintense, similar to fluid.[30]

Lumbar disc herniations have some unique imaging features based on their location and extent that deserve further discussion.

Disc Sequestration

MR is very sensitive in detecting sequestered (*free*) disc fragments, which are a subset of disc extrusion that has broken through the annulus and is no longer in continuity with the parent intervertebral disc. Sequestered fragments at the disc level in the spinal canal often have the appearance of two distinct fragments, which I refer to as a *double fragment sign* (***Figs. 22-21 and 22-22***). Herniated discs that penetrate the posterior longitudinal ligament (PLL) often represent sequestered fragments (*free fragments*) and can be diagnosed by a thin dark line between the free fragment and the parent disc, which implies a breach in the posterior longitudinal ligament. Not all free disc fragments represent nuclear material solely. Fragments of the annulus and the cartilaginous endplate are frequently included in the herniated disc material.[31] Free, sequestered disc fragments more commonly migrate inferior to the disc level rather than superior to the disc level, but both are common

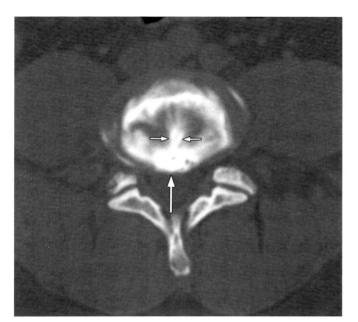

Figure 22-13 ► **Midline Posterior Disc Protrusion At L4-5 Level.** Axial post-discogram CT image from a different patient than shown in Figure 22-12. Injected contrast agent extends throughout most of the L4-5 intervertebral disc. A posterior midline annular fissure *(small arrows)* communicates with contrast in the midline focal disc protrusion *(long arrow)*. Mild coexistent generalized disc bulging is also demonstrated.

(Figs. 22-23 and 22-24). Sequestered discs can be located anterior or posterior to the PLL. Rarely, sequestered disc fragments extend posterolateral to the thecal sac.[32]

Sequestered disc fragments located above or below the disc level tend to be positioned off midline because of the presence of a midline fibrous septum between the posterior vertebral body periosteum and the posterior longitudinal ligament *(Fig. 22-25)*.[33] These disc fragments are often located anterior to the peridural membrane. The peridural membrane is a little known fibrovascular sheath surrounding the thecal sac. The space between the peridural membrane and the thecal sac is the epidural space. The peridural membrane contains many fenestrations that are traversed by veins of Batson's plexus.[34]

Intradural Disc Herniation

The intradural herniated disc represents a rare type of free fragment that penetrates the dura to reside within the thecal sac in the subarachnoid space adjacent to the cauda equina roots. The intradural disc fragment appears as a soft tissue mass within the thecal sac on T1-weighted or T2-weighted MR images, or on post-myelogram CT images *(Fig. 22-26)*. These can be misdiagnosed as intradural masses such as schwannomas.

Lumbar Traumatic Disc Herniation

Traumatic disc herniations can occur anywhere along the spine and are often associated with spine fracture or subluxation. In

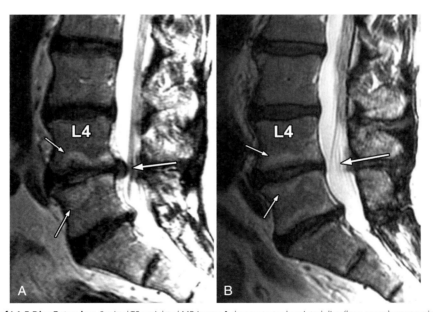

Figure 22-14 ► **Involution of L4-5 Disc Extrusion.** Sagittal T2-weighted MR image **A** demonstrates herniated disc *(long arrow)* compressing thecal sac. L4-5 intervertebral disc is markedly narrowed and is T2 "dark" due to disc degeneration. Note T2 hyperintense signal disturbance *(small arrows)* in vertebral bodies adjacent to L4-5 endplates secondary to reactive marrow response to disc degeneration (Modic Type 1). On sagittal T2-weighted MR image **B**, obtained 2 years after image **A**, the extruded disc fragment in the epidural space has involuted completely. Less reactive signal disturbance *(small arrows)* is located adjacent to L4-5 endplates. The L4-5 intervertebral disc height has increased slightly.

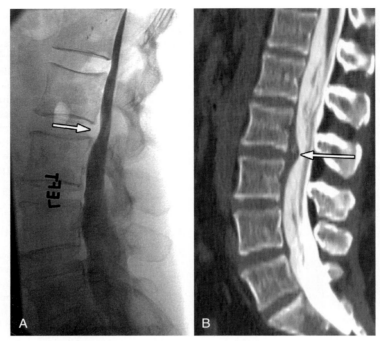

Figure 22-15 ▶ **Midline Disc Herniation L2-3 Level.** Lateral myelographic radiograph (image **A**) and corresponding post-myelogram sagittal CT (image **B**) show ventral indentation of the thecal sac caused by extrinsic indentation from herniated disc. The disc herniation *(arrow)* is directly seen on the CT image and its presence is inferred by ventral thecal sac deformity on the radiograph. In image **B**, the herniated disc *(arrow)* contains a tiny hyperdense focal calcification visible slightly above the intervertebral disc level.

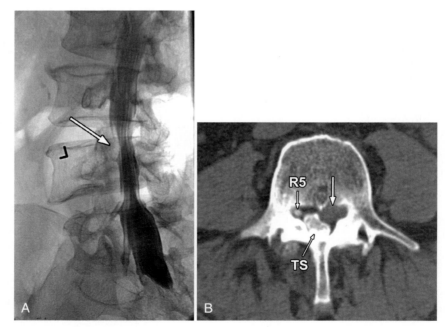

Figure 22-16 ▶ **Herniated Disc In Lateral Recess (Subarticular Zone) Just Inferior to L4-5 Intervertebral Disc Level.** Image **A,** a right anterior oblique (RAO) myelographic radiograph obtained with patient prone, shows intrathecal contrast, indentation of the thecal sac anterolaterally on the left *(arrow)*, and absent filling of left L5 nerve root sleeve (pouch) just below L4-5 disc level. The myelographic image gives indirect evidence of disc herniation. Image **B,** post myelogram CT image shows the herniated disc fragment *(arrow)* obscuring the left L5 nerve root pouch in the left lateral recess and deforming the anterolateral aspect of the contrast-filled thecal sac *(TS)*. Note right L5 nerve root pouch *(R5)* fills with contrast.

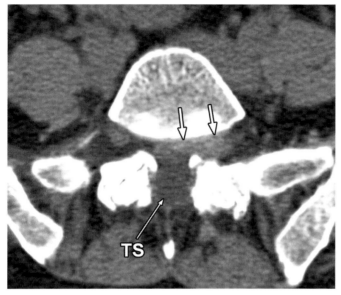

Figure 22-17 ► **Herniated Disc on Left at L5-S1 Level.** Axial unenhanced axial CT image. The herniated disc *(arrows)* is hyperdense relative to CSF in the thecal sac *(TS)*. The herniated disc *(arrows)* obscures the epidural fat ventral to the thecal sac on the left and also obscures the left L5-S1 intraforaminal fat adjacent to the left L5 nerve root.

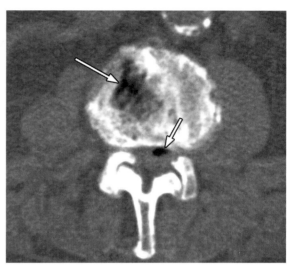

Figure 22-18 ► **Epidural Gas Communicating with Intradiscal Gas.** Axial CT image showing epidural gas *(short arrow)* in the left anterior epidural space, indicating a communication (fissure) between gas in the intervertebral disc *(long arrow)* and the epidural space. No hyperdense disc material seen adjacent to the epidural gas collection. Patient had vague low back pain but no radiculopathy.

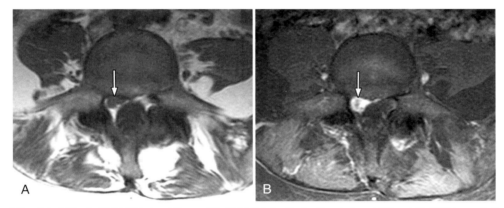

Figure 22-19 ► **Small Herniated Disc in Right L5 Lateral Recess (Right L4-5 Subarticular Zone).** On axial T1-weighted MR image **A,** the herniated disc *(arrow)* is slightly hyperintense relative to the intrathecal CSF. The herniated disc on this T1-weighted MR image is visible because it displaces the right anterior epidural fat. On corresponding contrast-enhanced fat-saturated T1-weighted MR image **B,** the herniated disc *(arrow)* enhances intensely except for a tiny central nonenhancing core.

adults traumatic herniations are more common in the cervical region following severe traumatic episodes and often are associated with vertebral fractures or subluxations. However, traumatic herniations may also occur in the lumbar region. (See chapters on traumatic disc herniation for more details.) Sometimes a traumatic disc fragment will migrate posterior to the subluxed vertebra. Traumatic herniations in older children or adolescents occur most often in the lumbar region or sometimes in the lower thoracic spine. Acute traumatic lumbar herniations in adolescents most often occur at the L4-5 and L5-S1 levels and usually disrupt and/or displace the ring apophysis. The disc herniation is commonly associated with a posterior vertebral rim fracture on CT or MR imaging, and this condition can cause intense low back pain.[35] The limbus vertebra represents the sequela of a traumatic herniated disc that had ruptured beneath the ring apophysis, in late childhood or adolescence.

Foraminal (Lateral) Disc Herniation

Herniated discs that extend into the neural foramen (intervertebral foramen) usually are not detected by myelography alone, because they cause minimal or no root pouch deformity and therefore require CT or MR for imaging detection. (See Chapter 16 for

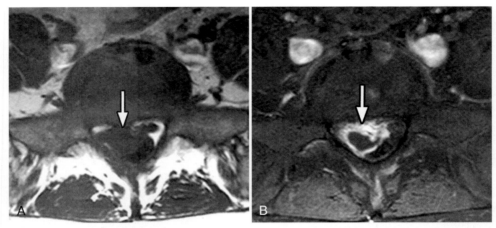

Figure 22-20 ▶ **Large Sequestered Disc Fragment Inferior to L5-S1 Intervertebral Disc.** Patient with severe right S1 radicular pain. On axial T1-weighted MR image **A,** a large disc fragment *(arrow)* obscures the anterior epidural fat on the right and deforms the thecal sac. On contrast-enhanced fat-saturated T1-weighted MR image **B,** intensely enhancing tissue *(arrow)* surrounds a nonenhancing central core.

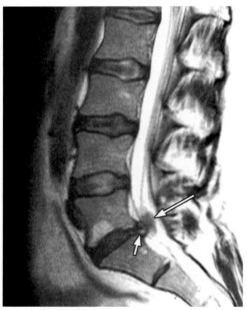

Figure 22-21 ▶ **Disc Sequestration at L5-S1 Intervertebral Disc Level.** *Double Fragment Sign.* Sagittal T2-weighted MR image. A small T2 hyperintense disc extrusion *(short arrow)* is in continuity with the parent intervertebral disc. A larger separate disc fragment *(long arrow)* is positioned more posterior to the smaller disc extrusion.

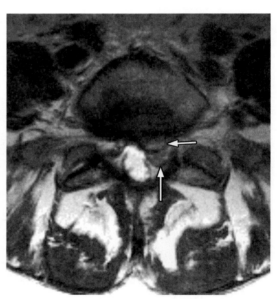

Figure 22-22 ▶ **Disc Sequestration at L5-S1 Intervertebral Disc Level.** *Double Fragment Sign.* Axial T2-weighted MR image at L5-S1 in same patient as in Figure 22-1. The smaller disc extrusion *(short arrow)* is in continuity with the posterior disc margin on the left. The larger sequestered fragment *(long arrow)* is positioned posterior to the smaller disc fragment. Both herniated discs produce left anterolateral thecal sac deformity.

further discussion of foraminal disc herniations.) However, it is not uncommon for foraminal and extraforaminal (far lateral) disc herniations to be overlooked, even with CT and MR imaging.[36,37] Lateral disc fragments compress the exiting nerve roots as they course below the pedicle at a given lumbar disc level. For example, a lateral disc herniation at the L4-5 level will produce L4 radiculopathy, whereas a posterolateral disc herniation compressing the thecal sac at the same level causes L5 radiculopathy. MR has advantages over CT in regard to detection of lateral disc herniation. Intraforaminal disc herniations are often readily visible on sagittal

and axial T1- weighted MR images because of intrinsic contrast provided by the presence of intraforaminal fat. Foraminal disc herniations can be confused with foraminal tumors such as schwannomas.

Schmorl's Node

Intravertebral disc herniations that extend through developmental or acquired defects in the vertebral endplates are called *Schmorl's*

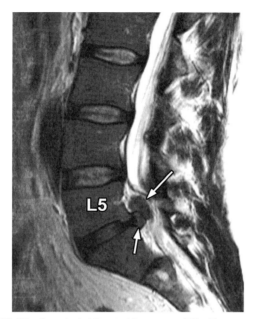

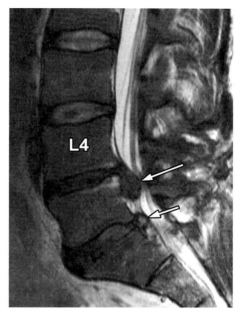

Figure 22-23 ▶ Superiorly Migrated Sequestered Disc Fragment at L5-S1 Level. *Double Fragment Sign.* Sagittal T2-weighted MR image shows a small disc extrusion *(short arrow)* at the disc level in continuity with the parent disc. A larger sequestered disc fragment *(long arrow)* is positioned superior to the intervertebral disc level and causes marked thecal sac deformity. Note that the L5-S1 Intervertebral disc is hypointense relative to normal discs above and disc height is diminished secondary to disc degeneration.

Figure 22-24 ▶ L4-5 Disc Herniation with Inferiorly Migrated Sequestered Disc Fragment. Sagittal T2-weighted MR image. A large disc fragment *(long arrow)*, hypointense relative to CSF, extends below the L4-5 intervertebral disc level into the epidural space posterior to the L4 vertebral body. This causes marked thecal sac deformity. Note small posterior disc herniation *(short arrow)* at L5-S1 level. Intervertebral disc degeneration at L4-5 and L5-S1.

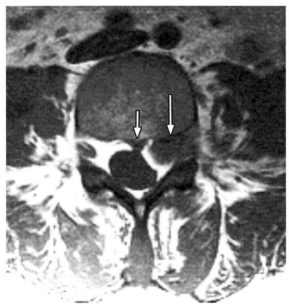

Figure 22-25 ▶ Sequestered, Inferiorly Migrated, L4-5 Disc Fragment. The herniated disc fragment is shown on left *(long arrow)* on axial T1-weighted MR image. The disc fragment compresses the left L5 nerve root. Note midline "septum" *(short arrow)* between L4 vertebral body and the anterior margin of the thecal sac.

nodes. Schmorl's nodes likely develop secondary to trauma, most often occurring in young adults or in adolescents. Acute Schmorl's nodes may be painful. In the acute stage, T2 hyperintense bone marrow edema and contrast enhancement are typically seen in the bone adjacent to the nodal defect. As the Schmorl's node evolves,

a thin rim of enhancement may be seen at the margin of the node, and later the nodal tissue itself will often enhance. The majority of Schmorl's nodes seen in adults are usually not symptomatic and are frequently seen as small endplate defects on MR images that typically do not enhance. Vertebral metastases adjacent to the endplate may sometimes be confused with a Schmorl's node. (See Chapter 59 for further discussion of Schmorl's node.)

DIFFERENTIAL DIAGNOSIS

1. **Epidural hematoma:** A small epidural hematoma may accompany an acute disc herniation and may contribute to the thecal sac or nerve root compromise. A post-traumatic or iatrogenic epidural hematoma, unrelated to disc herniation, might be confused with a herniated disc, if the hematoma is centered at a disc level.
2. **Postoperative epidural scar or granulation tissue:** There is nearly always enhancement along the peripheral margin of recurrent disc herniations. Postoperative scar and/or granulation tissue enhances homogeneously or nearly homogeneously after IV contrast administration. This can help to differentiate recurrent disc herniation from postoperative scar. The postoperative annular defect also typically enhances postoperatively.
3. **Epidural tumor:** In the lumbar spine, epidural tumor is often associated with vertebral metastases, except in some patients with epidural lymphoma. The vertebral and epidural tumor usually enhances heterogeneously with contrast.
4. **Neural foramen tumor:** Commonly schwannoma or rarely other tumors in the neural foramen can be confused with foraminal disc herniation. The foraminal schwannoma usually

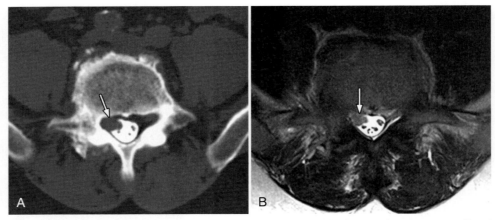

Figure 22-26 ▶ Intradural Disc Herniation. Patient with severe right L5 radicular pain. An intradural disc fragment *(arrow)* is seen as a filling defect within the contrast-filled thecal sac at the L5 level on axial post-myelogram CT image **A.** On corresponding axial T2-weighted MR image **B,** the intradural disc fragment *(arrow)* is outlined by T2 hyperintense CSF in the thecal sac. The intradural fragment originated from a disc herniation at L5-S1 level on the right.

enhances homogeneously with contrast, whereas the herniated disc within the neural foramen most often displays peripheral contrast enhancement.

TREATMENT

Pain and other symptoms associated with disc herniation may improve using conservative or surgical therapy and treatment is tailored to the individual patient.[12,38] Even patients with noncontained disc herniations (extruded discs) often do not require surgical therapy if they can tolerate their pain for 1 to 2 months.[21] The back pain and radicular pain associated with disc herniation often diminishes or resolves within 4 to 8 weeks with conservative therapy. This usually corresponds with slight diminution in the size of the herniated disc fragment. However, if lower extremity weakness develops during this time, prompt surgical intervention is indicated to prevent a permanent neurologic deficit. Development of cauda equina syndrome is an indication for urgent surgical intervention.

1. **Conservative therapy**: Most patients with lumbar disc herniations can be managed conservatively.[20] The type of conservative therapy should be tailored to the individual patient.[12,38] Conservative therapy includes bed rest, administration of nonsteroidal anti-inflammatory medications, and sometimes epidural steroid injections. A progressive paraspinal muscle strengthening exercise program is essential as the patient's symptoms subside. Some patients do not respond to conservative therapy. These tend to be patients with large disc extrusions or sequestered disc herniations. In these patients, surgery is usually indicated.

2. **Injections:** Selective nerve root injection or transforaminal epidural steroid injections can be very useful in patients with symptomatic disc herniations, especially in patients with a strong radicular pain component. A selective nerve root block will confirm the nerve root affected by the herniated disc fragment and will often provide excellent relief of pain.[39] This can be used to control the patient's pain for weeks by reducing peridiscal and radicular inflammation that commonly accompanies the disc herniation, allowing the disc fragment to undergo involution. In some cases, no further therapy is

required. Nerve root injection should not be used if the patient is developing leg weakness or a foot drop. Epidural steroid injection has been shown to be less effective than discectomy for relief of painful symptoms associated with large disc herniations.[40]

3. **Laminectomy (or laminotomy) and discectomy**: These procedures are still commonly performed today as treatment for lumbar disc herniation. Discectomy is effective for relief of low back pain and radicular pain associated with disc herniation.[41] Today laminectomy or laminotomy with discectomy is often reserved for patients with large disc extrusions or sequestered discs, in patients who fail conservative therapy, or patients who have a progressive neurologic deficit. Urgent surgical decompression is indicated if the patient has a cauda equina syndrome related to the disc herniation or if a foot drop develops.

4. **Disc herniation removal:** Surgical removal of disc herniations in the neural foramen or lateral recess usually require more extensive laminectomy and medial facetectomy, which may require instrumentation including anterior stabilization with intradiscal cage or spacer implants and posterior stabilization with bone graft material and instrumentation rods. Failure to remove a disc fragment in the lateral recess or neural foramen can result in *failed back syndrome*.[42]

5. **Automated percutaneous lumbar discectomy (APLD):** APLD is an alternative to open surgery and can be effective in treating some lumbar disc herniations.[43,44]

6. **Percutaneous laser disc decompression (PLDD):** PLDD is under investigation as a technique for treatment of contained disc herniations (disc protrusions).[45]

7. **Chemonucleolysis with chymopapain:** Percutaneous intradiscal chemonucleolysis using chymopapain has been used successfully to treat patients with small- to medium-sized nonsequestered disc herniations.[46] This procedure is no longer performed in the United States because of the occurrence of rare serious complications that have been reported with this procedure, including anaphylaxis and death.

8. **Chemonucleolysis with oxygen-ozone:** Percutaneous intradiscal chemonucleolysis performed by injecting oxygen-ozone combined with collagenase has been suggested as an alternative to surgery for treatment of noncontained (extruded) lumbar herniated discs.[47]

References

1. Dammers R, Koehler PJ. Lumbar disc herniation: level increases with age. *Surg Neurol.* 2002;58(3-4):209-212; discussion 12-3.
2. Varlotta GP, Brown MD, Kelsey JL, Golden AL. Familial predisposition for herniation of a lumbar disc in patients who are less than twenty-one years old. *J Bone Joint Surg Am.* 1991;73(1):124-128.
3. Zhang Y, Sun Z, Liu J, Guo X. Advances in susceptibility genetics of intervertebral degenerative disc disease. *Int J Biol Sci.* 2008;4(5):283-290.
4. Kawaguchi Y, Osada R, Kanamori M, et al. Association between an aggrecan gene polymorphism and lumbar disc degeneration. *Spine (Phila Pa 1976).* 1999;24(23):2456-2460.
5. Videman T, Leppavuori J, Kaprio J, et al. Intragenic polymorphisms of the vitamin D receptor gene associated with intervertebral disc degeneration. *Spine (Phila Pa 1976).* 1998;23(23):2477-2485.
6. Zortea M, Vettori A, Trevisan CP, et al. Genetic mapping of a susceptibility locus for disc herniation and spastic paraplegia on 6q23.3-q24.1. *J Med Genet.* 2002;39(6):387-390.
7. Roberts S, Caterson B, Menage J, et al. Matrix metalloproteinases and aggrecanase: Their role in disorders of the human intervertebral disc. *Spine (Phila Pa 1976).* 2000;25(23):3005-3013.
8. Adams MA, Bogduk N, Burton K, Dolan P. *The Biomechanics of Back Pain.* Edinburgh; New York: Churchill Livingstone, 2002.
9. Resnick D. Degenerative diseases of the vertebral column. *Radiology.* 1985;156(1):3-14.
10. Lindahl O. Hyperalgesia of the lumbar nerve roots in sciatica. *Acta Orthop Scand.* 1966;37(4):367-374.
11. Goupille P, Jayson MI, Valat JP, Freemont AJ. The role of inflammation in disk herniation-associated radiculopathy. *Semin Arthritis Rheum.* 1998;28(1):60-71.
12. Weber H. The natural history of disc herniation and the influence of intervention. *Spine (Phila Pa 1976).* 1994;19(19):2234-2238; discussion 3.
13. Modic MT, Ross JS. Lumbar degenerative disk disease. *Radiology.* 2007;245(1):43-61.
14. Nachemson A. Intradiscal measurements of pH in patients with lumbar rhizopathies. *Acta Orthop Scand.* 1969;40(1):23-42.
15. Crock HV. Internal disc disruption: A challenge to disc prolapse fifty years on. *Spine (Phila Pa 1976).* 1986;11(6):650-653.
16. Kang JD, Georgescu HI, McIntyre-Larkin L, et al. Herniated lumbar intervertebral discs spontaneously produce matrix metalloproteinases, nitric oxide, interleukin-6, and prostaglandin E2. *Spine (Phila Pa 1976).* 1996;21(3):271-277.
17. Saal JS, Franson RC, Dobrow R, et al. High levels of inflammatory phospholipase A2 activity in lumbar disc herniations. *Spine (Phila Pa 1976).* 1990;15(7):674-678.
18. Takahashi H, Suguro T, Okazima Y, et al. Inflammatory cytokines in the herniated disc of the lumbar spine. *Spine (Phila Pa 1976).* 1996;21(2):218-224.
19. Habtemariam A, Gronblad M, Virri J, et al. Comparative immunohistochemical study of group II (synovial-type) and group IV (cytosolic) phospholipases A2 in disc prolapse tissue. *Eur Spine J.* 1998;7(5):387-393.
20. Bush K, Cowan N, Katz DE, Gishen P. The natural history of sciatica associated with disc pathology: A prospective study with clinical and independent radiologic follow-up. *Spine (Phila Pa 1976).* 1992;21(10):1205-1212.
21. Ito T, Takano Y, Yuasa N. Types of lumbar herniated disc and clinical course. *Spine (Phila Pa 1976).* 2001;26(6):648-651.
22. Thornton MJ, Lee MJ, Pender S, et al. Evaluation of the role of magnetic resonance myelography in lumbar spine imaging. *Eur Radiol.* 1999;9(5):924-929.
23. Tsitouridis I, Sayegh FE, Papapostolou P, et al. Disc-like herniation in association with gas collection in the spinal canal: CT evaluation. *Eur J Radiol.* 2005;56(1):1-4.
24. Czervionke LF, Berquist TH. Imaging of the spine: Techniques of MR imaging. *Orthop Clin North Am.* 1997;28(4):583-616.
25. Ferreiro Perez A, Garcia Isidro M, et al. Evaluation of intervertebral disc herniation and hypermobile intersegmental instability in symptomatic adult patients undergoing recumbent and upright MRI of the cervical or lumbosacral spines. *Eur J Radiol.* 2007;62(3):444-448.
26. Czervionke LF, Haughton VM. Degenerative disease of the spine. In: Atlas SW, ed. *Magnetic Resonance Imaging of the Brain and Spine.* 3rd ed. Philadelphia: Lippincott Williams & Wilkins; 2002.
27. Lee HK, Lee DH, Choi CG, et al. Discal cyst of the lumbar spine: MR imaging features. *Clin Imaging.* 2006;30(5):326-330.
28. Chiba K, Toyama Y, Matsumoto M, et al. Intraspinal cyst communicating with the intervertebral disc in the lumbar spine: Discal cyst. *Spine (Phila Pa 1976).* 2001;26(19):2112-2118.
29. Gundry CR, Heithoff KB. Epidural hematoma of the lumbar spine: 18 surgically confirmed cases. *Radiology.* 1993;187(2):427-431.
30. Dorsay TA, Helms CA. MR imaging of epidural hematoma in the lumbar spine. *Skeletal Radiol.* 2002;31(12):677-685.
31. Brock M, Patt S, Mayer HM. The form and structure of the extruded disc. *Spine (Phila Pa 1976).* 1992;17(12):1457-1461.
32. Chen CY, Chuang YL, Yao MS, et al. Posterior epidural migration of a sequestrated lumbar disk fragment: MR imaging findings. *AJNR Am J Neuroradiol.* 2006;27(7):1592-1594.
33. Schellinger D, Manz HJ, Vidic B, et al. Disk fragment migration. *Radiology.* 1990;175(3):831-836.
34. Wiltse LL, Fonseca AS, Amster J, et al. Relationship of the dura, Hofmann's ligaments, Batson's plexus, and a fibrovascular membrane lying on the posterior surface of the vertebral bodies and attaching to the deep layer of the posterior longitudinal ligament: An anatomical, radiologic, and clinical study. *Spine (Phila Pa 1976).* 1993;18(8):1030-1043.
35. Beggs I, Addison J. Posterior vertebral rim fractures. *Br J Radiol.* 1998;71(845):567-572.
36. Lee IS, Kim HJ, Lee JS, et al. Extraforaminal with or without foraminal disk herniation: Reliable MRI findings. *AJR Am J Roentgenol.* 2009;192(5):1392-1396.
37. Osborn AG, Hood RS, Sherry RG, et al. CT/MR spectrum of far lateral and anterior lumbosacral disk herniations. *AJNR Am J Neuroradiol.* 1988;9(4):775-778.
38. Mirza SK. Either surgery or nonoperative treatment led to improvement in intervertebral disc herniation. *J Bone Joint Surg Am.* 2007;89(5):1139.
39. Narozny M, Zanetti M, Boos N. Therapeutic efficacy of selective nerve root blocks in the treatment of lumbar radicular leg pain. *Swiss Med Wkly.* 2001;131(5-6):75-80.
40. Buttermann GR. Treatment of lumbar disc herniation: epidural steroid injection compared with discectomy: A prospective, randomized study. *J Bone Joint Surg Am.* 2004;86-A(4):670-679.
41. Toyone T, Tanaka T, Kato D, Kaneyama R. Low-back pain following surgery for lumbar disc herniation: A prospective study. *J Bone Joint Surg Am.* 2004;86-A(5):893-896.
42. Burton CV, Kirkaldy-Willis WH, Yong-Hing K, Heithoff KB. Causes of failure of surgery on the lumbar spine. *Clin Orthop Relat Res.* 1981(157):191-199.
43. Onik G, Maroon J, Shang YL. Far-lateral disk herniation: Treatment by automated percutaneous diskectomy. *AJNR Am J Neuroradiol.* 1990;11(5):865-868.
44. Teng GJ, Jeffery RF, Guo JH, et al. Automated percutaneous lumbar discectomy: A prospective multi-institutional study. *J Vasc Interv Radiol.* 1997;8(3):457-463.
45. Steiner P, Zweifel K, Botnar R, et al. MR guidance of laser disc decompression: Preliminary in vivo experience. *Eur Radiol.* 1998;8(4):592-597.
46. Muralikuttan KP, Hamilton A, Kernohan WG, et al. A prospective randomized trial of chemonucleolysis and conventional disc surgery in single level lumbar disc herniation. *Spine (Phila Pa 1976).* 1992;17(4):381-387.
47. Wu Z, Wei LX, Li J, et al. Percutaneous treatment of non-contained lumbar disc herniation by injection of oxygen-ozone combined with collagenase. *Eur J Radiol.* 2008.

DISC HERNIATION
Recurrent vs. Postoperative Scarring

Douglas S. Fenton, M.D.

CLINICAL PRESENTATION

The patient is a 37-year-old man who presented with low back and right leg pain. He underwent a right L5-S1 microdiscectomy. He did well for about 5 years, but then developed recurrent symptoms. He currently describes right leg pain and numbness radiating down to the foot greater than low back pain. The pain is 60% in the right leg and 40% in the low back. There is no left leg pain or acute change in bladder function. Pain score ranges from 3/10 to 8/10. Straight leg raise is positive at 60 degrees on the right and negative to 90 degrees on the left.

IMAGING PRESENTATION

Axial T1-weighted pre-contrast and post-contrast magnetic resonance (MR) images at the L5-S1 level reveal a focal region of soft tissue along the right posterolateral aspect of the disc with peripheral enhancement. These findings are consistent with a recurrent disc herniation with surrounding granulation tissue in a patient with a previous right-sided laminectomy. The disc herniation causes posterior displacement of the traversing right S1 nerve root (*Fig. 23-1*).

DISCUSSION

Surgery for lumbar disc herniation is successful in 75% to 92% of patients.[1] This leaves 8% to 25% of patients with residual or recurrent low back pain and/or radicular pain. The success of a second operation depends on whether the initial surgical indication was correct and what the diagnosis is currently. The causes of failure include insufficient disc removal including sequestered disc, wrong site surgery, unrecognized second disc herniation, recurrent disc herniation, epidural fibrosis/scar, arachnoid adhesions, and traumatic injury to a nerve root. Recurrent herniations have been reported in 5% to 11% of patients and are therefore a major cause of surgical failure.[2-5] If the residual/recurrent pain is due to a retained or recurrent disc herniation, then these patients tend to show improvement with a second operation with a percentage showing improvement similar to that after a primary surgical procedure.[6] If, however, the surgical failure is due to scar formation, then these patients tend to show little improvement.[7] It has been suggested that the annulotomy created during the surgical procedure weakens the disc and that it is thereafter more susceptible to recurrent disc herniations. Disc herniations are usually ipsilateral to the annulotomy; however, up to 34% of patients have contralateral disc herniations.[4,8] Risk factors associated with recurrent disc herniations include young age, male gender, smoking, and traumatic events, particularly sports-related activities and lifting.[8]

The distinction between recurrent disc herniation and scar formation has been attempted with myelography, unenhanced computerized tomography (CT), enhanced CT, CT/discography, unenhanced magnetic resonance imaging (MRI), and enhanced MRI. Benoist and colleagues[9] demonstrated that myelography was not sensitive or specific for the differentiation of recurrent disc herniation and scar. Braun and colleagues[10] showed that enhanced CT was more sensitive than unenhanced CT. Prior to the advent of MRI, CT was the study of choice to evaluate the postoperative spine. Studies comparing enhanced CT imaging with unenhanced MR imaging evaluating the accuracy of diagnosing recurrent disc herniation versus scar demonstrated the superiority of MR imaging. MRI had a 79% accuracy for diagnosing scar and a 97.8% accuracy for recurrent disc herniation compared with CT's 42.2% accuracy in the diagnosis of scar and 71% accuracy for recurrent disc herniation.[11,12] Furthermore, enhanced CT requires a large volume of iodinated contrast and is only able to scan one level of the spine at a time. MRI does not have these drawbacks, and therefore MRI has become the preferred method in the evaluation of recurrent disc versus scar formation. A study by Bernard[13] demonstrated that CT/discography was more sensitive than enhanced MRI in predicting recurrent disc herniation. However, discography is an invasive procedure with significant risks to the patient, and therefore is not considered a preferred method in evaluation of recurrent disc herniation.

MRI, in patients without contraindications to MRI, has replaced other imaging modalities in the evaluation of the postoperative back. The differentiation of recurrent disc herniation and scar tissue is predicated on the fact that scar tissue enhances because it has a blood supply, a fenestrated capillary endothelium, and an extravascular space.[14] Disc material does not have a blood supply. Instead, contrast diffuses into the cartilaginous disc fragment. Scar tissue enhances maximally soon after injection of contrast and then begins to decrease 20 minutes after injection. Disc material demonstrates mild continuous enhancement over the first 45 minutes after injection, although enhancement is always less than that of adjacent scar tissue.[15]

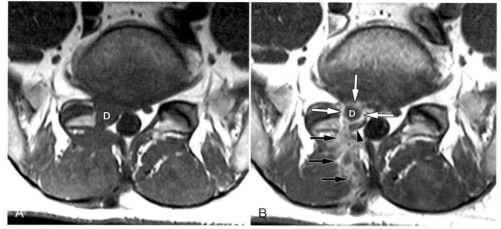

Figure 23-1 ▶ Recurrent Disc Herniation. Axial T1-weighted pre-contrast Image **A** and post-contrast Image **B**. Disc herniation identified with enhancing granulation tissue around the periphery of the herniated disc (*white arrows*). Similar enhancing granulation tissue extends along the patient's prior laminectomy defect (*black arrows*). Nerve root (*arrowhead*) is posteriorly displaced.

Studies have also suggested the utility of unenhanced MRI in the determination of scar tissue versus recurrent disc herniation. Hueftle and colleagues[16] reported 100% sensitivity, 71% specificity, and 89% accuracy of unenhanced MRI with 100% sensitivity, specificity, and accuracy after the administration of contrast media. Mullin and colleagues[17] evaluated postoperative patients with non-contrast MRI and obtained the correct diagnosis in 90% of cases. In the other 10% of the cases (nine patients) contrast was administered and three diagnoses were unchanged, two diagnoses were improved, and four diagnoses were made worse. The criteria used to diagnose recurrent disc herniation were based on signal characteristics and morphology. In the abstract of a study by Hochhauser and colleagues,[18] "the most reliable MR sign for recurrent herniated disk was the presence of a sharply marginated focal polypoid disk protrusion beyond the posterior margins of the adjacent vertebral bodies shown to best advantage on sagittal T1- and T2-weighted and axial T1-weighted spin-echo MR images. Disc herniations usually maintained isointensity with the intervertebral disc of origin, while extradural fibrosis exhibited variable signal intensity. The preoperative diagnosis of extradural fibrosis on MR was based primarily on its irregular configuration and extension." Other morphologic features that suggest scar include the absence of mass effect upon the thecal sac, absence of continuity with the parent disc, and retraction of the thecal sac at the level of the soft tissue mass. These authors suggest that suspected recurrent disc herniation could be evaluated with noncontrast MR examination and that contrast could be "reserved for difficult or unresolved cases."

The intervertebral disc, as well as other cartilage, has a large amount of glycosaminoglycans, which have fixed negative charges. These negative charges slow the diffusion of charged particles or ions through the cartilage.[14] Therefore, in principle, a paramagnetic contrast agent that has a charge should diffuse less readily into and through a disc as opposed to a contrast agent without a charge. Experiments have demonstrated that ionic contrast media diffuses through an intervertebral disc less well than a nonionic contrast medium.[14,15] In animal and human studies, discs enhanced twice as much using nonionic contrast media versus ionic media.[14,19] Therefore, if a patient is being evaluated for recurrent disc herniation, it is more appropriate to choose an ionic contrast agent so

that surrounding scar tissue is maximally enhanced and disc material is minimally enhanced.

Another method of separating recurrent disc herniation from scar tissue is through adjusting the dose of paramagnetic contrast. A concentration of 0.1 mmol/kg is typical for post-contrast imaging. Scar tissue is better enhanced at a concentration of 0.3 mmol/kg and is more clearly separated from a recurrent disc herniation than at 0.1 mmol/kg.[20] One has to weigh the slightly added benefit of additional contrast versus cost and the potential toxic effects of higher doses of gadolinium.

Lastly, over time, a disc herniation becomes vascularized. Scar tissue, over time, decreases in its enhancement. It is possible that if a patient waits to get imaged a few months after a disc herniation that it may be impossible to see a difference between scar tissue and disc herniation.

It appears that the best way to distinguish between scar tissue and disc herniation is with MR imaging using ionic paramagnetic contrast, preferably but not necessarily at a higher concentration, and within a few days to weeks of the beginning of symptoms.

IMAGING FEATURES

Recurrent Disc Herniation

A recurrent disc herniation has many of the same imaging characteristics of a nonoperated disc herniation. With CT imaging, the recurrent disc herniation will be seen as a mass-like region of soft tissue attenuation, similar to the parent disc, usually ventral or ventral lateral in location that may be connected with the parent disc (*Fig. 23-2*). There may be a decrease of complete obliteration of the normal epidural fat. If contrast is given, there may be peripheral enhancement around the disc herniation because of scar tissue. On MRI, the recurrent disc herniation will be isointense to the parent disc unless the fragment is calcified, in which case it would be of low T1 signal intensity (*Fig. 23-3, A*). The disc herniation is isointense to hyperintense on T2-weighted sequences (*Fig. 23-3, B*). The disc material will demonstrate no to minimal enhancement if imaged within the first 20 minutes after intravenous injection. There may be peripheral enhancement around the disc and in the laminectomy defect secondary to vascularized scar tissue (see **Figs.** 23-1, *B*, and **23-3, C**).

Scar Tissue

On CT, scar tissue is seen as nonspecific epidural and/or perineural soft tissue density, which may have density similar to the thecal sac and nerve roots. Very often, it can be difficult to separate fibrotic tissue from the thecal sac and nerve roots. On MRI, scar tissue is of intermediate T1 signal intensity and variable T2 signal intensity. Scar tissue enhances quickly after the intravenous injection of contrast *(Fig. 23-4)*. Enhancement of scar tissue may persist for years.

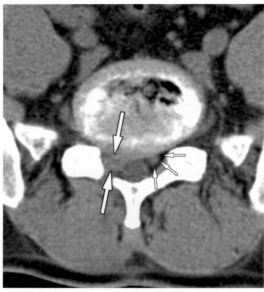

Figure 23-2 ▸ Axial CT Image. Soft tissue abnormality along the right posterolateral aspect of the disc (*large white arrows*) having similar density to the parent disc compatible with a disc herniation. There is obliteration of the epidural fat secondary to the disc herniation. Normal epidural fat identified surrounding the left nerve root (*small arrows*).

DIFFERENTIAL DIAGNOSIS

1. **Recurrent disc herniation**
2. **Epidural fibrosis/scar**
3. **Epidural abscess/phlegmon:** An epidural abscess can have imaging characteristics similar to a recurrent disc herniation and a phlegmon can look like scar tissue *(Fig. 23-5)*. However, these patients are usually sick and have typical chemistry abnormalities including elevated white blood cell counts, C-reactive protein, and sedimentation rates.
4. **Hematoma:** A hematoma is typically discovered in the immediate postoperative period and therefore needs to be clinically distinguished from recurrent/residual disc herniation. The imaging characteristics of a hematoma are typically quite different from a recurrent disc herniation. Hematomas are typically amorphic, nonfocal regions of decreased T2 signal intensity in the immediate postoperative period and exert mass effect on the thecal sac and/or nerve roots *(Fig. 23-6)*.
5. **Facet joint synovial cyst:** These are typically located along the ventral medial border of a degenerated facet joint. When they become large enough, they can contact the posterolateral disc making it difficult to distinguish its origin. The cyst can be of variable T2 signal intensity and can demonstrate peripheral enhancement. There may also be enhancement of the adjacent ligamentum flavum and periarticular soft tissues *(Fig. 23-7)*.

TREATMENT

Recurrent/Residual Disc Herniation

The treatment of recurrent or residual symptomatic disc herniation is identical to that of a primary disc herniation.

1. **Nonoperative treatment:** Typically treatment includes rest, nonsteroidal anti-inflammatory drugs, physical therapy, a short course of oral steroids, and percutaneous injection therapy of steroids.

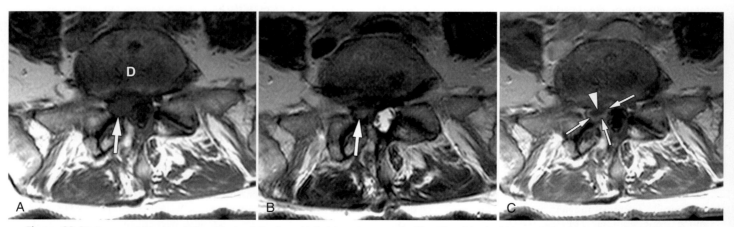

Figure 23-3 ▸ Recurrent Disc Herniation. Disc herniation (*arrow*) is isointense to parent disc (*D*) on T1-weighted axial image **A**. The disc herniation is of mildly increased T2 signal intensity (image **B**). The disc herniation (*arrowhead*) is surrounded by peripheral enhancement (*arrows*, image **C**) secondary to inflammatory/granulation tissue.

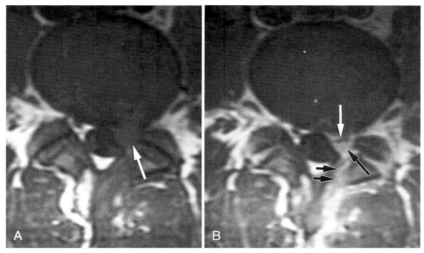

Figure 23-4 ▶ Enhancing Scar Tissue. Axial T1-weighted pre-contrast image **A** demonstrates an isointense soft tissue mass along the left posterolateral disc. On post-contrast T1-weighted image **B**, there is enhancement of the entire soft tissue abnormality (*long black arrow*) except for the traversing nerve root (*white arrow*). There is also enhancement through the laminectomy defect (*short black arrows*). Note the considerable mass effect that scar tissue can have on the thecal sac.

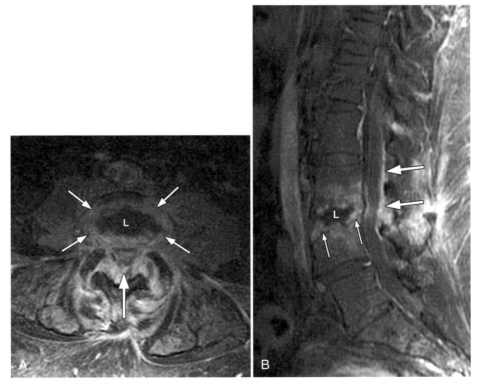

Figure 23-5 ▶ Discitis/Osteomyelitis with Epidural Phlegmon. Axial post-contrast T1-weighted image **A** and sagittal post-contrast T1-weighted image **B**. Enhancement of the L4-5 intervertebral disc (*small arrows*), liquefaction of the central disc (*L*), and enhancement in the epidural space (*large arrows*) are compatible with phlegmon. Phlegmon can have imaging characteristics similar to scar tissue; however, there should be no enhancement of the disc with scar tissue. Patients with an epidural phlegmon are typically ill with elevated temperatures and white blood cell counts.

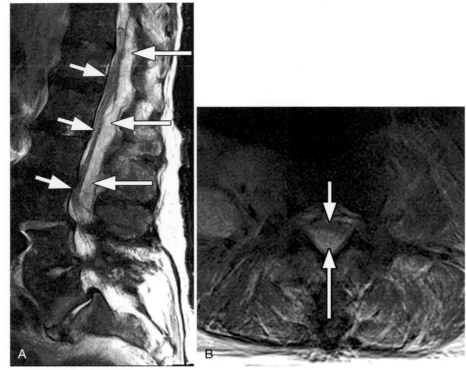

Figure 23-6 ► **Spinal Epidural Hematoma.** Long-segment region of intraspinal increased T2 signal intensity on sagittal image **A** (*long arrows*). The spinal cord and cauda equina (*short arrows*) are displaced anteriorly. Axial T2-weighted image **B** shows the hematoma posteriorly (*long arrow*) and the spinal cord ventrally (*short arrow*).

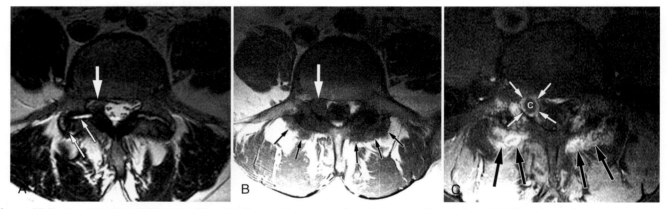

Figure 23-7 ► **Facet Joint Synovial Cyst.** Axial T2-weighted image **A** shows intermediate soft tissue signal intensity in the right L5 lateral recess (*large arrow*). Degenerated facet joint (*small white arrows*). Axial T1-weighted image **B** demonstrates an ovoid region of decreased signal intensity in the right L5 lateral recess (*large arrow*). Amorphic low signal intensity around the facet joints (*small black arrows*). Post-contrast, fat-saturated, T1-weighted image **C** reveals the more "cystic" nature of the lesion. There is exuberant enhancement around the facet joints bilaterally (*black arrows*) compatible with an inflammatory facet synovitis and enhancement (*white arrows*) around the synovial cyst (*C*).

2. Surgical treatment: Surgical removal of the recurrent disc herniation can be performed. Surgery is usually performed for symptomatic residual disc herniation.

Epidural Fibrosis/Scar

Patients with symptomatic epidural fibrosis/scar tissue are difficult to treat.

1. Nonoperative treatment: Includes physical therapy, oral pain medications, percutaneous injection of steroid, and spinal cord stimulator.

2. Surgical treatment: Surgical removal of scar tissue does not have very good results.

References

1. Law JD, Lehman RAW, Kirsch WM. Reoperation after lumbar intervertebral disc surgery. *J Neurosurg.* 1978;48:259-263.

2. Connolly ES. Surgery for recurrent lumbar disc herniation. *Clin Neurosurg.* 1992;39:211-216.

3. Jackson RK. The long-term effects of wide laminectomy for lumbar disc excision: A review of 130 patients. *J Bone Joint Surg Br.* 1971;53:609-616.

4. O'Sullivan MG, Connolly AE, Buckley TF. Recurrent lumbar disc protrusion. *Br J Neurosurg.* 1990;4:319-325.

5. Suk KS, Lee HM, Moon SH, Kim NH. Recurrent lumbar disc herniation: Results of operative management. *Spine.* 2001;26:672-676.

6. Jonsson B, Stromqvist B. Clinical characteristics of recurrent sciatica after lumbar discectomy. *Spine.* 1996;21:500-505.

7. Finnegan WJ, Fenlin JM, Marvel JP, et al. Results of surgical intervention in the symptomatic multiply-operated back patient. *J Bone Joint Surg Am.* 1979;61:1077-1082.

8. Cinotti G, Gumina S, Giannicola G, Postacchini F. Contralateral recurrent lumbar disc herniation: Results of discectomy compared with those in primary herniation. *Spine.* 1999;24:800-806.

9. Benoist M, Ficat C, Baraf P, Cauchoix J. Postoperative lumbar epiduroarachnoiditis. *Spine.* 1980;5:432-436.

10. Braun IF, Hoffman JC, Davis PC, et al. Contrast enhancement in CT differentiation between recurrent disk herniation and postoperative scar: Prospective study. *AJNR Am J Neuroradiol.* 1985;6:607-612.

11. Firooznia H, Kricheff II, Rafii M, Golimbu C. Lumbar spine after surgery: Examination with intravenous contrast-enhanced CT. *Radiology.* 1987;163:221-226.

12. Sotiropoulos S, Chafetz NI, Lang P, et al. Differentiation between postoperative scar and recurrent disk herniation: Prospective comparison of MR, CT, and contrast-enhanced CT. *AJNR Am J Neuroradiol.* 1989;10:639-643.

13. Bernard TN. Using computed tomography/discography and enhanced magnetic resonance imaging to distinguish between scar tissue and recurrent lumbar disc herniation. *Spine.* 1994;19:2826-2832.

14. Haughton V, Schreibman K, De Smet A. Contrast between scar and recurrent herniated disk on contrast-enhanced MR images. *AJNR Am J Neuroradiol.* 2002;23:1652-1656.

15. Nguyen CM, Ho KC, An H, et al. Ionic versus nonionic paramagnetic contrast media in differentiating between scar and herniated disk. *AJNR Am J Neuroradiol.* 1996;17:501-505.

16. Hueftle MG, Modic MT, Ross JS, et al. Lumbar spine: Postoperative MR imaging with Gd-DTPA. *Radiology.* 1988;167:817-824.

17. Mullin WJ, Heithoff KB, Gilbert TJ, Renfrew DL. Magnetic resonance evaluation of recurrent disc herniation: Is gadolinium necessary? *Spine.* 2000;25:1493-1499.

18. Hochhauser L, Kieffer SA, Cacayorin ED, et al. Recurrent postdiskectomy low back pain: MR-surgical correlation. *AJR Am J Roentgenol.* 1988;151:755-760.

19. Ibrahim MA, Haughton VM, Hyde JS. Enhancement of intervertebral disks with gadolinium complexes: Comparison of an ionic and nonionic medium in an animal model. *AJNR Am J Neuroradiol.* 1994;15:1907-1910.

20. Nguyen C, Haughton VM, Ho KC, An H. MRI contrast enhancement: An experimental study in post laminectomy epidural fibrosis. *AJNR Am J Neuroradiol.* 1993;14:997-1002.

DISC HERNIATION AND SPONDYLOSIS—CERVICAL

Douglas S. Fenton, M.D.

CLINICAL PRESENTATION

The patient is a 43-year-old female who presented with complaint of 8 days of right-sided upper back pain that radiates down the right arm. The patient gives a history of a left-sided disc herniation at C5-6. The right arm pain is characterized as an electric shock sensation down the medial portion of the right arm with subjective weakness. The pain is 6/10 in intensity and is exacerbated by activities such as carrying her purse or manipulating a steering wheel while driving. Over-the-counter pain medications can reduce her pain to 5/10. The patient does not recollect any history of trauma or inciting event. Upon physical examination, the patient has full strength in the deltoids, biceps, triceps, wrist extensors, wrist flexors, finger flexors, and intrinsic hand muscles bilaterally. She reports decreased sensation to pin prick in the right upper extremity in both the ulnar and median nerve distributions.

IMAGING PRESENTATION

Sagittal and axial T2-weighted magnetic resonance (MR) images were obtained and show a moderate-sized region of soft tissue signal intensity along the right posterolateral disc margin consistent with a disc herniation that compresses the right ventral aspect of the thecal sac with mild central spinal canal narrowing and severe narrowing of the right C6-7 neural foramen (*Fig. 24-1*).

DISCUSSION

Cervical radicular pain caused by cervical disc herniation or spondylosis is a common cause of neck and/or arm pain. Cervical radiculopathy can also occur from many other processes including vertebral fracture, spondylolisthesis, trauma, neoplasm, infection, and metabolic conditions. A 15-year study by Radhakrishnan and colleagues[1] of patients with cervical radicular pain concluded that the mean age at diagnosis was approximately 48 years of age. The annual age-adjusted rates per 100,000 were 83.2 for the total, 107.3 for males, and 63.5 for females. The male to female ratio was 1.7. A history of trauma immediately preceding the onset of radicular pain was seen in 14.8% of patients. The duration of symptoms before diagnosis had a mean of 40.6 days. The onset of symptoms was acute in 50%, subacute in 24%, and insidious in 26%. Neck and

arm symptoms occurred in nearly all patients (97.5%). Subjective weakness was present in only 15% of patients. Symptoms were unilateral in 98% of the patients. Pain with neck movement occurred in 90% of patients. The most common etiologies of the radicular pain found at surgery were spondylosis, disc herniation, or a combination in 68.4% and a disc protrusion in 21.9%. The age- and gender-specific annual incidence rates of cervical disc herniation causing radicular pain was greatest in the 50 to 54-year-old age group and rapidly declined after 60 years of age. A similar large review of patients with cervical radicular pain by Henderson and colleagues[2] demonstrated arm pain in 99.4%, sensory deficits in 85.2%, neck pain in 79.7%, reflex deficits in 71.2%, motor deficits in 68%, scapular pain in 52.5%, anterior chest pain in 17.8%, headaches in 9.7%, anterior chest and arm pain in 5.9%, and left-sided chest and arm pain in 1.3%.

It is important to distinguish a common misuse of the terms *radiculopathy* and *radicular pain*, which are often incorrectly interchanged. "Radiculopathy is the objective loss of sensory and/or motor function as a result of conduction block or loss of axons in a spinal nerve or its roots. There are typically symptoms of numbness and weakness in the distribution of the affected nerve. Radicular pain is caused by ectopic impulse generation. Radiculopathy relates to objective neurologic signs caused by a conduction block or loss of axons. The two conditions may coexist and may be caused by the same lesion."[3]

The most common cause of cervical nerve root compression is narrowing of the neural foramen secondary to spondylosis, typically from uncovertebral joint spurring, osteophytes, and/or degenerative spurring of the superior facet articulation from the more caudad vertebral body.[1,4] Cervical disc herniations are the second most common cause of nerve root compression in the cervical spine.[1,4] The most common level of nerve root compression by any etiology is C6-7 (~50% to 70%) followed by, C5-6 (~20%), C7-T1 (~10%), and C4-5 (~5%).[1,5] The most common levels of cervical disc herniation are C6-7 followed by C5-6.[5,6] Disc herniations are rare at or above C3-4.[6,7]

Post-traumatic cervical disc herniations are rare.[8] The vast majority of cervical disc herniations occur along with the degenerative disc cascade. Prior to the age of 20, few morphologic changes occur in the cervical disc.[8] Around 30 years of age, there is a progressive decrease in disc hydration. The cervical disc becomes more compressible and less elastic. The disc loses height and begins to bulge into the spinal canal. The adjacent vertebral bodies settle closer to each other, which begins a process

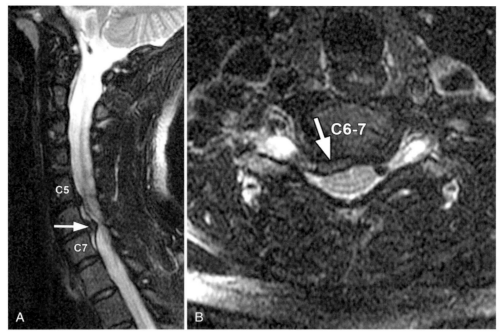

Figure 24-1 ► **Right Posterolateral Cervical Disc Herniation at C6-7.** On sagittal T2 image **A** and axial T2 image **B** (*arrow*). The right ventral cervical spinal cord is mildly flattened on the axial image. Smaller disc herniation seen at C5-6 on the sagittal image.

of osteophyte formation around the disc margin as well as the uncovertebral joints and facet joints, which can narrow the neural foramen and cause radiculopathy and radicular pain. The anatomy of the cervical disc is such that the anterior cervical annulus is very dense, but the posterior annulus has few fibers to contain the nucleus pulposus.[9] There is also no substantive annulus over the lateral uncovertebral regions.[9] This renders the patient with cervical discogenic degeneration susceptible to disc herniations posteriorly and laterally.

Pain is the most common finding in patients with an acute cervical radiculopathy. The pain diminishes as the condition becomes more chronic. The pain may be sharp, achy, or burning. Its location depends on which nerve root(s) are affected and can involve the neck, arm, or chest. The classic radiculopathy manifests as radiating pain in a myotomal distribution.[8] Radicular pain is often worsened with coughing, sneezing, Valsalva maneuvers, and certain movements of the neck.[8] Patients with high cervical disc protrusion may have nonfocal symptoms such as headache, dizziness, and tinnitus. Patients with C2-3 disc protrusions characteristically have suboccipital pain.[10]

The Spurling test can be used to aid in the diagnosis of cervical radicular pain. The test is positive if there is reproduction of the patient's typical pain with the Spurling maneuver (extension of the neck, rotation of the head to the side of the pain, and applying downward pressure on the head). The Spurling test has been found to be specific, but not sensitive, for cervical radiculopathy.[11]

Selective nerve root blocks (SNRBs) can be performed both for diagnosis and therapeutic treatment. Diagnostically, SNRBs are performed if there is a question of which cervical level(s) is/are causing symptoms when imaging demonstrates more than one level of abnormality. A single-level fluoroscopically guided transforaminal SNRB with 0.3 mL of local anesthetic can help in this determination. The amount of injectate is low enough so as not to spread to adjacent levels and potentially give a false-positive result. If the test is positive, the patient should experience complete pain relief in the myotomal distribution of the injected nerve root for up to 1 hour. It is important to realize that an SNRB does not discern the cause of the radicular pain, only the level. The nerve root pain can be caused by a disc herniation, osteophyte, uncovertebral spur, or facet joint compression. Also, an SNRB blocks a portion of the facet joint, and therefore, the cause of a patient's pain may in fact be facet-related as opposed to a compressive etiology at the neural foramen. We have found, in our institution, that inflammation of the cervical facet joint (facet synovitis) is a common cause of noncompressive radicular pain.

IMAGING FEATURES

Plain radiographic oblique views can give some information as to narrowing of particular foramen, but do not assist in the diagnosis of disc herniations. They are performed because they are inexpensive and render information about sagittal balance, instability, fractures, and congenital abnormalities.[8] Neural compression by disc herniation or osteophyte can be indirectly diagnosed with myelography *(Fig. 24-2)*; however, there are many occasions when it is difficult to distinguish between an osteophyte alone compressing the thecal sac or a combination osteophyte/disc complex. The most common cause of an extradural defect on the thecal sac is a disc herniation, osteophyte, or a combination of the two.

The addition of computerized tomography (CT) after myelography is much more sensitive to the cause of thecal sac compression *(Fig. 24-3)*. Myelography is notorious for its inability to diagnose a lateral disc herniation. Another major disadvantage of myelography is its invasive nature. Noncontrast CT allows for the direct visualization of the pathology causing neural compression.

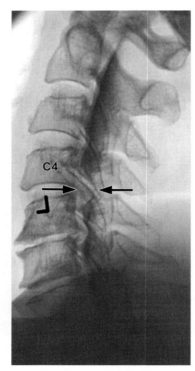

Figure 24-2 ▶ Filling Defect on the Thecal Sac. Lateral view from cervical myelography demonstrates a negative filling defect on the ventral surface of the thecal sac (*between arrows*). The cause of the negative defect is unknown based on myelography alone.

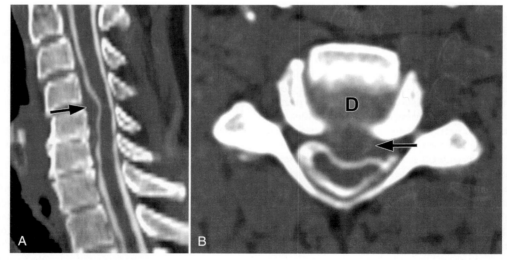

Figure 24-3 ▶ Left Paramidline Disc Herniation, CT. Same patient as in Figure 24-2. Reformatted sagittal image **A** and axial image **B** post-myelography. The negative defect on myelography represents a left paramidline disc herniation (*arrow*). The disc herniation has the same density as the parent disc (*D*).

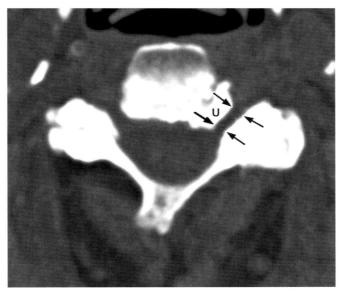

Figure 24-4 ▶ Uncovertebral Spur, CT. Axial CT of the cervical spine demonstrates a prominent left uncovertebral joint spur (*U*) causing moderate narrowing of the neural foramen (*bounded by arrows*).

The typical disc herniation is intermediate density (similar to the parent disc) that may be focally protruded or have a broad-based attachment to the parent disc (see Fig. 24-3). The thecal sac and neural elements may be displaced by the disc herniation. A vertebral osteophyte or uncovertebral spur has bone density and can cause central spinal stenosis, with possible myelopathic symptoms or foraminal stenosis with radicular symptoms (*Fig. 24-4*). Compared with myelography, CT uses less radiation; however, CT still emits radiation. The advantage of CT lies in its ability to distinguish between soft tissue and bone, which is a major advantage for surgical planning.

Magnetic resonance imaging (MRI) is the procedure of choice to detect disc herniations. Foraminal stenosis can be overestimated with MRI. It can be difficult to distinguish a foraminal uncovertebral spur from a disc herniation. The typical MR appearance of a cervical disc herniation is isointensity to the parent disc on T1-weighted acquisitions, variable signal intensity on T2-weighted acquisitions, depending on the age and hydration of the disc and iso- to increased signal intensity on gradient recall acquisitions (*Fig. 24-5*). The disc material does not enhance; however, there may be some peripheral enhancement in a subacute/chronic disc herniation from granulation tissue. An osteophyte or uncovertebral spur will usually be of low T1- and T2-weighted signal intensity (*Fig. 24-6*) except in the case of an osteophyte that gains a marrow cavity in which it may demonstrate increased T1 signal intensity.

DIFFERENTIAL DIAGNOSIS

1. **Osteophyte**: It is difficult to distinguish between an osteophyte and disc herniation by MR imaging alone. CT is a helpful adjunct; however, there are many times that central canal and foraminal narrowing are caused by a combination of a disc herniation and osteophyte.
2. **Ossification of the posterior longitudinal ligament:** Ossification has a flowing appearance along the posterior vertebral bodies (*Fig. 24-7*).
3. **Abscess**: Patients with an abscess are often sick with elevated white blood cell counts, sedimentation rates, and C-reactive proteins. There may be associated vertebral endplate destruction. An abscess cavity will have MRI characteristics similar to fluid, and there is often robust enhancement (*Fig. 24-8*).
4. **Hemorrhage:** Has variable MR signal intensity and is often elongated in the spinal canal. In the cervical spine, hemorrhage is typically posterior to the spinal cord (*Fig. 24-9*).

TREATMENT

1. **Rest**
2. **Cervical collar:** Not universally recommended but may be of some benefit in the acute stage.
3. **Nonsteroidal anti-inflammatory drugs (NSAIDs)**
4. **Exercise therapy**
5. **Narcotic medications**
6. **Transforaminal epidural steroid injections:** May reduce/ resolve the inflammation associated with neural compression and ameliorate the patient's pain.
7. **Surgery:** Usually indicated for patients with intractable pain, long-lasting pain, or motor weakness. There are various surgical options including anterior and posterior approaches.

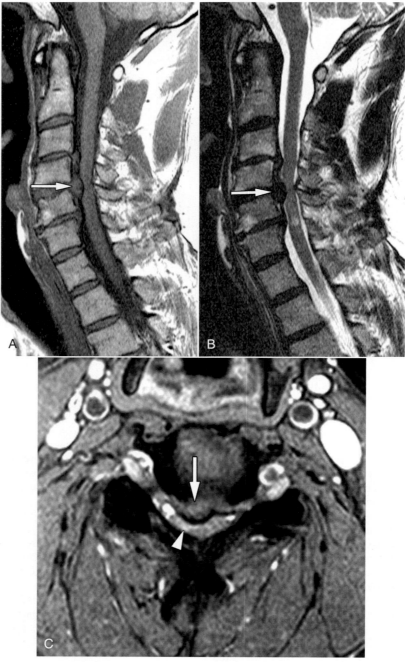

Figure 24-5 ▶ Cervical Disc Herniation, MRI. Sagittal T1 image **A**, sagittal T2 image **B**, and axial gradient recall image **C**. Moderate-sized central/right paramidline disc herniation (*arrow*) is shown. Focus of increased T2 signal in the right side of the cervical cord (*arrowhead,* image **C**) compatible with focus of cord ischemia or myelomalacia.

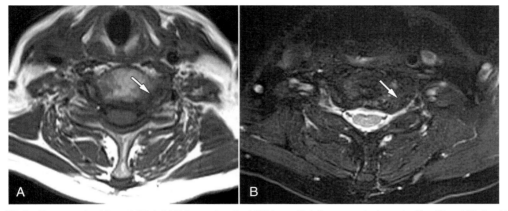

Figure 24-6 ► **Uncovertebral Spur, MRI.** Axial T1 image **A** and axial T2 image **B**. Left uncovertebral spur is of low T1 and T2 signal intensity (*arrow*).

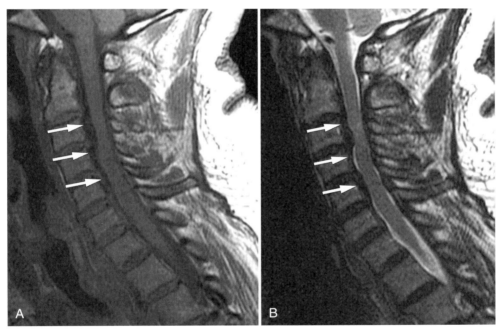

Figure 24-7 ► **Ossification of the Posterior Longitudinal Ligament.** Sagittal T1 image **A** and sagittal T2 image **B** reveal flowing decreased signal intensity along the posterior aspect of the vertebral bodies typically in the midline (*arrows*).

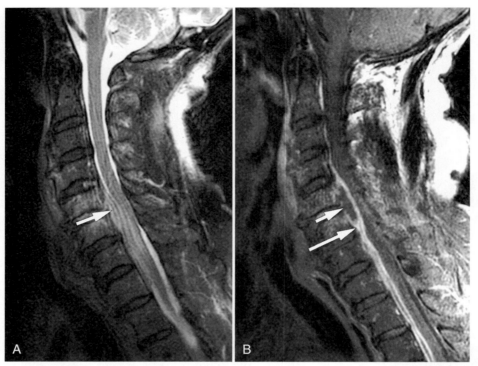

Figure 24-8 ► **Cervical Discitis with Abscess Formation.** Abnormal mixed signal intensity in the ventral epidural space spanning the C5 and C6 vertebral segments (*arrow*) as well as abnormal signal intensity within these vertebral bodies is shown on sagittal T2 image **A**. Post-contrast T1 image **B** shows a nonenhancing abscess cavity (*short arrow*) with surrounding enhancing phlegmon (*long arrow*).

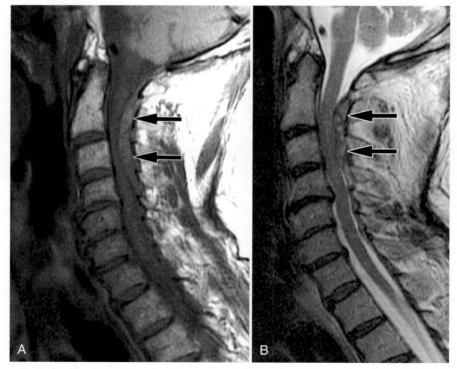

Figure 24-9 ► **Spontaneous Cervical Epidural Hematoma.** Dorsal intermediate T1 (image **A**) and T2 (image **B**) signal intensity epidural mass is shown extending from the skull base to the C4-5 level (*arrows*) causing mass effect with ventral displacement of the cervical spinal cord.

References

1. Radhakrishnan K, Litchy WJ, O'Fallon M, Kurland LT. Epidemiology of cervical radiculopathy: A population-based study from Rochester, Minnesota, 1976 through 1990. *Brain*. 1994;117:325-335.
2. Henderson CM, Hennessy RG, Shuey HM, Shackelford EG: Posterior-lateral foraminotomy as an exclusive operation technique for cervical radiculopathy: A review of 846 consecutively operated cases. *Neurosurgery*. 1983;13: 504-512.
3. Benzon HT. *Essentials of Pain Medicine and Regional Anesthesia*. 2nd ed. Philadelphia: Churchill Livingstone; 2005:350.
4. Kuijper B, Tans JTJ, Schimsheimer RJ, et al. Degenerative cervical radiculopathy: Diagnosis and conservative treatment. A review. *Europ J Neurol*. 2009;16:15-20.
5. Yoss RE, Corbin KB, Maccarty CS, Love JG. Significance of symptoms and signs in localization of involved root in cervical disk protrusion. *Neurology*. 1957;7:673-683.
6. Chirspin AR, Lees F. The spinal canal in cervical spondylosis. *J Neurol Neurosurg Psychiatry*. 1963;26:166-170.
7. Good DF, Couch JR, Wacaser L. Numb, clumsy hands and high cervical spondylosis. *Surg Neurol*. 1984;22:285-291.
8. Abbed KM, Coumans JVCE. Cervical radiculopathy: Pathophysiology, presentation, and clinical evaluation. *Neurosurgery*. 2007;60:S28-S34.
9. Mercer S, Bogduk N. The ligaments and annulus fibrosus of human adult cervical intervertebral discs. *Spine*. 1999;24:619-628.
10. Chen TY. The clinical presentation of uppermost cervical disc protrusion. *Spine*. 2000;25:439-442.
11. Viikari-Juntura E, Porras M, Laasonen EM: Validity of clinical tests in the diagnosis of root compression in cervical disc disease. *Spine*. 1989;14: 253-257.

DISC HERNIATION—THORACIC

Douglas S. Fenton, M.D.

CLINICAL PRESENTATION

The patient is a 75-year-old female who has presented with mid and low back pain and report of numbness and tingling in both legs for the past 4 weeks. The patient was on a three-step ladder putting away some dishes when she lost her balance and fell on her back. She was initially only sore from her fall; however, her back pain did not subside over the next several days, and she began to feel numbness and tingling in both legs that did not change character with a change in position. She has been incontinent of urine twice over the last 2 weeks and feels she is unsteady on her feet.

IMAGING PRESENTATION

Axial and sagittal reformatted computed tomography (CT) images of the thoracic spine demonstrate a calcified mass along a left posterior paramedian midthoracic disc, which impresses the left ventrolateral aspect of the thecal sac and displaces it to the right compatible with a calcified herniated disc (*Fig. 25-1*).

DISCUSSION

Thoracic disc herniations are rare when compared with lumbar and cervical herniations. Most series report an incidence of thoracic disc herniations in less than 2% of all operated discs[1,2] and symptomatic disc herniations composing less than 1% of spinal disc herniations. Autopsy studies have demonstrated an incidence of thoracic disc herniations of 7% to 15%.[3] It has been postulated that the low incidence of thoracic disc herniation is related to the limited mobility of the thoracic spine secondary to the small size of the thoracic discs, the restraint placed on the thoracic spine by the ribs, and the coronal orientation of the thoracic facet joints.[4] Most thoracic disc herniations are reported in the lower thoracic spine, with T11-12 being the most common;[3] 75% of all thoracic disc herniations occur below the T8 level.[3] Most surgical series demonstrate thoracic disc herniations to be central or paramidline and less likely posterolateral or lateral.[3,5,6] Multilevel disc herniations have been reported with an incidence of less than 5% of all patients.[1] Most studies show an equal distribution of thoracic disc herniations between men and women. Degenerative changes are likely the most common cause of thoracic disc herniations.[2]

The role of trauma as a cause of thoracic disc herniations has been widely debated. Most series demonstrate trauma to not be a significant etiology of thoracic disc herniations,[2,6] whereas others disagree and believe that the trauma may have been minor or too far in the past for the patient to recall.[3] One study demonstrated that men under the age of 40 had a 53% incidence of traumatic disc herniation, whereas all others had a 17% rate.[7] This suggests that younger men are a distinct group in regard to incidence of thoracic disc herniation.

Thoracic disc herniations can be difficult to diagnosis clinically because there are a myriad of clinical presentations. Unlike cervical or lumbar disc herniations where pain may be associated with an extremity, thoracic disc herniation pain may have vague symptoms that could easily be confused with cardiac, pulmonary, gastrointestinal, or genitourinary disorders. Patients with a lateral disc herniation at the C7-T1 or T1-2 level may present with Horner's syndrome. A disc herniation in the mid or lower thoracic spine can present as a Brown-Séquard syndrome or anterior spinal artery syndrome. A disc herniation at the thoracolumbar junction could present with a conus medullaris syndrome. Patients have incorrectly had abdominal surgery to alleviate their pain.[4]

However, most often, the patient demonstrates typical signs and symptoms of disc herniation. If the patient has a foraminal or lateral disc herniation, he or she will have back and radicular pain. If the patient has a central disc herniation, he or she may have pyramidal tract signs. The patient may describe decreased sensation over a dermatomal level.[2,3] The patient may demonstrate decreased abdominal and/or anal reflexes.[6]

It is extremely important, in the thoracic region, to make sure the imaging level is well defined. The thoracic spine has no good landmarks, as there are in the cervical or lumbar regions, and therefore a wrong level surgery could occur. It is important to have a sagittal scout image that extends either from C2 through the thoracic spine or a scout image that includes the lumbosacral junction. Although exact counting is preferred, the key is for the surgeon or interventionalist to understand what level(s) the radiologist is describing.

IMAGING FEATURES

Plain film radiography cannot be used to diagnose a thoracic disc herniation; however, radiographs can show intervertebral disc calcification, which is more common in people with thoracic disc herniations than in the normal population.[8] On CT, the disc herniation is often contiguous with the intradiscal calcification (*Fig. 25-2*). Some believe that the intradiscal calcification is

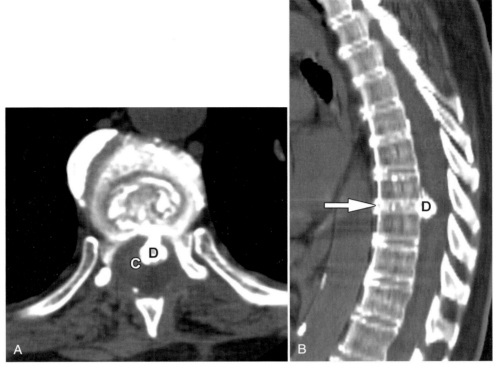

Figure 25-1 ► **Calcified Thoracic Disc Herniation.** Axial CT image **A**, through a midthoracic disc, demonstrates a calcified "mass" (*D*) along the left posterior disc margin compatible with a calcified disc herniation. The spinal cord (*C*) is displaced to the right. Sagittal reformatted image **B** shows the disc herniation (*D*) to be centered on the disc level (*arrow*).

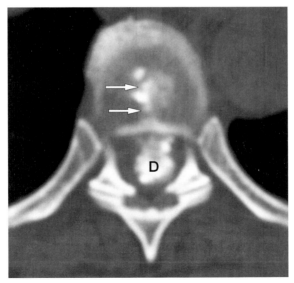

Figure 25-2 ► **Intradiscal Calcification.** Axial CT image through a thoracic disc level. Large calcified disc herniation (*D*) is contiguous with intrinsic disc matrix calcification (*arrows*).

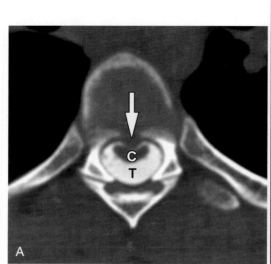 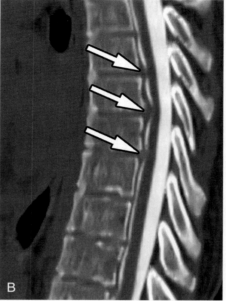

Figure 25-3 ▶ Thoracic Disc Herniations, CT Myelography. Axial CT image **A** and sagittal reformatted image **B**, post-myelography. Small thoracic disc herniations (*arrows*) are readily apparent as extradural defects upon the contrast-filled thecal sac (*T*) and spinal cord (*C*). The degree of compression of the spinal cord and thecal sac is easier to discern when there is contrast in the thecal sac because a disc herniation is low density, and the thecal sac and cord are also low density with routine imaging without myelographic contrast.

calcification along a radial fissure similar to radial fissures seen with lumbar discography. However, a normal thoracic radiograph does not preclude a thoracic disc herniation. Myelography without CT can demonstrate the mass effect that a disc herniation may have on a contrast-filled thecal sac resulting in central spinal stenosis or a nerve root amputation sign secondary to a foraminal soft tissue abnormality; however, the findings on myelography are not specific to disc herniations. Any extradural soft tissue mass can result in similar myelographic findings. Furthermore, myelography is more invasive than either CT or magnetic resonance imaging (MRI). A CT scan after myelography is more sensitive and specific for thoracic disc herniations *(Fig. 25-3)*.

MRI is used more frequently for the evaluation of thoracic disc herniations.[9,10] Although MRI has very high sensitivity for the detection of thoracic disc herniations, it has poor specificity. MRI often finds thoracic disc herniations in asymptomatic patients.[11] The typical MR appearance of a disc herniation is a focal or broad-based region of isointense to hypointense T1-weighted signal intensity that may extend from the parent disc *(Fig. 25-4)*. If the disc herniation is densely calcified, it may be of very low T1 signal and may be difficult to distinguish from the adjacent cerebrospinal fluid (CSF). T2 signal is variable secondary to the hydration state of the disc. Disc material does not demonstrate enhancement; however, there may be peripheral enhancement (so-called *wrapped disc*) from granulation tissue or a dilated epidural plexus.

DIFFERENTIAL DIAGNOSIS

1. **Osteophytes:** These have sharp margins and do not arise from the disc, but rather from the endplates.
2. **Hemorrhage:** More often posterior and elongated and can usually be distinguished by its CT density or variable MR signal intensity.
3. **Abscess/phlegmon:** Often associated with endplate destruction or disc infection *(Fig. 25-5)*.
4. **Neoplasm:** Appears as an irregular or infiltrative mass with homogeneous enhancement. The abnormality arises from bone and the disc is often spared *(Fig. 25-6)*.

TREATMENT

1. **Surgery:** The treatment of choice for symptomatic thoracic disc herniations is surgery. There are several different approaches including transthoracic, transpedicular, transfacet sparing the pedicle, and lateral approaches, each with their specific morbidity and mortality. Surgical failure can occur if the surgery is at the wrong level, if the thoracic cord is injured, or if a migrated fragment is missed.
2. **Conservative management:** If the patient does not have symptoms of myelopathy, then conservative management

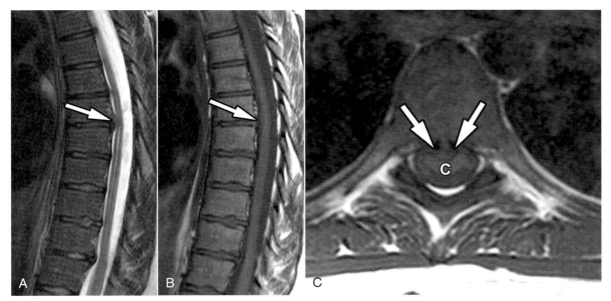

Figure 25-4 ▶ Thoracic Disc Herniations, MRI. Same patient as in Figure 25-3. Sagittal T2-weighted image **A** demonstrates a small, intermediate signal intensity disc herniation (*arrow*) in the midthoracic spine causing mild ventral impression on the thecal sac. This disc herniation is barely perceptible on sagittal T1-weighted image **B** (*arrow*) due to its low signal intensity adjacent to the low signal intensity CSF. The effect of the disc herniation is better appreciated on axial T1-weighted image **C** with the disc hernia-tion (*arrows*) causing extrinsic compression of the spinal cord (*C*).

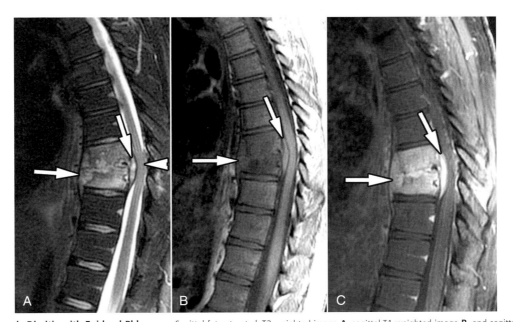

Figure 25-5 ▶ Thoracic Discitis with Epidural Phlegmon. Sagittal fat-saturated, T2-weighted image **A**, sagittal T1-weighted image **B**, and sagittal fat-saturated, post-contrast, T1-weighted image **C**. Diffuse abnormal low T1 signal, increased T2 signal, and enhancement throughout two adjacent thoracic vertebrae and intervening disc are compatible with discitis. There is soft tissue anterior and posterior to the vertebral bodies (*arrows*) compatible with phlegmon. Phlegmon in the ventral epidural space compresses the spinal cord (*arrowhead*, image **A**), which displays subtle increased signal intensity consistent with cord ischemia.

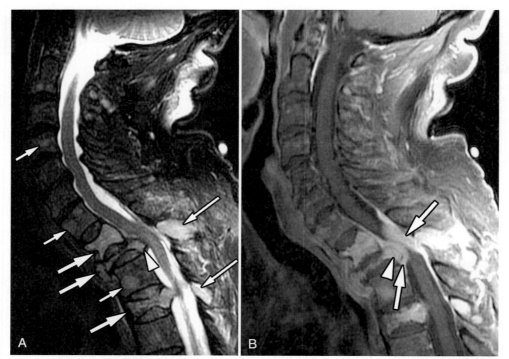

Figure 25-6 ▶ **Neoplasm.** Sagittal fat-saturated, T2-weighted image **A**. Several compressed vertebral bodies with complete marrow replacement (*large arrows*) as well as several ovoid regions of marrow signal intensity (*small short arrows*). Posterior elements are also involved (*small long arrows*). Abnormal epidural soft tissue from collapsed vertebral body (*arrowhead*) compresses the spinal cord. Sagittal fat-saturated, post-contrast, T1-weighted image **B** demonstrates the enhancing retropulsed T2 vertebrae (*arrowhead*) and the abnormal enhancing ventral and dorsal epidural soft tissue (*arrows*).

including physical therapy, activity modification, and anti-inflammatory medication can be attempted.

References

1. Alvarez O, Roque CT, Pampati M. Multilevel thoracic disk herniations: CT and MR studies. *J Comput Assist Tomogr.* 1988;12:649-652.
2. Arce CA, Dorhmann GJ. Thoracic disc herniation: Improved diagnosis with computed tomographic scanning and a review of the literature. *Surg Neurol.* 1985;23:356-361.
3. Arseni C, Nash F. Protrusion of thoracic intervertebral discs. *Acta Neurochir.* 1963;11:3-33.
4. Blumenkopf B. Thoracic intervertebral disc herniations: Diagnostic value of magnetic resonance imaging. *Neurosurgery.* 1988;23:36-40.
5. Albrand OW, Corkill G. Thoracic disc herniation: Treatment and prognosis. *Spine.* 1979;4:41-46.
6. Love JG, Schorn VG. Thoracic-disk protrusions. *JAMA.* 1965;191:627-631.
7. Russell T. Thoracic intervertebral disc protrusion: Experience of 67 cases and review of the literature. *Br J Neurosurg.* 1989;3:153-160.
8. McAllister VL, Sage MR. The radiology of thoracic disc protrusions. *Clin Radiol.* 1976;27:291-299.
9. Francavilla TL, Powers A, Dina T, Rizzoli HV. Case report: MR imaging of thoracic disk herniations. *JCAT.* 1987;11:1062-1065.
10. Ross JS, Perez-Reyes N, Masaryk TJ, et al. Thoracic disk herniation: MR imaging. *Radiology.* 1987;165:511-515.
11. Williams MP, Cherryman GR, Husband JE. Significance of thoracic disc herniation demonstrated by MR imaging. *JCAT.* 1989;13:211-214.

TRAUMATIC DISC HERNIATION—ADOLESCENT

Leo F. Czervionke, M.D.

CLINICAL PRESENTATION

The patient is a 19-year-old college basketball player with a 4-month history of progressively worsening low back pain, radiating into the thoracic region and also into the right buttock and thigh. The pain is not relieved by rest, aspirin, or nonsteroidal anti-inflammatory agents. Back strengthening exercises over the past 6 weeks have not relieved his pain whatsoever. He reports a tingling sensation in both feet when recumbent at night. No lower extremity weakness on examination.

IMAGING PRESENTATION

Magnetic resonance (MR) imaging of the lumbar spine reveals evidence of L4-5 intervertebral disc degeneration and a moderate-sized midline L4-5 disc herniation that causes ventral thecal sac deformity (*Figs. 26-1 and 26-2*). A lumbar spine computed tomography (CT) scan was obtained because of deformity of the posteroinferior corner of the L4 vertebral body and probable avulsion fracture of posterior margin of the L4 vertebral body seen on the MR scan. The CT scan confirms an avulsion fracture of the posteroinferior corner of the L4 vertebral body associated with L4-5 disc herniation (*Figs. 26-3 and 26-4*).

DISCUSSION

In children and adolescents, traumatic disc herniations usually involve the unused ring apophysis. Traumatic disc herniations and ring apophyseal injuries in young persons more commonly occur in the lumbar region, although occasionally they may occur in the cervical or thoracic spine. The injury most commonly involves the inferior rim of the L4 endplate or the superior rim of the S1 endplate (*Figs. 26-1 to 26-8*). Most traumatic herniations in children or adolescents occur in athletes or those who perform activities that subject the spine to repetitive stress.[3] Some have suggested that there may be a congenital insufficiency of the ring apophysis that predisposes one to this injury.[4] Motor vehicle accidents or other acute traumatic events can also damage the ring apophysis.[5]

In normal persons younger than 6 years, the ring apophysis is a cartilaginous ring that develops in an annular depression along the superior and inferior margins of the vertebral body peripherally. The cartilaginous ring apophysis develops separate from the vertebral epiphysis, and this ring may be lacking posteriorly.[6] The outer annular fibers of the intervertebral disc (Sharpey's fibers) and some fibers of both the anterior longitudinal ligament (ALL) and posterior longitudinal ligament (PLL) attach to this cartilaginous ring. Because Sharpey's fibers, the ALL, and the PLL normally exert tractional forces on the ring apophysis, it is sometimes referred to as a *traction apophysis*.[6] The radiolucent cartilaginous ring apophysis begins to calcify at age 6, begins to ossify at age 13, and begins to fuse to the vertebral body at age 17. Complete fusion of the ring apophysis to the vertebral body occurs between the ages of 18 and 20 years.[6] Trauma to the outer discovertebral margin results in accentuation of the traction forces upon the apophyseal ring, which can cause an avulsion fracture, or at the very least, can hamper or prevent fusion of the ossified ring apophysis to the vertebral body.

Alternatively, forced flexion and rotation of the spine can produce radial (shearing) forces that disrupt the ring apophysis.[7-8] This mechanism is believed by some to be the most common mechanism of injury in anterior ring apophysis injury and is most common in athletes, especially gymnasts and wrestlers.[9] This can cause anterior vertebral rim compression deformities of variable size or a tiny triangular-shaped ring apophyseal fragment that are commonly referred to as a *limbus vertebra* (*Figs. 26-9 and 26-10*). These may be located in the lumbar, thoracic, or cervical spine.[3,7] Larger anterior ring apophyseal fragments are more likely to be caused by avulsion of the ring apophysis, and most commonly occur in the lumbar region.[9] These can be produced by traumatic anterior vertebral compression or by anterior disc herniations.

The most common symptom associated with traumatic disc herniation is acute low back pain, although sciatica may also be present. Many conditions in the pediatric patient or young adult can cause back pain including trauma, scoliosis, a degenerative condition, developmental disorder, metabolic derangement, inflammatory spondyloarthropathy, discovertebral infection, and tumors of the spine or spinal cord.[3] Stress injury involving the pars interarticularis with subsequent development of pars interarticularis defects (spondylolysis), and spondylolisthesis is a common cause of back pain in young patients.[10] Paravertebral ligamentous injury or muscle strain can also cause back pain. The presence of back pain in a young person should always initiate a search for the etiology because potentially serious conditions may be the cause of the pain. With traumatic disc herniation in the low thoracic or lumbar region, a cauda equina syndrome may be present resulting in low back pain, sacral pain, or pelvic pain and bladder or bowel dysfunction depending on the location of the disc herniation.

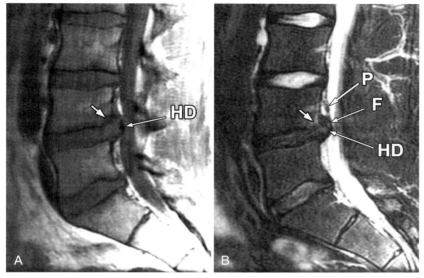

Figure 26-1 ▸ Traumatic Disc Herniation L4-5. 19-year-old basketball player with vertebral apophysis avulsion. A herniated disc (*HD*) at L4-5 is demonstrated on sagittal T1-weighted MR image **A** and sagittal T2-weighted image **B**. Note deformity of the posteroinferior margin of the L4 vertebral body (*small arrow* in image **A** and **B**). Avulsed apophyseal cortical bone fragment (*F*) is T2 hypointense on sagittal T2-weighted image **B**, but difficult to visualize on sagittal T1-weighted image **A**. The posterior longitudinal ligament (*P*) is displaced posteriorly by the avulsed bone fragment. Note diminished intradiscal T2 signal intensity in L4-5 intervertebral disc on image **B**, consistent with disc degeneration.

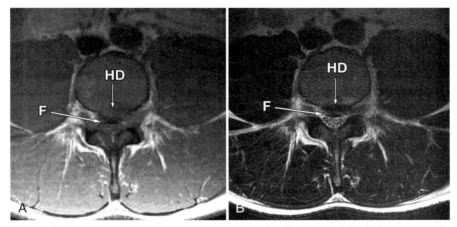

Figure 26-2 ▸ Traumatic Disc Herniation L4-5. Same patient as in Figure 26-1. A focal midline herniated disc (*HD*) causes posterior displacement of a T1 and T2 hypointense bone fragment (*F*) as seen on axial T1-weighted MR image **A** and T2-weighted image **B**. The herniated disc causes ventral effacement of the thecal sac.

IMAGING FEATURES

Radiographs and CT images of the spine are valuable in the detection of acute vertebral fractures, in detection of pars interarticularis defects, for assessment of vertebral alignment, and to evaluate the interspinous distances. Bone trauma in general is best demonstrated with CT. These bone abnormalities may also be visible on MR, which is the procedure of choice for evaluating for possible cord compression, cord contusion, and epidural hematoma. Paraspinal ligamentous disruption is best demonstrated with MR imaging using T2 fat-saturated or short tau inversion recovery (STIR) imaging sequences. Disruption or displacement of the anterior and posterior longitudinal ligaments and disruption of the interspinous ligament is well shown using these imaging techniques.

Apophyseal ring fractures, occurring in older children, adolescents, or young adults, are well demonstrated on CT and MR imaging, but easier to see on CT.[2,11] Posteriorly directed traumatic disc herniations at this age frequently avulse the posterior ring apophysis or posterior corner of the vertebral body, displacing a vertebral marginal bone fragment posteriorly. Posterior ring apophyseal injuries most commonly occur at the L4-5 or L5-S1 level and can involve the adjacent superior or inferior endplate, although most commonly involve the inferior L4 rim or superior

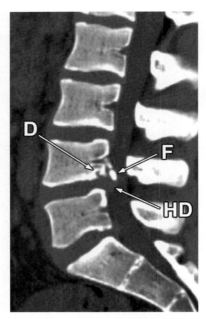

Figure 26-3 ▶ Apophyseal Avulsion Fracture. Same patient as in Figures 26-1 and 26-2. Sagittal CT image confirms presence of apophyseal avulsion fracture. The herniated disc (*HD*) has caused an avulsion fracture (*F*) of the posterior L4 vertebral cortex by disrupting the posteroinferior vertebral apophysis. An irregular vertebral endplate defect (*D*) is demonstrated where the inferior L4 endplate joins the vertebral apophysis.

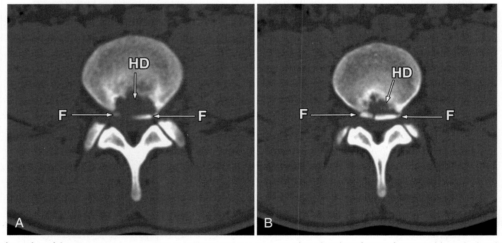

Figure 26-4 ▶ Apophyseal Avulsion Fracture. Same patient as in Figures 26-1 to 26-3. Apophyseal avulsion fracture fragments (*F*) are displaced posteriorly by the herniated disc (*HD*) as demonstrated on contiguous axial CT images **A** and **B** obtained just above the L4-5 intervertebral disc level. Image **B** is slightly superior to image **A**.

S1 rim.[1,2] The displaced bone fragment is hypointense on MR images and hyperdense on CT (see Figs. 26-1 to 26-8). The herniated disc material is T2 hyperintense and interposed between the hypointense vertebral body and the displaced apophyseal rim fragment. In the acute phase, T2 hyperintense marrow edema is often present in the adjacent vertebral body. This is replaced in the later stages of healing by sclerotic bone, which is T1 and T2 hypointense on MRI and hyperdense on CT.

Traumatic injuries to the anterior discovertebral junction in patients under the age of 20 either impede or prevent fusion of the anterior ring apophysis, or cause anterior vertebral marginal avulsion fractures. The tiny anterior avulsion fracture of the unfused anterior apophysis may be nondisplaced or minimally displaced. Anterior apophyseal injuries may involve the superior or inferior vertebral body rim. This can occur secondary to anterior disc herniation[11] but is more commonly due to compressive (axial loading) force or combined flexion and rotational forces upon the anterior ring apophysis.[7] Traumatic apophyseal injuries are believed to be the cause of the so called *limbus vertebra* seen on radiographs,[12] CT, or MRI (see Figs. 26-9 and 26-10). The limbus vertebra classically

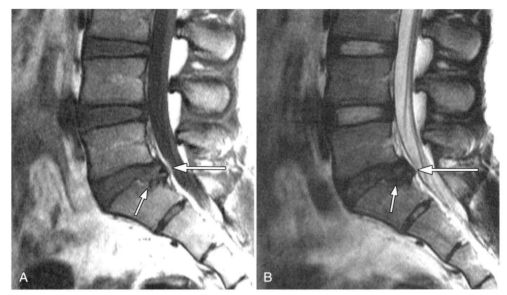

Figure 26-5 ▶ Traumatic Disc Herniation L5-S1. 17-year-old patient actively involved in wrestling and weightlifting. Two-month history of severe low back pain and right leg pain. Traumatic disc herniation (*long arrow*) associated with posterosuperior endplate defect (*short arrow*) is demonstrated on sagittal T1-weighted MR image **A** and T2-weighted image **B**. The disc herniation (*long arrow*) causes mild ventral thecal sac deformity. Diminished intradiscal T2 signal intensity in L5-S1 disc due to disc degeneration is shown in image **B**.

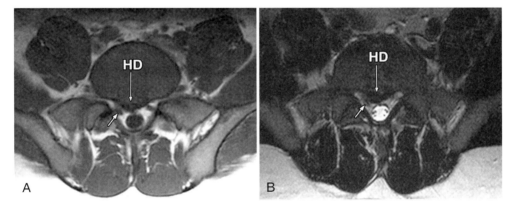

Figure 26-6 ▶ Traumatic Disc Herniation L5-S1. Axial T1-weighted MR image **A** and T2-weighted image **B** in same patient as in Figure 26-5. The focal herniated disc (*HD*) is centered to the right of midline, encroaches on the ventral epidural fat, and causes posterior displacement of right S1 nerve root (*short arrow*).

has a tiny triangular or arcuate fragment of the bone at the anterior margin of the vertebral body in the expected location of the ring apophysis. Limbus vertebrae may be seen in the lumbar, thoracic, or cervical spine *(see Figs. 26-9 to 26-11).*

Anterior discovertebral trauma occurring in young persons can with time produce anterior vertebral endplate depressions that persist into adulthood and are commonly seen on radiographs, CT, or MR images.[13] These anterior vertebral endplate depressions are often referred to as *anterior Schmorl's nodes.*

Occasionally, traumatic disc herniations occur in the cervical or thoracic spine in young persons. In the cervical spine, avulsion of the superior apophysis occurs with hyperflexion injury, whereas hyperextension injury causes avulsion of the inferior ring apophysis.[14] In patients with cervical or thoracic vertebral fractures, the spinal cord should always be carefully evaluated with MR imaging, especially if there is clinical evidence of cord compression. Posterior traumatic disc herniations or associated epidural hematomas commonly cause cord compression. If cord edema is present, this is typically T1 isointense or slightly hypointense and T2 hyperintense. Acute post-traumatic epidural hematomas are slightly T1 hyperintense or have mixed signal intensity on T1- and T2-weighted images. Epidural hematomas usually cause thecal sac deformity and

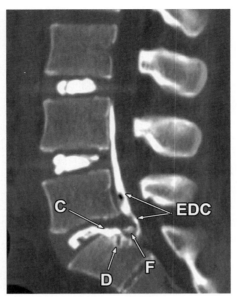

Figure 26-7 ► **Traumatic Disc Herniation L5-S1.** Sagittal post discogram CT in same patient as in Figure 26-6. Following contrast agent (*C*) injected into the L5-S1 intervertebral disc, the patient reported severe low back pain highly concordant with his usual pain in distribution and intensity. The injected intradiscal contrast agent (*C*) extends into the defect (*D*) in the posterior aspect of the superior S1 endplate. A bone fragment (*F*) is displaced from the vertebral apophysis posteriorly. The herniated disc is outlined posteriorly by anterior epidural contrast (*EDC*) that leaked from the intervertebral disc through a fissure in the posterior annulus.

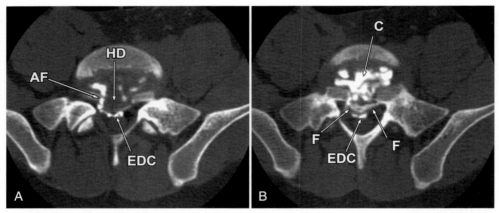

Figure 26-8 ► **Traumatic Disc Herniation L5-S1.** Same patient as in Figure 26-7. Axial post discogram CT image **A** obtained at the disc level and CT image **B** obtained slightly below the disc level. On image **A**, the intradiscal contrast agent extends through a right posterior paramidline annular fissure (*AF*). Epidural contrast (*EDC*) outlines the posterior margin of the herniated disc (*HD*). On image **B**, injected intradiscal contrast (*C*) is demonstrated in the intervertebral disc. Epidural contrast (*EDC*) resides posterior to an arcuate-shaped, bone fragment (*F*) that has been avulsed from the S1 apophyseal region.

possibly cord compression over several vertebral levels. Subacute epidural hematomas are classically T1 and T2 hyperintense.

Discography will define the annular fissures associated with traumatic anterior or posterior disc herniations and confirm whether the injury is symptomatic or not. The injected iodinated contrast agent will extend from the nucleus pulposus through the annular fissure and into the herniated disc fragment between the vertebral body and detached apophyseal ring fragment (see Figs. 26-7 and 26-8).[12,15]

Radionuclide bone scanning can be particularly useful in young patients with back pain if the radiographs, CT, or MR images do not reveal the source of the pain. These imaging studies can also be used to confirm the location of a symptomatic lesion. A focus of increased activity is typically present at the site of the apophyseal injury. Other stress-related injuries of the spine including pars stress fractures or sacral stress fractures may be detected with bone scanning.[16] Discovertebral infection and spine tumors will also display increased uptake on bone scans.

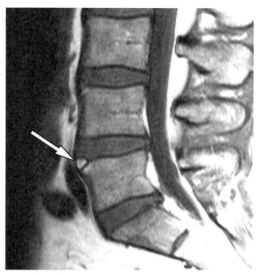

Figure 26-9 ▶ L5 Limbus Vertebra. Sagittal T1-weighted MRI. A corticated triangular-shaped fragment of bone (*arrow*) is located adjacent to the blunted anterosuperior corner of the L5 vertebral body.

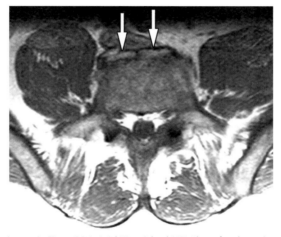

Figure 26-10 ▶ L5 Limbus Vertebra. Same patient as in Figure 26-9. Axial T1-weighted MRI. The unfused anterior apophyseal "fragment" is actually composed of two separate cylindrical fragments of bone (*arrows*).

DIFFERENTIAL DIAGNOSIS

1. **Calcified disc herniation:** The posterior margin of the annulus may calcify and be displaced posteriorly by a disc protrusion. This calcification must be differentiated from an apophyseal region avulsion fracture. In the case of avulsion fracture, an arcuate marginal bone fragment is separated from the vertebral body margin, resulting in a characteristic defect along the corner of the vertebral body. This is best demonstrated with CT.[3]

2. **Posterior vertebral osteophyte:** This may have an appearance similar to a displaced ring apophyseal fragment.

3. **Compression fractures of the anterior vertebral endplate:** These commonly occur in adults after the ring apophysis has fused. The superior endplate is most commonly involved resulting in an anterior vertebral body wedge deformity. This type of fracture can be traumatic in nature at any age or can represent an insufficiency fracture occurring in bone weakened by osteoporosis, radiotherapy, chronic steroid usage, osteomalacia, or some other bone metabolic disturbance.

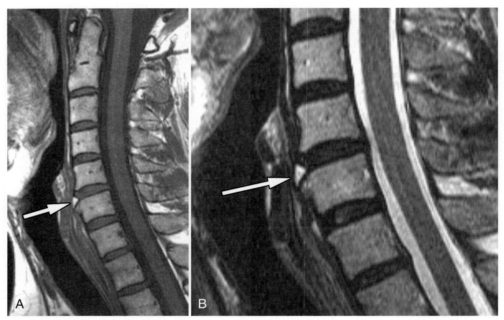

Figure 26-11 ▶ C6 Limbus Vertebra. Sagittal T1-weighted MR image **A** and sagittal T2-weighted image **B**. Sharply marginated triangular-shaped fragment of bone (*arrow* in images **A** and **B**) is associated with blunting of the anterosuperior corner of the C6 vertebral body.

TREATMENT

1. **Posterior traumatic disc herniations:** These injuries associated with displaced apophyseal fragments are usually highly symptomatic and usually do not respond well to conservative therapy. Laminectomy or laminotomy with removal of the herniated disc fragment and displaced bone fragment is the treatment of choice.

2. **Symptomatic anterior discovertebral injuries (limbus vertebra):** Conservative therapy is usually sufficient for these injuries. This includes rest, wearing a back brace during limited activity, and analgesic medications.[17] The back pain usually resolves within a few months.

References

1. Ikata T, Morita T, Katoh S, et al. Lesions of the lumbar posterior end plate in children and adolescents: An MRI study. *J Bone Joint Surg Br.* 1995;77(6):951-955.
2. Epstein NE, Epstein JA. Limbus lumbar vertebral fractures in 27 adolescents and adults. *Spine (Phila Pa 1976).* 1991;16(8):962-966.
3. Khoury NJ, Hourani MH, Arabi MM, et al. Imaging of back pain in children and adolescents. *Curr Probl Diagn Radiol.* 2006;35(6):224-244.
4. Martinez-Lage JF, Poza M, Arcas P. Avulsed lumbar vertebral rim plate in an adolescent: Trauma or malformation? *Childs Nerv Syst.* 1998;14(3):131-134.
5. Talha A, Cronier P, Toulemonde JL, Namour A. Fracture of the vertebral limbus. *Eur Spine J.* 1997;6(5):347-350.
6. Bick EM, Copel JW. The ring apophysis of the human vertebra: Contribution to human osteogeny. II. *J Bone Joint Surg Am.* 1951;33-A(3):783-787.
7. Sward L, Hellstrom M, Jacobsson B, et al. Acute injury of the vertebral ring apophysis and intervertebral disc in adolescent gymnasts. *Spine (Phila Pa 1976).* 1990;15(2):144-148.
8. Roaf R. Spinal injuries. *Burma Med J.* 1960;8:139-143.
9. Sward L, Hellstrom M, Jacobsson B, Karlsson L. Vertebral ring apophysis injury in athletes: Is the etiology different in the thoracic and lumbar spine? *Am J Sports Med.* 1993;21(6):841-845.
10. Morita T, Ikata T, Katoh S, Miyake R. Lumbar spondylolysis in children and adolescents. *J Bone Joint Surg Br.* 1995;77(4):620-625.
11. Banerian KG, Wang AM, Samberg LC, et al. Association of vertebral endplate fracture with pediatric lumbar intervertebral disk herniation: Value of CT and MR imaging. *Radiology.* 1990;177(3):763-765.
12. Ghelman B, Freiberger RH. The limbus vertebra: an anterior disc herniation demonstrated by discography. *AJR Am J Roentgenol.* 1976;127(5):854-855.
13. Henales V, Hervas JA, Lopez P, et al. Intervertebral disc herniations (limbus vertebrae) in pediatric patients: report of 15 cases. *Pediatr Radiol.* 1993;23(8):608-610.
14. Jonsson K, Niklasson J, Josefsson PO. Avulsion of the cervical spinal ring apophyses: Acute and chronic appearance. *Skeletal Radiol.* 1991;20(3):207-210.
15. Goldman AB, Ghelman B, Doherty J. Posterior limbus vertebrae: A cause of radiating back pain in adolescents and young adults. *Skeletal Radiol.* 1990;19(7):501-507.
16. Connolly LP, Drubach LA, Connolly SA, Treves ST. Young athletes with low back pain: Skeletal scintigraphy of conditions other than pars interarticularis stress. *Clin Nucl Med.* 2004;29(11):689-693.
17. Curtis C, d'Hemecourt P. Diagnosis and management of back pain in adolescents. *Adolesc Med State Art Rev.* 2007;18(1):140-164, x.

TRAUMATIC DISC HERNIATION—ADULT

Leo F. Czervionke, M.D.

CLINICAL PRESENTATION

The patient is a 38-year-old man who was thrown from a motorcycle during a motor vehicle collision and presented in the emergency department with severe neck pain, right upper extremity pain, and bilateral lower and upper extremity weakness, right more than left. Bowel and bladder function are intact.

IMAGING PRESENTATION

Radiographs and computed tomography (CT) scan (not shown) demonstrated anterior subluxation of C4 vertebral body on C5, widening of C4-5 intervertebral disc space posteriorly, and bilaterally subluxed C4 facets relative to C5. Magnetic resonance (MR) imaging confirms C4 on C5 subluxation and further reveals traumatic disc herniation compressing the spinal cord at the C4-5 level, right more than left (*Figs. 27-1 to 27-3*).

DISCUSSION

The vast majority of disc herniations in adults cannot be related to a specific traumatic episode. A traumatic disc herniation is one that occurs with a traumatic event. Most traumatic herniations are diagnosed in the acute post-traumatic setting with MR imaging. Commonly associated injuries include vertebral fracture, vertebral subluxation, epidural hematoma, traumatic cord compression, cord contusion, and paraspinal ligamentous disruption. Concomitant brain contusions or intracranial hemorrhage may also be present.

Herniated discs commonly occur with acute cervical spine trauma. In one series, traumatic disc herniations were demonstrated by MR imaging in 42% of patients with acute cervical spine trauma.[1] In the same series, traumatic disc herniations occurred in 80% of patients presenting with bilateral locked facets and 100% of patients with anterior cord syndrome.[1] In adults, traumatic disc herniations most commonly occur in the cervical spine but also occur in the thoracic or lumbar spine.

Most believe traumatic disc herniations occur because of excessive mechanical force on the disc. During normal axial loading, the normal nucleus and inner annulus is compressed slightly in the craniocaudal dimension, which in turn causes an increase in radially directed (shear) force, which causes slight circumferential annular expansion. Sharpey's outer annular fibers, composed of dense type II collagen, resist these outward shear forces. When traumatic compressive, rotational, or radial forces are exerted upon the spine and intervertebral discs, the shear force upon the annulus is likely far greater than normal and the annulus ruptures allowing nuclear and inner annular tissue to escape into the anterior epidural space or neural foramen. Pre-existing internal disc derangement, such as degenerative annular fissures, likely renders the disk more susceptible to herniation when the intervertebral disc is subjected to traumatic axial loading (compressive) forces or radial (shear) forces.

Small traumatic disc herniation may or may not be symptomatic. However, the vast majority of traumatic disc herniations are symptomatic. Commonly, the patient has neck or low back pain and often radicular pain depending on the location of the disc herniation. In one series of patients with symptomatic traumatic disc herniations, 63% had radiculopathy, 30% had both radiculopathy and myelopathy, and 7% had only myelopathy.[2]

Cervical hyperflexion or hyperextension injuries may cause traumatic disc herniations (*Figs. 27-4 and 27-5*).[3,4] Traumatic disc herniations may occur with or without vertebral fractures (*Figs. 27-6 to 27-8*). If the traumatic disc fragment is large and compresses the cord, or if there is an associated epidural hematoma, there is a high incidence of anterior cord syndrome resulting from compression of the anterior spinal artery. The anterior spinal artery supplies the anterior two thirds of the spinal cord so a large portion of the anterior spinal cord is at risk for traumatic or ischemic injury. In anterior cord syndrome, the patient experiences considerable weakness if the anterior horns are involved. Pain and temperature sensation may be disturbed. Dorsal column function including fine touch and proprioception are often intact.

Acute central cord syndrome is most commonly associated with hyperextension injury in the cervical spine and is the most common syndrome associated with incomplete injury to the spinal cord. Acute central cord syndrome is more common in patients with advanced cervical spondylosis deformans and may occur with or without traumatic disc herniation. The cervical cord typically becomes compressed between a posterior vertebral osteophytic ridge and/or traumatic disc herniation anteriorly and a thickened or buckled ligamentum flavum posteriorly (*Fig. 27-9*).[5] The central cord syndrome is characterized by disproportionately greater upper than lower extremity weakness, bladder dysfunction, and varying degrees of sensory loss below the level of injury.[5]

If the traumatic disc herniation is off midline and injures the right or left half of the cord, a Brown-Séquard syndrome may

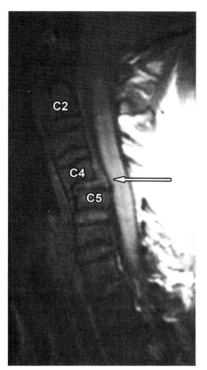

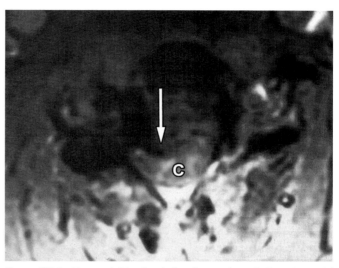

Figure 27-2 ▶ Traumatic Disc Herniation. Same patient as in Figure 27-1. Axial gradient echo image at C4-5 intervertebral disc level. The herniated disc causes (*arrow*) causes spinal cord (*C*) compression anteriorly on the right.

Figure 27-1 ▶ Traumatic Disc Herniation. A herniated disc (*arrow*) extends posterior to anteriorly subluxed C4 vertebra on sagittal T1-weighted image. The herniated disc causes mild cord compression. The adjacent cervical cord is mildly enlarged. Note narrowing of anterior portion of C4-5 intervertebral disc space. C2 = C2 vertebral body.

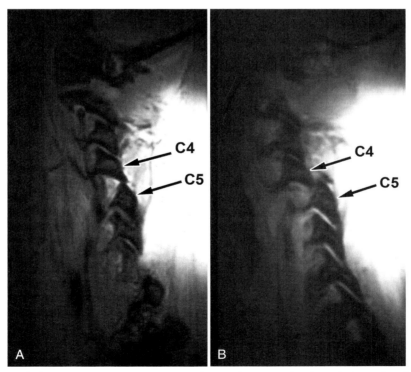

Figure 27-3 ▶ Traumatic Disc Herniation. Same patient as in Figures 27-1 and 27-2. Left parasagittal gradient echo image through left articular pillars (image **A**) and right articular pillars (image **B**). The left C4 articular pillar is anteriorly subluxed and the C4 inferior facet is "perched" on top of the C5 superior facet in image **A**. The right C4 articular pillar is anteriorly dislocated and the inferior C4 facet is "locked" anterior to the right superior C5 facet.

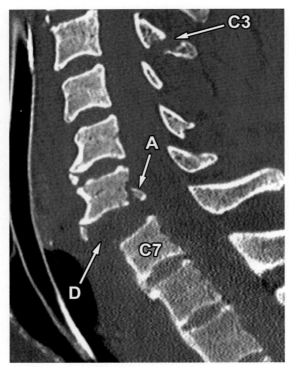

Figure 27-4 ▶ 62-year-old male near-drowning victim who suffered hypoxic ische-mic brain injury and multiple cervical spine fracture while body surfing in the ocean. Sagittal CT image. The C6-7 intervertebral disc (*D*) is disrupted resulting in widening of the C6-7 intervertebral disc space. The C6 vertebral body is anteriorly subluxed relative to C7. A posteroinferior vertebral body apophyseal (*A*) avulsion fracture is demonstrated. Note fracture of C3 posterior spinous process and apparent disruptions of anterior C5-6 and C6-7 osteophytes. C7 = C7 vertebral body.

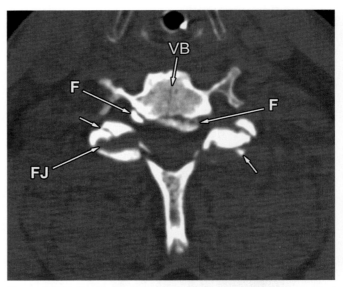

Figure 27-5 ▶ **Facet Joint Disruption and Vertebral Fractures.** Same patient as shown in Figure 27-4. Axial CT images at inferior C6 vertebral body level. Posterior apophyseal avulsion fractures (*F*) and bilateral facet fractures (*small arrows*) are shown. The right C6-7 facet joint is widened due to disruption of the facet joint. Note tiny sagittal nondisplaced fracture through inferior C6 vertebral body (*VB*).

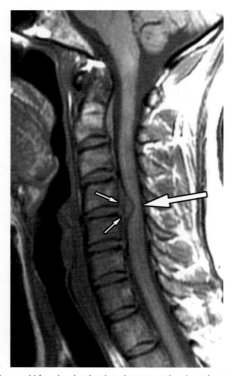

Figure 27-6 ▶ **Traumatic Disc Herniation, C4-5.** 36-year-old female who developed severe neck pain and acute myelopathy immediately following chiropractic manipula-tion. Sagittal T1-weighted image demonstrates a large herniated disc (*small arrows*) at the C4-5 level causing cord compression (*large arrow*).

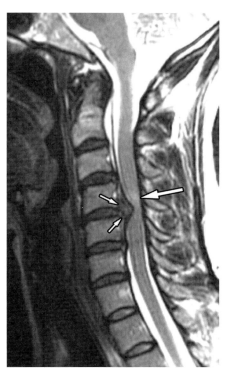

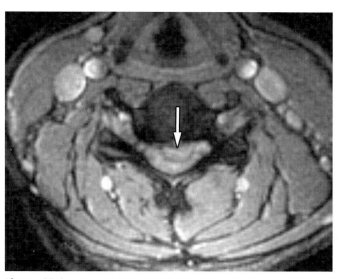

Figure 27-8 ▶ Traumatic Disc Herniation, C4-5. Same patient as in Figures 27-6 and 27-7. Axial gradient echo image at C4-5 level. A large, focal, relatively hyperintense disc fragment (*arrow*) is centered to the left of midline and causes severe cord compression.

Figure 27-7 ▶ Traumatic Disc Herniation, C4-5. Same patient as in Figure 27-6. Sagittal T2-weighted image reveals large C4-5 disc herniation (*small arrows*) which causes cord compression and T2 hyperintense edema (*large arrow*) in the spinal cord at the C4 level.

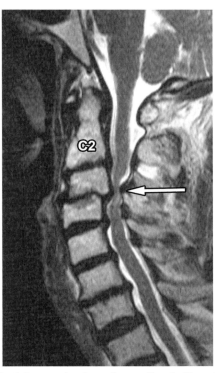

Figure 27-9 ▶ Severe Central Canal Stenosis and Cord Compression Secondary to Chronic C3 on C4 Traumatic or Degenerative Subluxation. The spinal cord surface anteriorly is deformed due to C3 retrolisthesis relative to C4, C3-4 bulging disc and thickened posterior longitudinal ligament. Posterior thecal sac impingement secondary to ligamentum flavum buckling and thickening (*arrow*). C2 = C2 vertebral body.

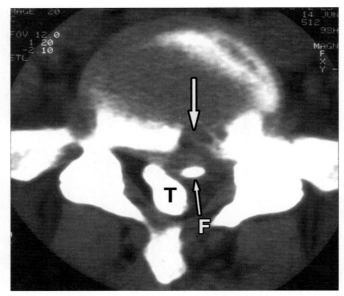

Figure 27-10 ▶ Avulsion Fracture, Traumatic Disc Herniation L5-1. Axial post myelogram CT image at L5-S1 level in patient with acute left lower extremity pain immediately after a fall from height. Left posterior disc herniation causes deformity of anterolateral margin of the contrast filled thecal sac (*T*). The acute traumatic disc herniation has disrupted the posterior vertebral body margin (*long arrow*) causing displacement of a vertebral bone fragment (*F*) posteriorly.

result, including ipsilateral weakness and loss of touch sensation and contralateral loss of temperature and pain sensation. The presenting symptoms may include features of both anterior cord syndrome and Brown-Séquard syndrome.

Traumatic disc herniations may also occur in the thoracic or lumbar spine. For example, acute lumbar hyperflexion injuries with lumbosacral dislocation may be associated with traumatic lumbar disc herniation (*Fig. 27-10*).[6] With traumatic disc herniation in the low thoracic or lumbar region, a cauda equina syndrome may be present resulting in low back pain, sacral pain or pelvic pain, and bladder or bowel dysfunction depending on the location of the disc herniation.

IMAGING FEATURES

CT has replaced plain radiography as the procedure of choice for detecting and evaluating acute vertebral fractures, to assess vertebral alignment, bilateral articular pillar alignment, and to evaluate the interspinous distances. Special attention should be given to the relationship of the articular facets, because facet subluxation or dislocation may be present (see Figs. 27-2 and 27-3). If there is widening of the interspinous space, this suggests possible disruption of the interspinous ligament, and this should be confirmed with MR imaging. Herniated discs are not visible on plain radiographs of the spine but may be evident on CT images as a slightly hyperdense focal soft tissue density at the disc level causing deformity of the thecal sac. If there is evidence of traumatic disc herniation by CT, MR imaging should be obtained to confirm this diagnosis and to evaluate the spinal cord and paraspinal ligaments.

Bony trauma is best demonstrated with CT but also may be well demonstrated on MR imaging including vertebral fractures, vertebral subluxation, and facet subluxation/dislocation. Furthermore, MR is the procedure of choice for evaluating soft tissue injuries associated with the spine including traumatic disc herniation, cord

compression, cord contusion, and epidural hematoma (see Figs. 27-1, 27-2, and 27-6 to 27-9).[7] Paraspinal ligamentous disruption or ligamentous separation from the vertebral body (ligamentous "stripping") are best demonstrated with MR imaging using fat-saturated, T2-weighted images, short tau inversion recovery (STIR) imaging or gradient-echo imaging (*Fig. 27-11*).[8] The anterior and/or posterior longitudinal ligaments or the interspinous ligaments may be involved.

MRI is the modality of choice for detecting all types of disc herniations, including traumatic disc herniations, and for assessing the extent of the displaced disc fragment and its effect upon adjacent structures such as the nerve roots or spinal cord. Traumatic disc herniations are well demonstrated with MR and often have the same appearance as nontraumatic disc herniations. Herniated discs are focal contour abnormalities, where the disc margin extends beyond the margin of the annulus, but involve less than one quarter of the disc circumference (less than 90%) (see Figs. 27-6 to 27-8). Herniated discs are said to be *disc extrusions* if they have a relatively narrow neck on axial or sagittal images, or disc protrusions if they have a wider neck. Herniated discs of all types are usually slightly T1 hyperintense and T2 hypointense relative to the thecal sac, although the signal intensity characteristics can vary.

The spinal cord should be carefully evaluated for possible cord compression or intrinsic signal abnormalities in patients with spine trauma (see Figs. 27-6 to 27-8). Cord edema may be seen with traumatic disc herniation. Cord edema is visible on the T2-weighted images as a region of increased signal intensity in the cord, with or without cord swelling (see Fig. 27-7). Cord edema is not usually seen on T1-weighted images (see Fig. 27-6).[2]

Acute post-traumatic epidural hematomas may accompany traumatic disc herniations, sometimes obscuring the herniated disc fragment. Epidural hematomas are slightly hyperintense or of mixed intensity on T1- and T2-weighted images, and usually cause thecal sac deformity and possibly cord compression over several vertebral levels. Subacute epidural hematomas are classically T1 and T2 hyperintense (*Fig. 27-12*).

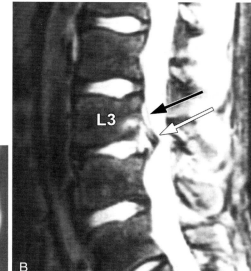
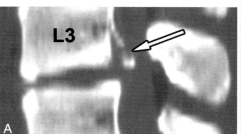

Figure 27-11 ▶ Traumatic Disc Herniation, Vertebral Avulsion Fracture. Sagittal CT reformatted image **A** in a patient with posterior traumatic disc herniation at L3-4 level. Avulsion fracture fragment (*arrow*) in apophyseal region caused by the herniated disc. On corresponding sagittal gradient echo MR image **B**. The vertebral fragment (*white arrow*) is hypointense and the posterior longitudinal ligament (*black arrow*) has been "stripped" from the L3 vertebral body margin.

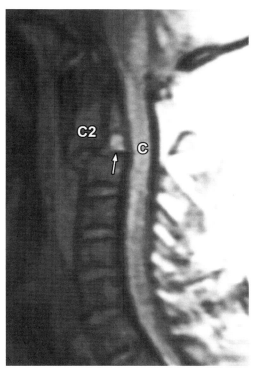

Figure 27-12 ▶ Hangman's Fracture, Traumatic Disc Herniation C2-3. Sagittal T1-weighted MR image. The C2 vertebral body is subluxed 60% anteriorly relative to C3. Hyperintense tissue (*arrow*) behind C2 vertebral body likely represents small subacute hematoma in or adjacent to posterior C2-3 intervertebral disc fragment. Minimal associated anterior deformity of the spinal cord (*C*) deformity at C2-3 level.

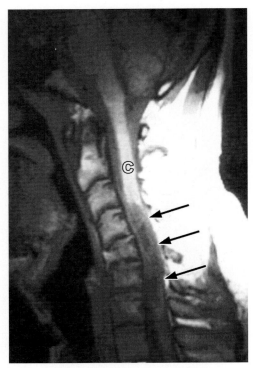

Figure 27-13 ► Chronic Post Traumatic Cervical Spinal Cord Myelomalacia Following Old C5 Vertebral Fracture. Extensive region of spinal myelomalacia (*arrows*) is T1 hypointense relative to the normal spinal cord (*C*) on this sagittal T1-weighted MRI.

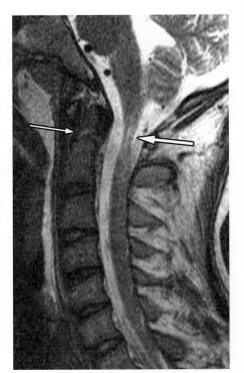

Figure 27-14 ► Chronic Post-Traumatic Localized Cervical Spinal Cord Atrophy and Myelomalacia. Atrophic, myelomalacic spinal cord (*large thick arrow*) at C1-2 level is secondary to old C2 odontoid fracture is demonstrated on this sagittal T2-weighted MR image. The cord myelomalacia at the C1-2 level is T2 hyperintense. The odontoid fracture line (*small thin arrow*) is still visible as a subtle region of T2 hyperintensity at the base of the odontoid process.

Chronic cord compression secondary to chronic disc herniation or chronic vertebral fracture-subluxation often results in spinal cord myelomalacia and atrophy. Post-traumatic spinal cord myelomalacia is heterogeneous but predominantly hypointense on T2-weighted images and hyperintense on T2-weighted images (*Figs. 27-13 and 27-14*).

DIFFERENTIAL DIAGNOSIS

1. **Disc herniation:** A disc herniation, unrelated to trauma, may have an identical appearance on MR and CT as a traumatic disc herniation and can also cause acute myelopathy or paraplegia.[9,10] Acute myelopathy in the setting of acute trauma with presence of bilateral locked facets or anterior cord syndrome is highly suggestive of a traumatic disc herniation.[1]
2. **Nontraumatic epidural hematoma, abscess, or tumor:** These all may have a similar appearance as traumatic epidural hematoma.

TREATMENT

There are differing opinions as to how patients with traumatic disc herniations should be managed.

1. **Conservative therapy:** Some prefer a conservative approach to cervical spine injuries, using closed traction reduction to reduce vertebral subluxations in cervical spine trauma. However, closed cervical traction with a halo should be used with great caution, because traction can accentuate or produce cord compression after traumatic disc herniation or vertebral fracture-subluxation.[5,11,12]
2. **Surgical Decompression:** Surgery may be necessary to alleviate cord compression. This approach is preferred if there is significant cord compression secondary to a traumatic disc herniation causing anterior or central cord syndrome.[5] Anterior discectomy without bone fusion is the preferred method of treatment by some.[2] If the traumatic herniation occurs with facet dislocation, anterior discectomy and fusion is the preferred method of treatment.[12]
3. **Evacuation:** Associated epidural hematomas causing cord compression are usually evacuated to alleviate cord compression
4. **Fusion:** Surgical stabilization by fusion is usually required if unstable fractures are present.

References

1. Rizzolo SJ, Piazza MR, Cotler JM, et al. Intervertebral disc injury complicating cervical spine trauma. *Spine (Phila Pa 1976)*. 1991;16(6 Suppl): S187-S189.
2. Bucciero A, Carangelo B, Cerillo A, et al. Myeloradicular damage in traumatic cervical disc herniation. *J Neurosurg Sci*. 1998;42(4):203-211.
3. Hayes KC, Askes HK, Kakulas BA. Retropulsion of intervertebral discs associated with traumatic hyperextension of the cervical spine and absence of vertebral fracture: An uncommon mechanism of spinal cord injury. *Spinal Cord*. 2002;40(10):544-547.

4. Marar BC. Hyperextension injuries of the cervical spine: The pathogenesis of damage to the spinal cord. *J Bone Joint Surg Am.* 1974;56(8):1655-1662.
5. Dai L, Jia L. Central cord injury complicating acute cervical disc herniation in trauma. *Spine.* 2000;25(3):331-335; discussion 6.
6. Tohme-Noun C, Rillardon L, Krainik A, et al. Imaging features of traumatic dislocation of the lumbosacral joint associated with disc herniation. *Skeletal Radiol.* 2003;32(6):360-363.
7. Katzberg RW, Benedetti PF, Drake CM, et al. Acute cervical spine injuries: prospective MR imaging assessment at a level 1 trauma center. *Radiology.* 1999;213(1):203-212.
8. Benedetti PF, Fahr LM, Kuhns LR, Hayman LA. MR imaging findings in spinal ligamentous injury. *AJR Am J Roentgenol.* 2000;175(3):661-665.
9. Song KJ, Lee KB. Non-traumatic acute myelopathy due to cervical disc herniation in contiguous two-level disc spaces: A case report. *Eur Spine J.* 2005;14(7):694-697.
10. Ueyama T, Tamaki N, Kondoh T, et al. Non-traumatic acute paraplegia associated with cervical disc herniation: A case report. *Surg Neurol.* 1999;52(2):204-206; discussion 6-7.
11. Vaccaro AR, Falatyn SP, Flanders AE, et al. Magnetic resonance evaluation of the intervertebral disc, spinal ligaments, and spinal cord before and after closed traction reduction of cervical spine dislocations. *Spine.* 1999;24(12):1210-1217.
12. Doran SE, Papadopoulos SM, Ducker TB, Lillehei KO. Magnetic resonance imaging documentation of coexistent traumatic locked facets of the cervical spine and disc herniation. *J Neurosurg.* 1993;79(3):341-345.

EPIDURAL ABSCESS

Leo F. Czervionke, M.D.

CLINICAL PRESENTATION

The patient is a 51-year-old male with 3-week history of mid back pain with radiation initially to the right side, but more recently the pain has migrated to the left side. The pain is moderate to severe in intensity. He has become weak in the legs in the past 36 hours, and over the past 12 hours he has become unable to move his lower extremities. He has no bladder or bowel dysfunction. The patient has a sensory deficit (absent pin prick sensation) at and below the T6 level. He has had intermittent fever for the past 3 weeks. Blood cultures confirmed presence of methicillin-resistant *Staphylococcus aureus* (MRSA) septicemia.

IMAGING PRESENTATION

Magnetic resonance (MR) imaging revealed a fusiform right posterolateral epidural fluid collection with peripheral enhancement, extending from the T6 to T8 level *(Figs. 28-1 to 28-3)*. The MR appearance is consistent with epidural abscess. The abscess is displacing the spinal cord anteriorly and to the left (see Fig. 28-2). A decompressive laminectomy was performed from T6 to T8 levels to débride and evacuate the thoracic epidural abscess. The patient was placed on intravenous antibiotics for 6 weeks, which was administered via a peripherally inserted central catheter (PICC) line.

DISCUSSION

Spinal epidural abscess (epidural empyema) is an infection in the epidural space. This begins as a phlegmon that cavitates and fills with infectious liquid and necrotic debris. These abscesses most commonly arise in the anterior epidural space in the lower thoracic or lumbar region secondary to disc space infection and vertebral osteomyelitis (spondylodiscitis). Epidural abscess may also occur in the cervical or upper thoracic spinal canal secondary to spondylodiscitis or hematogenous dissemination *(Figs. 28-4 and 28-5)*.[1,2] Cervical epidural abscesses more commonly occur in the anterior epidural space, whereas thoracic epidural abscesses more commonly arise posteriorly (see Figs. 28-1 to 28-3).

Anterior epidural abscesses associated with spondylodiscitis are usually centered at an intervertebral disc level, but may extend over one to several vertebral levels.[3] Posterior epidural abscesses occur by direct extension from paraspinal infections, hematogenous spread, or via the paravertebral venous plexus *(Figs. 28-6 and 28-7)*. Posterior epidural abscesses may occur by direct extension after surgery, spinal anesthesia, or percutaneous spinal injections.[4,5] Anterior or posterior epidural abscesses may arise from infections in the oral cavity, neck soft tissues, lungs, gastrointestinal (GI) tract (diverticulitis), genitourinary (GU) tract (bladder infection or pyelonephritis), from endocarditis, or secondary to septicemia. Spinal epidural infections may disseminate through the spinal canal diffusely along the leptomeninges.

Epidural abscess may occur at any age, but is more common in the older age groups. Diabetics, patients with chronic renal failure, other chronically ill patients, IV drug abusers, chronic alcoholics, and immunocompromised patients, including patients receiving steroid therapy and patients with HIV infection, have an increased incidence of developing spinal infections.[4-6] Patients often present with acute or subacute onset of back pain and usually fever. Symptoms of myelopathy are present if cord compression exists or if the infection has spread to the spinal cord. Bowel/bladder dysfunction may be present if the abscess is located in the lower thoracic or lumbar region, because of compression of the conus medullaris or cauda equina. The ESR (erythrocyte sedimentation rate) and C-reactive protein and white blood cell count are usually elevated. The patient may develop hyponatremia.[7]

Paraparesis and paralysis may be manifesting clinical findings or may develop if the cord compression is not alleviated by surgical evacuation of the epidural abscess in timely fashion. Children with epidural abscess have a better prognosis than older patients. Prognosis is dependent upon the degree of the clinical onset of symptoms, length of symptoms, whether or not cord compression exists, and length of time between diagnosis and surgical evacuation of the abscess. Persistent neurologic deficit or death may occur if there is a delay in surgical decompression.

The most common pathogens causing epidural abscess are *Staphylococcus aureus* followed by *Mycobacterium tuberculosis*, which recently has been seen with increasing frequency.[1,3,6] Gram-negative bacilli may also be the cause of the abscess and should be considered if the patient has diabetes, a urinary tract infection, diverticulitis, an aortic graft, or gram-negative sepsis. Granulomatous spine infections can be caused by tuberculosis, *Brucella*, *Salmonella*, and fungal organisms. Fungal infections are more common in immunocompromised patients, in diabetics, alcoholics, or those suffering from other chronically debilitating disease.[3,6] The most common fungal organisms causing spine infections are *Candida albicans* and *Aspergillus*.[5] Spinal echinococcosis (hydatid disease)

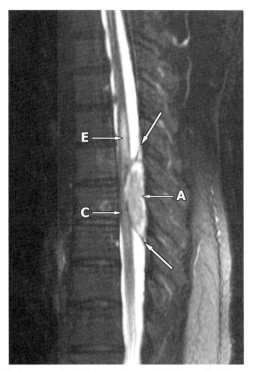

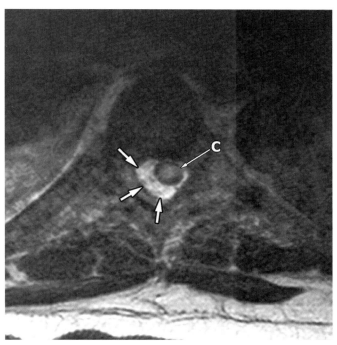

Figure 28-1 ►Posterior Epidural Abscess, Mid-Thoracic Spine. Sagittal fat saturated T2-weighted image. The abscess (A) is predominantly T2 hypointense centrally with surrounding fluid. The dura (*obliquely oriented arrows*) is displaced anteriorly by the posterior epidural abscess. The spinal cord (C) is displaced anteriorly and contains T2 hyperintense edema (E).

Figure 28-2 ►Posterior Epidural Abscess, Mid-Thoracic Spine. Same patient as in Figure 28-1. The epidural abscess (*arrows*) is predominantly T2 hyperintense on axial gradient echo image. The abscess displaces the spinal cord (C) anteriorly and to the left.

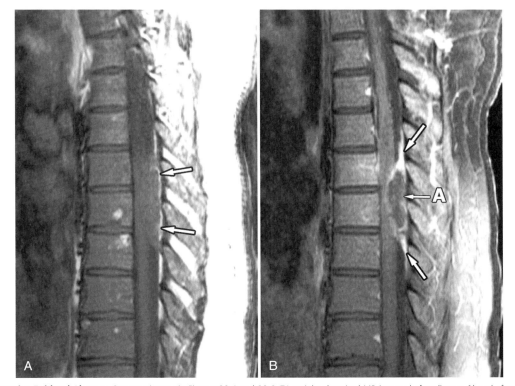

Figure 28-3 ►Posterior Epidural Abscess. Same patient as in Figures 28-1 and 28-2. T1-weighted sagittal MR images before (image **A**) and after (image **B**) IV contrast administration. The abscess is T1 isointense (*arrows in image* **A**) with respect to the spinal cord and displaces the cord anteriorly. In image **B**, the abscess (A) does not enhance centrally but enhances at its margin. There is also enhancement in the adjacent epidural space and dura (*arrows*).

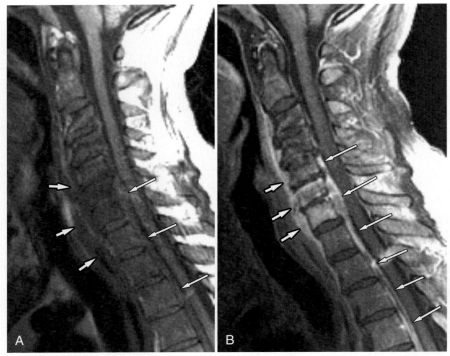

Figure 28-4 ▶ **C6-7 Discitis, Osteomyelitis, and Anterior Paraspinal Phlegmon.** On sagittal T1-weighted MR image **A**, the prevertebral phlegmon (*short arrows*) and anterior epidural phlegmon (*long arrows*) are relatively isointense compared to the spinal cord. On sagittal contrast-enhanced image **B**, the prevertebral phlegmon (*short arrows*) enhances diffusely. The enhancing anterior epidural phlegmon (*long arrows*) extends inferiorly into the upper thoracic anterior epidural space, displacing the spinal cord posteriorly.

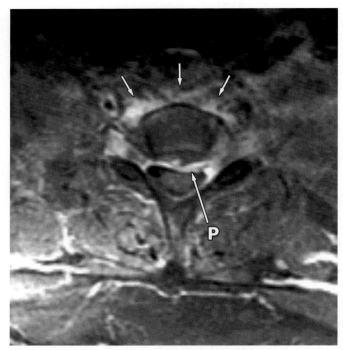

Figure 28-5 ▶ **C6-7 Discitis, Osteomyelitis, and Anterior Paraspinal Phlegmon.** Axial contrast enhanced image at C6-7 level. The phlegmon (*P*) in the anterior epidural space deforms the ventral aspect of the thecal sac and spinal cord. The anterior paraspinal phlegmonous tissue displays ill defined enhancement (*short arrows*).

is a rare manifestation of this parasitic disease that can cause vertebral, paraspinal, intradural, or epidural infection.[6]

IMAGING FEATURES

Paraspinal or psoas abscesses most commonly occur by direct extension from spinal infections but can occur secondary to hematogenous spread from infections elsewhere in the body (see Fig. 28-7, *B*). The presence of a psoas abscess should raise concern of a mycobacterial infection, because the majority of patients with tuberculous or atypical mycobacterial spinal infections develop a paraspinal or psoas abscess. However, psoas or paraspinal abscesses can be produced by other organisms including *Staphylococcus aureus* (*Fig. 28-8*), *Escherichia coli*, other gram-negative bacilli, and fungi. Fungal paraspinal or psoas abscesses are more common in immunocompromised patients. The presence of a calcification in or adjacent to the abscess is characteristic of tuberculous abscess.

With anterior epidural abscesses, on radiographs and computed tomography (CT) images, there are usually classic findings of discitis/osteomyelitis with indistinct or destroyed adjacent vertebral endplates and often reduction in vertebral stature.[1,6] The anterior epidural abscess may spread into the posterior epidural space (see Figs. 28-6 and 28-7). An epidural soft tissue mass may be visible on plain CT images as a relatively hyperdense region in the epidural space.[4]

MR imaging is now the procedure of choice for imaging spinal infections. MR imaging should be performed using fat saturation techniques with T2-weighted images or T1-weighted images after IV contrast enhancement with paramagnetic agents. Short tau

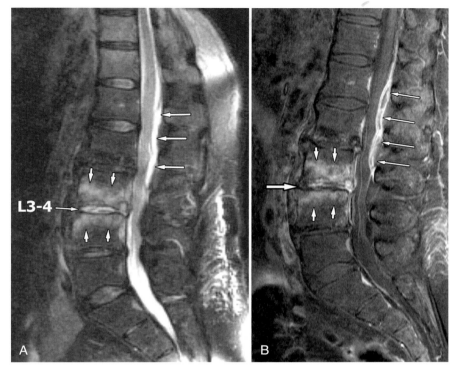

Figure 28-6 ▸ L3-4 Discitis, Osteomyelitis, Paraspinal Phlegmon, and Posterior Epidural Abscess. Infecting organism *Streptococcus viridans*. On unenhanced T2-weighted image **A**, the fluid and inflammation in the L3-4 disc is T2 hyperintense. The adjacent vertebral marrow edema and inflammation is T2 hyperintense (*short arrows in image* **A**). On contrast-enhanced fat-saturated T1-weighted MR image **B**, the vertebral marrow (*short arrows*) adjacent to the L3-4 disc enhances. Tissue within the L3-4 intervertebral disc (*long arrow in image* **B**) enhances with contrast. The posterior epidural abscess, which extends superiorly from the L3-4 level, is T2 hyperintense (*long arrows in image* **A**) and the abscess contains nonenhancing liquid spaces and enhances intensely at its margin (*long arrows in image* **B**).

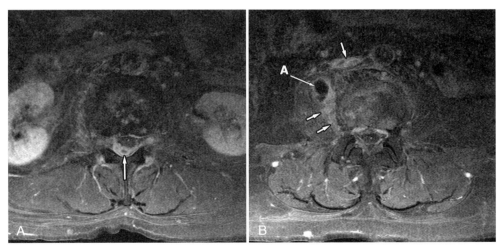

Figure 28-7 ▸ L3-4 Discitis, Osteomyelitis, Paraspinal Phlegmon, and Posterior Epidural Abscess. Same patient as in Figure 28-6. Axial fat-saturated contrast-enhanced MR images **A** and **B**. The abscess (*arrow in image* **A**) is positioned posteriorly and along the right lateral margin of the thecal sac. The abscess contains nonenhancing liquid. In image **B**, at the L3-4 level, there is a right anterior and lateral enhancing phlegmonous tissue (*small arrows*) containing a small nonenhancing abscess (*A*).

inversion recovery (STIR) imaging results are equivalent to fat-saturated, T2-weighted images. With MRI, vertebral endplate cortical bone erosion or bone destruction and usually loss of vertebral height are evident. With MRI, marrow edema in the bone adjacent to the vertebral endplates usually is seen as a region of T1 hypointensity, T2 hyperintensity, or STIR hyperintensity in the vertebral body on either side of the infected disc (see Fig. 28-6).[1] T1-weighted images are more reliable than T2-weighted images

for assessing the vertebral endplate destruction on MRI (see Figs. 28-4 and 28-6). The characteristic T2 signal hyperintensity in the endplates and adjacent bone marrow in spondylodiscitis may be absent in some patients.[8] Areas of restricted diffusion are usually observed within the regions of osteomyelitis and in the epidural phlegmon or abscess.[9]

Contrast-enhanced MR images, after IV administration of a paramagnetic contrast agent, should be obtained in all patients

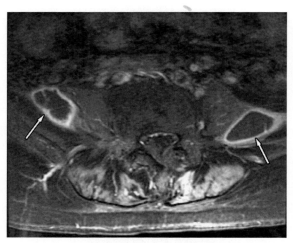

Figure 28-8 ▶ Atypical Mycobacterial Infection. Axial fat-saturated T1-weighted MRI shows peripherally enhancing abscesses (*arrows*) in both psoas muscles secondary to Mycobacterium abscessus spondylodiscitis, which originated from spondylodiscitis at the L2-3 level (*not shown*).

with suspected spinal infection. Enhancement in the region of the abnormal vertebral marrow signifies inflammation and hence osteomyelitis in this setting.[8] The disc is usually T2 hyperintense and enhances to a variable degree with IV contrast administration, especially in suppurative bacterial spine infections (see Figs. 28-4 to 23-6). The T2 hyperintensity in the disc may be lacking in patients with tuberculous or fungal infections because the abscess may contain granulation tissue rather than purulent material.[1] The epidural phlegmon that may accompany the spondylodiscitis is characteristically T1 hypointense or isointense relative to the spinal cord and of intermediate to high signal intensity on T2-weighted images (see Fig. 28-6, A).[1,2,8] The epidural phlegmon enhances intensely with IV contrast (see Fig. 28-4, B).

Contrast-enhanced images are needed to differentiate phlegmon from abscess.[8] A phlegmon will enhance homogeneously or slightly heterogeneously (see Fig. 28-4, B).[3] When frank abscess formation occurs, the abscess is a nonenhancing region that develops within enhancing phlegmonous tissue. The adjacent dura and epidural venous plexus usually enhance intensely (see Figs. 28-4, B and 28-5).[3] A frank abscess typically displays intense peripherally enhancing tissue surrounding a heterogeneous nonenhancing central zone of necrosis, pus, or granulation tissue (see Figs. 28-3, B, 28-6, B, 28-7, B, and 28-8).[3,4,8]

In tuberculous spondylitis, endplate destruction and intradiscal T2 signal hyperintensity may be lacking, especially in the early stages of the disc infection. The appearance in this situation may simulate severe degenerative discogenic vertebral osteochondrosis. The disc infected by tuberculosis or fungal infections may lack the usual T2 signal hyperintensity if water in the infected disc is absent and instead contains infected granulation tissue.[1]

The epidural phlegmon and/or abscess typically compresses the thecal sac and spinal cord, displacing the cord posteriorly. T2 signal hyperintensity may develop in the cord representing cord edema, myelitis, or ischemia secondary to cord compression.[1] Direct invasion or hematogenous spread of the infectious process into the spinal cord may occur but this is rare. In this instance, an enhancing focus develops within the cord, and eventually an intramedullary cord abscess may form that is a clinically devastating complication.[6]

Epidural abscess may arise secondary to infectious arthritis of the facet joints, which is an exceedingly rare condition. Noninfectious inflammatory facet arthropathy (facet synovitis) is exceedingly common and may be associated with enhancing inflammatory tissue in and adjacent to the facets, in the adjacent neural foramen, or in the adjacent epidural space. This noninfectious inflammatory tissue may enhance after IV contrast, but central necrosis and abscess formation does not occur unless this tissue becomes secondarily infected, which is believed to be exceedingly rare.

Radionuclide scanning with Gallium-67 is usually positive in the region of the phlegmon or abscess.[10] A white blood cell scan with Indium-111 may be useful in detecting a frank abscess.[11]

After surgical drainage of the abscess, enhancing tissue may remain in the epidural space representing granulation tissue or residual inflammation. The patients should be followed with serial MR imaging and with serial ESR (erythrocyte sedimentation rate) and/or serum C-reactive protein.

DIFFERENTIAL DIAGNOSIS

1. **Subdural abscess (subdural empyema):** This is a rare condition that can have the same clinical presentation as an epidural abscess. In the case of a subdural abscess, the phlegmon or abscess is located in the subdural space, which is the potential space between the dura and arachnoid. On sagittal images there is a thin linear rim of T1 isointense and T2 hyperintense tissue along the margin of the thecal sac, which enhances with contrast. The fluid in the abscess does not enhance. On axial images, the subdural abscess has a ring or crescent configuration along the margin of the thecal sac. This encroaches upon the cerebrospinal fluid (CSF) within the thecal sac, appearing to narrow the volume of the sac. The adjacent epidural fat is usually spared. Subdural abscesses more commonly occur in the immunocompromised patient or those suffering from diabetes or some chronic debilitating disorder. These abscesses can arise from hematogenous spread or secondary to trauma, surgery, or spinal percutaneous needle procedure, such as after a lumbar puncture. Subdural abscess can occur with spinal pachymeningitis or epidural abscess. *Staphylococcus aureus* is the organism most commonly responsible for development of subdural abscess, but gram-negative organisms can also cause subdural abscess. Treatment usually requires surgical drainage and IV antibiotics. Without aggressive surgical and antibiotic treatment, the mortality rate is high with subdural abscess.

2. **Epidural (ED) hematoma:** The clinical presentation is vital in differentiating ED hematoma from epidural abscess.[6] Epidural hematoma may closely simulate an epidural abscess on unenhanced MR images, especially if it is located in the posterior epidural space.[6] ED hematomas are usually heterogeneous in signal intensity and predominantly isointense on T1-weighted images with islands of T1 hyperintensity. They tend to be heterogeneous with variable signal intensity on T2-weighted images, usually containing regions of T2 hyperintensity or loculated fluid collections with fluid/fluid levels. Subtle contrast enhancement may be seen along the margin of an epidural hematoma, but intense contrast enhancement as seen in a phlegmon or abscess is lacking. No imaging features of spondylodiscitis are present. Epidural hematomas may rarely become secondarily infected and transform into abscesses.

3. **Epidural metastasis:** The neoplastic epidural mass is nearly always secondary to vertebral metastases. Vertebral tumor causes bone destruction or marrow infiltration in the adjacent vertebral bodies, pedicles, or posterior vertebral arch.

4. **Herniated disc extrusion:** If an extruded disc fragment migrates above or below the disc level, the imaging appearance may resemble an epidural abscess. Indeed there is typically contrast enhancement adjacent to the disc fragment caused by the presence of adjacent inflammation or enhancement of adjacent epidural veins. Findings of spondylodiscitis are absent with disc herniation.

5. **Tophaceous gout:** Gout may cause urate deposits at the discovertebral junction, resulting in vertebral endplate erosions, bone destruction, and abnormal signal in the intervertebral disc simulating discitis and osteomyelitis (i.e., spondylodiscitis). These patients usually present with back pain. Approximately 80% of patients with vertebral involvement have polyarticular gout and hyperuricemia.[12] Gouty tophus may extend into the epidural space, where its imaging appearance can mimic an anterior epidural abscess in every respect. The tophus is typically T1 hypointense and T2 hyperintense, and there is peripheral contrast enhancement at the margin of the epidural tophus, believed to be caused by the presence of vascularized fibrous tissue at the margin of the urate crystalline deposits.[12,13] The facet joint and adjacent soft tissues may also be involved by gout representing a rare type of facet synovitis.[13] Pathologic fracture, vertebral ankylosis, and spinal deformity may result from gouty involvement of the vertebrae.[13]

TREATMENT

1. **Surgical intervention:** Emergent surgical evacuation of the epidural abscess is the treatment of choice.[6] Delay in surgical intervention may result in permanent neurologic deficit or death. Mortality rate may be as high as 30%. A more conservative approach using IV antibiotics alone can be considered if the patient has a small phlegmon with no significant neurologic deficit, but these patients must be frequently observed and followed for symptoms of neurologic deterioration.[6]

2. **Antibiotic therapy:** Early intravenous antibiotic therapy should be initiated as soon as possible with broad-spectrum antibiotic targeting gram-positive cocci, gram-negative bacilli, and anaerobic organisms. Ideally the organism should be identified by percutaneous needle aspiration so the optimal antibiotic agent can be chosen. However, initiation of antibiotic therapy should not be delayed until the organism is identified.

3. **Surgical débridement:** If a psoas abscess develops, surgical débridement, drainage, and IV antibiotic therapy are usually required.

References

1. Kricun R, Shoemaker EI, Chovanes GI, Stephens HW. Epidural abscess of the cervical spine: MR findings in five cases. *AJR Am J Roentgenol.* 1992;158:1145-1149.
2. Lang IM, Hughes DG, Jenkins JP, et al. MR imaging appearances of cervical epidural abscess. *Clin Radiol.* 1995;50:466-471.
3. Numaguchi Y, Rigamonti D, Rothman MI, et al. Spinal epidural abscess: evaluation with gadolinium-enhanced MR imaging. *Radiographics.* 1993;13:545-559; discussion 559-560.
4. Goris H, Wilms G, Hermans B, Schillebeeckx J. Spinal epidural abscess complicating epidural infiltration: CT and MR findings. *Eur Radiol.* 1998;8:1058.
5. Saigal G, Donovan Post MJ, Kozic D. Thoracic intradural Aspergillus abscess formation following epidural steroid injection. *AJNR Am J Neuroradiol.* 2004;25:642-644.
6. Tali ET, Gultekin S. Spinal infections. *Eur Radiol.* 2005;15:599-607.
7. Kose M, Arslan D, Altunay L, et al. Cervicothoracolumbar spinal epidural abscess and cerebral salt wasting. *Spine J.* 2009;9:e1-e5.
8. Dagirmanjian A, Schils J, McHenry M, Modic MT. MR imaging of vertebral osteomyelitis revisited. *AJR Am J Roentgenol.* 1996;167:1539-1543.
9. Eastwood JD, Vollmer RT, Provenzale JM. Diffusion-weighted imaging in a patient with vertebral and epidural abscesses. *AJNR Am J Neuroradiol.* 2002;23:496-498.
10. Tzen KY, Yen TC, Yang RS, et al. The role of 67Ga in the early detection of spinal epidural abscesses. *Nucl Med Commun.* 2000;21:165-170.
11. Bedont RA, Datz FL. In-111-labeled leukocyte scan demonstrating septic meningitis complicating a spinal epidural abscess. *Clin Nucl Med.* 1985;10:112-113.
12. Bonaldi VM, Duong H, Starr MR, et al. Tophaceous gout of the lumbar spine mimicking an epidural abscess: MR features. *AJNR Am J Neuroradiol.* 1996;17:1949-1952.
13. Yen PS, Lin JF, Chen SY, Lin SZ. Tophaceous gout of the lumbar spine mimicking infectious spondylodiscitis and epidural abscess: MR imaging findings. *J Clin Neurosci.* 2005;12:44-46.

EPIDURAL HEMATOMA

Leo F. Czervionke, M.D.

CLINICAL PRESENTATION

The patient is a 71-year-old female who had a relatively abrupt onset of moderately severe mid and right-sided neck pain, difficulty lifting her right arm, and mild loss of balance. These symptoms began 12 days before presentation. No history of trauma. Patient is taking Coumadin for atrial fibrillation.

IMAGING PRESENTATION

Magnetic resonance (MR) imaging of the cervical spine reveals a heterogeneous epidural fluid collection causing compression of the right posterolateral aspect of the thecal sac and spinal cord from the C3 to C5 level on the right consistent with epidural hematoma (*Figs. 29-1 to 29-3*).

DISCUSSION

Spinal epidural hematoma (EDH) is a collection of blood that accumulates in the spinal canal outside of the dural sac, usually from epidural venous hemorrhage.[1] EDH most commonly occurs after spinal trauma or surgery and may arise in the anterior or posterior epidural space, but is more common posteriorly in the postoperative setting (*Fig. 29-4*). Postoperative epidural hematomas more commonly occur when multilevel spine surgery has been performed or in patients with a coagulopathy.[2-4] Epidural hematomas may be associated with traumatic or pathologic vertebral fractures as well.[5]

Spontaneous epidural hematomas are those that occur in the absence of trauma or any invasive iatrogenic procedure.[6] Spontaneous epidural hematomas (SEDH) most commonly occur in patients on anticoagulant therapy or patients with a coagulopathy or bleeding diathesis, but can occur secondary to presence of tumor, vascular malformation, epidural hemangioma, or epidural varix.[1,6] Coughing episodes or Valsalva maneuver also may cause spontaneous epidural hematomas, probably by rupture of epidural veins. There is an increased incidence of epidural hematoma during the third trimester of pregnancy when blood volume is high and engorged veins may be more prone to rupture.[7]

Small epidural hematomas frequently arise adjacent to herniated discs, especially extruded disc fragments, most common in the lumbar region, likely caused by rupture of epidural veins.[8,9] These small epidural hematomas that may accompany disc extrusions often are overlooked and therefore go unreported. Spinal epidural hematomas may occur in association with epidural metastases, leukemia, and lymphoma.[10,11] Some have hypothesized that alteration in intracranial pressure may predispose one to spontaneous spinal epidural hematoma development in rare cases.[12] In some cases of spontaneous epidural hematoma, no etiology is found.

Spontaneous ED hematomas more commonly arise posterior to the thecal sac and are more common in the cervical or upper thoracic region (see Figs. 29-1 to 29-3). Spontaneous epidural hematomas can occur in the anterior epidural space as well (*Figs. 29-5 and 29-6*).

Patients most commonly present with acute neck pain or back pain, with history of no or minimal trauma. Acute onset myelopathy may occur if there is cord compression. Patients may also present with rapidly progressive radiculopathy, sensory deficit, or bladder/bowel dysfunction, depending on the location of the ED hematoma; 75% of spontaneous ED hematomas occur in males. The ED hematoma usually arises secondary to rupture of the epidural venous plexus that may occur after an episode of sneezing or Valsalva maneuver. A higher incidence of ED hematoma occurs during pregnancy, in patients with Paget's disease, and in patients with leukemia. There is a higher association of ED hematoma with disc herniation and with spinal atrioventricular (AV) malformations.

IMAGING FEATURES

Spontaneous epidural hematomas usually manifest as fusiform, lens-shaped collections of blood that extend over several vertebral levels within the spinal canal and usually displace adjacent epidural fat.[13] EDH may be seen on plain computed tomography (CT) images as slightly hyperdense tissue adjacent to the thecal sac, causing cord compression if sufficiently large. The hyperdense epidural hematoma may be visible over several vertebral levels. At myelography, epidural hematomas produce extradural extrinsic compression of the contrast-filled thecal sac or if large, can cause a complete "myelographic" block appearance.

With MR, an epidural hematoma typically obscures the adjacent epidural fat and one may observe extradural displacement of the thecal sac dura, both of which are useful signs that help distinguish an epidural hematoma from a subdural hematoma. The use of a T1-weighted sequence with fat-suppression technique may help differentiate epidural hematoma from epidural fat (see Figs. 29-3 and 29-5).[14] If the epidural hematoma compresses the cord,

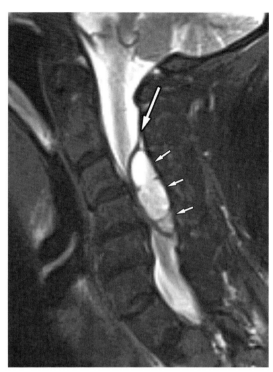

Figure 29-1 ▶ Posterior Cervical Epidural Hematoma. Right parasagittal T2-weighted image, cervical spine. Heterogeneous, predominantly T2 hyperintense posterior epidural hematoma (*short arrows*) compresses the thecal sac and displaces the spinal cord. Note obtuse angle superiorly caused by extrinsic dural sac displacement (*long arrow*) by the epidural hematoma.

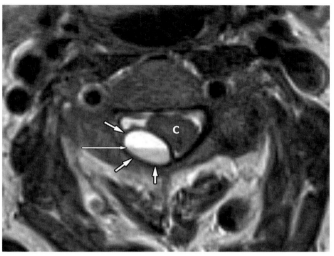

Figure 29-2 ▶ Posterior Cervical Epidural Hematoma. Same patient as in Figure 29-1. Axial T2-weighted image C3-4 level. The epidural hematoma (*short arrows*) is located along the right posterolateral aspect of the thecal sac and displaces the spinal cord (*C*) anteriorly and to the left. Note fluid/fluid level (*long thin arrow*) in the hematoma.

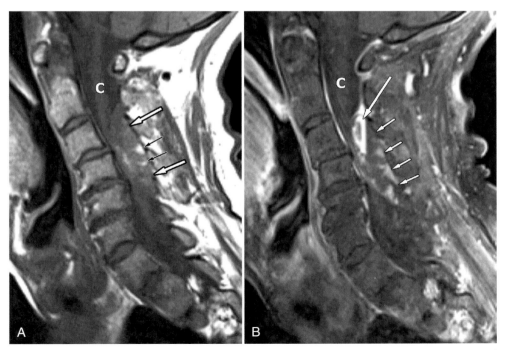

Figure 29-3 ▶ Posterior Cervical Epidural Hematoma. Right parasagittal T1-weighted image **A** and contrast-enhanced image **B** at same slice location as in Figure 29-1. In image **A**, the hematoma (*white arrows*) is predominantly T1 isointense relative to the spinal cord (*C*) and contains focal areas of T1 hyperintensity (*tiny black arrows*) representing regions of extracellular methemoglobin within the hematoma. In image **B**, there are heterogeneous areas of enhancement within the hematoma (*short arrows*). Intense area of enhancement (*long arrow*) in anterosuperior portion of hematoma represents contrast leakage into fluid space within hematoma (note vertical fluid/fluid level) consistent with active bleeding.

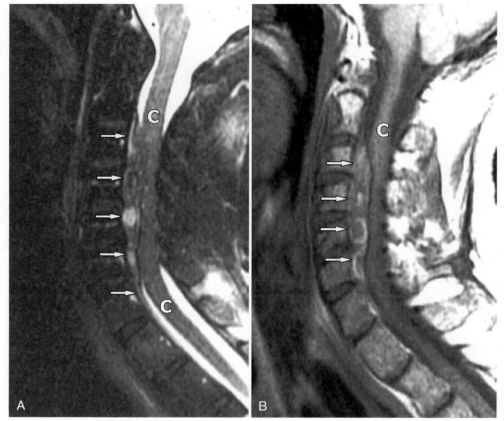

Figure 29-4 ► Cervical Anterior Epidural Hematoma. The epidural hematoma is heterogeneous on both sagittal T2-weighted fat-saturated image **A** and corresponding T1-weighted image **B**, due to blood products in different stages of metabolism within the hematoma. The spinal cord (*C*) is compressed and displaced posteriorly in the canal.

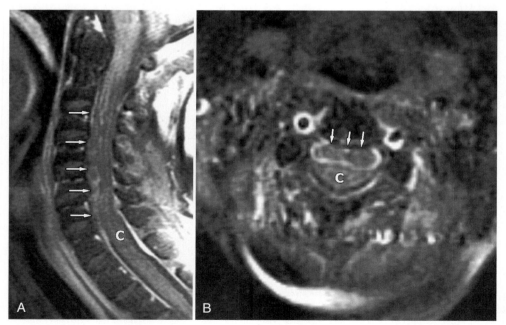

Figure 29-5 ► Cervical Anterior Epidural Hematoma. Same patient as in Figure 29-4. No appreciable contrast enhancement seen within the hematoma (*arrows*) on sagittal contrast-enhanced fat-saturated image **A** and axial contrast-enhanced fat-saturated image **B**. Contrast enhancement is seen along the margin of the hematoma, best shown on image **B**. The spinal cord (*C*) and the central portion of the hematoma have nearly the same signal intensity on the contrast enhanced images.

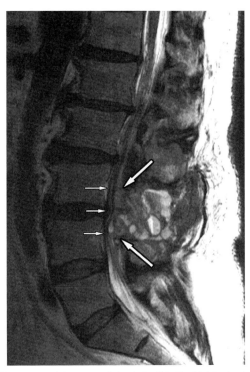

Figure 29-6 ► **Postoperative Lumbar Epidural Hematoma.** A hematoma is located within the L3-4 laminectomy defect and in the posterior epidural space. Sagittal T2-weighted MR image. The heterogeneous epidural hematoma (*long arrows*) impinges upon the posterior margin of the thecal sac. Marked AP diameter flattening of the thecal sac (*short arrows*) due to ED hematoma posteriorly and L3-4 bulging disc anteriorly.

edema may be observed as T2 hyperintense signal in the cord.[15] Unless there is active bleeding into the epidural hematoma (see Fig. 29-3, *B*), the epidural hematoma usually does not enhance appreciably, although there is commonly enhancement of the peripheral margin of the hematoma because of hypervascularity of the hematoma pseudocapsule or enhancement of adjacent epidural veins (Fig. 29-6).

MR imaging is the modality of choice for evaluating epidural hematoma, but its signal intensity varies with age.[14] Epidural hematomas hopefully are detected early and surgically evacuated in a timely fashion, but the epidural hematoma may not always manifest in a hyperacute or acute stage of development. Hematomas in the brain and spinal canal undergo similar stages of evolution. In reality, the stages of hematoma evolution as demonstrated with MR imaging are not always visualized as distinct stages because blood by-products in the hematoma may metabolize and form at different rates in different patients. The imaging appearance of a given hematoma may contain blood metabolites of varying stages, the resulting hematoma having a heterogeneous or mixed signal intensity MR appearance.

Hyperacute Hematoma (less than 12 hours old)

In the hyperacute stage, the hematoma may be difficult to visualize on MR imaging because it is isointense or hypointense on T1-weighted images and hyperintense on T2-weighted images, which may be nearly identical to the appearance of cerebrospinal fluid (CSF). Hyperacute hemorrhage contains oxyhemoglobin that is a very weak paramagnetic substance. Contrast enhancement

may be seen within the hyperacute hematoma if active bleeding is occurring (see Fig. 29-3, *B*).

Acute Hematoma (1-3 days old)

Intracellular deoxyhemoglobin predominates in the hematoma, but some intracellular methemoglobin may also be accumulating in the hematoma. Intracellular deoxyhemoglobin is a substance that causes selective T2 shortening.[16] The signal intensity of the EDH in this phase is isointense to hypointense on T1-weighted images and usually T2 hypointense on T2-weighted images because of the presence of intracellular deoxyhemoglobin, clot retraction, fibrin production, and concentration of red blood cells in the clot. On gradient echo images, the EDH in this stage is usually hyperintense but may contain T2 hypointense areas if intracellular deoxyhemoglobin is present.

Early Subacute Hematoma (3-7 days old)

Intracellular methemoglobin predominates in the hematoma, which can impart a heterogeneous signal intensity that is sometimes difficult to characterize. The signal intensity of the hematoma in this phase is usually T1 isointense to hyperintense and T2 isointense to hypointense (see Fig. 29-5). Contrast enhancement may be seen along the margin of the hematoma because of hypervascularity of the developing hematoma pseudocapsule or in the case of spinal epidural hematomas, also because of enhancement of adjacent epidural veins (see Fig. 29-6).

Late Subacute Hematoma (1-4 weeks)

The hematoma predominantly contains lysed red blood cells and extracellular methemoglobin, which is exposed to abundant free (extracellular) water that allows proton-electron dipole-dipole (PEDD) interactions to occur.[16] As a result, the hematoma is both T1 and T2 hyperintense in this stage.

Chronic Stage (greater than 4 weeks)

In the chronic stage, significant extracellular methemoglobin may persist, rendering the hematoma T1 hyperintense, which may persist indefinitely depending on the local metabolic environment. The T1 hyperintensity tends to diminish slowly over time. The T1 and T2 signal intensity in a chronic hematoma tends to become increasingly hypointense with time because of accumulation of hemosiderin and ferritin, which is ingested by macrophages that die along the margin of the hematoma, leaving deposits of hemosiderin and ferritin at the hematoma periphery. Hemosiderin and ferritin are substances that cause selective T2 shortening, so they are hypointense on T2-weighted images.[16] On gradient echo imaging, substances with high magnetic susceptibility, such as hemosiderin, are markedly hypointense because of T2* effects. Eventually, as the hematoma ages and becomes very old, these substances also accumulate within the hematoma itself, imparting a T1 hypointense and T2 hypointense appearance to the entire old hematoma. The hematoma often contracts to a smaller volume in this very late stage (residual hematoma "cleft" formation), which is commonly seen in very old hematomas in the brain. Marginal contrast enhancement of chronic hematomas may occur because of the presence of reactive hypervascularity in the hematoma pseudocapsule or adjacent dura.[17]

DIFFERENTIAL DIAGNOSIS

1. **Spinal subdural hematoma (SDH):** Occurs between the dura and arachnoid, usually in the thoracolumbar or lumbosacral spinal canal. Spontaneous subdural hematomas are rare. SDH may also cause acute back pain, radiculopathy, or bladder/bowel dysfunction. It may be difficult to differentiate an epidural from a subdural hematoma with imaging. SDH is rare in the cervical region. Subdural hematomas most commonly occur after lumbar percutaneous needle procedure (e.g., lumbar puncture) in a patient with a bleeding diathesis. Subdural hematomas may extend over many vertebral levels, and usually adjacent epidural fat remains visible. A lumbar puncture should not be performed if the patient's INR (international normalized ratio) is greater than 1.5. Both SDH and EDH have similar CT density (slightly hyperdense), are usually heterogeneous in intensity on MRI, and typically display heterogeneous contrast enhancement on MRI, depending on the age of the subdural blood collection.
2. **Epidural abscess:** More commonly occurs in the ventral epidural space, where it nearly always is associated with discitis/osteomyelitis. ED abscess is a T1 hypointense or T1 isointense and T2 hyperintense collection of fluid. Intense peripheral contrast enhancement is common. Typical findings are spondylodiscitis that is present when the epidural abscess is anteriorly located. Posterior epidural abscess may occur after surgery or percutaneous procedures in which the spinal canal is entered. Sepsis can also be the cause of an epidural abscess.
3. **Epidural lipomatosis:** Most common in the thoracic or lumbar epidural space. ED lipomatosis has the MR signal intensity of fat on all pulse sequences and suppresses using fat-saturation techniques. Fat does not enhance after contrast administration. Usually this does not present a diagnostic dilemma.
4. **Disc herniation:** An extruded disc fragment that migrates above or below the disc level might be confused with a small epidural hematoma in the anterior lumbar epidural space.[18] Small epidural hematomas are also known to occur adjacent to extruded disc fragments.[8,9,18]

TREATMENT

1. **Conservative therapy:** Recommended if no significant neurologic deficit exists or if neurologic symptoms are improving. The ED hematoma may resolve spontaneously.[12] Any underlying coagulopathy should be corrected if present.
2. **Intravenous dexamethasone:** May help reduce associated cord swelling and inflammation in the acute setting.
3. **Surgery:** Decompressive laminectomy and drainage of the ED hematoma is indicated if there is a significant or progressive neurologic deficit or if neurologic symptoms do not improve. The chance of clinical improvement is better if surgery is performed soon after onset of symptoms, preferably before 24 hours from onset of symptoms. If the neurologic deficit is severe or prolonged, the patient may not recover full neurologic function.[19]

References

1. Holtas S, Heiling M, Lonntoft M. Spontaneous spinal epidural hematoma: Findings at MR imaging and clinical correlation. *Radiology*. 1996;199: 409-413.
2. Kou J, Fischgrund J, Biddinger A, Herkowitz H. Risk factors for spinal epidural hematoma after spinal surgery. *Spine*. 2002;27:1670-1673.
3. Lee SC, Lee ST, Lui TN. Epidural hematoma of the cervical spine after cervical laminectomy in a patient with ventriculo-peritoneal shunt. *J Clin Neurosci*. 2004;11:302-304.
4. Wong YW, Luk KD. Spinal epidural hematoma in a scoliotic patient with long fusion: A case report. *Spine J*. 2008;8:538-543.
5. Tashjian RZ, Bradley MP, Lucas PR. Spinal epidural hematoma after a pathologic compression fracture: An unusual presentation of multiple myeloma. *Spine J*. 2005;5:454-456.
6. Akutsu H, Sugita K, Sonobe M, Matsumura A. A case of nontraumatic spinal epidural hematoma caused by extradural varix: Consideration of etiology. *Spine J*. 2003;3:534-538.
7. Steinmetz MP, Kalfas IH, Willis B, et al. Successful surgical management of a case of spontaneous epidural hematoma of the spine during pregnancy. *Spine J*. 2003;3:539-542.
8. Dorsay TA, Helms CA. MR imaging of epidural hematoma in the lumbar spine. *Skeletal Radiol*. 2002;31:677-685.
9. Gundry CR, Heithoff KB. Epidural hematoma of the lumbar spine: 18 surgically confirmed cases. *Radiology*. 1993;187:427-431.
10. Lin HS, Chen SJ. Metastatic carcinoma related long segment thoracic spinal epidural hematoma: A case report. *Spine*. 2009;34:E266-E268.
11. Vazquez E, Lucaya J, Castellote A, et al. Neuroimaging in pediatric leukemia and lymphoma: Differential diagnosis. *Radiographics*. 2002;22: 1411-1428.
12. Hung KS, Lui CC, Wang CH, et al. Traumatic spinal subdural hematoma with spontaneous resolution. *Spine*. 2002;27:E534-E538.
13. Boukobza M, Haddar D, Boissonet M, Merland JJ. Spinal subdural haematoma: A study of three cases. *Clin Radiol*. 2001;56:475-480.
14. Braun P, Kazmi K, Nogues-Melendez P, et al. MRI findings in spinal subdural and epidural hematomas. *Eur J Radiol*. 2007;64:119-125.

15. Gonzalez CM, Matheus G, Solander S, Castillo M. Transient edema of the spinal cord as a result of spontaneous acute epidural hematoma in the thoracic spine. *Emerg Radiol.* 2004;11:53-55.

16. Gomori JM, Grossman RI, Goldberg HI, et al. Intracranial hematomas: Imaging by high-field MR. *Radiology.* 1985;157:87-93.

17. Vazquez-Barquero A, Abascal F, Garcia-Valtuille R, et al. Chronic nontraumatic spinal epidural hematoma of the lumbar spine: MRI diagnosis. *Eur Radiol.* 2000;10:1602-1605.

18. Watanabe N, Ogura T, Kimori K, et al. Epidural hematoma of the lumbar spine, simulating extruded lumbar disk herniation: Clinical, discographic, and enhanced magnetic resonance imaging features: A case report. *Spine.* 1997;22:105-109.

19. Matsumura A, Namikawa T, Hashimoto R, et al. Clinical management for spontaneous spinal epidural hematoma: Diagnosis and treatment. *Spine J.* 2008;8:534-537.

EPIDURAL LIPOMATOSIS

Douglas S. Fenton, M.D.

CLINICAL PRESENTATION

The patient is a 66-year-old male with a 7-year history of low back and bilateral hip pain. The pain is most evident when he is walking. His pain has been progressive over the last several years and now he can only walk 20 yards before he has to stop because of bilateral buttock and hip pain. The patient has been significantly obese since he was 35 years old and presently weighs 298 pounds with a height of 6'1".

IMAGING PRESENTATION

Sagittal and axial T1-weighted magnetic resonance (MR) images demonstrate lobulated increased signal intensity in the posterior epidural space throughout the lumbar spine, which is most prominent at the disc levels and causes ventral displacement and narrowing of the thecal sac compatible with epidural lipomatosis (*Fig. 30-1*).

DISCUSSION

Spinal epidural lipomatosis (SEL) is characterized by unencapsulated fat in the epidural space of the spinal canal. The vast majority of cases of SEL are in patients that are either morbidly obese, on chronic steroid therapy, or suffering from Cushing's syndrome or other endocrinopathy.[1-3] SEL occurs more commonly in men than women (3:1), with a mean age of approximately 43 years. The youngest reported case was in a 6-year-old boy receiving high-dose steroids.[4] Approximately 75% of the cases of SEL are associated with exogenous steroid use.[5] The quantity of exogenous steroid necessary to cause SEL ranges from 30 to 100 mg daily with a duration of use from 5 to 11 years.[6] However, there have been reported cases of SEL developing in patients using steroids for only a few months at low dosages.[6] There have been varying reports as to the location of SEL. There have been reports that SEL occurs most commonly in the thoracic spine with between 58% and 61% of cases, followed by lumbar involvement in 39% to 42%.[6] Cervical epidural lipomatosis has not been reported. Others have reported that there is no difference in the incidence between thoracic and lumbar SEL.[7]

In general, epidural fat that has a thickness greater than 7 mm has been reported to be diagnostic of SEL. A more specific classification was observed by Borre and colleagues[8] as it pertained to lumbar spinal epidural lipomatosis (Table 30-1).

The most common symptom with SEL is back pain, which often manifests long before other symptoms. Other common symptoms include slowly progressive lower extremity weakness and sensory changes with numbness, paresthesias, or radicular symptoms. Although bowel and bladder complications have been reported, these tend to be rare. The location of symptoms is, of course, related to the level of the SEL.

IMAGING FEATURES

SEL cannot be diagnosed by plain film radiography. Prior to MR imaging, the diagnosis of SEL was based on myelography and computed tomography (CT) imaging. Myelography may reveal obstruction to the normal flow of contrast if the spinal canal is blocked or may demonstrate the typical extradural defects on the thecal sac if there is partial obstruction. Myelography, alone, does not lead to the diagnosis of SEL because this will only reveal the level and space of the narrowing or obstruction, not the cause. Plain CT, or post-myelogram CT, has the advantage of being able to measure the density of the cause of the obstruction. Fatty tissue has a density ranging between −80 and −120 Hounsfield units on CT scan, which differentiates it from other tissues (*Fig. 30-2*). MRI has replaced CT as the study of choice for the evaluation of SEL. MRI readily demonstrates the level and degree of obstruction caused by a mass lesion—in this particular case, an abnormal quantity of epidural fat. Secondly, fat has specific T1- and T2-weighting, being of increased signal intensity on T1-weighting and intermediate to increased signal intensity on T2-weighting (Figs. 30-1 and *30-3*). Blood, extracellular methemoglobin, in the epidural space can have a similar T1- and T2-weighted appearance; however, through the use of fat-saturation or fat-suppression MR techniques, these two entities can be easily distinguished. As its name implies, if a fat-saturated or fat-suppressed technique is used, the fat becomes dark or gray with T1- or T2-weighting, whereas the signal of blood remains the same (*Fig. 30-4*).

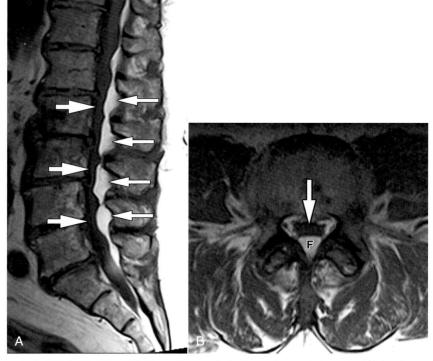

Figure 30-1 ▶ Epidural Lipomatosis, MRI. Sagittal T1-weighted image **A** in a patient with prominent posterior epidural fat (*small arrows*) displacing the thecal sac (*large arrows*) ventrally and causing narrowing of the central spinal canal. Axial T1-weighted image **B** shows pronounced posterior epidural fat (*F*) with moderate narrowing of the thecal sac (*arrow*) and its contents.

TABLE 30-1 Classification of Lumbar Spinal Epidural Lipomatosis (LEL) by MRI Grading

MRI Grade	AP Diameter (thecal sac/ epidural fat)	AP Diameter (epidural fat/ spinal canal)
Normal	≥1.5	≤0.40
LEL I (mild)	1.49	0.41-0.50
LEL II (moderate)	0.99-0.34	0.51-0.74
LEL III (severe)	≤0.33	≥0.75

From Borre DG, Borre GE, Aude F, Palmieri GN. *Eur Radiol* 2003;13:1709-1721.
AP, Anteroposterior; *MRI*, magnetic resonance imaging.

DIFFERENTIAL DIAGNOSIS

1. **Intradural lipoma:** Appears as a more focal, often well-circumscribed mass usually seen in the thoracic or cervicothoracic region *(Fig. 30-5).*
2. **Epidural hematoma:** May have "fat" signal intensity on T1-weighted images, but is heterogeneous on T2-weighted acquisitions. The T1 hyperintensity will not suppress with fat-suppression technique. Patients with an epidural hematoma often have a sudden onset of symptoms. CT imaging can easily distinguish fat density (− Hounsfield units) from blood (+ Hounsfield units).

3. **Epidural metastases or primary neoplasm:** Often appear hypointense to the normal epidural fat on both T1- and nonfat-saturated, T2-weighted acquisitions and demonstrate enhancement *(Fig. 30-6).* When a T2-weighted fat-saturation sequence is used, a metastatic lesion is typically of increased signal intensity, whereas fat becomes dark.

TREATMENT

1. **Weight loss:** The first-line treatment for idiopathic epidural lipomatosis is weight loss and exercise therapy.[9]
2. **Steroid withdrawl:** Weaning patients off their exogenous steroids and weight loss have been successful conservative treatments in a number of cases.[6,9]
3. **Evaluation of corticosteroid overproduction:** Patients who are not receiving exogenous steroids or are not obese should be evaluated for a possible endogenous etiology of corticosteroid overproduction.
4. **Surgery:** Surgical therapy with decompressive laminectomy and resection of the epidural fat is most commonly used for steroid-induced SEL that did not respond to weight loss or weaning off of steroids. Surgery is often successful and has low perioperative risk. However, the concomitant medical problems and comorbidities that are often associated with the typical SEL patient can lead to delayed complications and morbidity. One study demonstrated a 22% mortality rate within 1 year of the surgical decompression.[6]

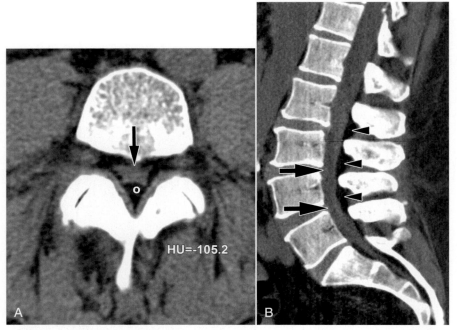

Figure 30-2 ▶ Epidural Lipomatosis, CT. Axial (**A**) and reformatted sagittal (**B**) CT images. Small circle (*o*) in the posterior epidural space, **A**, refers to a Hounsfield unit measurement of −105.2 and is consistent with fat (*arrowheads*, **B**). Thecal sac (*arrows*) is moderately narrowed.

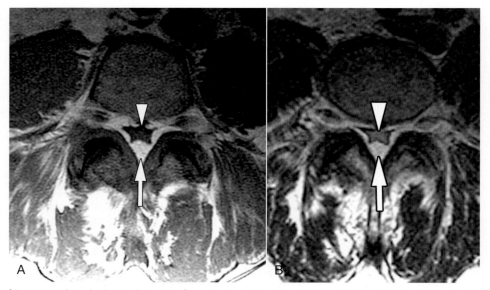

Figure 30-3 ▶ Epidural Fat. *Arrow* shows bright signal intensity of prominent posterior epidural fat on axial T1-weighted image **A** and axial T2-weighted image **B**. The thecal sac (*arrowhead*) is diffusely narrowed.

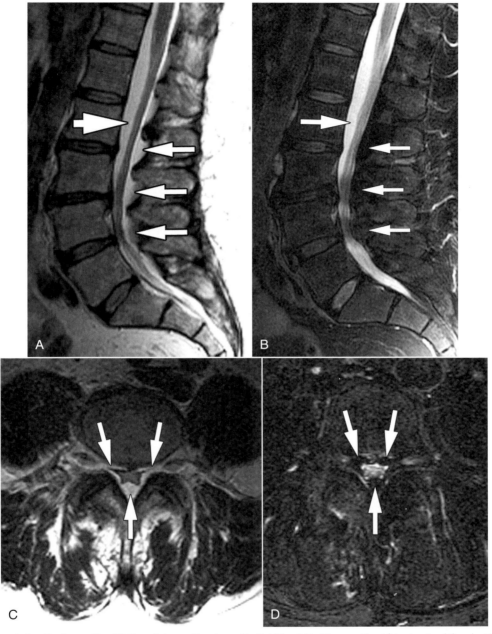

Figure 30-4 ▶ Differentiating Fat from other T2 Hyperintense Structures. Sagittal T2-weighted image without fat saturation (**A**) and with fat saturation (**B**). The posterior epidural fat (**A**, *small arrows*) has bright signal intensity similar to CSF (**A**, *large arrow*). Using a fat-saturated sequence (**B**), the posterior epidural fat becomes dark (*small arrows*) and the CSF remains bright (*large arrow*). Axial T2 without fat saturation (**C**) demonstrates the bright signal of posterior and ventrolateral epidural fat (*arrows*), which becomes low signal intensity with fat saturation (**D**).

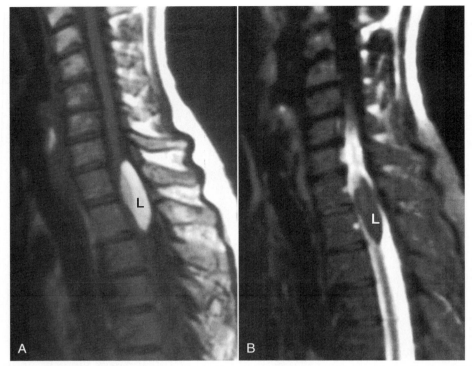

Figure 30-5 ▶ Intradural Lipoma. Well-defined intradural T1 hyperintensity (*L*) on sagittal image **A** compatible with a lipoma. The lipoma (*L*) is of low signal intensity on fat-saturated T2 image **B**.

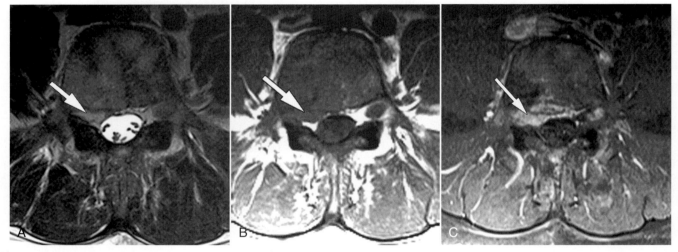

Figure 30-6 ▶ Epidural Metastasis. The metastasis (*arrow*) is of increased signal intensity on axial fat-saturated T2 image **A**, intermediate to a slight decrease signal on T1-weighted image **B,** and shows homogeneous enhancement on image **C**.

References

1. Badami JP, Hinck VC. Symptomatic deposition of epidural fat in a morbidly obese woman. *AJNR AM J Neuroradiol.* 1982;3:664-665.
2. Haddad SF, Hitchon PW, Godersky JC. Idiopathic and glucocororticoid-induced spinal epidural lipomatosis. *J Neurosug.* 1991;74:38-42.
3. Toshniwal PK, Glick RP. Spinal epidural lipomatosis: Report of a case secondary to hypothyroidism and review of literature. *J Neurol.* 1987;234:172-176.
4. Perling LH, Laurent JP, Cheek WR. Epidural hibernoma as a complication of corticosteroid treatment: Case report. *J Neurosurg.* 1988;69:613-616.
5. Stern JD, Quint DJ, Sweasey TA, Hoff JT. Spinal epidural lipomatosis: Two new idiopathic cases and a review of the literature. *J Spinal Disord.* 1994;7:343-349.
6. Fessler RG, Johnson DL, Brown FD, et al. Epidural lipomatosis in steroid-treated patients. *Spine.* 1992;17:183-188.
7. Fogel GR, Cunningham PY 3rd, Esses SI. Spinal epidural lipomatosis: Case reports, literature review and metaanalysis. *Spine J.* 2005;5:202-211.
8. Borre DG, Borre GE, Aude F, Palmieri GN. Lumbosacral epidural lipomatosis: MRI grading. *Eur Radiol.* 2003;13:1709-1721.
9. Beges C, Rousselin B, Chevrot A, et al. Epidural lipomatosis: Interest of magnetic resonance imaging in a weight-reduction treated case. *Spine.* 1994;19:251-254.

CHAPTER
31

EPIDURAL AND VERTEBRAL METASTASES

Douglas S. Fenton, M.D.

CLINICAL PRESENTATION

The patient is a 75-year-old female with complaints of generalized pain and pleural effusions. The patient began experiencing dyspnea on exertion 5 months ago and was discovered to have a large pleural effusion. This was drained and then a month later a recurrent effusion was drained. Over the next few months she began to experience left-sided pain in the region of the chest tube and subxiphoid pain. Over the past 2 weeks, the patient has noticed a mildly tender left-sided neck mass. Since last night, the patient has been noticing a sensation of pins and needles in her legs while trying to stand up, with significant leg weakness and imbalance.

IMAGING PRESENTATION

Sagittal and axial fat-saturated, post-contrast, T1-weighted images reveal abnormally enhancing soft tissue in the epidural space that is compressing the thecal sac. Two vertebrae reveal pathologic enhancement. The findings are compatible with metastatic disease to bone and epidural neoplasm (*Fig. 31-1*).

DISCUSSION

Spinal cord compression from spinal epidural metastasis (SCCSEM) is a common complication of malignancy affecting approximately 5% of cancer patients.[1] SCCSEM is a medical emergency that if left untreated will invariably lead to paraplegia. However, with early diagnosis and treatment, the effects of spinal cord compression can be prevented or reversed in most patients.[2] SCCSEM is second only to brain metastasis as the cause of neurologic dysfunction caused by metastasis.[3]

Metastatic spinal disease can arise from three different locations: the vertebral body (85%), the paravertebral region (10%-15%), and although rarely, the epidural space itself (less than 5%).[4,5] Prostate, breast, and lung cancers each account for 15% to 20% of all spinal metastases and SCCSEM cases. Non-Hodgkins is lymphoma, renal cell carcinoma, and multiple myeloma each account for 5% to 10% of cases, and the remainder are primarily due to colorectal cancers, thyroid cancer, and sarcomas.[3,6,7] The location of SCCSEM appears to be related to the relative bone mass and blood flow to each segment of the spine, with 60% of SCCSEM occurring in the thoracic spine, 25% in the lumbar spine,

and 15% in the cervical spine.[3,6,7] Spinal epidural metastases are reported to be multiple in 17% to 30% of patients.[8]

Most cases of SCCSEM (85%) occur through entrance into the epidural space from a vertebral metastasis. Historically, it was thought that metastatic disease to the vertebral body occurred through the Batson's plexus, the valveless venous system of the spine.[9] However, there has been more recent work that suggests that arterial embolization is the most common and important route of vertebral metastasis.[10]

SCCSEM can damage the spinal cord through, most importantly, vascular compromise and secondarily by direct compression. Anterior spinal cord compression can result in occlusion of Batson's plexus resulting in vasogenic edema. If compression continues, and arterial flow to the spinal cord becomes impaired, the cord may undergo ischemic change and eventually infarction.[11]

Pain is the most common manifesting symptom with SCCSEM, occurring in approximately 90% of patients.[6,12] Local spine pain is confined to the region of metastatic disease and is thought to be due to periosteal stretching and/or a local neoplastic inflammatory process.[13] Local pain is often made worse by recumbency caused by the lengthening of the spine and distention of the epidural venous plexus.[3] Radicular pain is often made worse with Valsalva maneuvers. Mechanical back pain is often secondary to a vertebral body compression. These fractures tend to be associated with spinal instability, made worse with movement, and relieved with recumbency.[3]

Weakness is the second most common symptom of SCCSEM, seen in 60% to 85% of patients at the time of diagnosis.[12] Two-thirds of patients with SCCSEM are nonambulatory at the time of diagnosis.[14] Bowel and bladder symptoms are seen in 50% to 60% of patients with SCCSEM at the time of diagnosis and parallel the degree of generalized weakness.[6,15] Sphincter problems are a poor prognostic sign for the preservation or improvement of ambulation.[3,6,15]

The diagnosis of SCCSEM begins with clinical suspicion. Any new-onset back or neck pain in a patient with a known history of cancer, especially of the prostate, breast, or lung, should prompt an evaluation for SCCSEM. This is even more concerning in a patient with thoracic back pain because the thoracic spine is much less commonly involved by degenerative back pain such as in the cervical and lumbar spine. A study by Kienstra and colleagues[16] indicated that identifying patients at risk for SCCSEM was not possible with the standard neurologic checkup and therefore imaging, particularly MRI of the entire spine should be performed.

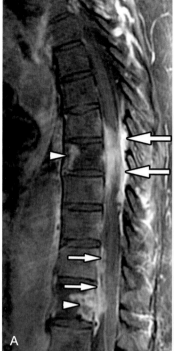
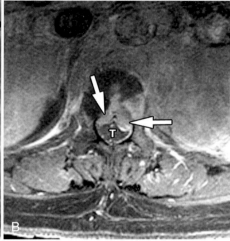

Figure 31-1 ▶ Metastatic Disease to the Epidural Space and Bone. Sagittal fat-saturated, post-contrast, T1-weighted image **A** and axial post-contrast, T1-weighted image **B** reveal regions of vertebral body enhancement (*arrowheads*) compatible with metastatic disease to the bone. Two regions of enhancing soft tissue (*large and small arrows*) are compatible with epidural metastatic disease. The epidural metastatic disease is seen to compress the thecal sac (*T*).

IMAGING FEATURES

MRI is the imaging method of choice for evaluating metastatic disease and SCCSEM because it is nonionizing and can survey the entire spine quickly. Computed tomography (CT), particularly CT post-myelography, is still used in patients with contraindications to MR examination. Sagittal T1-weighted and sagittal fat-saturation or water excitation T2-weighted acquisitions of the cervicothoracic and thoracolumbar spine can be initially performed. Axial acquisitions and potentially contrast-enhanced acquisitions can then be performed at localized areas of abnormality. Typically, SCCSEM appears as a region of decreased T1 signal, increased T2 signal, and enhancement *(Fig. 31-2)*. MRI is able to depict the relationship of the tumor to the spinal cord and neural foramen and whether or not there is abnormal increased T2 signal intensity in the spinal cord to suggest compressive edema, ischemia, or infarction *(Fig. 31-3)*. MRI also adds information that is often not detected by CT, and for 40% of patients, the MRI information changes the radiation fields being used in treatment.[17] CT can detect vertebral body destruction by metastatic disease and associated soft tissue masses as well as intraspinal and paraspinal metastases, although not as well as MRI *(Fig. 31-4)*. The addition of intrathecal contrast during myelography with a follow-up CT scan has a higher sensitivity for intraspinal abnormalities. Vertebral metastases and epidural metastases are of low to intermediate density. Nuclear medicine positron emission tomography (PET) imaging can detect regions of metastatic disease, and when fused with CT data, can localize the abnormality. A bone scan is able to detect only bone metastasis and not the adjacent soft tissue abnormalities. Plain film radiographs should not be used as a primary diagnostic test for SCCSEM because they are falsely negative in

10% to 17% of cases and greater than 50% of the bone must be destroyed before an abnormality can be detected.[6]

DIFFERENTIAL DIAGNOSIS

1. **Primary bone tumor**: Primary bone tumors can look identical to vertebral metastasis with epidural extension *(Fig. 31-5)*. With metastasis, there is often more than one site of involvement and there may be a known primary.
2. **Epidural hematoma**: Hematomas do not enhance or may have only some mild peripheral enhancement as opposed to the avid enhancement of metastatic disease *(Fig. 31-6)*.
3. **Epidural lipomatosis**: Epidural lipomatosis measures as fat density (approximately −50 to −100 Hounsfield units). On MRI, it demonstrates fat signal intensity. Imaging using both routine and fat-saturation sequences makes the diagnosis of fat straightforward *(Fig. 31-7)*. Metastatic disease is of intermediate CT density and intermediate to low signal on T1-weighted imaging.
4. **Epidural abscess**: Patients with epidural abscess are often sick and have elevated white blood cell counts and sedimentation rates. The abscess is commonly in the ventral epidural space and often associated with spondylodiscitis *(Fig. 31-8)*.
5. **Lymphoma:** Appearance can be identical to epidural metastatic disease. One should evaluate for other vertebral body lesions to differentiate lymphoma from metastatic epidural neoplasm.
6. **Intervertebral disc herniation**: A disc herniation is often connected to the parent disc, and there may be some parent

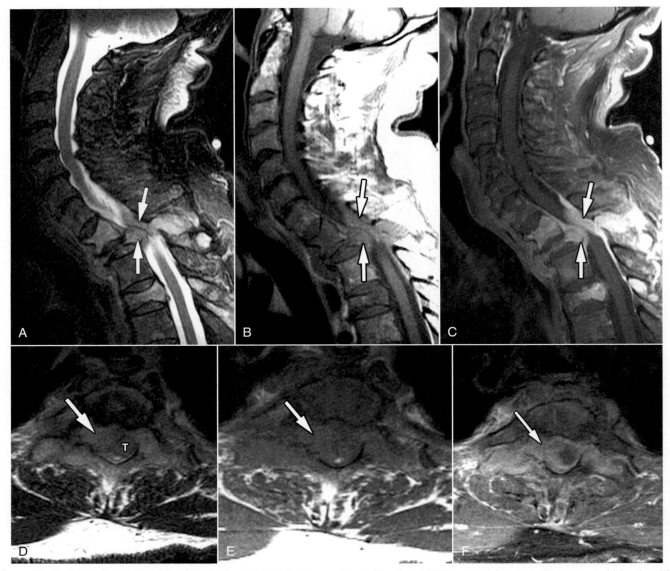

Figure 31-2 ▶ **Spinal Cord Compression from Epidural Metastatic Disease.** Sagittal (**A**) and axial (**D**) T2-weighted, fat-saturated images, sagittal (**B**) and axial (**E**) T1-weighted images, sagittal (**C**) and axial (**F**) fat-saturated, post-contrast, T1-weighed images. Classic appearance of epidural metastatic disease. Epidural tumor (*arrows*) demonstrates decreased T1 signal, increased T2 signal, and enhancement. Mass effect from the epidural tumor displaces and compresses the thecal sac (*T*).

disc height loss. The disc herniation has similar signal intensity to the parent disc and may show some peripheral enhancement *(Fig. 31-9).*

TREATMENT

1. **Combination surgery/radiotherapy**: In the past, before radiotherapy, SCCSEM was treated with simple laminectomy. However, this treatment alone had a low success rate because most epidural metastases arose from vertebral bodies and was thus anterior to the spinal cord. Radiotherapy had better success rates than laminectomy. Combination laminectomy and radiotherapy was attempted; however, the success of this combined procedure was no different than radiotherapy alone.[18] Another study was performed using an anterior or

anterolateral surgical approach with direct removal of the tumor, circumferential decompression, and postoperative radiotherapy compared to radiotherapy alone. This combined surgical/radiotherapy approach had far superior results compared to radiotherapy alone, with a greater percentage of patients continuing to be able to ambulate after the procedure and for a significantly longer period of time, regaining the ability to ambulate, decreasing their need for opiates and steroids, maintaining muscle strength and functional status for longer periods of time, and having longer survival times.[19]

2. **Pain relief with narcotics**: Pain relief with narcotics can be attempted, however, this may cause constipation and therefore an aggressive bowel regimen should also be instituted to decrease constipation-related straining, which could lead to aggravation of the patient's mechanical back pain.[20]

Text continued on page 235

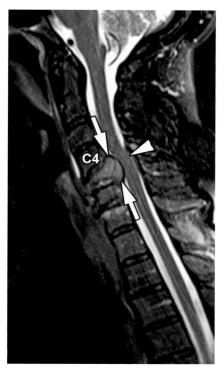

Figure 31-3 ► **Abnormal T2 Spinal Cord Signal Secondary to Compression.** Sagittal fat-saturated, T2-weighted image. Epidural tumor from the posterior C5 vertebral body (*between arrows*) compresses the spinal cord. There is subtle increased T2 signal intensity in the spinal cord (*arrowhead*) compatible with cord ischemia.

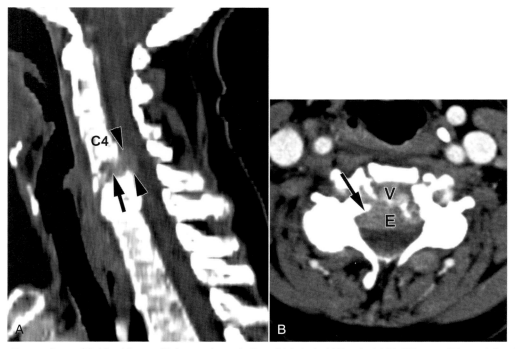

Figure 31-4 ► **Bone Destruction and Epidural Tumor, CT.** Same patient as in Figure 31-3. Sagittal (**A**) and axial (**B**) CT images. CT better defines bone destruction and replacement with abnormal soft tissue both in the vertebral body (*arrow* image **A,** *V* image **B**) and in the epidural space (*between arrows* image **B**; *E,* image **B**). *Arrow* in image **B** shows the only remaining normal posterior vertebral cortex.

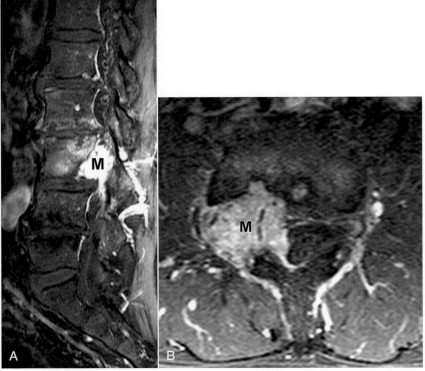

Figure 31-5 ▶ **Primary Bone Tumor, Hemangioblastoma.** Sagittal post-contrast, T1-weighted image **A** and axial post-contrast T1-weighted image **B**. Large right epidural and foraminal mass (*M*) with widening of the neural foramen and destruction of the right posterior vertebral body.

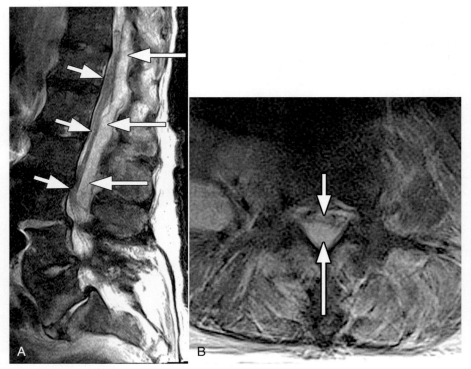

Figure 31-6 ▶ **Epidural Hematoma.** Sagittal (image **A**) and axial (image **B**) T2-weighted images demonstrate a long segment region of abnormal increased T2 signal intensity in the posterior epidural space (*long arrows*). The conus medullaris and cauda equina (*short arrows*) are displaced anteriorly.

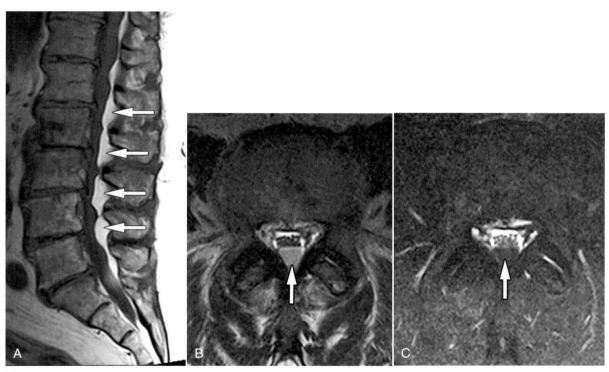

Figure 31-7 ▸ **Epidural Lipomatosis.** Sagittal T1-weighted image **A** reveals an undulating region of increased signal intensity in the posterior epidural space (*arrows*) with anterior displacement of the thecal sac. Axial T2-weighted image **B** also shows focal increased T2 signal intensity (*arrow*) impressing the thecal sac. The fat-saturated, T2-weighted image **C** causes the increased signal intensity on the standard T2 image to decrease (*arrow*), confirming the diagnosis of epidural lipomatosis.

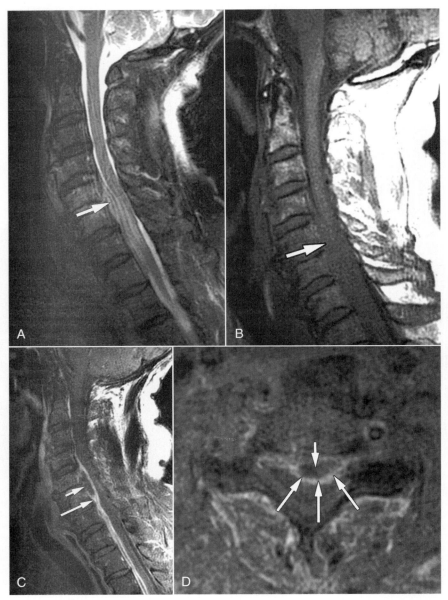

Figure 31-8 ▶ Cervical Discitis with Abscess Formation. Abnormal mixed signal intensity in the ventral epidural space spanning the C5 and C6 vertebral segments (*arrow*) as well as abnormal signal intensity within these vertebral bodies on sagittal T2 image **A** and sagittal T1 image **B**. Post-contrast T1 image **C** shows a nonenhancing abscess cavity (*short arrow*) with surrounding enhancing phlegmon (*long arrow*).

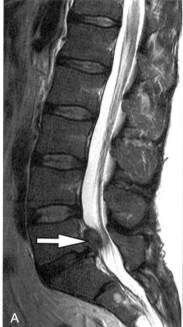
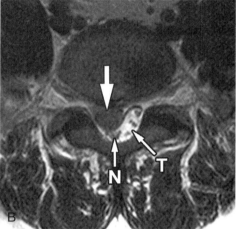

Figure 31-9 ▶ Disc Herniation. Sagittal T2-weighted image **A** and axial T2-weighted image **B**. Large right L5-S1 disc herniation extruded superiorly behind the L5 vertebral body (*arrow*) with preferential compression of the right ventral thecal sac (*T*) and posterior displacement of the intrathecal nerve roots (*N*).

3. **Corticosteroids:** Corticosteroids are also important in the treatment of SCCSEM. Steroids have been shown to help alleviate the pain related to bone metastases, spinal cord compression, and edema of the spinal cord. Steroids have also been shown to improve the patient's overall clinical outcome.[21,22] However, there is no definitive regimen regarding longer-term, low-dose or shorter-term, high-dose steroids.

References

1. Barron KD, Hirano A, Araki S, Tery RD. Experiences with metastatic neoplasms involving the spinal cord. *Neurology.* 1959;9:91-106.
2. Abrahm JL, Banffy MB, Harris MB. Spinal cord compression in patients with advanced metastatic cancer. *JAMA.* 2008;299:937-946.
3. Cole JS, Patchell RA. Metastatic epidural spinal cord compression. *Lancet Neurol.* 2008;7:459-466.
4. Byrne TN. Spinal cord compression from epidural metastases. *New Engl J Med.* 1992;327:614-619.
5. Gerszten PC, Welch WC. Current surgical management of metastatic spinal disease. *Oncology.* 2000;14:1013-1024.
6. Bach F, Larsen BH, Rohde K, et al. Metastatic spinal cord compression, occurrence, symptoms, clinical presentations and prognosis in 398 patients with spinal cord compression. *Acta Neurochir.* 1990;107:37-43.
7. Constans JP, De Divitiis E, Donzelli R, et al. Spinal metastases with neurologic manifestations: review of 600 cases. *J Neurosurg.* 1983;59:111-118.
8. Van der Sande JJ, Boogerd W. Multiple spinal epidural metastases: An unexpectedly frequent finding. *J Neurol Neurosurg Psychiatry.* 1990;53:1001-1003.
9. Batson OV. The function of the vertebral veins and their role in the spread of metastases. *Ann Surg.* 1940;112:138-149.
10. Arguello F, Baggs RB, Duerst RE, et al. Pathogenesis of vertebral metastasis and epidural spinal cord compression. *Cancer.* 1990;65:98-106.
11. Kato A, Ushio Y, Hayhakawa T, et al. Circulatory disturbance of the spinal cord with epidural neoplasm in rats. *J Neurosurg.* 1985;63:260-265.
12. Helweg-Larsen S, Sorensen P. Symptoms and signs in metastatic spinal cord compression: A study from first symptom until diagnosis in 153 patients. *Eur J Cancer.* 1994;30:396-398.
13. Gokaslan ZL. Spine surgery for cancer. *Curr Opin Oncol.* 1996;8:178-181.
14. Husband DJ. Malignant spinal cord compression: Prospective study of delays in referral and treatment. *BMJ.* 1998;317:18-21.
15. Gilbert RW, Kim JH, Posner JB. Epidural spinal cord compression from metastatic tumor: Diagnosis and treatment. *Ann Neurol.* 1978;3:40-51.
16. Kienstra GEM, Terwee CB, Dekker FW, et al. Prediction of spinal epidural metastases. *Arch Neurol.* 2000;57:690-695.
17. Colletti PM, Siegal HJ, Woo MY, et al. The impact on treatment planning of MRI of the spine in patients suspected of vertebral metastasis: An efficacy study. *Comput Med Imaging Graph.* 1996;20:159-162.
18. Greenberg HS, Kim JH, Posner JB. Epidural spinal cord compression from metastatic tumor: results with a new treatment protocol. *Ann Neurol.* 1980;8:361-366.
19. Patchell RA, Tibbs PA, Regine WF, et al. Direct decompressive surgical resection in the treatment of spinal cord compression caused by metastatic cancer: A randomised trial. *Lancet.* 2005;366:643-648.
20. Schiff D. Spinal cord compression. *Neurol Clin N Am.* 2003;21:67-87.
21. Cantu RC. Corticosteroids for spinal metastases. *Lancet.* 1968;2:912.
22. Delattre JY, Arbit E, Rosenblum MK, et al. High dose versus low dose dexamethasone in experimental epidural spinal cord compression. *Neurosurgery.* 1988;22:1005-1007.

EWING'S SARCOMA

Douglas S. Fenton, M.D.

CLINICAL PRESENTATION

The patient is a 42-year-old male with a chief complaint of left leg pain for approximately 1 year. One year ago, he developed increasing left radicular type pain in the S1 distribution with radiation to the posterior aspect of the thigh and leg to the ankle. This became more frequent. He had a magnetic resonance image (MRI) performed 10 months ago that demonstrated a soft tissue mass in an enlarged S1 lateral recess. The possibility of a schwannoma or neuroma was raised. The patient underwent conservative treatment with painkillers and had a repeat MRI scan along with a computed tomography (CT) myelogram 3 months later that showed the mass to be unchanged. He then developed increasing symptoms with numbness in his left foot.

IMAGING PRESENTATION

Sagittal and axial T1-weighted images demonstrate a large intermediate signal intensity soft tissue mass in an enlarged left S1 lateral recess displacing the thecal sac to the right. The L5-S1 disc is of normal height, which would not be expected if this were a massive disc herniation. This was found to be a Ewing's sarcoma at surgery (*Fig. 32-1*).

DISCUSSION

Ewing's sarcoma (ES) is a malignant tumor that occurs mainly in children and adolescents. Ewing's sarcoma can be divided into skeletal Ewing's with its origin in bone and extraskeletal Ewing's. Extraskeletal Ewing's sarcoma has been reported to arise from numerous sites including the scalp, larynx, nasal fossa, neck, lung, extremities, paravertebral soft tissues, and the epidural space.[1] Chromosomal and structural evaluation of both types of Ewing's sarcoma strongly suggests that they are identical tumor types.[2] ES is part of a group of blue, round cell tumors that include primitive neuroectodermal tumor (PNET), lymphoma, Langerhans cell granulomatosis, and neuroblastoma. It is believed that ES and PNET share a common origin from a precursor neural cell.

Skeletal ES is the second most common cancer of bone in children and adolescents and has an incidence of 2.1 per million children in the United States.[3] Involvement of the vertebrae with ES is usually the result of metastatic disease. Primary ES of the vertebrae is much rarer, comprising 3.5% to 10% of all cases of osseous ES.[4] Skeletal ES manifests between the ages of 5 and 30 years of age in 90% of cases, with its peak incidence in the second decade of life.[5,6] ES is uncommon in children of African or Asian descent.[7] ES has a male predominance of approximately 1.5:1.[6,8] Extraskeletal ES manifests at a slightly older age (average 20 years) and occurs equally in both sexes.[9] Unlike osteosarcoma, ES does not appear to be caused by exposure to radiation.[7] ES most commonly occurs in the sacrum, slightly less commonly in the lumbar and thoracic regions, and least commonly in the cervical spine.[10] Most lesions occur in the vertebral body, although lesions can extend into the posterior elements.[11]

The most common manifesting symptom in patients with spinal ES is pain.[4] The pain can be local or radiate to one or both extremities.[10] A common misdiagnosis is lumbar disc disease; however, unremitting pain and/or pain at night should raise the suspicion for tumor.[4] At initial presentation, 58% to 80% of patients will present with a neurologic deficit or radiculopathy.[4,11,12] Cord compression is common.[2,13] Other symptoms include swelling or a palpable mass and systemic symptoms including fever, which may mistakenly lead to a diagnosis of underlying infection.[7,14] Approximately 20% of patients present with gross metastatic disease, but there is a high incidence of micrometastases.[7] Because ES metastasizes to bone and lung, evaluation for metastatic disease should include nuclear medicine technetium bone scan and CT of the chest.[7,10] Serum lactic dehydrogenase is the only reliable marker of tumor burden and should be closely monitored.[7]

IMAGING FEATURES
Extraskeletal Ewing's Sarcoma

Extraskeletal ES of the spine arises in the epidural space. Plain radiographs may be of assistance only when one sees smooth enlargement of a neural foramen. CT will demonstrate a mass of intermediate density in the epidural space. Depending on the location of the mass, the neural foramen may be enlarged with smooth borders. One may see the effect of the mass on the thecal sac with myelography, plain CT, or post-myelogram CT (*Fig. 32-2*). On MRI, the tumor is typically low to intermediate T1 signal intensity, high T2 signal intensity, and exhibits heterogeneous enhancement (*Fig. 32-3*).

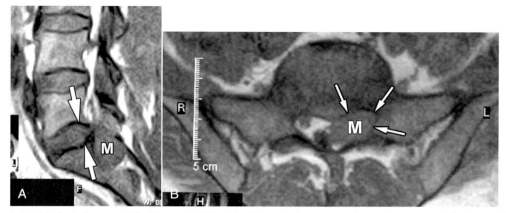

Figure 32-1 ▶ Extraskeletal Ewing's Sarcoma. Off-midline sagittal T1-weighted image **A** demonstrates a large soft tissue mass (*M*) inferior to the L5-S1 disc. The disc height (*between arrows*) is normal. Axial T1-weighted image demonstrates the mass (*M*) in the left SI lateral recess. The lateral recess is enlarged (*arrows*) from chronic pressure erosion.

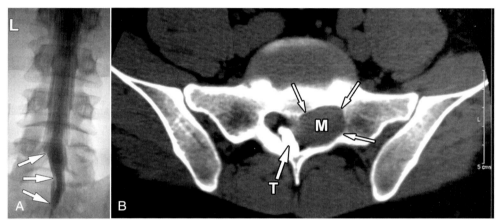

Figure 32-2 ▶ Extraskeletal Ewing's Sarcoma, Myelogram and CT. Same patient as in Figure 32-1. Frontal radiograph from a lumbar myelogram, image **A**. Smooth extradural defect on the thecal sac (*arrows*) displacing the thecal sac to the right. Axial CT post-myelogram image **B** shows an intermediate density mass (*M*) in the left SI lateral recess displacing and compressing the thecal sac (*T*) to the right.

Skeletal Ewing's Sarcoma

Plain radiographs demonstrate imaging findings late in skeletal ES, often after neurologic signs have appeared. The most common finding in skeletal ES is lytic bone destruction of the vertebrae, which can vary from the more common focal tiny perforation-like lytic lesions to vertebra plana.[14] A small proportion of ES may show reactive sclerotic change. CT can demonstrate the extent of bone involvement and any soft tissue component. On CT, ES appears as a permeative intramedullary mass with a possible extraosseous soft tissue mass (*Fig. 32-4*). There may be heterogeneous enhancement of both the intraosseous and extraosseous components of the mass and also areas of central necrosis.[15] CT can be important diagnostically to separate ES from osteogenic sarcoma because the latter often has a matrix of bone that can be seen on CT and occasionally on plain radiographs.[15] Magnetic resonance imaging (MRI) is superior to CT in demonstrating the relationship of the tumor to the spinal canal and its contents, the adjacent vasculature, and the extent of bone marrow abnormality. The tumor exhibits signal abnormality that is typical of most malignant tumors: intermediate signal intensity on T1-weighted images and intermediate to high T2-weighted signal intensity.[15] The tumor demonstrates moderate enhancement that may appear homogeneous or heterogeneous depending on intrinsic regions of tumor necrosis (*Fig. 32-5*).

MRI can also be helpful in following the success or failure of treatment and for preoperative treatment planning (*Fig. 32-6*). Similarly, a nuclear medicine bone scan can be used to evaluate for metastatic disease to bone or assessing treatment response (*Fig. 32-7*).

DIFFERENTIAL DIAGNOSIS

1. **Primitive neuroectodermal tumor (PNET):** Radiographically indistinguishable from ES. Histologic evaluation is necessary to distinguish between them.

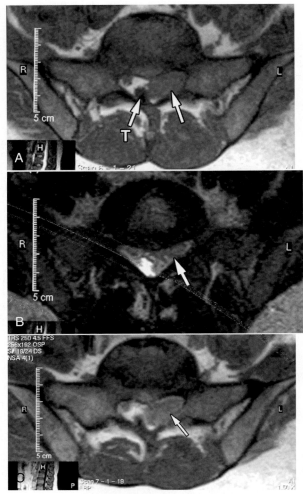

Figure 32-3 ▶ Extraskeletal Ewing's Sarcoma. Same patient as in Figures 32-1 and 32-2. Axial T1-weighted image **A**, axial T2-weighted image **B**, axial post-contrast, T1-weighed image **C**. The mass (*arrow*) is of intermediate T1 signal intensity, increased T2 signal intensity, and demonstrates only mild enhancement. Again identified is rightward displacement and compression of the thecal sac (*T*).

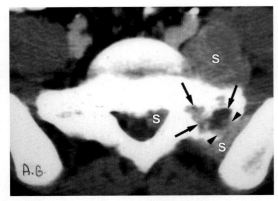

Figure 32-4 ▶ Skeletal Ewing's Sarcoma. Axial CT scan shows bone destruction of a portion of the left SI sacral ala (*arrows*). Extraosseous soft-tissue mass (*S*) is seen both ventral and dorsal to the sacral ala as well as a small amount in the left SI lateral recess. (Courtesy of Steven M. Weindling, M.D.)

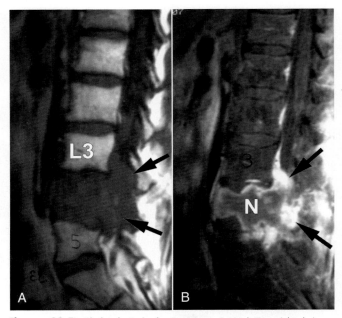

Figure 32-5 ▶ Skeletal Ewing's Sarcoma. Sagittal T1-weighted image **A** and fat-saturated, post-contrast, T1-weighted image **B**. The soft tissue mass is of homogeneous low T1 signal intensity throughout the L4 vertebral body and extends posteriorly into the epidural space (*arrows*). Post-contrast image **B** reveals a large central region of tumor necrosis (*N*). (Courtesy of Steven M. Weindling, M.D.)

2. **Osteogenic sarcoma:** Can have the same appearance as ES. One should look for mineralization of the tumor matrix, which is seen in 80% of osteogenic sarcomas.

3. **Langerhans cell histiocytosis (LCH):** Can be radiographically identical to ES. LCH has less of a propensity than ES to form a large soft tissue mass.

4. **Osteomyelitis:** ES can extend across the disc. Osteomyelitis is centered on the intervertebral disc. The disc is often hyperintense on T2-weighted images *(Fig. 32-8)*. Patients with osteomyelitis have elevated white blood cell counts, sedimentation rates, and C-reactive proteins.

5. **Disc herniation:** Can have an appearance similar to extraskeletal ES *(Fig. 32-9)*. A disc herniation is often attached to the parent disc and does not typically enhance. Disc herniation is rarely seen in patients less than 15 years of age.

6. **Schwannomas/neurofibromas:** Can have an appearance identical to extraskeletal ES *(Fig. 32-10)*.

TREATMENT

1. **Combined radiation and chemotherapy:** A combination of radiation therapy and multiagent chemotherapy is necessary to treat ES because of its high rate of micrometastases. There have been three Intergroup Studies of Ewing's Sarcoma studying patients over a 5-year period. The last study used a combination of vincristine, dactinomycin, cyclophosphamide, doxorubicin, and etoposide-ifosfamide with a significant improvement in survival among patients with localized disease.[16,17] The 3-year survival rate was 80% with this six-drug

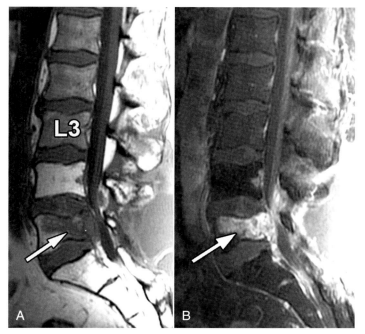

Figure 32-6 ▶ Skeletal Ewing's Sarcoma. Sagittal T1-weighted image **A** and fat-saturated, post–contrast, T1-weighted image **B**. Hyperintensity of L4 through the sacrum on image **A** are secondary to radiation change. However, there is abnormal decreased T1 signal intensity and enhancement within the L5 vertebral body (*arrow*) and epidural space consistent with recurrent and/or residual tumor.

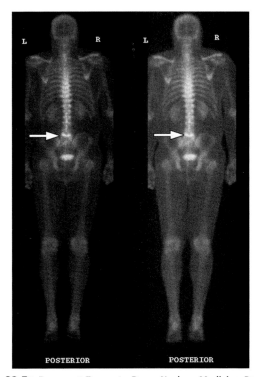

Figure 32-7 ▶ Recurrent Tumor to Bone, Nuclear Medicine Bone Scan. Same patient as in Figure 32-6. Region of increased radiotracer activity in the L5 vertebral body (*arrow*) compatible with increased bone turnover suggesting recurrent tumor.

regimen as opposed to 56% before the addition of etoposide and ifosfamide in patients with only local disease.[16,17] Neither regimen improved survival in the 25% of patients that had metastatic disease at diagnosis.[16,17] Patients with metastatic disease remain a therapeutic challenge, with only 20% not having a relapse/recurrence at 5 years.

2. **Surgery**: The role of surgery for local control continues to be debated because there is a high rate of postlaminectomy kyphosis and deformity.[7] However, given the 20% failure of local control of tumor with radiation and chemotherapy, gross tumor debulking with negative margins may have a survival benefit.[7] Dini and colleagues[14] state their indications for surgery are for "epidural decompression in patients with neurologic decompensation, stabilization for primary instability or cases with extensive bony involvement of tumor where instability is likely to occur after tumor resection, in patients with a poor response to the initial treatment with chemotherapy and/or radiotherapy and for residual disease."

Progonostically, the size of the tumor at presentation is an important factor, with those with larger tumors having worse outcomes.[10] Patients with metastatic disease limited to the lungs seemed to have better outcomes than those with metastatic disease at other sites.[17] A major concern of the intensive treatment of Ewing's sarcoma is the development of a treatment-related second malignancy. The risk of developing leukemia is 2% and that of developing a radiation-induced sarcoma is 5% at 10 years.[7] There is also a risk of developing cardiomyopathy from the chemotherapy.[3]

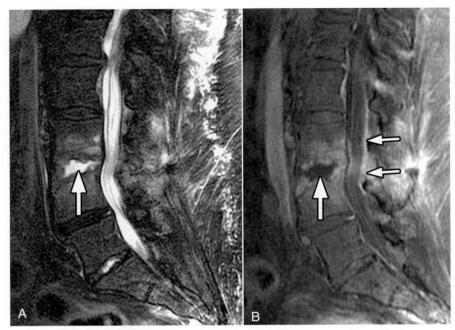

Figure 32-8 ▶ Discitis/Osteomyelitis with Epidural Phlegmon. Sagittal fat-saturated, T2-weighted image **A** and sagittal post-contrast, T1-weighted image **B**. Fluid signal intensity (increased T2, decreased T1) within the L3-4 disc (*large arrow*). Abnormal increased T2 signal intensity and enhancement of the adjacent vertebral endplates as well as enhancement in the epidural space (*small arrows*).

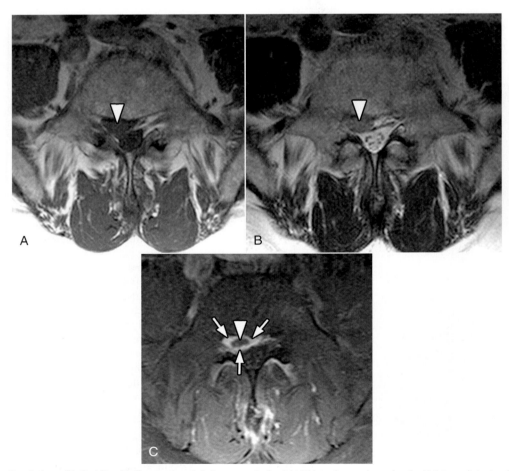

Figure 32-9 ▶ Disc Herniation with Peridiscal Inflammation. Soft-tissue mass in the right S1 lateral recess (*arrowhead*) with intermediate signal intensity on T1 (image **A**), T2 (image **B**), and postcontrast T1 (image **C**). Rind of inflammatory enhancement (*arrows, image **C***) surrounds this extruded disc.

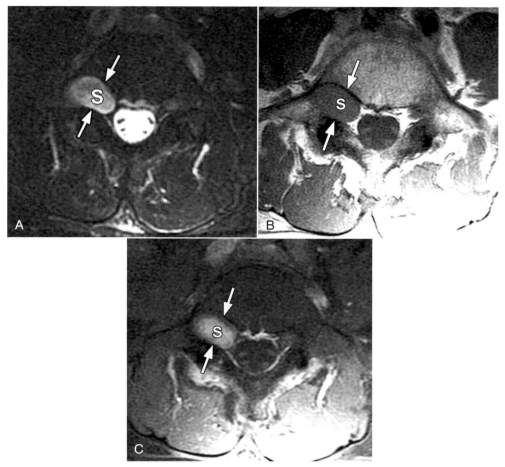

Figure 32-10 ▶ **Schwannoma.** Large ovoid soft tissue mass in the right neural foramen (*S*), widening the neural foramen (*between arrows*) and causing chronic pressure erosion of the right posterior vertebral body. The mass has characteristic increased T2 signal (image **A**), intermediate to decreased T1 signal (image **B**) and avid enhancement (image **C**).

References

1. Kaspers GJ, Kamphorst W, van de Graaff M, et al. Primary spinal epidural extraosseous Ewing's sarcoma. *Cancer.* 1991;68:648-654.
2. Turc-Carel C, Aurias A, Mugneret F, et al. Chromosomes in Ewing's sarcoma. I. An evaluation of 85 cases and remarkable consistency of t(11;22) (q24;12). *Cancer Genet Cytogenet.* 1988;32:229-238.
3. Arndt CAS, Crist WM. Common musculoskeletal tumors of childhood and adolescence. *N Engl J Med.* 1999;341:342-352.
4. Grubb MR, Currier BL, Pritchard DJ, Ebersold MJ. Primary Ewing's sarcoma of the spine. *Spine.* 1994;19:309-313.
5. Diel J, Ortiz O, Losada RA, et al. The sacrum: Pathologic spectrum, multimodality imaging, and subspecialty approach. *Radiographics.* 2001;21:83-104.
6. Motamedi K, Ilaslan H, Seeger LL. Imaging of the lumbar spine neoplasms. *Semin Ultrasound CT MRI.* 2004;25:474-489.
7. Sundaresan N, Rosen G, Boriani S. Primary malignant tumors of the spine. *Orthop Clin N Am.* 2009;40:21-36.
8. Smorenburg CH, van Groeningen CJ, Meijer OWM, et al. Ewing's sarcoma and primitive neuroectodermal tumours in adults: Single-centre experience in the Netherlands. *Neth J Med.* 2007;65:132-136.
9. Stuart-Harris R, Wills EJ, Philips J, et al. Extraskeletal Ewing's sarcoma: A clinical, morphological and ultrastructural analysis of five cases with a review of the literature. *Eur J Cancer Clin Oncol.* 1986;22:393-400.
10. Venkateswaran L, Rodriquez-Galindo C, Merchant TE, et al. Primary Ewing tumor of the vertebrae: Clinical characteristics, prognostic factors, and outcome. *Med Pediatr Oncol.* 2001;37:30-35.
11. Pilepich MV, Vietti TJ, Nesbit ME, et al. Ewing's sarcoma of the vertebral column. *Int J Radiat Oncol Biol Phys.* 1981;7:27-31.
12. Knoeller SM, Uhl M, Gahr N, et al. Differential diagnosis of primary malignant bone tumors in the spine and sacrum: The radiological and clinical spectrum. *Neoplasma.* 2008;55:16-22.
13. Marco RAW, Gentry JB, Rhines LD, et al. Ewing's sarcoma of the mobile spine. *Spine.* 2005;30:769-773.
14. Dini LI, Mendonça R, Gallo P. Primary Ewing's sarcoma of the spine. *Arq Neuropsiquiatr.* 2006;64:654-659.
15. Erlemann R. Imaging and differential diagnosis of primary bone tumors and tumor-like lesions of the spine. *Eur J Radiol.* 2006;58:48-67.
16. Grier H, Krailo M, Link M, et al. Improved outcome in nonmetastatic Ewing's sarcoma and PNET of bone with the addition of ifosfamide and etoposide to vincristine, adriamycin, cyclophophamide, and actinomycin: A Children's Cancer Group and Pediatric Oncology Group report. *Proc Am Soc Clin Oncol.* 1994;13:421.
17. Miser JS, Krailo MD, Tarbell NJ, et al. Treatment of metastatic Ewing's sarcoma or primitive neuroectodermal tumor of bone: Evaluation of combination ifosfamide and etoposide—a children's cancer group and pediatric oncology group study. *J Clin Oncol.* 2004;22:2873-2876.

ATLANTOAXIAL FACET OSTEOARTHRITIS
Inflammatory Facet Arthropathy C1-2 Level

Leo F. Czervionke, M.D.

CLINICAL PRESENTATION

The patient is an 86-year-old man with prostate carcinoma who presented with history of several months of progressive right upper neck pain and recent development of suboccipital headaches. No pain or numbness reported in the upper extremities. Limited range of motion was observed in the right upper extremity. Otherwise, the physical examination was normal.

IMAGING PRESENTATION

Radionuclide bone scan reveals focal area of increased activity in right upper cervical spine region (*Fig. 33-1*). Otherwise the bone scan is normal. Magnetic resonance (MR) imaging obtained both without and with intravenous contrast enhancement reveals abnormal T1 and T2 signal intensity in and adjacent to the right C1-2 facets. Contrast enhancement is demonstrated in the C1-2 facets and adjacent bone marrow, in the periarticular soft tissues, and within the right C1-2 facet joint (*Figs. 33-2 to 33-4*). Findings indicate active right C1-2 inflammatory facet arthropathy (facet synovitis).

DISCUSSION

Osteoarthritis commonly occurs in the cervical zygapophyseal (facet) joints in patients with advancing age. Any cervical level may be affected by facet osteoarthritis. Osteoarthritis has been reported to involve the atlantoaxial (C1-2) facet joints (also called the *lateral atlantoaxial joints*) in approximately 4% of patients overall, and the prevalence increases significantly after the fifth decade of life.[1,2]

Osteoarthritis involving the C1-2 facet joints can produce a distinct clinical syndrome characterized by limitation of neck rotation, severe upper neck pain, and occipital headaches.[3] The patient may have suboccipital pain trigger points, suboccipital crepitus upon palpation, and a rotational head tilt deformity may be present.[1] Upper neck pain and occipital neuralgia can also be secondary to osteoarthritis involving the atlantal-odontoid joint (anterior C1-2 joint).[4] Lateral and anterior C1-2 osteoarthritis commonly coexist (see Figs. 33-3 and 33-4).

The joints between the lateral masses of C1 and C2 anatomically are considered to be zygapophyseal (facet) joints. These joints have some unique anatomic features that are not present in the lower cervical facet joints. The inferior C1 (atlas) articular facet is relatively flat, and this articulates with the relatively convex C2 (axis) superior articular facet. This incongruent configuration of the C1-2 articular facets results in a rather wide (3 to 5 mm) atlantoaxial facet joint space anteriorly and posteriorly.[5] The shape of these joints and the relatively loose capsule that normally surrounds these joints imparts greater joint mobility to these joints than is possible at other cervical levels. The greatest degree of neck rotation occurs at this level.[6]

Meniscus-like synovial folds are present within the C1-2 facet joints during infancy, but these folds usually involute and are not present in older children and young adults. As the atlantoaxial joints age or degenerate, meniscus-like synovial folds again develop that fill the incongruous spaces within the C1-2 joints. These folds are believed to provide stability to these joints.[6] Such meniscal folds also develop in degenerated facet joints elsewhere in the spine.[7]

The earliest findings in degeneration of the lateral atlantoaxial joints is superficial flaking of the articular cartilage.[5] Thinning and fibrillation of the articular cartilage with associated facet cortical sclerosis and irregularity also occur as in any other degenerating facet joint.[5] Eventually the joint space narrows and hypertrophic bone arises at the bone margins of the joint (*Figs. 33-5 to 33-8*).

As the C1-2 facet joints degenerate, fluid may accumulate in these joints resulting in distension of the lax facet capsules. This joint distention can be localized or diffuse and is often referred to as a C1-2 *synovial cyst* (*Figs. 33-9 and 33-10*). These cysts probably form as a result of joint degeneration, excessive stress, or repeated microtrauma.[8] Synovial cysts can develop when atlantoaxial subluxation occurs, which likely places excessive stress on the joint.[8] Atlantoaxial subluxation with associated synovial cyst formation may occur in patients with severe osteoarthritis, rheumatoid arthritis, or with os odontoideum.[9] Rarely, localized C1-2 synovial cysts can extend into the epidural space ventrally, where they may cause cord compression. When this occurs, these patients often present with myelopathy. Rarely, a synovial cyst in the epidural space can communicate with the subarachnoid space.[9]

So called *atlantoaxial rotary fixation* likely occurs as a result of chronic inflammation or prior trauma in this region resulting in severe degenerative disease of the C1-2 joints (see Chapter 12). Presumably the joint becomes fixated because of intracapsular and pericapsular adhesions and capsular infolding into the joint that limit mobility of the C1-2 facet joint.[6]

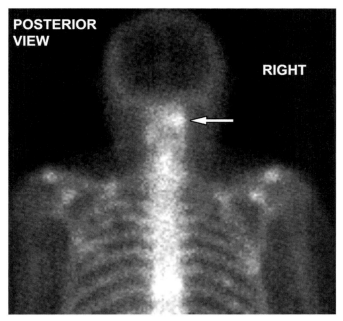

Figure 33-1 ▶ Active Inflammatory Facet Arthropathy (Facet Synovitis), C1-2 level. Technetium-99m methylene-diphosphonate (MDP) bone scan. Posterior view. A focal area of increased uptake (*arrow*) overlies right upper cervical spine.

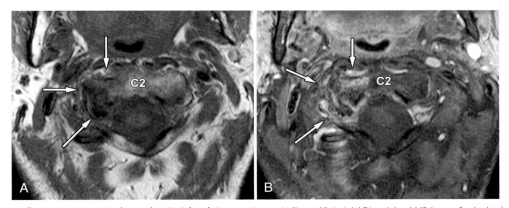

Figure 33-2 ▶ Active Inflammatory Facet Arthropathy, C1-2 level. Same patient as in Figure 33-1. Axial T1-weighted MR image **A**, obtained at the C2 level, reveals irregularity and T1 hypointensity of the right C2 superior articular facet (*arrows*). On contrast-enhanced fat-saturated T1-weighted MR image **B**, the right C2 facets, right C2 lateral mass, and tissues adjacent to the right C2 facets (*arrows*) enhance with contrast.

IMAGING FEATURES

On radiographs and computed tomography (CT), the osteoarthritic C1-2 facet joint is usually narrowed (see Figs. 33-5, 33-6, and 33-8). However, if a joint effusion is present, the C1-2 joint space may be widened. Intra-articular gas formation may also be located in the degenerated facet joint. The cortical articular surfaces of the C1-2 facets are typically irregular and sclerotic, and this sclerosis may extend into the adjacent marrow (see Fig. 33-5). Hypertrophic osteophytes typically develop along the margins of the osteoarthritic lateral C1-2 facets (see Figs. 33-4 to 33-6).

Concomitant atlantal-odontoid (anterior atlantoaxial joint) osteoarthritis is often present along with osteoarthritis of the C1-2 facets. Anterior atlantoaxial joint osteoarthritis commonly presents with anterior C1-2 joint space narrowing and adjacent cortical

marginal sclerosis and osteophyte formation.[10] Gas may be present in the degenerated anterior C1-2 joint space. The adjacent odontoid process is frequently hypertrophic.[11] In advanced degeneration of the anterior atlantoaxial joint, a *horseshoe-shaped* or *crown-shaped* osteophytic ridge often "crowns" the dens, visible on coronal or sagittal CT images (see Fig. 33-9).[4]

C1-2 facet joint effusions are well demonstrated with MR imaging and may be visible, which may be associated with joint space widening. Joint effusion can be seen in the setting of active or chronic indolent osteoarthritis. The absence of MR T2 signal abnormality in the adjacent articular facets in the presence of a facet joint effusion usually indicates that the effusion is chronic (Figs. 33-10 and *33-11*). If intra-articular effusion distends the C1-2 facet joint capsules, these are sometimes referred to as C1-2 synovial

Text continued on page 247

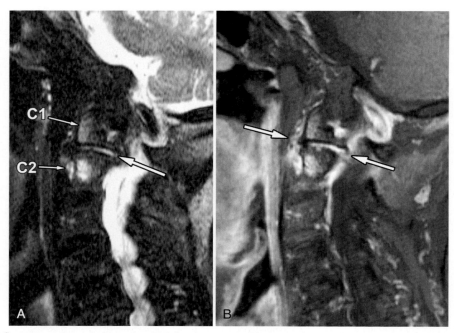

Figure 33-3 ▶ Active Inflammatory Facet Arthropathy, C1-2 level. Parasagittal fat-saturated T2-weighted MR image **A** and contrast-enhanced fat-saturated T1-weighted MR image **B**, in same patient as in Figures 33-1 and 33-2. The C1-2 facet joint (*arrow* in **A**) is narrowed and T2 hyperintense due to presence of joint effusion. T2 hyperintense marrow is located in the articular facets and lateral masses of C1 and C2 on the right (*small arrows* in image **A**). In image **B**, inflammatory tissue, in and adjacent to the right C1-2 facet joint, enhances with contrast. The bone marrow of the right lateral masses of C1 and C2 and periarticular soft tissues (*arrows* in **B**) also enhance with contrast.

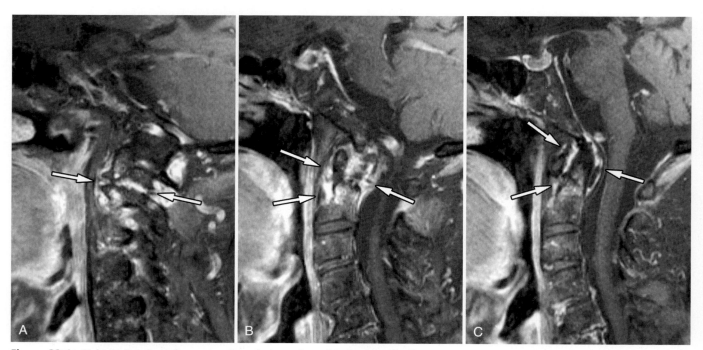

Figure 33-4 ▶ Right C1-2 Active Inflammatory Facet Arthropathy and Peri-Odontoid Inflammation. Same patient as in Figures 33-1 to 33-3. In parasagittal image **A**, which is lateral to Figure 33-3B, the right C1-2 facet joint is widened and tissues in the facet joint (*between arrows*) enhance with contrast. Note small osteophytes arising anteriorly at C1-2 level (*arrows*). On parasagittal image **B**, which is medial to Figure 33-3B, the ligaments and tissues adjacent to C1-2 on the right enhance with contrast indicating presence of inflammation. On sagittal midline image **C**, the dens has been eroded and the prevertebral soft tissue and ligaments anterior and posterior to the dens (*arrows*) enhance indicating inflammation of these tissues.

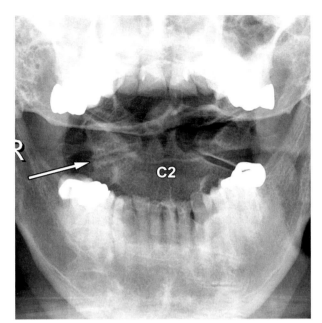

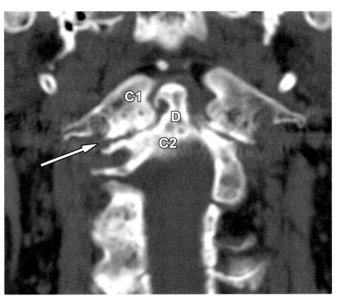

Figure 33-5 ▶ Right C1-2 Facet Osteoarthritis. Anteroposterior (AP) "Open mouth" radiograph shows marked narrowing of right C1-2 facet (zygapophyseal) joint (*arrow*) with sclerosis of adjacent articular facets. Left C1-2 facet joint space is mildly narrowed medially but relatively normal in size laterally.

Figure 33-6 ▶ Right C1-2 Facet Osteoarthritis. Coronal CT image corresponding to AP radiograph in Figure 33-5. The right C1-2 facet joint (*arrow*) is markedly narrowed, and adjacent articular facets are irregular due to subchondral erosions. Adjacent articular processes are sclerotic. Note large erosion along right lateral margin of dens (*D*). The left C1-2 facet joint is narrowed medially and adjacent facets are slightly sclerotic due to relatively mild osteoarthritis on the left.

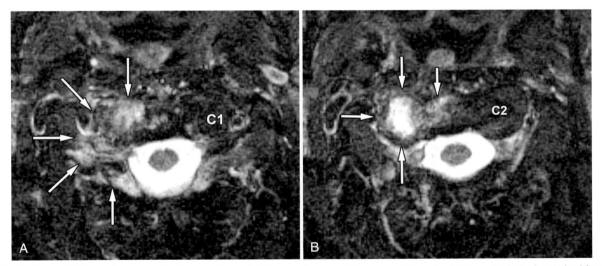

Figure 33-7 ▶ Right C1-2 Facet Osteoarthritis, Marrow Edema in Adjacent Bone. Axial fat-saturated T2-weighted MR images obtained at C1 level (image **A**) and C2 level (image **B**). Heterogeneous T2 hyperintense signal intensity, consistent with marrow edema, is located within the right C1 inferior facet/lateral mass (*arrows* in image **A**) and in the right C2 superior facet/lateral mass (*arrows* in image **B**). T2 hyperintense signal (*arrows* in image **B**) is located in the right C2 lateral mass and body of C2 on the right consistent with marrow edema.

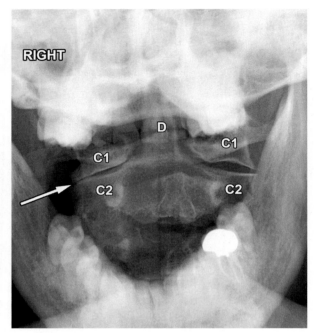

Figure 33-8 ▶ Right C1-2 Facet Osteoarthritis. Anteroposterior (AP) radiograph, "open mouth" view. The right C1-2 joint space is markedly narrowed and the adjacent articular facets are smooth and slightly sclerotic. Osteophytes (*arrow*) arise from the lateral margins of the facets.

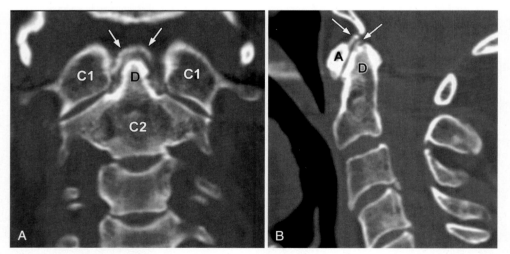

Figure 33-9 ▶ Pri-Odontoid Osteophytic. "Horseshoe-shaped" or "crown" osteophytic ridge (*arrows*) adjacent to the dens (*D*) demonstrated on coronal CT image **A**. C1 = lateral mass of C1 in image **A**. Crown osteophytes (*arrows*) arise from the superior margins of the anterior arch of C1 and the dens as demonstrated on sagittal CT image **B**. *A* = anterior arch of C1 in image **B**. C2 = C2 vertebral body.

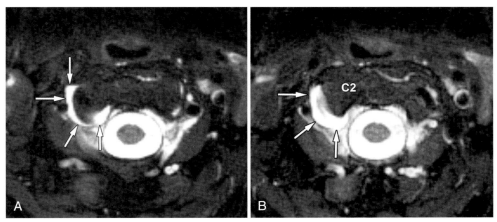

Figure 33-10 ▶ Right C1-2 Joint Effusion in Asymptomatic Patient. This condition is sometimes referred to as a C1-2 "synovial cyst." The right C1-2 facet capsule (*arrows*) is distended circumferentially by intra-articular synovial fluid on contiguous axial fat-saturated T2-weighted images **A** and **B**, obtained at C1-2 level. Note normal intensity of right C2 lateral mass. No evidence of active inflammatory facet arthropathy affecting adjacent bone.

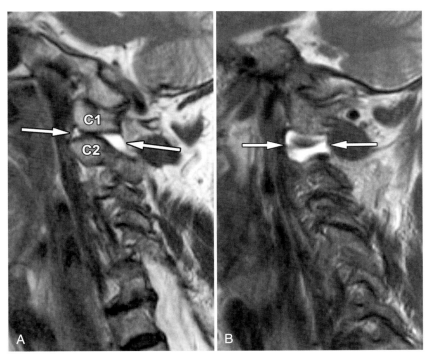

Figure 33-11 ▶ Right C1-2 Joint Effusion in Asymptomatic Patient. Same patient as in Figure 33-9. Contiguous right parasagittal T2-weighted images through right C1-2 facets. The facet capsule is distended by intra-articular fluid (*arrows*) anterior and posterior to the facet joint in more medial image **A**, and lateral to the facet joint (*arrows*) in more lateral image **B**. Note normal signal intensity in adjacent facets and lateral mass of C1 and C2.

cysts. The distended facet capsule typically protrudes into the tissues lateral or anterolateral to the facet joint (see Figs. 33-10 and 33-11). If the cyst is large and extends medially into the epidural space, the synovial cyst may compress and displace the spinal cord.[8]

On MR images, cortical irregularity is usually visible along the margins of the osteoarthritic facets; the signal intensity in the adjacent marrow of the C1 lateral mass and C2 articular pillar are either T1 or T2 hypointense (if sclerotic) or T2 hyperintense if marrow edema is present (see Figs. 33-2, 33-3, 33-7; *Figs. 33-12 and 33-13*). The presence of marrow edema and/or contrast enhancement in the bone marrow adjacent to the C1-2 facets indicates the presence

of active inflammation involving the C1-2 facet joint, similar to that seen with active inflammatory facet arthropathy (facet synovitis) elsewhere in the spine (see Figs. 33-3 and 33-7). This can be seen on fat-saturated, T2-weighted images, although it is best demonstrated on fat-saturated, contrast-enhanced, T1-weighted images (see Figs. 33-2, 33-3, 33-4, 33-12, and 33-13). This appearance is most often due to a noninfectious inflammatory arthropathy, because infectious facet arthropathy is exceedingly rare.

Radionuclide bone scans nearly always show increased uptake in the upper cervical region in patients with active C1-2 facet arthropathy (facet synovitis) (see Fig. 33-1). However, bone

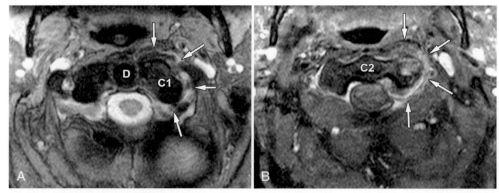

Figure 33-12 ▶ Left C1-2 Osteoarthritis and Facet Synovitis. In axial gradient-recalled echo (GRE) image **A**, the left C1 lateral mass and inferior facet are hypertrophic and surrounded by heterogeneous predominantly hyperintense tissue (*arrows*), which causes slight deformity of the left lateral aspect of the thecal sac. On fat-saturated T2-weighted MR image **B**, the left C2 lateral mass and superior C2 facet contains an enhancing erosion or geode and is surrounded by enhancing inflammatory tissue (*arrows*).

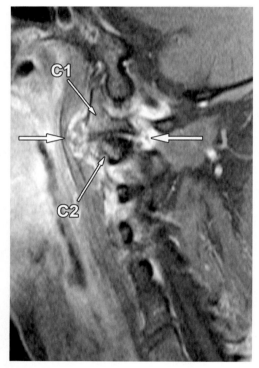

Figure 33-13 ▶ Left C1-2 Osteoarthritis and Facet Synovitis. Same patient as in Figure 33-12. Left parasagittal fat-saturated T1-weighted MR image obtained through left C1-2 facets. Demonstrated is C1-2 joint space narrowing and enhancing hypertrophic inflammatory tissue (*arrows*) anterior and posterior to the facet joint.

scanning is also positive in patients with facet synovitis at other cervical facet levels and in cases with active inflammation involving the atlanto-occipital joints. It may be difficult on bone scan images to determine the precise level of abnormal uptake. Therefore, fat-saturated MR imaging is recommended to define the precise level of joint involvement.

DIFFERENTIAL DIAGNOSIS

1. **Septic arthritis** involving any facet joint is exceedingly rare and the C1-2 level is no exception. However, infection may involve the atlantoaxial articulations and may result in paraspinal phlegmon and abscess formation (*Figs. 33-14 and 33-15*). If there is evidence of cortical bone destruction, exuberant periarticular contrast enhancement, or systemic signs of infection, a C1-2 joint aspiration biopsy may be necessary to evaluate for possible infection. If infection is suspected, intra-articular steroid injection should not be performed pending culture of the joint aspirate.

2. **Neoplasm** involving the lateral mass of C1 or C2 is usually not confused with active inflammatory facet arthropathy, because bone destruction is usually present with neoplasm. Furthermore, active inflammation of the C1-2 joints usually manifests with abnormal signal and/or contrast enhancement

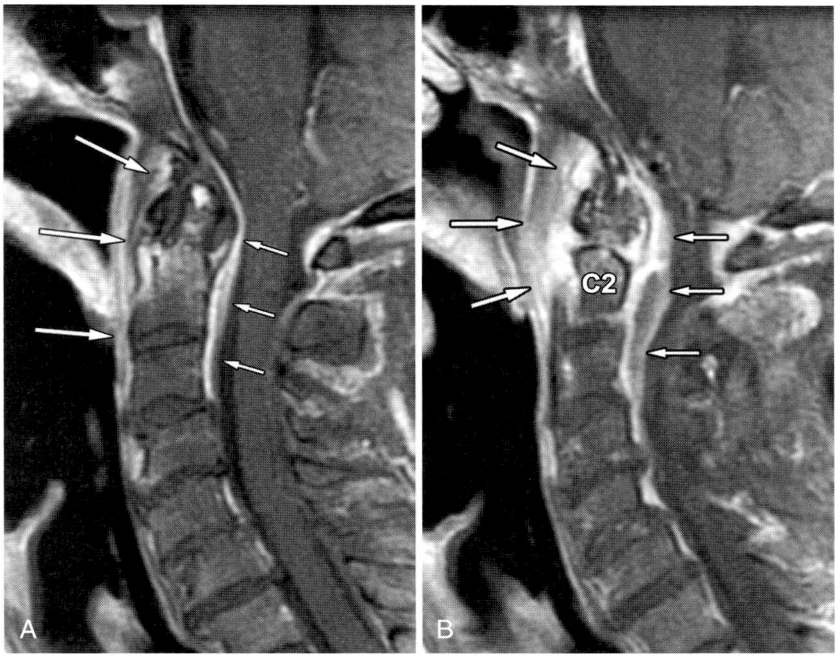

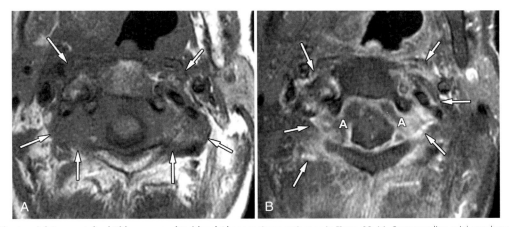

Figure 33-14 ▶ **Atlantoaxial Paravertebral Phlegmon and Epidural Abscess.** Sagittal midline contrast-enhanced fat-saturated T1-weighted MR image **A** and right parasagittal image **B**. Enhancing inflammatory tissue is seen in the epidural space (*short arrows* in **A**) and in the prevertebral soft tissues (*long arrows* in **A** and **B**). Areas of hypointensity in ventral epidural space (*small arrows* in **B**) represent areas of abscess formation within the epidural phlegmon.

Figure 33-15 ▶ **Atlantoaxial Paravertebral Phlegmon and Epidural Abscess.** Same patient as in Figure 33-14. Corresponding axial unenhanced T1-weighted image **A** and contrast-enhanced fat-saturated image **B** at the C2 level. Paravertebral phlegmonous inflammatory tissue (*arrows*) surrounds the C2 vertebra in image **A**, and this tissue enhances heterogeneously in image **B**. Relatively homogeneous inflammatory tissue surrounds the thecal sac on unenhanced image **A**. The hypointense, nonenhancing areas adjacent to the thecal sac in image **B** represent areas of abscess formation (*A*) within the phlegmon in the epidural space.

on both sides of the joint, which would be highly unlikely with a neoplasm.

TREATMENT

1. **Percutaneous C1-2 facet joint injection with anesthetic-steroid agents** can provide effective pain relief and is used to confirm that the pain is actually originating in the C1-2 facet joint *(Figs. 33-16 and 33-17)*.[12] Repeated injections may be necessary to control the neck pain or headaches commonly associated with this condition.

2. **Radiofrequency denervation** can be effective for treatment of recurrent pain related to C1-2 facet arthritis. However, denervation does not treat the ongoing inflammatory process.

3. **Surgical C1-2 fusion** may be necessary if repeated injections fail to provide sufficient or long-term relief.[3,13]

4. **Synovial cysts** causing cord compression may be treated by resection of the cyst and surgical fusion. Synovial cysts occurring at the C1-2 level may regress spontaneously after cervical fusion alone.[8,9,14]

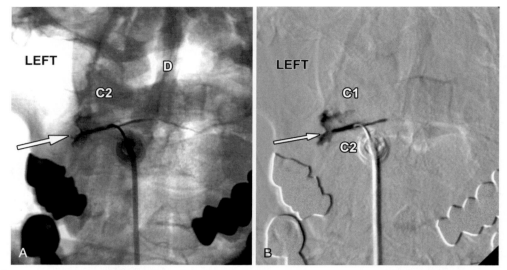

Figure 33-16 ▶ **Left C1-2 Facet Joint Injection.** Procedure performed on patient described in Figures 33-12 and 33-13. Patient is prone, and the needle has been inserted using a posterior approach. The injected iodinated contrast agent is within the left C1-2 facet joint demonstrating the position of the facet joint in posteroanterior (PA) radiograph (image **A**) and in posteroanterior (PA) subtracted radiograph (image **B**). C1 = left lateral mass of C1. C2 = left lateral mass of C2. D = Dens.

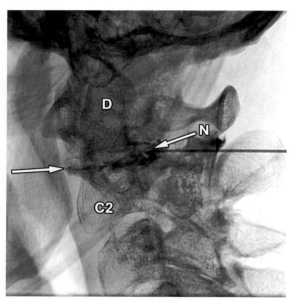

Figure 33-17 ▶ **Facet Joint Injection for Symptomatic C1-2 Facet Osteoarthritis.** Contrast agent has been injected into the C1-2 facet joint in using a posterior approach similar to that shown in Figure 33-16. The C1-2 intra-articular contrast agent is positioned between the needle tip (*N*) and the arrow anteriorly. Note that the C1-2 intra-articular contrast agent overlies the upper body of C2 in this projection.

References

1. Halla JT, Hardin JG Jr. Atlantoaxial (C1-C2) facet joint osteoarthritis: A distinctive clinical syndrome. *Arthritis Rheum.* 1987;30(5):577-582.
2. Zapletal J, de Valois JC. Radiologic prevalence of advanced lateral C1-C2 osteoarthritis. *Spine.* 1997;22(21):2511-2513.
3. Star MJ, Curd JG, Thorne RP. Atlantoaxial lateral mass osteoarthritis: A frequently overlooked cause of severe occipitocervical pain. *Spine.* 1992;17 (6 Suppl):S71-S76.
4. Zapletal J, Hekster RE, Straver JS, Wilmink JT. Atlanto-odontoid osteoarthritis: Appearance and prevalence at computed tomography. *Spine.* 1995;20(1):49-53.
5. Berlemann U, Laubli R, Moore RJ. Degeneration of the atlanto-axial joints: A histological study of 9 cases. *Acta Orthop Scand.* 2002;73(2):130-133.
6. Chang H, Found EM, Clark CR, et al. Meniscus-like synovial fold in the atlantoaxial (C1-C2) joint. *J Spinal Disord.* 1992;5(2):227-231.
7. Yu SW, Sether L, Haughton VM. Facet joint menisci of the cervical spine: Correlative MR imaging and cryomicrotomy study. *Radiology.* 1987;164(1):79-82.
8. Okamoto K, Doita M, Yoshikawa M, et al. Synovial cyst at the C1-C2 junction in a patient with atlantoaxial subluxation. *J Spinal Disorders Techniques.* 2004;17(6):535-538.
9. Morio Y, Yoshioka T, Nagashima H, et al. Intraspinal synovial cyst communicating with the C1-C2 facet joints and subarachnoid space associated with rheumatoid atlantoaxial instability. *Spine.* 2003;28(23):E492-E495.
10. Genez BM, Willis JJ, Lowrey CE, et al. CT findings of degenerative arthritis of the atlantoodontoid joint. *AJR Am J Roentgenol.* 1990;154(2):315-318.

11. Sato K, Senma S, Abe E, et al. Myelopathy resulting from the atlantodental hypertrophic osteoarthritis accompanying the dens hypertrophy: Two case reports. *Spine.* 1996;21(12):1467-1471.

12. Dreyfuss P, Rogers J, Dreyer S, Fletcher D. Atlanto-occipital joint pain: A report of three cases and description of an intraarticular joint block technique. *Reg Anesth.* 1994;19(5):344-351.

13. Wertheim SB, Bohlman HH. Occipitocervical fusion: Indications, technique, and long-term results in thirteen patients. *J Bone Joint Surg.* 1987;69(6):833-836.

14. Chang H, Park JB, Kim KW. Synovial cyst of the transverse ligament of the atlas in a patient with os odontoideum and atlantoaxial instability. *Spine.* 2000;25(6):741-744.

CHAPTER 34

FACET OSTEOARTHRITIS AND SYNOVITIS—CERVICAL

Leo F. Czervionke, M.D.

CLINICAL PRESENTATION

The patient is an 80-year-old female with severe neck pain, neck stiffness, right C4 radiculopathy, and suboccipital headaches. The patient has limited range of neck rotation.

IMAGING PRESENTATION

Radiographs of the spine revealed multilevel cervical spondylosis deformans, disc space narrowing. There is also narrowing of left C1-2 facet joint and multilevel facet and uncinate process hypertrophy. Bone scan reveals increased activity in the upper cervical spine on the left and mid cervical spine on the right *(Fig. 34-1)*. Magnetic resonance (MR) imaging reveals a small effusion in the left C1-2 facet joint, thickened parafacetal soft tissues at C3-4 on the right, and enhancement of the parafacetal soft tissues posterior to the left C1-2 facets, surrounding the right C3-4 facets and in the right C3-4 neural foramen *(Figs. 34-2 to 34-6)*.

DISCUSSION

The cervical facet (zygapophyseal) joints are true diarthrodial joints, containing synovial fluid and lined by hyaline cartilage *(Fig. 34-7)*. The cervical facets are oriented in an oblique coronal plane, which helps prevent translation of the cervical vertebrae along the anteroposterior axis *(Figs. 34-7 and 34-8)*. The degree of orientation of the cervical facet joints in the oblique coronal plane varies according to the cervical level (see Fig. 34-7). The C2 vertebra is unique because of the odontoid process but also because the lateral arch of C2 anatomically is like no other vertebra. The lateral atlantoaxial joint, that is, the C1-2 facet joint, is positioned more anteriorly than the cervical facets below the C1-2 level (see Fig. 34-7). The superior articular facet of C2 is nearly horizontally oriented and is positioned relatively far forward and superior to the inferior articular process of C2. The lateral arch of C2 is very unique because it is in reality an elongated articular pillar that embodies both the C2 pedicle and C2 pars interarticularis. The cervical neural foramen is located anterior to the cervical articular pillars and superior articular process and is bounded anteromedially by the uncinate process (see Fig. 34-8). The cervical neural foramen

contains a ventral nerve root, the dorsal root ganglion, foraminal veins, and a small amount of fat. The vertebral artery traverses the anterior portion of the cervical neural foramen; at the vertebral body level, the vertebral artery courses through the transverse foramen. The dorsal root ganglion lies in a small concave depression along the anterior surface of the superior articular process. The cervical facet joints have a relatively thick capsule laterally (see Fig. 34-8). The cervical neural foramina are bounded superiorly and inferiorly by pedicles *(Fig. 34-9)*.

The cervical facets undergo osteoarthritic degeneration in a similar manner as the lumbar facet joints and other synovial-lined joints. Abnormal acute or repeated stress upon the facet joint initiates a series of biomechanical events that cause an inflammatory process that involves the synovial lining of the joint, eventually leading to erosion of the facet articular cartilage, cortical facet erosions, facet joint narrowing, and cortical thickening *(Fig. 34-10)*.[1] Cystic erosions or geodes may occur in the facets similar to those that occur in other joints involved by osteoarthritis (see Fig. 34-10; *Fig. 34-11*). Eventually the facet capsules become thickened and redundant. In the cervical region, joint capsular inflammation and capsular thickening occurs, which is most obvious in the lateral facet capsule. Pain-sensitive nerve endings (nociceptors) exist in the facet capsules and synovium.[2,3] Simultaneously, bony spurs develop along the margins of the facet joint and the articular processes enlarge overall, as a reactive response to the chronic inflammatory osteoarthritic process (see Figs. 34-10 and 34-11).[1,3]

These enlarged facets are readily visible on routine radiographs, computed tomography (CT) and MR images (Figs. 34-10 to 34-13). The enlarged (hypertrophic) cervical facets contribute to cervical foraminal stenosis along with uncinate process enlargement related to degeneration of the uncovertebral joints *(Figs. 34-12 and 34-13)*.[3] Hypertrophic facets and uncinate processes can also narrow the transverse foramen and thereby cause localized narrowing of the vertebral arteries (see Fig. 34-12).[4] Enlarged cervical facets do not encroach significantly upon the vertebral (central) canal as is commonly the situation in the lumbar region. Therefore, cervical facet hypertrophy does not contribute appreciably to cervical central canal stenosis. Cervical *central canal* stenosis occurs in the anteroposterior (AP) dimension and is secondary to disc bulging or protrusion, posterior vertebral osteophytes, thickened posterior longitudinal ligament, and thickened ligamentum flava.

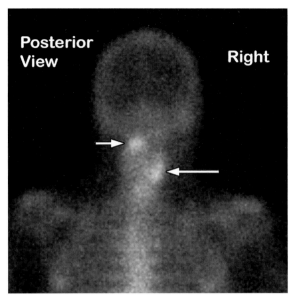

Figure 34-1 ▶ Cervical Facet Synovitis Left C3-4 and Right C1-2. 99mTc—methylene diphosphonate (MDP) radionuclide bone scan, posterior view. Increased activity is demonstrated in the upper left (*short arrow*) and mid-right (*long arrow*) cervical spine.

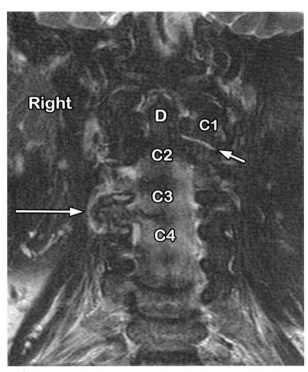

Figure 34-2 ▶ Cervical Facet Synovitis Left C3-4 and Right C1-2. Same patient as in Figure 34-1. Coronal fat-saturated T2-weighted MRI of the cervical spine. T2 hyperintense facet joint effusion (*short arrow*), left C1-2 level. Right C3-4 facet hypertrophy and T2 hyperintense signal is demonstrated in and adjacent to the right C3-4 facets (*long arrow*). C1 = left lateral mass of C1. C2, C3, and C4 vertebral bodies labeled. D = Dens.

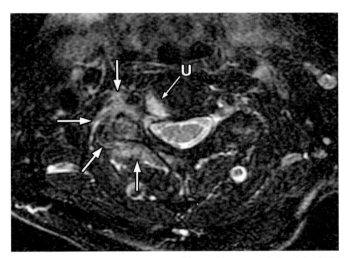

Figure 34-3 ▶ Right C3-4 Facet Synovitis. Axial fat-saturated T2-weighted MRI at the C3-4 level in same patient as in Figures 34-1 and 34-2. T2 hyperintense signal is demonstrated in the right C3-4 facets, right parafacetal soft tissues (*arrows*) and right uncinate process (*U*), representing edema and/or active inflammation.

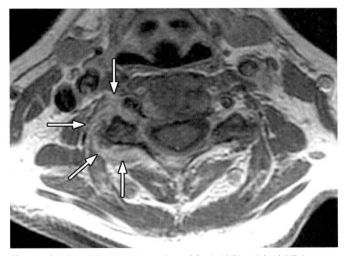

Figure 34-4 ▶ Right C3-4 Facet Synovitis. Axial T1-weighted MR image at C3-4 level, corresponding to Figure 34-3, shows thickened right parafacetal soft tissues (*arrows*) surrounding irregular hypertrophic right C3-4 facets.

Clinical Presentation of Facetogenic Pain

The classic facet syndrome is manifested clinically by unilateral or bilateral back or neck pain that is greater with extension, twisting, or rotation. The pain may be exacerbated upon moving from a sitting to standing position, and may be relieved with spine flexion, standing, walking, rest, or repeated activity. Primary facetogenic pain is generally nonradicular, but may occur if enlarged facets compress the nerve root in the neural foramen or if parafacetal inflammation can extend into the neural foramen, producing a noncompressive inflammatory radiculopathy.

There is poor correlation between neural foraminal stenosis and symptomatic cervical radiculopathy. The cervical neural foramina commonly become stenotic with advancing age and yet relatively few of these stenotic neural foramina are associated with neck pain or radiculopathy, except intermittently. Severely stenotic cervical neural foraminal are more likely to be associated with radicular symptoms, but even severely narrowed cervical neural foramina may be asymptomatic.

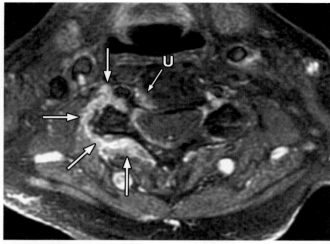

Figure 34-5 ▶ **Right C3-4 Facet Synovitis.** Axial contrast-enhanced fat-saturated T1-weighted MRI at C3-4 level corresponding to Figures 34-3 and 34-4. The thickened parafacetal soft tissues (*arrows*) enhance intensely representing inflammation. Enhancing inflammatory tissue is also located in the right C3-4 neural foramen. The right uncinate process (*U*) also enhances and therefore is involved with the inflammatory process.

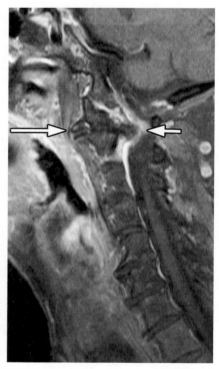

Figure 34-6 ▶ **Left C1-2 Osteoarthritis and Active Left C1-2 Facet Synovitis.** Left parasagittal contrast-enhanced fat-saturated T1-weighted MRI through cervical spine in same patient as in Figures 34-1–34-5. The left C1-2 zygapophyseal (facet) joint is narrowed and hypertrophic bone is visible along its anterior (*long arrow*) and posterior margin (*short arrow*). The posterior C1-2 parafacetal soft tissues enhance intensely (*short arrow*).

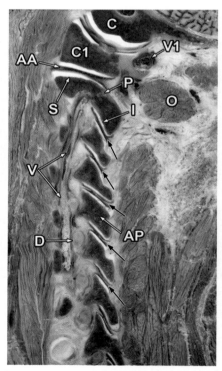

Figure 34-7 ▶ Sagittal Cryomicrotome Image of Cadaver Specimen, Obtained Through Level of Cervical Articular Pillars. A thin layer of pearly white hyaline cartilage lines the articulating surfaces of the cervical facet joints (*black arrows*). A thick layer of hyaline cartilage lines the margins of the lateral atlantoaxial joint (*AA*) and the occipital-atlantal joint, located between the occipital condyle (*C*) and the lateral mass of C1. The lateral atlantoaxial joint (*AA*) is positioned more anteriorly than the cervical facets below the C1-2 level. The superior articular facet (*S*) of C2 is nearly horizontally oriented and is positioned anterosuperior to the inferior articular process (*I*) of C2. The lateral arch of C2 is an elongated articular pillar (*P*) which embodies the C2 pedicle and C2 pars interarticularis. *AP* = articular pillar of C6. D = C7 dorsal root ganglion, which lies in concave depression along anterior surface of C7 superior articular process. V = vertebral artery located anterior to cervical dorsal root ganglia. V1 = vertebral artery at C1 level. O = obliquus capitis inferior muscle.

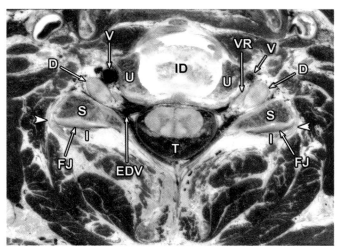

Figure 34-8 ▶ Axial Cryomicrotome Image in Cadaver, C4-5 Neural Foramen and Intervertebral Disc Level. The cervical facet joints (*FJ*) are lined by hyaline cartilage and have a relatively thick cord-like capsule laterally (*arrowheads*). The cervical neural foramen is bounded posteriorly by the superior articular process (*S*) and the uncinate process (*U*) anteromedially. The neural foramen contains the dorsal root ganglion (*D*), ventral nerve root (*VR*), intraforaminal veins, and a minimal amount of fat. The vertebral artery (*V*) forms the anterior boundary of the cervical neural foramen laterally. ID = intervertebral disc, I = inferior articular facet, T = CSF within thecal sac. EDV = epidural veins.

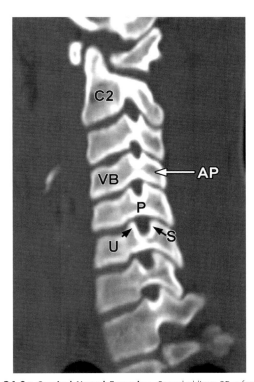

Figure 34-9 ▶ Cervical Neural Foramina. Curved oblique 3D reformatted CT image through the medial portion of the left cervical neural foramina. The cervical neural foramen medially is bounded by the uncinate process (*U*) anteriorly, the superior articular process (*S*) posteriorly and by a pedicle (*P*) above and below. AP = articular pillar of C4. C2 = C2 vertebral body.

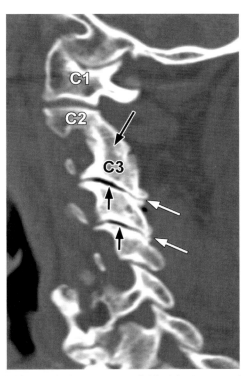

Figure 34-10 ▶ Cervical Facet Osteoarthritis, Joint Degeneration. Sagittal CT image through left cervical lateral C1 and C2 lateral masses, cervical articular pillars and facet joints. Marked narrowing of C2-3 facet joint (*long black arrow*) secondary to advanced degenerative joint disease. Narrowed C3-4 and C4-5 facet joints contain gas (*short black arrows*). Osteophytes are seen (*white arrows*) along posterior margin of C3-4 and C4-5 facet joints.

Traditionally, the diagnosis of facet-related pain has been based on clinical history and physical findings, and the level or levels ultimately selected for facet injection have been based primarily on clinical data and secondarily on gross morphologic imaging data. In effect, this allowed one to select the level of facet injection using a "best guess" approach. The morphologic configuration of the cervical spine, as displayed on radiographs, CT images, and conventional MR images, provide little if any useful information regarding which facets are actively inflamed, and therefore most likely to be the source of acute facetogenic pain. Attempts at predicting the response of facet injection based solely on the morphologic appearance of the facets on images have proven unsuccessful.

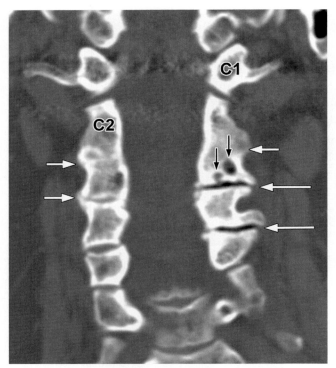

Figure 34-11 ► **Cervical Facet Osteoarthritis, Joint Degeneration.** Same patient as in Figure 34-10. Coronal CT image through cervical articular pillars. Markedly narrowed bilateral C2-3 and right C3-4 facet joint spaces (*short white arrows*). Intra-articular gas (*long arrows*) is located within the narrowed left C3-4 and C4-5 facet joints. Gas is also located within erosions or geodes (*black arrows*) in the inferior articular process of C3 on the left. C1 = left lateral mass of C1.

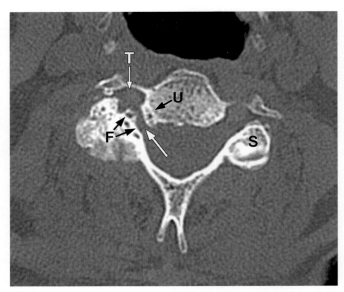

Figure 34-12 ► **Cervical Facet and Uncinate Process Hypertrophy.** Axial CT image C4-5 neural foramen. Severe right neural foraminal stenosis (*white arrow*) compared to relatively normal sized left neural foramen. The foraminal stenosis is due to uncinate process hypertrophy (*U*) and facet hypertrophy (*F*). The hypertrophic facet is also encroaching slightly upon the vertebral artery in the right transverse foramen (*T*). S = minimally hypertrophic left superior articular process.

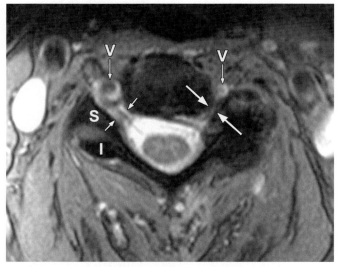

Figure 34-13 ► **Cervical Facet and Uncinate Process Hypertrophy.** Axial gradient-echo (GRE) MRI at the C4-5 level. Marked left facet hypertrophy and moderate left uncinate process hypertrophy result in severe left C4-5 neural foraminal stenosis (*between long arrows*). Relatively normal sized right C4-5 neural foramen (*between short arrows*). S = superior articular process C5. I = inferior articular process C4. V = vertebral arteries.

Pain relief after cervical facet joint injection does not correlate with the morphologic appearance of the facets as seen on CT.[5] This is because the majority of enlarged (hypertrophic) facets visible on radiographs, CT, and MR are not acutely inflamed and therefore not likely to respond to facet injections. These hypertrophic facets are the result of chronic, cyclica inflammation involving the facet joints and adjacent bone. The majority of these hypertrophic facets are in a relatively inactive or indolent phase at the time of imaging.

Current cervical MR imaging techniques should not only provide morphologic information regarding the cervical facets but also allow the MR study interpreter to identify actively inflamed "symptomatic" facets. This can be achieved with currently available MR imaging using fat-saturation techniques (see Figs. 34-2, 34-3, and 34-5). Fat-saturated MR imaging of some type should always be obtained in all routine MR imaging of the cervical, thoracic, and lumbar spine. Otherwise the "symptomatic" facets will go undetected. The use of fat-suppression techniques for skeletal imaging is not new and has been shown to be a valuable technique for the diagnosis of other inflammatory conditions involving bone including vertebral spondylodiscitis,[6,7] and for the diagnosis of bursitis,[8] osteoarthritis,[9] and synovitis[10] in the joints of the extremities. More recently, this same technique has been applied for evaluating active inflammatory facet arthropathy in the lumbar region.[11-14]

We have used fat-saturated MR imaging for routine spine MR imaging for nearly 10 years to detect active inflammatory conditions of the spine including facetogenic inflammation. We use this technique not only to identify inflamed facets but also to help direct our approach for therapeutic facet injections. We inject the facets that are not necessarily enlarged but that display active inflammation based on fat-saturated MR images and therefore have a high likelihood of being symptomatic.

For unknown reasons, facet synovitis in the cervical spine is most commonly observed on MR images in the upper cervical region, most commonly at the C3-4 level. Active inflammatory

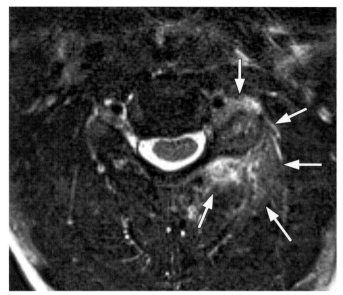

Figure 34-14 ▶ **Infectious Left C3-4 Facet Synovitis.** Infection secondary to methicillin-resistant *Staphyloccus aureus* (MRSA) septicemia. Axial T2-weighted MR image demonstrates diffuse T2 hyperintense signal in the left C3-4 facets and adjacent soft tissues (*arrows*).

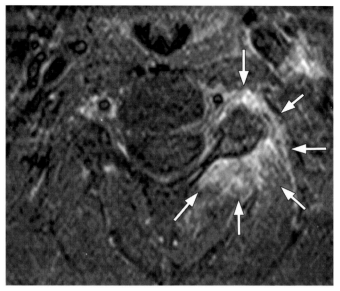

Figure 34-15 ▶ **Infectious Left C3-4 Facet Synovitis.** Same patient as in Figure 34-14. Infectious left C3-4 facet synovitis secondary to methicillin-resistant *Staphyloccus aureus* (MRSA) septicemia. Axial contrast-enhanced fat-saturated T1-weighted MR image shows subtle enhancement of the facets on the left and intense enhancement of the parafacetal soft tissues (*arrows*) secondary to facet and parafacetal inflammation.

facet arthropathy is also quite commonly observed at the C2-3 level and also at the C1-2 level (lateral atlantoaxial joint) (see Fig. 34-6). It is interesting to note here that the greatest degree of cervical facet hypertrophy is most commonly observed in the mid and lower cervical levels, especially at C4-5, C5-6, and C6-7. However, cervical facet synovitis is also observed on fat-saturated MR imaging in the lower cervical region. Facet synovitis also occurs occasionally in the thoracic facets and very commonly involves the lumbar facets (see Chapter 30, "Facet Osteoarthritis and Synovitis: Lumbar"). Cervical facet synovitis is commonly associated with neck pain and cervical radiculopathy. Patients with upper cervical facet synovitis commonly present with suboccipital headaches.

Active inflammatory facet osteoarthropathy is nearly always a noninfectious condition and is encountered in routine everyday MR imaging practice when fat-saturation MR techniques are used. In a retrospectively examined series of 100 patients who had cervical MR imaging for neck or radicular pain at our institution, 26% had active inflammatory facet arthropathy detected on fat-saturated MR imaging. It is important to emphasize that septic facet arthritis can have an identical MR appearance to the exceedingly common noninfectious facet synovitis presented in this case. Facet joint infection is exceedingly rare in our experience. We have encountered only one case of infectious facet synovitis in the past 10 years in a patient who had septicemia with MRSA (methicillin-resistant *Staphylococcus aureus*) **(Figs. 34-14 and 34-15)**. If there is clinical suspicion of septic facet synovitis, needle aspiration biopsy should be obtained before therapeutic facet injection with steroidal agents.

IMAGING FEATURES

Cervical facet enlargement and neural foraminal stenosis are well demonstrated on oblique plain radiographs of the cervical spine **(Fig. 34-16)**. Cervical radiographs remain a valuable adjunct imaging procedure for evaluating the cervical spine, especially

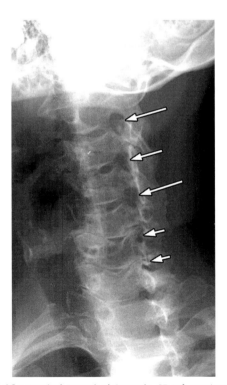

Figure 34-16 ▶ **Cervical Foraminal Stenosis, CT.** Left anterior oblique (LAO) radiograph of the cervical spine in patient with normal sized left C2-3 and C4-5 neural foramina (*long arrows*), mild left C3-4 neural foraminal stenosis (*intermediate-length arrow*), and severe left C5-6 and C6-7 neural foraminal stenosis (*short arrows*).

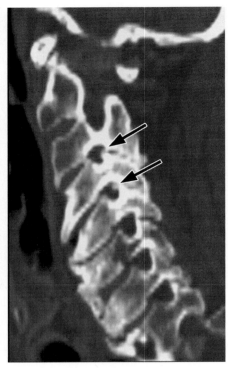

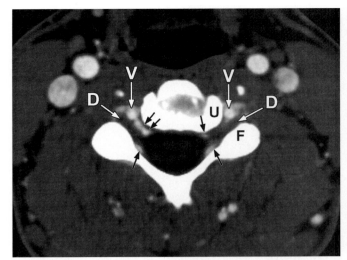

Figure 34-18 ▶ **Normal Contrast Enhanced Axial CT Image from Soft Tissue Neck Study.** Normally enhancing epidural and foraminal veins (*black arrows*) surround the thecal sac and nerve root sheaths in the neural foramen. The dorsal root ganglia (*D*) and vertebral arteries (*V*) are also surrounded by enhancing veins. U = uncinate process. F = facet.

Figure 34-17 ▶ Oblique 3D CT image showing left cervical neural foramina in patient with multilevel spondylosis deformans and moderate neural foraminal stenosis (*arrows*) at C3-4 and C4-5 levels on the left.

when interpreted along with MR studies of the cervical spine.[15] However, the cervical neural foraminal size is more accurately assessed using two-dimensional (2D) axial or three-dimensional (3D) CT imaging. The neural foraminal dimensions and configuration are most accurately demonstrated by generating oblique-reformatted 3D-reformatted images through the neural foramina (see Fig. 34-9; **Fig. 34-17**).[16] However, axial 2D CT images are adequate for assessing the degree of foraminal stenosis (see Fig. 34-12). Myelography with post-myelogram CT scanning or MR myelography[17] are most useful for evaluating the nerve roots as they traverse the thecal sac, where hypertrophic uncinate process or facet may impinge upon the nerve roots. However, CT and radiographs are not optimal for directly evaluating the cervical soft tissues, intervertebral discs, ligaments, and paraspinal soft tissues, which are more optimally demonstrated with MR imaging; 2D or 3D MR imaging techniques can be used to evaluate the cervical neural foramina.[18]

MR can be used to assess cervical foraminal stenosis, but caution must be used in assessing cervical foraminal stenosis with MR, because there is a tendency to overestimate the degree of foraminal narrowing on MR images. However, with experience, an accurate assessment of the cervical neural foramen can be made with MR (see Fig. 34-13). T1-weighted MR images of the cervical spine are useful for assessing the gross morphologic configuration of the vertebrae, intervertebral discs, and spinal cord and are least susceptible to artifact from motion and paramagnetic susceptibility. Contrast between bone and soft tissue in the cervical spine is generally poor on T1-weighted images. The intensity of the disc, vertebral marrow, and tissues within the vertebral (central) canal and neural canal (neural foramen) is very similar in intensity on T1-weighted images, unless intravenous paramagnetic contrast

agent is administered. This is in part due to the cervical vertebral and neural canals containing little if any epidural or intraforaminal fat, which acts as a contrasting tissue on T1-weighted images. In the lumbar spine, epidural and intraforaminal fat is abundant, which makes T1-weighted imaging more useful for evaluating the lumbar spine.

In the cervical region, the epidural space is largely filled by an extensive venous plexus that envelops the thecal sac and surrounds the nerve root sheaths in the cervical neural foramina (*Fig. 34-18*). These veins are not optimally visualized on T1-weighted or T2-weighted images in the cervical spine unless an intravenous (IV) contrast agent is given.[11,14,19] Gradient-recalled echo (GRE) images are useful in the cervical region because they render the epidural and intraforaminal veins visible and are routinely obtained in the cervical region for evaluating the neural foramen and also the intervertebral disc. GRE images provide excellent contrast between hypointense bone and relatively hyperintense disc and foraminal tissues.[19] Unfortunately, paramagnetic susceptibility artifacts are greater on GRE images, making bone appear larger than reality. Therefore, the cervical neural foramina appear more stenotic on GRE images than on conventional T1-weighted MR images, so caution must be exercised when evaluating GRE images. However, with experience, gradient-recalled echo images can be used as a reliable screening assessment of cervical neural foraminal size (see Fig. 34-13). Alternatively, short tau inversion recovery (STIR) imaging can be used to evaluate the cervical spine.[19] STIR imaging is also excellent for evaluating the paraspinal ligaments, and is especially useful for evaluating the cervical spine with MR in the setting of trauma.

The epidural and foraminal tissues, cervical neural and foraminal configuration, are best demonstrated with MR imaging when intravenous (IV) paramagnetic contrast agents are used with conventional T1-weighted imaging (see Figs. 34-5 and 34-15). This is because the abundant cervical epidural and intraforaminal veins enhance with this technique. In the past, IV contrast has not been widely used to evaluate the cervical spine in the traditional MR "screening" studies of the cervical spine.

By applying fat-suppression techniques, the signal intensity of fat in normal bone marrow and in normal soft tissues adjacent to the facets is suppressed. On T2-weighted MR images, abnormal tissues will display T2 hyperintensity, which is rendered more conspicuous by applying a fat-saturation technique (see Figs. 34-3 and 34-14). Alternatively, STIR imaging obtained with an inversion pulse to suppress fat, can also be effective in identifying actively inflamed facets. The most sensitive MR imaging technique for detection of the actively inflamed facet is fat-saturated, T1-weighted, spin echo MR imaging obtained after IV contrast administration. After contrast enhancement, inflamed facets or adjacent tissues will enhance relative to normal soft tissue and bone. This abnormal enhancement is augmented by the use of a fat-saturation technique (see Figs. 34-5 and 34-15).

In the case of active cervical facet inflammation, T1 hypointensity and T2 hyperintensity are typically seen in the bone marrow adjacent to the actively inflamed facets, which is visible on sagittal images obtained through the articular pillars *(Fig. 34-19)*. A facet joint effusion may or may not be present. Increased T2 signal intensity or contrast enhancement is frequently observed in the facet joint, facet joint capsule, bone adjacent to the facets, and in other parafacetal soft tissues (see Fig. 34-19; *Fig. 34-20*). The

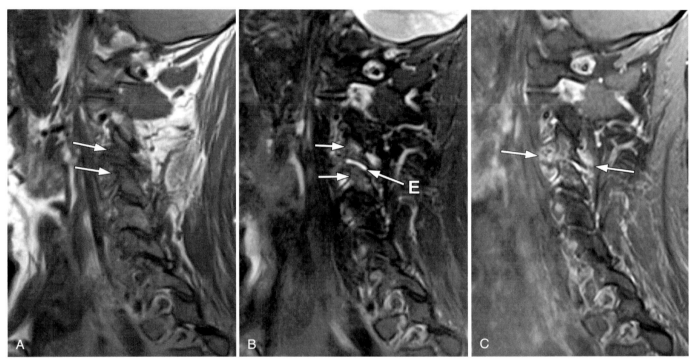

Figure 34-19 ▶ Left C3-4 Facet Synovitis. Sagittal MR images through the left articular pillars. The marrow in the articular processes adjacent to the left C3-4 facet joint is T1 hypointense on T1-weighted MR image **A** and T2 hyperintense on T2-weighted image **B**. A joint effusion (*E*) is demonstrated in the C3-4 facet joint in image **B**. Enhancement of the marrow and soft tissues (*arrows*) adjacent to the C3-4 facet joint is demonstrated on contrast-enhanced fat-saturated T1-weighted MR image **C**.

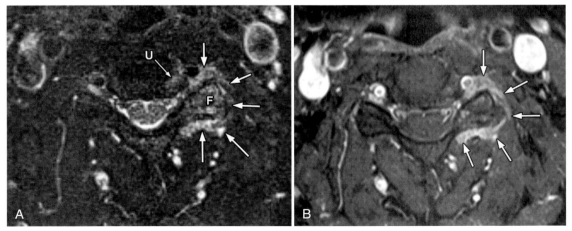

Figure 34-20 ▶ Left C3-4 Facet Synovitis. Patient with left C4 radicular pain and neck pain. The left C3-4 facets (*F*), left C4 uncinate process (*U*) and perifacetal soft tissues are hyperintense on axial T2-weighted MR image **A**. The left C3-4 facets and perifacetal soft tissues enhance (*arrows*) on axial contrast-enhanced fat-saturated T1-weighted MR image **B**. Abnormal enhancing tissue is also located within left C3-4 neural foramen.

inflammation may also involve the neural foraminal soft tissues, ligamentum flavum, and soft tissues adjacent to the lamina and spinous process at the level of the involved facets.[11] The MR signal abnormality or abnormal contrast enhancement represents either edema and/or inflammation extending into the adjacent bone or soft tissues.

A grading system can be used to characterize the degree of cervical inflammatory facet arthropathy similar to the grading system discussed in Chapter 30.[11] Patients with cervical inflammatory facet arthropathy most commonly present with grade 3 or grade 4 facet synovitis, and these patients are nearly always symptomatic. The periarticular inflammatory process adjacent to the facets commonly extends into the cervical neural foramen where the inflammation may encase the nerve roots and causes an inflammatory radiculopathy (see Figs. 34-3 and 34-20).

Radionuclide Imaging and Facet Disease

The radionuclide bone scan, which is an indicator of active bone turnover, often reveals increased radiotracer uptake in one or more of the posterior vertebral elements in patients with facetogenic pain (see Fig. 34-1). In a minority of cases, the bone scan may be normal at a given level that is positive for facet synovitis on fat-saturated MR imaging. Bone scan images have relatively poor spatial resolution and often do not provide enough anatomic detail for accurately determining what portion of the vertebra is affected or even what vertebral level is involved. This is especially problematic in the cervical spine. For this reason, standard reports of bone scans, showing nonspecific increased activity off-midline in the spine, frequently mention increased activity probably secondary to *degenerative disease* or *arthritis* but do not usually mention that the activity could be arising from the facets.[20] Degenerative processes in the spine can also be seen with F18-fluorodeoxy-D-glucose (FDG) positron emission tomography (PET) imaging and is believed to be the result of active inflammation in the involved portions of the spine.[21]

DIFFERENTIAL DIAGNOSIS OF FACET SYNOVITIS

1. **Infectious facet synovitis:** The MR findings of facet synovitis may be identical in active inflammation secondary to sterile synovitis or infectious synovitis. Noninfectious inflammatory facet arthropathy, as mentioned above, is exceedingly common. Septic facet arthritis is exceedingly rare, but should always be considered, especially when bone destruction is present or if the parafacetal inflammatory response in the adjacent soft tissues is greater than expected (see Figs. 34-14 and 34-15). In these patients, a percutaneous needle aspiration biopsy of the facet joint and surrounding tissues should be obtained. Laboratory studies including white blood cell count, erythrocyte sedimentation rate (ESR), and/or C-reactive protein should also be obtained before facet injection with steroidal agents, if an infected facet joint is suspected.

2. **Metastatic neoplasm:** Marrow infiltrating disorders such as vertebral metastases can also have abnormal T2 signal hyperintensity on fat-saturated MR images. The possibility of metastatic neoplasm should always be considered in patients with facet synovitis. We have often observed that patients with spinal metastases also have coexisting lumbar or cervical facet synovitis, which may be an additional factor contributing to their back pain. This empirical observation does not suggest that facet synovitis is more prevalent in patients with spinal metastases, but rather that facet synovitis is detected more frequently in this population, because fat-saturation techniques are widely used in the evaluation of patients with metastatic disease. It is likely exceedingly rare for metastasis to involve the articular facet joints alone, without associated involvement of the adjacent pedicle, lamina, or vertebral body. Typically, multiple sites of vertebral involvement are seen in patients with spinal metastatic disease, and therefore the distinction between facet synovitis and metastatic neoplasm is usually not problematic.

3. **Primary vertebral tumors:** Primary tumors of the spine or other skeletal structures will also enhance using fat-suppression techniques and produce T2 signal hyperintensity and contrast enhancement of the involved bone. The MR appearance of osteoid osteoma in the hip has been reported using a fat-saturation technique.[24] An osteoid osteoma arising in the posterior vertebral arch or osteoblastoma could be mistaken for facet synovitis, and therefore correlation with the clinical presentation is crucial. It is also theoretically possible that a facet joint synovial sarcoma could have an MR appearance similar to facet synovitis. However, we have never encountered a proved case of facet synovial sarcoma in our practice.

TREATMENT: ACTIVE INFLAMMATORY FACET ARTHROPATHY (FACET SYNOVITIS)

1. **Nonsteroidal analgesics and/or physical therapy:** Patients are often treated initially with nonsteroidal analgesics and/or physical therapy, which provide little if any short-term relief of pain. Physical activity often exacerbates the patient's symptoms in the acute phase of facet joint inflammation. Physical therapy is very important for the long-term therapy of patients with facetogenic and other types of back pain, after the acute inflammatory phase, when symptoms are subsiding or have resolved.

2. **Facet injection with anesthetic/steroidal agents:** Percutaneous facet injection with anesthetic/steroidal agents is the recommended procedure for treatment of acute facetogenic back and neck pain. Patients with MR imaging evidence of facet synovitis are most often symptomatic and usually respond favorably to facet injections for relief of neck pain and radicular symptoms. It is important to perform intra-articular and para-articular injections in these patients, especially patients with radicular pain secondary to facet synovitis. A detailed description of the methodology of facet injection can be found elsewhere.[14] Repeated facet injections may be necessary to diminish the pain. A program of long-term physical therapy is vital in these patients to improve paraspinal muscle strength and flexibility and to facilitate long-term pain relief.

3. **Radiofrequency denervation:** Patients who respond well repeatedly to facet injections can be considered for radiofrequency denervation, but have symptoms that continually recur. These patients have recurrent symptoms at shorter intervals after each subsequent facet injection. It is important to remember that denervation procedures ablate the nerves and relieve pain, but do not affect the osteoarthritic inflammatory condition, which continues to involve the facets and will likely continue to cause progressive degeneration of the facets.

The subject of radiofrequency denervation is beyond the scope of this chapter, but a detailed description of this topic can be found elsewhere.[22]

4. **Posterior cervical fusion:** A last resort therapeutic option for intractable primary facetogenic pain is posterior cervical fusion. This is rarely performed for facetogenic pain alone. Fusion of the cervical facets results in markedly limited neck mobility.

5. **Laminectomy:** Decompressive laminectomy with anterior or posterior fusion may be performed in patients with intractable radicular pain, myelopathy, or spinal instability.[23]

References

1. Fletcher G, Haughton VM, Ho KC, Yu SW. Age-related changes in the cervical facet joints: Studies with cryomicrotomy, MR, and CT. *AJR Am J Roentgenol.* 1990;154(4):817-820.
2. Giles LG, Taylor JR. Human zygapophyseal joint capsule and synovial fold innervation. *Br J Rheumatol.* 1987;26(2):93-98.
3. Resnick D. Degenerative diseases of the vertebral column. *Radiology.* 1985;156(1):3-14.
4. Prescher A. Anatomy and pathology of the aging spine. *Eur J Radiol.* 1998;27(3):181-195.
5. Hechelhammer L, Pfirrmann CW, Zanetti M, et al. Imaging findings predicting the outcome of cervical facet joint blocks. *Eur Radiol.* 2007;17(4):959-964.
6. Longo M, Granata F, Ricciardi K, et al. Contrast-enhanced MR imaging with fat suppression in adult-onset septic spondylodiscitis. *Eur Radiol.* 2003;13(3):626-637.
7. Georgy BA, Hesselink JR. Evaluation of fat suppression in contrast-enhanced MR of neoplastic and inflammatory spine disease. *AJNR Am J Neuroradiol.* 1994;15(3):409-417.
8. Skaf AY, Boutin RD, Dantas RW, et al. Bicipitoradial bursitis: MR imaging findings in eight patients and anatomic data from contrast material opacification of bursae followed by routine radiography and MR imaging in cadavers. *Radiology.* 1999;212(1):111-116.
9. Link TM, Steinbach LS, Ghosh S, et al. Osteoarthritis: MR imaging findings in different stages of disease and correlation with clinical findings. *Radiology.* 2003;226(2):373-381.
10. Barakat MS, Schweitzer ME, Morisson WB, et al. Reactive carpal synovitis: Initial experience with MR imaging. *Radiology.* 2005;236(1):231-236.
11. Czervionke LF, Fenton DS. Fat-saturated MR imaging in the detection of inflammatory facet arthropathy (facet synovitis) in the lumbar spine. *Pain Med.* 2008;9(4):400-406.
12. D'Aprile P, Tarantino A, Jinkins JR, Brindicci D. The value of fat saturation sequences and contrast medium administration in MRI of degenerative disease of the posterior/perispinal elements of the lumbosacral spine. *Eur Radiol.* 2007;17(2):523-531.
13. Czervionke LF, Haughton VM. Degenerative Disease of the Spine. In: Atlas SW, ed. *Magnetic Resonance Imaging of the Brain and Spine.* 3rd ed. Philadelphia: Lippincott Williams & Wilkins; 2002.
14. Czervionke LF, Fenton DS. Facet joint injection and medial branch block. In: Fenton DS, Czervionke LF, eds. *Image-Guided Spine Intervention.* Philadelphia: Saunders; 2002.
15. Brown BM, Schwartz RH, Frank E, Blank NK. Preoperative evaluation of cervical radiculopathy and myelopathy by surface-coil MR imaging. *AJR Am J Roentgenol.* 1988;151(6):1205-1212.
16. Roberts CC, McDaniel NT, Krupinski EA, Erly WK. Oblique reformation in cervical spine computed tomography: A new look at an old friend. *Spine (Phila Pa 1976).* 2003;28(2):167-170.
17. Birchall D, Connelly D, Walker L, Hall K. Evaluation of magnetic resonance myelography in the investigation of cervical spondylotic radiculopathy. *Br J Radiol.* 2003;76(908):525-531.
18. Yousem DM, Atlas SW, Goldberg HI, Grossman RI. Degenerative narrowing of the cervical spine neural foramina: Evaluation with high-resolution 3DFT gradient-echo MR imaging. *AJNR Am J Neuroradiol.* 1991;12(2):229-236.
19. Czervionke LF, Berquist TH. Imaging of the spine: Techniques of MR imaging. *Orthop Clin North Am.* 1997;28(4):583-616.
20. Oppenheim BE, Cantez S. What causes lower neck uptake in bone scans? *Radiology.* 1977;124(3):749-752.
21. Rosen RS, Fayad L, Wahl RL. Increased 18F-FDG uptake in degenerative disease of the spine: Characterization with 18F-FDG PET/CT. *J Nucl Med.* 2006;47(8):1274-1280.
22. Fenton DS, Czervionke LF. Facet denervation. In: Fenton DS, Czervionke LF, eds. *Image-Guided Spine Intervention.* Philadelphia: Saunders; 2002.
23. Grob D. Surgery in the degenerative cervical spine. *Spine (Phila Pa 1976).* 1998;23(24):2674-2683.
24. Liu PT, Chivers FS, Roberts CC, Schultz CJ, Beauchamp CP. Imaging of osteoid osteoma with dynamic gadolinium-enhanced MR imaging. *Radiology.* 2003;27(3):691-700.

FACET OSTEOARTHRITIS AND SYNOVITIS—LUMBAR

Leo F. Czervionke, M.D.

CLINICAL PRESENTATION

The patient is a 46-year-old male with low back pain on the right and pain in the right buttock and right hip. No objective physical findings found on examination.

IMAGING PRESENTATION

Magnetic resonance (MR) imaging reveals right L4-5 facet hypertrophy and abnormal T2 signal and contrast enhancement in and around the right L4-5 facets compatible with active inflammatory facet arthropathy (facet synovitis) (*Figs. 35-1 to 35-3*). Bone scan was initially reported as normal, but reveals minimal increase in activity in the lower lumbar spine on the right (*Fig. 35-4*).

DISCUSSION

The zygapophyseal (facet) joints are diarthrodial synovial joints that allow the spine to bend and twist. At any given level, the articular facets are the ovoid surfaces of the inferior and articular processes. Each opposing facet "faces" the joint space, and the facet is composed of a thin layer of dense cortical bone and an overlying layer of hyaline cartilage (*Fig. 35-5*). The facet joint contains a small amount of fluid normally and is lined by a thin layer of synovium. Synovial lined joints are contained by a fibroelastic capsule. The facet joint capsule is comprised of two layers, an outer fibrous layer made of parallel bundles of collagen and an inner layer of elastic fibers similar to the ligamentum flavum (see Fig. 35-5).[1] The facet joint capsule is thicker where it surrounds the inferior portion of the lumbar facet joint compared with the middle and superior portions of the joint. A band of tendinous fibers reinforce the medial portion of the joint capsule. These tendinous fibers are contiguous with the deep layer of the multifidus muscle and run from the posterolateral margin of the lamina at a given level to the posteromedial margin of the lamina one level above.[1]

Nociceptive and proprioceptive nerve endings are found in the facet capsules and in the synovium.[1,2] The nociceptive endings are found mainly in the middle-lateral and inferior portions of the joint capsule.[1] Normally nociceptors have a high threshold, firing only when subjected to extreme mechanical stress. When the capsule becomes inflamed, these nociceptors are sensitized by inflammation-induced chemicals that cause the nociceptors to fire at a lower threshold.[3] Hence, pain is generated at a lower threshold in the presence of facet capsular and synovial inflammation. Spinal extension tends to constrict the inferior portion of the facet capsule and therefore is likely to elicit more factogenic pain than spinal flexion.[1]

Arthritis may affect any synovial joint and the facet joints are no exception. Osteoarthritis (degenerative joint disease) is the most common arthritic process that affects the facet joints. Facet joints that are oriented in the sagittal plane are more prone to developing osteoarthritis and are commonly associated with degenerative spondylolisthesis.[4] Facet joint osteoarthritis is a common finding associated with low back pain in a community-based practice. The prevalence of lumbar facet osteoarthritis increases with advancing age, is slightly greater in women, and is most common at the L4-5 level, followed by L5-S1 and L3-4.[5]

The transition between a normally aging facet joint and a "degenerated" facet joint is not clearly defined. Multiple etiologic processes interact or may contribute to the end result we know as *facet degeneration* or *osteoarthritis*, including age, a genetic predisposition, trauma (acute or repeated microtrauma), metabolic factors, repeated biomechanical stress, and sometimes infection.

The histopathologic events that cause osteoarthritis in any synovial joint are usually cyclic, and if symptoms occur with this process, these tend to be episodic as well. In an *active* phase, something triggers an inflammatory response within the synovial joint. The synovial lining of the joint becomes inflamed, thickened, and redundant, and the cells in the synovium malfunction resulting in a joint effusion. The inflammation usually extends to involve the adjacent articular capsular tissues and adjacent bone. The capsules and adjacent tissues become inflamed, thickened, and redundant as well. As a result of this process, articular cartilage becomes degraded and erosions develop in the articular cartilage and subsequently in the adjacent bone (*Fig. 35-6*).

A reactive inflammatory response occurs in the adjacent bone. Eventually, when the inflammation becomes quiescent, the cartilage and adjacent bone heal to some extent but not completely. The intra-articular effusion may or may not resolve. Erosions in the cartilage and adjacent bones may heal or persist, and the bone enlarges slightly and becomes sclerotic in this reparative phase. Simultaneously, inflammation in the adjacent joint capsules subsides, but the capsules often remain slightly thickened and weakened. When the same process occurs repeatedly over time, the damage to the synovium, facet capsule, and articular facet bone becomes more extensive. Eventually, as a result of this chronic osteoarthritic process, the synovium becomes thickened and redundant, the articular cartilage becomes degraded and thinned,

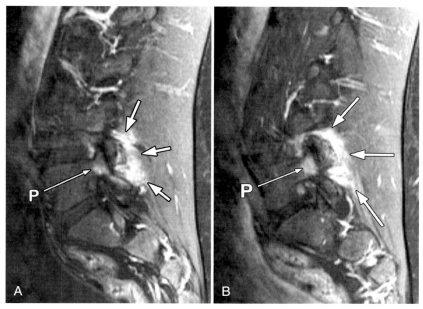

Figure 35-1 ► **Active Inflammatory Facet Arthropathy (Facet Synovitis).** Right L4-5 level. Contrast-enhanced fat-saturated T1-weighted parasagittal MR image **A** and more lateral parasagittal image **B**. Intense contrast-enhancement of the L4-5 facets, parafacetal soft tissues (*arrows*) and right pedicle (P) of L5.

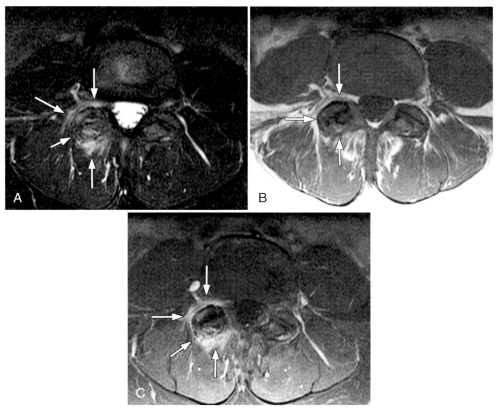

Figure 35-2 ► **Active Inflammatory Facet Arthropathy (Facet Synovitis).** Same patient as in Figure 35-1. On axial T2-weighted MR image **A**, hyperintensity is demonstrated in the right C4-5 facets and parafacetal soft tissues (*arrows*). Corresponding axial T1-weighted image **B** shows mild left and moderate right facet hypertrophy (*arrows*). On corresponding contrast-enhanced fat-saturated T1-weighted MR image, intense enhancement is present in the right parafacetal soft tissues (*arrows*).

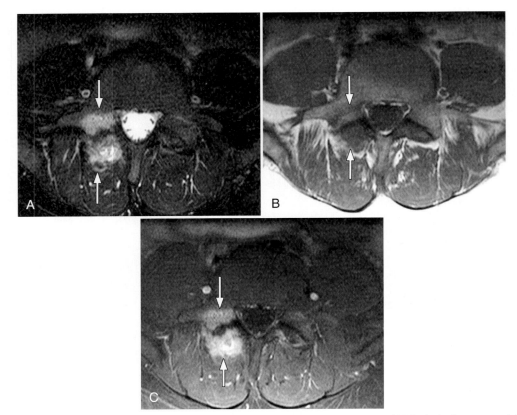

Figure 35-3 ► **Active Inflammatory Facet Arthropathy (Facet Synovitis).** Some patient as in Figures 35-1 and 35-2, obtained at more caudal level through inferior portion of L4-5 facets. The facets and adjacent bone (*arrows*) are hyperintense on fat-saturated T2-weighted MR image **A**, slightly hypointense relative to normal marrow on T1-weighted image **B**, and enhance intensely with contrast on contrast-enhanced fat-saturated T1-weighted MR image **C**.

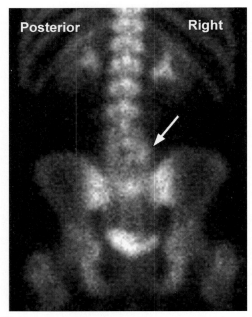

Figure 35-4 ► **Radionuclide Bone Scan Image, Posterior View.** Same patient as in Figures 35-1 to 35-3. Minimal increased uptake (*arrow*) is demonstrated in the lower lumbar spine on the right at the L4-5 level.

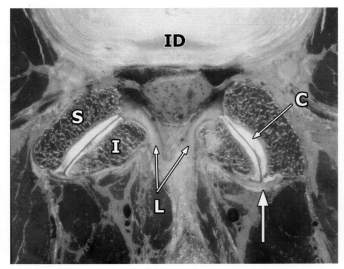

Figure 35-5 ► **Normal Lumbar Facets at L3-4 Level.** Axial cryomicrotome photograph of cadaver specimen. The superior articular process/facet (*S*) of L4 is anterior to the inferior articular process/facet (*I*) of L3. The normal articular cartilage (*C*), on either side of the facet joint, is smooth and intact. Note relatively thick but normal posterior facet capsule on the left (*long arrow*). L = Ligamentum Flavum. ID = Intervertebral Disc.

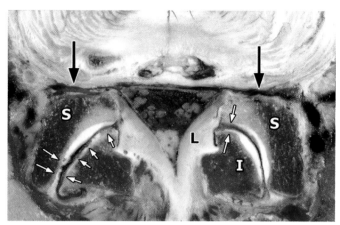

Figure 35-6 ▶ Lumbar Facet Degeneration. Axial cryomicrotome photograph of cadaver specimen. The facet cortical bone is nonuniform and the facet articular hyaline cartilage is eroded in multiple locations (*small white arrows*). Bilateral neural foraminal stenosis (*black arrows*) is due to generalized disc bulging and hypertrophy of the superior articular processes (S). L = Ligamentum Flavum. I = Inferior articular process.

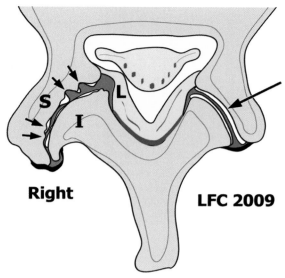

Figure 35-7 ▶ Illustration of Normal Lumbar Facets on Left and Osteoarthritic Facets on Right in Axial Plane. The normal articular facets are smooth and the hyaline cartilage (*long arrow*) is smooth and uniform in thickness. The osteoarthritic superior (*S*) and inferior (*I*) articular processes on the right are enlarged (hypertrophic). On the right, the articular cartilage is irregular due to multiple erosions and subchondral erosions involve the bony facets (*small arrows*) in multiple locations. The anteromedial portion of the facet capsule is distended; the facet capsule is thickened, as is adjacent ligamentum flavum (*L*).

permanent articular and bone erosions occur, and subchondral cysts or geodes form in the articular facets *(Fig. 35-7)*. The facet capsules become thickened, yet weakened and lax. The chronically inflamed facet joint capsules and adjacent ligamentum flavum become thickened and encroach upon the paraspinal soft tissues, central vertebral canal, and neural foramen (see Fig. 35-7; *Fig. 35-8*). Cystic outpouchings of the facet joints, called *synovial cysts,* may form. In the late stages of this episodic inflammatory process, the facet joint often becomes unstable resulting in facet subluxation or dislocation. (See Chapter 75 for more discussion of synovial cysts.)

Facet joint effusions form in the active stage of the disease and may persist long after acute inflammation subsides in a chronic degenerated facet joint *(Fig. 35-9)*. The facet joint fluid may also become replaced by gas (the *vacuum facet phenomenon*) *(Fig. 35-10)*. The facet joint spaces are typically widened when acute or chronic inflammatory effusions are present, but the facet joint space is often narrowed with an undulating, irregular margin in severe chronic facet degeneration *(Fig. 35-11)*.

As facet hypertrophy becomes pronounced, the hypertrophic bone encroaches upon adjacent structures, contributing to neural foraminal stenosis, central canal stenosis, and lateral recess stenosis. Superior facet hypertrophy is the primary cause of lateral recess stenosis. Facet hypertrophy, along with ligamentum flavum thickening, also contributes to central canal stenosis. Facet hypertrophy tends to encroach upon the lower portion of the lumbar neural foramen initially. Because the lumbar nerve roots are positioned in the superior portion of the neural foramen, severe facet hypertrophy is usually required to cause significant foraminal nerve root impingement.[6] At any given lumbar level, foraminal stenosis is typically caused by disc bulging or protrusion, posterolateral vertebral osteophyte formation and hypertrophy of the superior articular process/facet (see Figs. 35-6 and 35-8). The L5 nerve root is the most commonly affected nerve by neural foraminal narrowing secondary to bulging or protruding disc, posterolateral vertebral osteophytes, and facet hypertrophy.[7] The L5 nerve root is also the most common nerve to be affected by lateral recess stenosis. (See Chapters 71 and 72 for further discussion of spinal stenosis and lateral recess stenosis).

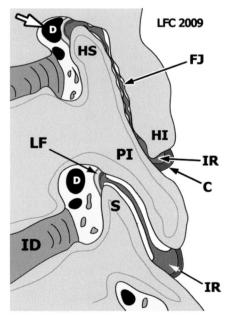

Figure 35-8 ▶ Illustration of Normal (Inferior) and Osteoarthritic (Superior) Lumbar Facets in Sagittal Plane at Level of Lumbar Neural Foramen. On either side of the osteoarthritic facet joint (*FJ*), hypertrophic superior articular process (*HS*) and hypertrophic inferior articular process (*HI*) are illustrated. The hypertrophic superior articular process (*HS*), and thickened synovium, facet capsule and ligamentum flavum compress the dorsal root ganglion (*D*) within the superior portion of the neural foramen. Compare with normal sized neural foramen at more inferior level. C = posteroinferior facet capsule. S = normal superior articular process at level below. ID = Intervertebral Disc. IR = inferior recess.

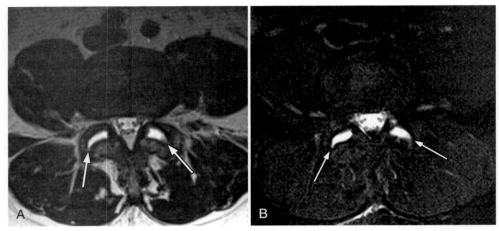

Figure 35-9 ► **Chronic Bilateral Facet Joint Effusions, L4-5 Level.** T2 hyperintense fluid (*arrows*) is located in both facet joints shown on axial T2-weighted MR image **A** and fat-saturated T2-weighted image **B**. Absence of abnormal T2 signal hyperintensity in the adjacent articular facets makes active inflammation highly unlikely.

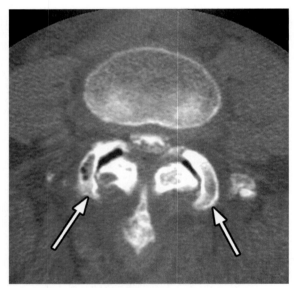

Figure 35-10 ► **Severe Face Osteoarthritis, L3-4 Level.** Axial CT image shows hypertrophic superior articular processes (*arrows*) overriding the posterior portion of the facet joints. Articulating surfaces of facets are irregular. Bilateral intra-articular gas formation ("*vacuum facets*").

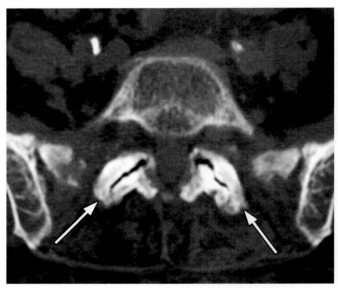

Figure 35-11 ► **Severe Facet Osteoarthritis, L5-S1 Level.** Axial CT image shows hypertrophic superior and inferior articular processes (*arrows*). Note irregular undulating margins of the articulating surfaces of the facets with intra-articular gas formation bilaterally.

At the same time the osteoarthritic process is occurring in the facets, other degenerative processes are occurring elsewhere in the spine including intervertebral disc degeneration, vertebral osteochondrosis, and spondylosis deformans.[8] Although disc degeneration and vertebral osteophyte formation are considered degenerative processes, osteoarthritis is not causing these other degenerative conditions because the disc is not a synovial joint. Yet these coexistent degenerative processes likely alter the biomechanical stresses placed upon various spinal articulations and as a result may accelerate the degenerative process in these other articulations.

The osteoarthritic process involving the facets described above may be asymptomatic or accompanied by a varying degree of *stiffness* or *pain*. Pain accompanying facet osteoarthritis is often related to active inflammation (facet synovitis). It is inflammation that likely sensitizes the nociceptors in the facet capsule and synovium. Facetogenic pain is caused by any stress placed upon the inflamed facet capsule, so facetogenic pain is often worse while sitting or twisting or bending the spine. Facetogenic pain may be referred into the buttocks, groin, or thigh but usually does not extend below the knee, although there are exceptions to this.

Patients with facet joint instability develop vertebral subluxations (spondylolisthesis). Spinal instability is commonly associated with back pain. Degenerative lumbar vertebral spondylolisthesis is most commonly related to facet instability secondary to longstanding facet osteoarthritis at that level of the vertebral subluxation. The facet joints in patients with degenerative spondylolisthesis tend to be oriented in the sagittal plane.[4] When the spine becomes unstable, back pain is often produced as a result of the spinal instability.

IMAGING FEATURES

Radiographs of the lumbar spine should be obtained in spine flexion and extension to assess for lumbar vertebral instability. Patients with vertebral instability often report back pain related to this unstable situation. Facet enlargement and related spinal stenosis may be visible on radiographs, but are demonstrated to better advantage with computed tomography (CT) or MR imaging (*Figs. 35-12 and 35-13*).

Facet overgrowth (hypertrophy), facet joint widening, and intra-articular joint gas formation (*vacuum facets*) are easiest to visualize with CT (see Figs. 35-10 and 35-11), but can be visible with MR imaging as well.[9] A grading system, based on the morphologic appearance of the facets and the degree of facet joint narrowing seen on CT scans, has been proposed by Pathria and colleagues.[10] However, the morphologic grade of facet osteoarthritis correlates poorly with facetogenic pain.

Conventional radiographs and CT and MR imaging techniques provide secondary morphologic information regarding abnormalities of the articular facets and facet joints (see Figs. 35-10 to 35-13). Facet morphology is well demonstrated on conventional T1- and T2-weighted MR images of the spine (see Figs. 35-2 and 35-13). T2*-weighted gradient echo sequences and short tau inversion

recovery (STIR) sequences are also well suited for assessing bone configuration. Using these imaging sequences, bone has low signal intensity, and intra-articular fluid, cortical erosions, and fracture lines have high signal intensity.[11,12]

Morphologic information regarding the configuration of the facets is useful for assessing the contribution of facet hypertrophy in spinal stenosis including central canal stenosis, neural foraminal stenosis, and lateral recess stenosis. However, there is poor correlation between the morphologic appearance of the facets and the state of the inflammatory process in the facet joints that has caused these structural abnormalities. The morphologic appearance of the facet joints does not correlate well with the patient's symptoms. Large, hypertrophic facets may contribute to spinal stenosis but are often asymptomatic.

MR images should be obtained in all patients using fat-suppression techniques to identify facetogenic signal intensity alterations corresponding to active inflammation within and surrounding the facet joints, in the adjacent vertebral bone, and surrounding ligaments (*Figs. 35-14*).[13,14] MR imaging, using these techniques, can provide important additional information by identifying facets that are actively inflamed and thereby likely to be symptomatic. Although we use a frequency-selective fat-saturation technique to evaluate our patients,[15] STIR imaging or water excitation techniques are equally effective.[14,16,17] Fat-saturated MR imaging has also been shown to be a valuable tool in the detection and characterization of other inflammatory bone and joint conditions including vertebral discitis/osteomyelitis as well as synovitis and bursitis involving the joints of the extremities.[18-22]

In our practice, this MR imaging information, along with clinical findings, is used to select the most appropriate levels and approach for therapeutic facet injections in patients with facetogenic pain.

Figure 35-12 ▶ Severe Central Stenosis and Bilateral Neural Foraminal Stenosis. Axial CT image through L4-5 intervertebral disc level. The bilateral hypertrophic facets (*long arrows*), diffusely bulging disc (*tiny arrows*), and thickened ligamentum flavum cause central canal stenosis. The bulging disc and hypertrophic superior articular facet produce narrowing of the neural foramen bilaterally (*intermediate length arrows*).

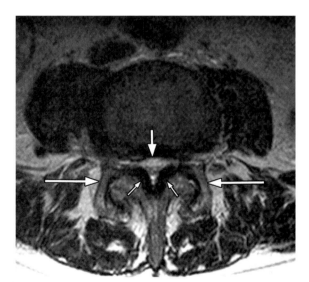

Figure 35-13 ▶ Spinal Stenosis, L3-4 Level. Axial T2-weighted MR image. Demonstrated is central canal stenosis secondary to disc bulging (*intermediate length arrow*), bilateral facet hypertrophy (*long arrows*), and ligamentum flavum thickening (*tiny arrows*). Bilateral neural foraminal stenosis is also demonstrated.

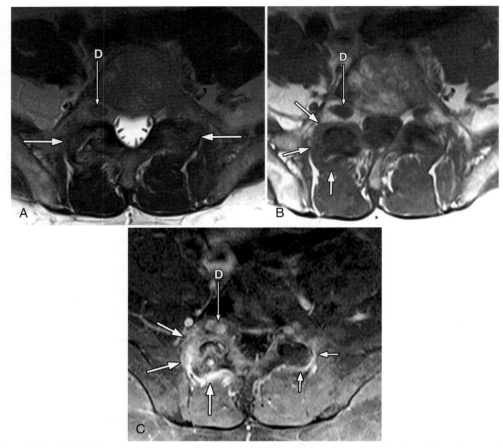

Figure 35-14 ▸ **Bilateral Active L5-1 Inflammatory Facet Arthropathy.** Patient with low back pain and severe right L5 radicular pain. On axial T2-weighted MR image **A**, bilateral facet hypertrophy is demonstrated (*arrows*). On axial T1-weighted MR image **B**, the tissues surrounding the right L5-S1 facets are thickened (*arrows*). On axial contrast-enhanced fat-saturated T1-weighted MR image **C**, intensely enhancing tissue (*large arrows*) surrounds the right L5-S1 facets. Enhancing inflammatory tissue also extends into the right L5-S1 neural foramen and encases the dorsal root ganglion (*D*). The right L5 dorsal root ganglion (*D*) is enlarged in images **A**, **B**, and **C**. Note there is mild parafacetal contrast enhancement adjacent to the left L5-S1 facets (*tiny arrows*) consistent with facet synovitis on the left.

MRI Appearance of Active Inflammatory Facet Arthropathy (Facet Synovitis)

Facet synovitis is not readily visible on conventional MR images obtained without the use of fat suppression, water excitation, or STIR techniques. Facet synovitis may be detected on bone scanning as a nonspecific focal area of increased activity off midline (*Fig. 35-15*). On MR images obtained without fat suppression, subtle T2 signal hyperintensity may or may not be visible in the articular facets or in the facet joints (see Fig. 35-14).

A facet joint effusion may or may not be present in patients with facet synovitis. The presence of joint fluid alone is not a reliable indicator of symptomatic facet disease, because chronic facet joint effusions are common in chronic asymptomatic osteoarthritic facet joints (see Figs. 35-9 to 35-11).

In active inflammatory facet arthropathy, signal hyperintensity is observed on fat-saturated, T2-weighted images in the articular facets consistent with presence of marrow edema due to active inflammation.[23] This is best seen on axial (Figs. 35-2, 35-3, and *35-16*) or parasagittal images through the facets (*Fig. 35-17*). The presence of facet synovitis on MR imaging is commonly associated with back pain.[14] The T2 signal hyperintensity may be seen in the articular facets, adjacent facet joint capsules, and frequently in adjacent bone structures including the articular pillars, lamina, and pedicles (*Fig. 35-18*). This periarticular inflammatory process correlates highly with facetogenic pain, based on our clinical experience.[14] Fat-saturated, T1-weighted, gadolinium-enhanced images are the most sensitive for detecting inflammation secondary to facet synovitis (see Figs. 35-1, 35-2, 35-3, 35-14, 35-17, and 35-18). However, facet synovitis is seen in a high percentage of cases on unenhanced fat-saturated, T2-weighted (or STIR) MR images because of the presence of marrow edema in the articular facets or other adjacent bone structures (see Figs. 35-2, 35-3, 35-16, and 35-17). The earliest signal abnormalities with facet synovitis occur in the posteroinferior portion of the facet capsule and may be visible only on contrast-enhanced, fat-saturated, T1-weighted MR images (*Fig. 35-19*).[14]

The periarticular facetogenic inflammatory process can have a profound effect on the surrounding bone, ligaments, and other periarticular tissues. The associated inflammatory process may infiltrate the tissues within the adjacent neural foramen producing a noncompressive radiculopathy (see Fig. 35-14). Posterior extension of the inflammatory process may involve the anterior or paraspinal soft tissues, sometimes resulting in severe myofascial pain, which clinically may be difficult to distinguish from other types of low back pain (*Fig. 35-20*). Facet synovitis can produce a

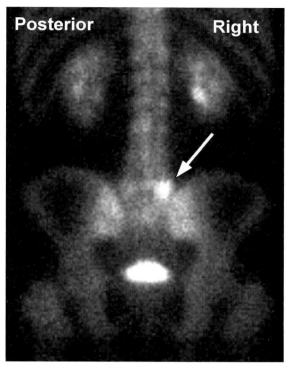

Figure 35-15 ▶ Bilateral Active L5-1 Inflammatory Facet Arthropathy. Same patient as in Figure 35-14. Technetium-99m methylene diphosphonate (MDP) radionu-clide bone scan. Intense focus of increased activity (*arrow*) in the spine on the right at L5-S1 level corresponding to right L5-S1 facet synovitis shown in Figure 35-14. No appreciable abnormal uptake on the left at this level, even though MR imaging shows active inflammatory facet arthropathy on the left at L5-S1 as well.

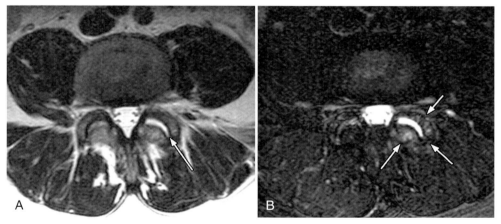

Figure 35-16 ▶ Active Left L4-5 Facet Synovitis, Facet Joint Effusion. On axial T2-weighted MR image **A**, fluid (*arrow*) is located in the left L4-5 facet joint. On fat-saturated image **B**, abnormal T2 hyperintensity is seen in the articular facets (*arrows*) adjacent to the effusion consistent with active inflammatory facet arthropathy (facet synovitis).

denervation response causing T2 hyperintense signal in the ipsilateral multifidus muscle *(Fig. 35-21)*. The same appearance can be seen after radiofrequency denervation for treatment of patients with facet disease. Facet synovitis is commonly associated with active inflammation in the interspinous ligaments (Baastrup's disease).[23] (See Chapter 39 for further discussion of Baastrup's disease.)

Septic facet arthritis can mimic noninfectious arthritis. Isolated septic facet arthritis is extremely rare, whereas noninfectious inflammatory facet arthropathy is exceedingly common, seen in

daily MR imaging practice.[14] In the 10 years our practice has used fat-saturated MR imaging techniques for spine imaging, we have observed only one case of facet joint infection, and this occurred in a patient with spondylodiscitis and diffuse paravertebral infection (see *Figs. 35-22 and 35-23*). However, the presence of pronounced periarticular inflammation on fat-saturated MR images is nearly always noninfectious in nature (see Fig. 35-20), but should always raise suspicion of possible septic facet arthritis, which can have a similar appearance (see Figs. 35-22 and 35-23). If infection is suspected, appropriate laboratory studies should be obtained,

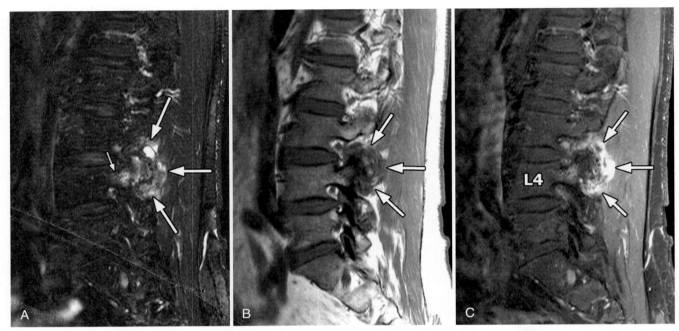

Figure 35-17 ▸ Facet Synovitis, Sagittal Plane. Patient with severe low back pain and active L3-4 inflammatory facet arthropathy. Sagittal imaging series obtained through the right L3-4 facets. On fat-saturated T2-weighted image **A** the right L3-4 facets (*large arrows*) are markedly T2 hyperintense compared to adjacent facets above and below. The right L4 pedicle (*small arrow*) is also hyperintense. On T1-weighted image **B**, the right L3-4 facets are hypertrophic and T1 hypointense and surrounded by thick soft tissue (*arrows*). On contrast-enhanced fat-saturated T1-weighted MR image **C**, the right parafacetal soft tissues enhance intensely and subtle enhancement is present in the right L3-4 facets and right L4 pedicle.

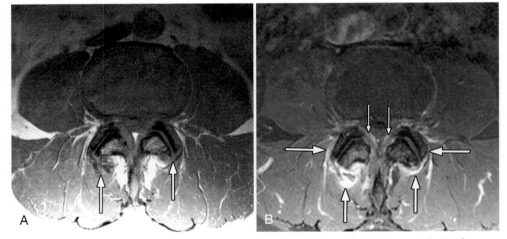

Figure 35-18 ▸ Bilateral Facet Synovitis, Axial Plane. Same patient as in Figure 35-17. On axial T1-weighted MR image **A**, the L3-4 facets are moderately hypertrophic bilaterally and posterior parafacetal soft tissues (*arrows*) are thickened. On axial contrast-enhanced fat-saturated T1-weighted MR image **B**, the parafacetal soft tissues enhance (*large arrows*), right more than left, and diffuse enhancement is also seen in the neural foramina bilaterally and along the margins of the ligamentum flavum (*small arrows*).

including white blood cell count (WBC), erythrocyte sedimentation rate (ESR), and C-reactive protein (CRP), to assess for possible infection. Percutaneous needle aspiration biopsy may be necessary to obtain tissue for microbial culture in some cases.

Bone Scanning and Facet Synovitis

Unilateral or bilaterally symmetric focal areas of radiotracer uptake are most commonly seen on bone scan images in patients with active inflammatory facet arthropathy. The most common level of increased uptake seen on bone scans secondary to facet disease in one study was L5-S1.[24] Facet synovitis by MR imaging correlates well with increased radiotracer uptake on bone scans (see Fig. 35-15). Unfortunately, bone scan uptake is disease nonspecific and not reliable for characterizing the exact vertebral site or even level of the abnormal uptake, because bone scan images suffer from relatively poor spatial resolution. Occasionally, the bone scan may be negative or show minimal uptake at levels where fat-saturated MR images show evidence of facet synovitis (see Fig. 35-4).

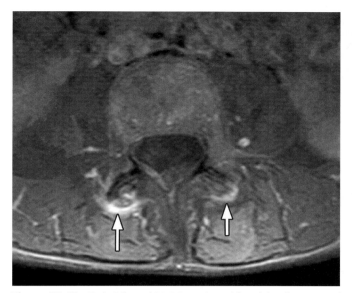

Figure 35-19 ▶ Early Bilateral L4-5 Facet Synovitis. Subtle enhancement of the posterior facet capsules (*arrows*), right more than left. Grade 1 Facet synovitis on the left. Grade 2 facet synovitis on the right.

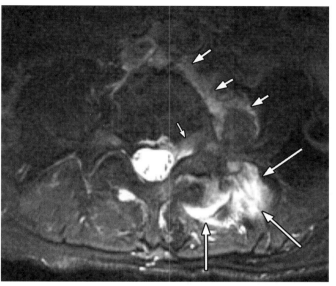

Figure 35-20 ▶ Severe Grade 4 Noninfectious Facet Synovitis. Axial fat-saturated T2-weighted MR image, L4-5 level. Subtle T2 hyperintensity in the left L4-5 facets and left L4 lamina is demonstrated. Extensive T2 hyperintense tissue (*arrows*) surrounds the left L4-5 facets and involves the left posterior paraspinal muscles. Enhancing tissue is also seen in left anterolateral paraspinal soft tissue (*shorter arrows*) and also in the left L4-5 neural foramen (*tiny arrow*). Biopsy was negative for infection. Patient had normal C-reactive protein and ESR. Patient responded favorably to anesthetic/steroid facet/parafacetal injections.

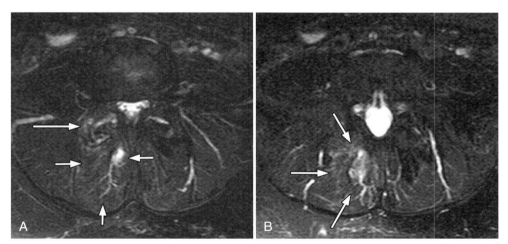

Figure 35-21 ▶ Grade 3 Facet Synovitis, Associated Denervation Response Affecting Right Posterior Paraspinal Muscles. In axial fat-saturated T2-weighted MR image **A**, T2 hyperintensity is seen in and adjacent to the right L4-5 facets (*long arrow*) and the facet joint is slightly widened. Subtle T2 hyperintensity is demonstrated in right multifidus muscle (*short arrows*) posterior to inflamed facets. On axial fat-saturated T2-weighted image **B**, obtained at a level inferior image **A**, the right multifidus muscle and adjacent tissues are T2 hyperintense (*arrows*).

Classification of Facet Synovitis

Noninfectious inflammatory facet arthropathy (facet synovitis) is an exceedingly common condition observed in daily imaging practice when fat-suppression techniques are routinely employed. In our practice, we have observed imaging findings of facet synovitis on MR imaging in 36% of patients presenting with neck or back pain overall, and in 41% of patients with low back pain.[14] We assess the degree of facet involvement on MR imaging using the following grading system.

Grade

0 = No facet synovitis

1 = Signal abnormality confined to the posterior facet capsule (see Fig. 35-19)

2 = Periarticular signal abnormality involving less than 50% of the facet joint perimeter (see Fig. 35-19)

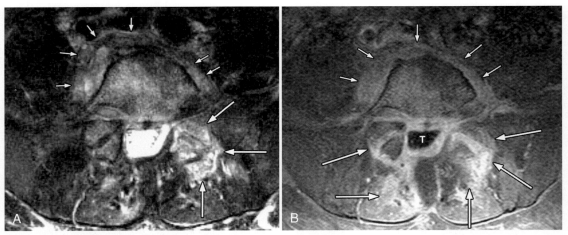

Figure 35-22 ▸ **Bilateral Septic Facet Synovitis in Patient With L5-S1 Spondylodiscitis.** On fat-saturated T2-weighted MR image **A**, the left L5-S1 facets and adjacent tissues (*long arrows*) are T2 hyperintense as is tissue within left L5-S1 facet joint. A T2 hyperintense anterior paraspinal phlegmon (*small arrows*) is located adjacent to the T2 hyperintense L5 vertebral body. On axial contrast-enhanced fat-saturated T1-weighted MR image **B**, intense enhancing phlegmonous tissue (*small arrows*) surrounds the enhancing L5 vertebral body. Enhancing phlegmonous tissue also encases the thecal sac (*T*) and is seen in both L5-S1 facet joints and parafacetal soft tissue (*long arrows*) and posterior paraspinal muscles bilaterally.

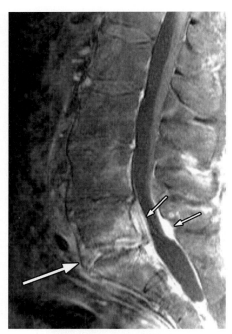

Figure 35-23 ▸ **L5-S1 Discitis, Osteomyelitis and Paraspinal Phlegmon.** Same patient as in Figure 35-22. Sagittal contrast-enhanced fat-saturated T1-weighted MRI. Enhancement of the L5 and S1 vertebral bodies, L5-S1 intervertebral disc (*long arrow*), and paravertebral tissues is demonstrated. Enhancing anterior and posterior epidural tissue (*small arrows*).

3 = Periarticular signal abnormality involving greater than 50% of the facet joint perimeter (see Fig. 35-20)
4 = Periarticular signal abnormality with extension into the neural foramen (see Figs. 35-1, 35-14, 35-18, and 35-20)

Note that signal abnormalities are often seen in the adjacent bone in grades 3 and 4 facet synovitis; however, the presence or absence of bone involvement is not used as a criterion for grading the degree of facet synovitis.

DIFFERENTIAL DIAGNOSIS

1. **Infectious facet synovitis:** The MR findings of facet synovitis can be seen in sterile synovitis or infectious synovitis. Infectious facet synovitis is extremely rare (Figs. 35-22 and 35-23). Sterile, noninfectious facet synovitis is exceedingly common, encountered in routine daily MR imaging practice. When MR imaging findings show evidence of periarticular inflammatory facet arthropathy, serum laboratory studies should be obtained to assess for possible infection. These tests should include WBC, ESR, and CRP. If these tests are positive or if there is a strong clinical suspicion of infectious synovitis, needle aspiration biopsy should be performed prior to facet injection with steroidal agents.

2. **Metastatic neoplasm:** Metastatic neoplasm should always be considered in patients with facet synovitis, particularly when the bone adjacent to the facets displays abnormal signal. We have frequently observed that patients with vertebral metastases commonly have coexistent facet synovitis, which may be an additional factor contributing to their back pain. Neoplastic conditions are best demonstrated on MR imaging using fat-saturation MR techniques as well.[19]

3. **Primary vertebral tumors:** Osteoid osteoma in the posterior vertebral arch could conceivably be mistaken for facet synovitis on MR imaging.[25] Other primary tumors of the vertebral arch such as osteoblastoma, aneurysmal bone cyst, or giant cell tumor tend to cause bony expansion and are not likely to be confused with facet synovitis.

TREATMENT

1. **Conservative therapy:** The widely held belief that low back pain usually resolves spontaneously if the patient is able to rest and can tolerate the pain for 6 to 8 weeks is the basis for recommending conservative therapy. Nonsteroidal anti-inflammatory agents (NSAIDs) are often administered initially but may not provide lasting relief of facetogenic pain.

The administration of short-term oral steroids can be beneficial in some patients. As pain subsides, it is important to introduce a physical rehabilitation program. Improving and maintaining normal paraspinal muscular strength and correcting postural abnormalities are essential for patients recovering from facetogenic pain.

2. **Percutaneous facet injection:** The procedure of first choice for treating active inflammatory facet arthropathy is percutaneous facet injection. Treatment will often provide effective relief of pain in the acute phase of facetogenic pain. The facet joints to be injected are selected based on clinical examination and the fat-saturated MR images. Intra-articular injection alone is performed in diagnostically identified facets first to confirm that a given facet joint is the source of pain. Therapeutic facet injections are performed by injecting a mixture of anesthetic and steroidal agents into the affected facet joint and also into the affected periarticular soft tissues. Patients who receive facet joint injections have a variable length of pain relief, which usually ranges from weeks to a few months.[26] Repeat facet injections may be necessary. Details describing the technique for performing facet injections can be found elsewhere.[17]

3. **Radiofrequency denervation:** Radiofrequency (RF) denervation should be considered if the patient's pain is relieved but returns after repeated facet injections. Before performing the RF denervation, medial branch blocks or intra-articular facet steroid injections should be performed to prove that the patient would benefit from denervation of the facet. Details describing the technique of RF denervation can be found elsewhere.[27]

4. **Surgical fusion:** If spinal instability is related to facet osteoarthritis, these patients can receive temporary pain relief from facet injections, but long-term relief is usually not achieved. Surgical fusion is the procedure of choice for vertebral instability.

References

1. Yamashita T, Minaki Y, Ozaktay AC, et al. A morphological study of the fibrous capsule of the human lumbar facet joint. *Spine (Phila Pa 1976).* 1996;21(5):538-543.
2. Giles LG, Taylor JR. Human zygapophyseal joint capsule and synovial fold innervation. *Br J Rheumatol.* 1987;26(2):93-98.
3. Cavanaugh JM, Ozaktay AC, Yamashita HT, King AI. Lumbar facet pain: Biomechanics, neuroanatomy and neurophysiology. *J Biomech.* 1996;29(9):1117-1129.
4. Fujiwara A, Tamai K, An HS, et al. Orientation and osteoarthritis of the lumbar facet joint. *Clin Orthop Relat Res.* 2001;(385):88-94.
5. Kalichman L, Li L, Kim DH, et al. Facet joint osteoarthritis and low back pain in the community-based population. *Spine (Phila Pa 1976).* 2008;33(23):2560-2565.
6. Cinotti G, De Santis P, Nofroni I, Postacchini F. Stenosis of lumbar intervertebral foramen: Anatomic study on predisposing factors. *Spine (Phila Pa 1976).* 2002;27(3):223-229.
7. Jenis LG, An HS, Gordin R. Foraminal stenosis of the lumbar spine: A review of 65 surgical cases. *American journal of orthopedics Belle Mead, NJ.* 2001;30(3):205-211.
8. Oegema TR Jr, Bradford DS. The inter-relationship of facet joint osteoarthritis and degenerative disc disease. *Br J Rheumatol.* 1991;30(Suppl 1):16-20.
9. Weishaupt D, Zanetti M, Boos N, Hodler J. MR imaging and CT in osteoarthritis of the lumbar facet joints. *Skeletal Radiol.* 1999;28(4):215-219.
10. Pathria M, Sartoris DJ, Resnick D. Osteoarthritis of the facet joints: Accuracy of oblique radiographic assessment. *Radiology.* 1987;164(1):227-230.
11. Czervionke LF, Haughton VM. Degenerative Disease of the Spine. In: Atlas SW, ed. *Magnetic Resonance Imaging of the Brain and Spine.* 3rd ed. Philadelphia: Lippincott Williams & Wilkins; 2002.
12. Czervionke LF, Berquist TH. Imaging of the spine: Techniques of MR imaging. *Orthop Clin North Am.* 1997;28(4):583-616.
13. Schellinger D, Hatipoglu H, Olivario P, Davis B. Spinal facet arthropathy: MR imaging depiction of facet related pathologies by the use of fat suppression. 38th Annual Meeting of the American Society of Neuroradiology. *Atlanta.* Georgia, 2000.
14. Czervionke LF, Fenton DS. Fat-saturated MR imaging in the detection of inflammatory facet arthropathy (facet synovitis) in the lumbar spine. *Pain Med.* 2008;9(4):400-406.
15. Chan TW, Listerud J, Kressel HY. Combined chemical-shift and phase-selective imaging for fat suppression: Theory and initial clinical experience. *Radiology.* 1991;181(1):41-47.
16. Lakadamyali H, Tarhan NC, Ergun T, et al. STIR sequence for depiction of degenerative changes in posterior stabilizing elements in patients with lower back pain. *AJR Am J Roentgenol.* 2008;191(4):973-979.
17. Czervionke LF, Fenton DS. Facet joint injection and medial branch block. In: Fenton DS, Czervionke LF, eds. *Image-Guided Spine Intervention.* Philadelphia: Saunders; 2002.
18. Barakat MS, Schweitzer ME, Morisson WB, et al. Reactive carpal synovitis: Initial experience with MR imaging. *Radiology.* 2005;236(1):231-236.
19. Georgy BA, Hesselink JR. Evaluation of fat suppression in contrast-enhanced MR of neoplastic and inflammatory spine disease. *AJNR Am J Neuroradiol.* 1994;15(3):409-417.
20. Link TM, Steinbach LS, Ghosh S, et al. Osteoarthritis: MR imaging findings in different stages of disease and correlation with clinical findings. *Radiology.* 2003;226(2):373-381.
21. Longo M, Granata F, Ricciardi K, et al. Contrast-enhanced MR imaging with fat suppression in adult-onset septic spondylodiscitis. *Eur Radiol.* 2003;13(3):626-637.
22. Skaf AY, Boutin RD, Dantas RW, et al. Bicipitoradial bursitis: MR imaging findings in eight patients and anatomic data from contrast material opacification of bursae followed by routine radiography and MR imaging in cadavers. *Radiology.* 1999;212(1):111-116.
23. D'Aprile P, Tarantino A, Jinkins JR, Brindicci D. The value of fat saturation sequences and contrast medium administration in MRI of degenerative disease of the posterior/perispinal elements of the lumbosacral spine. *Eur Radiol.* 2007;17(2):523-531.
24. Kim CK, Park KW. Characteristic appearance of facet osteoarthritis of the lower lumbar spine on planar bone scintigraphy with a high negative predictive value for metastasis. *Clin Nucl Med.* 2008;33(4):251-254.
25. Liu PT, Chivers FS, Roberts CC, et al. Imaging of osteoid osteoma with dynamic gadolinium-enhanced MR imaging. *Radiology.* 2003;227(3):691-700.
26. Boswell MV, Colson JD, Sehgal N, Dunbar EE, Epter R. A systematic review of therapeutic facet joint interventions in chronic spinal pain. *Pain Physician.* 2007;10(1):229-253.
27. Fenton DS, Czervionke LF. Facet denervation. In: Fenton DS, Czervionke LF, eds. *Image-Guided Spine Intervention.* Philadelphia: Saunders; 2002.

36

GIANT CELL TUMOR

Leo F. Czervionke, M.D.

CLINICAL PRESENTATION

The patient is a 35-year-old male who has a 3-month history of low back pain and difficulty emptying his bladder.

IMAGING PRESENTATION

Pelvic radiograph reveals an ill-defined destructive lesion involving the upper half of the sacrum. Computed tomography (CT) scan demonstrates an osteolytic expansile lesion that is destroying the anterior cortex of the sacrum, extending into the presacral soft tissues. A small portion of the tumor extends into the posterior sacral arch on the left *(Figs. 36-1 and 36-2)*.

DISCUSSION

The entity that has become known as *giant cell tumor* was first described by Coopers and Travers in 1818.[1] *Giant cell tumor of bone* was a term introduced by Jaffe and Lichtenstein in 1940.[2] A giant cell tumor (GCT) is an expansile, osteolytic primary bone neoplasm containing giant cells. Giant cell tumors represent approximately 5% to 7% of all bone tumors.[1,3] The majority of giant cell tumors arise in the ends of the long bones, the knee being the most common site; 3% to 7% of giant cell tumors occur in the spine, and 90% of spinal giant cell tumors arise in the sacrum (see Figs. 36-1 and 36-2).[3,4] Most vertebral giant cell tumors originate in the vertebral body as solitary lesions, but 80% extend into the posterior vertebral arch. Rarely, a GCT may arise in the posterior vertebral arch.[5]

Most patients with spinal or sacral giant cell tumors present between the ages of 20 and 50 with back pain.[3,4] If the tumor extends into the epidural space or neural foramen, the patient may have myelopathic or radicular symptoms. Patients with cord compression may exhibit hyperreflexia.[3] Sacral or pelvic giant cell tumors often manifest with low back pain and bilateral lower extremity pain.[6] A female preponderance for GCT exists.[4] About one-third of patients have an associated pathologic fracture that can also be the source of back pain and can cause spinal instability.

Histologically, giant cell tumors are comprised of sheets of stromal mononuclear spindle cells containing uniformly distributed multinucleated osteoclastic giant cells.[4] Hemorrhage and necrosis may be present in the tumor. Approximately 15% of giant cell tumors contain areas of aneurysmal bone cyst formation.[7]

The vast majority of giant cell tumors are benign neoplasms, although they are locally aggressive tumors that recur in up to 50% of cases.[6-8] Approximately 5% to 10% of giant cell tumors are malignant.[7,9] Some of these tumors have histologic features of the giant cell subtype of osteosarcoma, except that osteoid formation is characteristically absent in malignant giant cell tumors. Malignant giant cell tumor of the tendon sheath (pigmented villonodular synovitis) may also occur.[10] Malignant giant cell tumors have a poor prognosis and may metastasize to the liver, lungs, spine, and other portions of the skeleton; 1% to 5% of giant cell tumors metastasize to the lungs.[7,8,11]

Rarely, "benign" giant cell tumors may metastasize to the lungs, the pulmonary lesions being histologically benign. Benign giant cell tumors also rarely manifest as multicentric (multisynchronous) vertebral tumors. Benign or malignant giant cell tumors commonly recur at their initial site of presentation,[8] but rarely also can recur as multicentric benign (metachronous) or malignant (metastatic) tumors.[1] Again rarely, giant cell tumors of the spine or sacrum may have the same histology as appendicular giant cell tumors of the tendon sheath (pigmented villonodular synovitis).[10,12,13] Such tumors can be benign or malignant. Sacral giant cell tumors of the tendon sheath may extend into the L5 vertebra to involve the vertebral L5 vertebral body or L5-S1 facet joints. Vertebral giant cell tumors of the tendon sheath are rare but usually involve the facet joints.[13]

IMAGING FEATURES

Giant cell tumors in the spine are seen on radiographs or CT images as osteolytic, expansile lesions that have a thin shell of cortical bone at their margins (Figs. 36-1, 36-2, and **36-3**).[4,14] The cortical margin of the tumor is usually not sclerotic. Cortical marginal breakthrough may occur even with benign giant cell tumors *(Figs. 36-2 to 36-5)*. There is a narrow zone of transition between the expansile mass and the normal adjacent bone. The soft tissue component of the mass within the zone of osteolysis typically does not contain osteoid and therefore clumps of new bone formation are typically absent, although there may be islands of normal trabeculae in this region.[9] On radiographs, sacral giant cell tumors may be difficult to visualize, especially if overlying bowel gas obscures the sacrum, so CT and magnetic resonance (MR) imaging are the imaging modalities of choice for detecting these lesions (see Figs. 36-1 and 36-3).

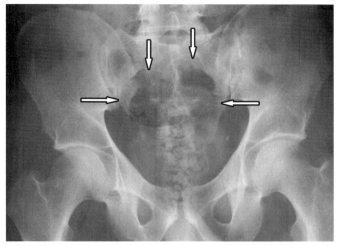

Figure 36-1 ▶ **Sacral Giant Cell Tumor.** Anteroposterior (AP) radiograph of the pelvis. Large destructive lesion of the sacrum (*arrows*) is partially obscured by bowel gas.

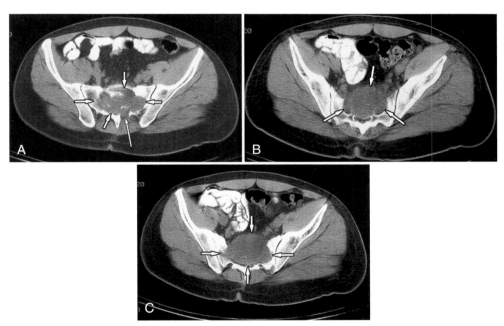

Figure 36-2 ▶ **Sacral Giant Cell Tumor.** Osteolytic, expansile, destructive lesion in the sacrum (*short arrows* in CT images **A, B** and **C**). The tumor is centered in the sacral vertebral bodies but extends into the sacral ala bilaterally. The anterior cortical margin of the sacral vertebral bodies is destroyed as is the left L2 lamina (*long arrow* in image **A**). No tumoral bone formation is demonstrated in the osteolytic lesion.

Giant cell tumors are usually heterogeneous lesions that are predominantly T1 hypointense or isointense and may be T2 hypointense but usually are T2 hyperintense (see Fig. 36-4).[4] Heterogeneous contrast enhancement is usually present due to hypervascularity of the tumor. Intratumoral necrosis or hemorrhage is commonly present in the tumor. The tumor may be solid or contain cystic areas, which resemble aneurysmal bone cysts within the tumor. Focal areas of hemorrhage with fluid-fluid levels are often visible in the cystic portions of the tumor, similar to those seen with aneurysmal bone cysts. MR imaging is especially valuable for assessing paraspinal, foraminal, or epidural extension of the tumor.

GCT is a hypervascular tumor, and this vascularity is well demonstrated at angiography, but conventional angiography is not routinely performed today for diagnosis of these tumors.[6] Embolization is often performed to devascularize the tumor prior to surgery, or therapeutic embolization may be performed for palliation in some cases.[15]

Radionuclide bone scanning reveals uptake in the involved portions of the skeleton and is most useful for detection of multisynchronous or metastatic skeletal lesions. Giant cell tumors of the sacrum may exhibit a photopenic center similar to aneurysmal bone cysts.[7]

Percutaneous needle aspiration may be helpful in the diagnosis of spinal or sacral giant cell tumors, because more common tumors involving the spine or sacrum such as metastasis, plasmacytoma, or lymphoma may have a similar imaging appearance and presentation.[16]

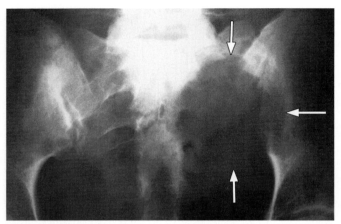

Figure 36-3 ▶ Sacral Giant Cell Tumor. In a 25-year-old female patient with vague lumbosacral and left hip pain. Anteroposterior (AP) radiograph reveals a large ovoid radiolucent region (*arrows*) in the left sacral wing representing an osteolytic lesion.

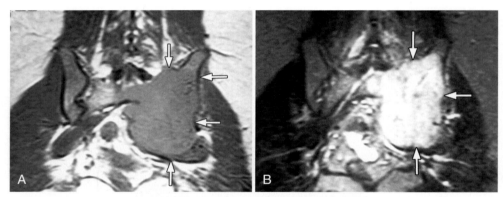

Figure 36-4 ▶ Sacral Giant Cell Tumor. (Same patient as in Fig. 36-3.) On coronal T1-weighted MR image **A**, the mass (*arrows*) is T1 hypointense and nearly homogeneous. On corresponding coronal T2-weighted MR image **B**, the left sacral wing and a portion of the left iliac wing are replaced by a heterogeneous T2 hyperintense soft tissue mass (*arrows*), which obliterates the left sacroiliac joint.

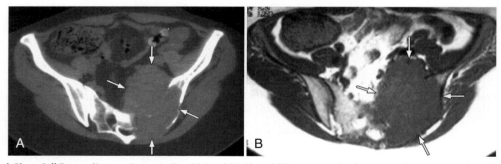

Figure 36-5 ▶ Sacral Giant Cell Tumor. (Same patient as in Figs. 36-3 and 36-4.) Axial CT image reveals a large expansile mass (*arrows*), which destroys the left half of the sacrum and medial portion of the left iliac bone. The mass is nearly homogeneous in density, similar to that of muscle. Cortical breakthrough is evident anteriorly and posteriorly. A large exophytic portion (*anterior arrows*) of the mass extends into the pelvic soft tissues. On corresponding axial T1-weighted MR image **B**, the mass (*arrows*) is nearly homogeneous in intensity. The mass is T1 hypointense relative to bone marrow and slightly T1 hyperintense relative to muscle. The mass obliterates the left sacroiliac joint.

DIFFERENTIAL DIAGNOSIS

1. **Aneurysmal bone cyst:** Expansile bone lesion arising in the vertebral arch and secondarily extending into the vertebral body. Sacral aneurysmal bone cysts may look very similar or identical to sacral giant cell tumors (*Figs. 36-6 and 36-7*). Approximately 15% of giant cell tumors contain aneurysmal bone cysts.[7]

2. **Malignant fibrous histiocytoma:** May involve the sacrum and may resemble giant cell tumors. Aggressive malignant fibrous histiocytomas usually have a wider zone of transition between the tumor and normal bone and may have thick, sclerotic expanded cortical margins (*Figs. 36-8 and 36-9*).

3. **Vertebral or sacral metastasis:** Aggressive malignant neoplasm usually with poorly defined margins and bone destruction. Usually multiple lesions are present in the spine.

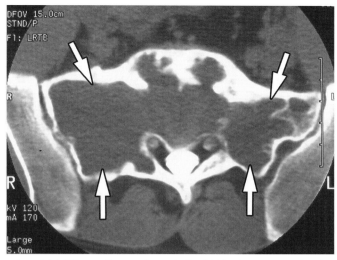

Figure 36-6 ► **Sacral Aneurysmal Bone Cyst.** Axial CT image. (Same patient as in Fig. 36-3.) A homogeneous, hypodense lesion (*arrows*) occupies almost the entire sacral contents, sparing the cortical margins of the sacrum. The sacroiliac joints and adjacent cortex remain intact.

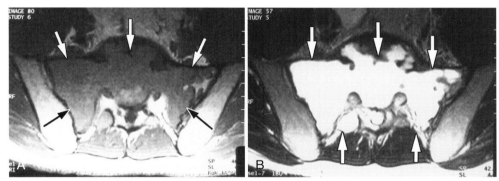

Figure 36-7 ► **Sacral Aneurysmal Bone Cyst.** (In same patient as in Fig. 36-6.) Corresponding axial T1-weighted MR image **A** and T2-weighted image **B**. The sacrum (*arrows*) is uniformly T1 hypointense relative to the iliac bones on image **A** and markedly T2 hyperintense on image **B**, relative to the iliac wings. T2 hyperintense liquid (*arrows*) has replaced nearly the entire contents of the sacrum.

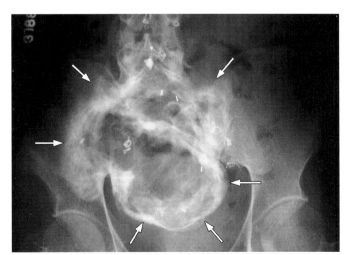

Figure 36-8 ► **Malignant Fibrous Histiocytoma.** Anteroposterior (AP) radiograph of pelvis. A large centrally radiolucent, expansile mass (*arrows*) with thick, sclerotic margins has replaced the sacrum.

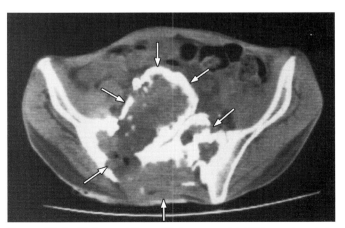

Figure 36-9 ► **Malignant Fibrous Histiocytoma.** Axial CT image through the sacrum and pelvis. (In same patient as in Fig. 36-9.) An expansile mass involves the entire sacrum (*arrows*). The lesion is predominantly hypodense centrally and has thick, sclerotic peripheral margins.

4. **Myeloma/plasmacytoma:** Osteolytic bone mass associated with cortical expansion may have an appearance similar to GCT, except that plasmacytomas usually occur in older patients with multiple myeloma.

5. **Lymphoma:** Osteolytic tumor involving the sacrum that is highly radiosensitive. This may have the same imaging appearance as GCT.

6. **Osteoblastoma:** Osteolytic expansile lesion often arises in the posterior vertebral arch, but often involves the vertebral body secondarily. These tumors typically contain areas of new bone formation.

7. **Giant cell reparative granuloma:** This condition is not neoplastic, but is believed to be a reparative response to intraosseous hemorrhage, sometimes but not always secondary to trauma. Osteoid production and hemorrhage is typically present within this granulomatous lesion.[7] A brown tumor of hyperparathyroidism should be excluded, because this can have a similar appearance.

8. **Osteosarcoma, giant cell type:** This type of osteosarcoma contains tissue with many giant cells.[4,17] An osteosarcoma is a destructive vertebral mass lesion with moth-eaten or permeative vertebral bone destruction and poorly defined margins. Most osteosarcomas contain areas of bone formation.

9. **Chordoma:** May occur in the sacrum or vertebrae. These are osteolytic, expansile lesions, sometimes with sclerotic margins, and often an associated epidural mass is present; 50% to 70% of sacral chordomas contain calcification.[18] Vertebral chordomas arise in the posterior portion of the vertebral body and have a strong tendency to extend along the posterior disc margin to involve adjacent vertebral bodies. (See Chapter 11.)

10. **Brown tumor:** Histologically, brown tumors have a more irregular distribution of giant cells but otherwise appear identical to giant cell tumor histologically and with images.[3] Serum calcium and parathyroid hormone are elevated in patients with brown tumors.

TREATMENT

1. **Intralesional resection/bone curettage:** This is the standard treatment for most spinal or sacral giant cell tumors.[6] However, this procedure alone is usually not sufficient to prevent recurrence, so curettage is usually performed along with adjuvant radiotherapy, cryotherapy, phenol therapy, or thermoablation.[3,11,19] The postcurettage bone cavity is usually filled with bone graft (autograft) or cement.[11,20]

2. **Spondylectomy:** Vertebral and sacral giant cell tumors are optimally treated with spondylectomy with a wide marginal excision of the tumor when feasible, which has the lowest rate of recurrence.[8,14] This is followed by stabilization with local autograft and spinal instrumentation.[3,21] En bloc removal of cervical and sacral giant cell tumors is difficult or impossible in many cases.[14,19,22] Wide resection of vertebral and sacral tumors is associated with increased morbidity, spinal instability, and a higher rate of recurrence.[8,22,23] Preprocedural arterial embolization is useful to eliminate vascularity to minimize bleeding.[3]

3. **Radiation therapy:** Usually reserved for tumors that cannot be completely excised. Giant cell tumors have a strong tendency to recur with or without radiotherapy.[8] Many believe that adjuvant radiotherapy is helpful in reducing the likelihood of recurrence.[3,14] Sarcomatous transformation of recurrent giant cell tumors is known to occur in some cases treated with radiotherapy, usually occurring more than 5 years after radiotherapy.[6,8,24] However, the incidence of postradiation sarcoma may be less after use of newer mega-voltage radiotherapy.[25]

4. **En bloc resection:** Malignant giant cell tumors are treated with en bloc resection with a wide surgical margin when possible. Adjuvant chemotherapy and radiation therapy are usually given.

5. **Therapeutic embolization:** Has been used as the only treatment in some cases or for palliative therapy in metastatic malignant giant cell tumors.[6,15]

References

1. Meyer A, Bastian L, Bruns F. Benign giant cell tumor of the spine: An unusual indication for radiotherapy. *Arch Orthop Trauma Surg.* 2006;126(8): 517-521.
2. Jaffe HL, Lichtenstein L. Giant cell tumor of bone: Its pathologic appearance, grading, supposed variants and treatment. *Arch Pathol.* 1940;30:993-1031.
3. Refai D, Dunn GP, Santiago P. Giant cell tumor of the thoracic spine: Case report and review of the literature. *Surg Neurol.* 2009;71(2):228-233; discussion 33.
4. Rodallec MH, Feydy A, Larousserie F, et al. Diagnostic imaging of solitary tumors of the spine: What to do and say. *Radiographics.* 2008;28(4): 1019-1041.
5. Kudawara I, Ueda T, Yoshikawa H. Giant cell tumor arising from the spinous process of the sacrum. *Eur Radiol.* 2000;10(7):1202.
6. Randall RL. Giant cell tumor of the sacrum. *Neurosurg Focus.* 2003;15(2): E13.
7. Murphey MD, Nomikos GC, Flemming DJ, et al. From the archives of AFIP. Imaging of giant cell tumor and giant cell reparative granuloma of bone: Radiologic-pathologic correlation. *Radiographics.* 2001;21(5): 1283-1309.
8. Leggon RE, Zlotecki R, Reith J, Scarborough MT. Giant cell tumor of the pelvis and sacrum: 17 cases and analysis of the literature. *Clin Orthop Relat Res.* 2004;(423):196-207.
9. Murphey MD, Andrews CL, Flemming DJ, et al. From the archives of the AFIP. Primary tumors of the spine: Radiologic pathologic correlation. *Radiographics.* 1996;16(5):1131-1158.
10. Oda Y, Takahira T, Yokoyama R, Tsuneyoshi M. Diffuse-type giant cell tumor/pigmented villonodular synovitis arising in the sacrum: Malignant form. *Pathol Int.* 2007;57(9):627-631.
11. Althausen PL, Schneider PD, Bold RJ, et al. Multimodality management of a giant cell tumor arising in the proximal sacrum: Case report. *Spine.* 2002;27(15):E361-E365.
12. Doita M, Miyamoto H, Nishida K, et al. Giant-cell tumor of the tendon sheath involving the thoracic spine. *J Spinal Disord Tech.* 2005;18(5): 445-448.
13. Dingle SR, Flynn JC, Flynn JC, Jr., Stewart G. Giant-cell tumor of the tendon sheath involving the cervical spine: A case report. *J Bone Joint Surg Am.* 2002;84-A(9):1664-1667.
14. Junming M, Cheng Y, Dong C, et al. Giant cell tumor of the cervical spine: a series of 22 cases and outcomes. *Spine.* 2008;33(3):280-288.
15. Lin PP, Guzel VB, Moura MF, et al. Long-term follow-up of patients with giant cell tumor of the sacrum treated with selective arterial embolization. *Cancer.* 2002;95(6):1317-1325.
16. Saikia B, Goel A, Gupta SK. Fine-needle aspiration cytologic diagnosis of giant-cell tumor of the sacrum presenting as a rectal mass: A case report. *Diagn Cytopathol.* 2001;24(1):39-41.
17. Ilaslan H, Sundaram M, Unni KK, Shives TC. Primary vertebral osteosarcoma: imaging findings. *Radiology.* 2004;230(3):697-702.
18. Nguyen TP, Burk DL, Jr. Musculoskeletal case of the day: Giant cell tumor of the sacrum. *AJR Am J Roentgenol.* 1995;165(1):201-202.
19. Michalowski MB, Pagnier-Clemence A, Chirossel JP, et al. Giant cell tumor of cervical spine in an adolescent. *Med Pediatr Oncol.* 2003;41(1): 58-62.
20. Ozaki T, Liljenqvist U, Halm H, et al. Giant cell tumor of the spine. *Clin Orthop Relat Res.* 2002;(401):194-201.

21. Samartzis D, Foster WC, Padgett D, Shen FH. Giant cell tumor of the lumbar spine: Operative management via spondylectomy and short-segment, 3-column reconstruction with pedicle recreation. *Surg Neurol.* 2008;69(2):138-141; discussion 41-42.

22. Guo W, Ji T, Tang X, Yang Y. Outcome of conservative surgery for giant cell tumor of the sacrum. *Spine.* 2009;34(10):1025-1031.

23. Yang SC, Chen LH, Fu TS, et al. Surgical treatment for giant cell tumor of the thoracolumbar spine. *Chang Gung Med J.* 2006;29(1):71-78.

24. Sanjay BK, Sim FH, Unni KK, et al. Giant-cell tumours of the spine. *J Bone Joint Surg Br.* 1993;75(1):148-154.

25. Nair MK, Jyothirmayi R. Radiation therapy in the treatment of giant cell tumor of bone. *Int J Radiat Oncol Biol Phys.* 1999;43(5):1065-1069.

HANGMAN'S FRACTURE

Douglas S. Fenton, M.D.

CLINICAL PRESENTATION

The patient is a 52-year-old male who was the driver of a jet ski on a private lake over the 4th of July weekend. Observers say that he was driving approximately 40 miles per hour when another boat pulling children on a tube crossed in front of him. The patient swerved so as not to hit the children, and he slammed head on into a boat dock. The patient was brought unconscious to the emergency department.

IMAGING PRESENTATION

Lateral radiograph and axial computed tomography (CT) images reveal fractures through the C2 pedicles with anterior displacement of C2 with respect to C3 consistent with a traumatic spondylolisthesis, also known as a *Hangman's fracture*. There are bone fragments in the region of the left vertebral artery foramen, which should be considered if there is suspicion of traumatic injury to the left vertebral artery *(Figs. 37-1 and 37-2)*.

DISCUSSION

The first cervical fracture-dislocation injury caused by hanging was described in 1913.[1] The term *traumatic spondylolisthesis* of the axis was described in 1964 in patients with fractures of the C2 pedicles after motor vehicle accidents.[2] The term *hangman's fracture* was attributed to Schneider, who in 1965 described the similarity of judicial hanging fractures to traumatic fractures of the axis.[3] The mechanism of a hanging fracture is one of distraction and hyperextension.[4] Today's hangman's fractures are typically deceleration injuries caused by motor vehicle accidents, diving, and falls in which the mechanism of injury is vertical compression and hyperextension, which causes the neural arch of C2 to be separated from the C2 vertebral body. Head injuries are highly associated with this type of hangman's fracture. The odontoid process remains intact. Fractures of the ring of the axis can occur through several areas of C2 including the laminae, pedicles, superior or inferior articular facets, pars interarticularis, and posterior wall of the vertebral body *(Fig. 37-3)*.[5] The fractures are often bilateral but not symmetric.[6]

Hangman's fractures can be classified into three types based on their displacement and mechanism of injury.[6] In type 1 injury (axial loading and hyperextension), the C2 vertebral body is nonangulated. The C2 body may be nondisplaced or minimally displaced (less than 2-3 mm) with a normal C2-3 intervertebral disc. In type 2 injuries, the C2 vertebral body is anteriorly displaced or angulated and there is disruption of the C2-3 disc. In type 3 injuries (primary flexion and rebound extension), there is anterior displacement and hyperflexion of the C2 vertebral body along with unilateral or bilateral facet dislocation. Type 2 has been subdivided into type 2 and type 2a.[7] This distinction is important because their mechanisms of injury are different and therefore their treatments are different. Type 2 fractures result from hyperextension and rebound flexion and type 2a is a flexion distraction injury. Hangman's fractures are typically treated with traction; however, treating a type 2a fracture with traction will lead to further distraction of the injury.[5]

Type 1 fractures are the most common (65%), followed by type 2 (28%), and type 3 (7%).[6] Type 1 fractures are considered stable. Types 2, 2a, and 3 are unstable fractures. In one study of all types of cervical fractures, 19% were fractures of the axis, with 4% being the hangman's type.[8] The incidence of spinal cord and nerve root injury is reported to be low, which may be related to the relatively spacious intracanalicular diameter at C2, which affords some protection against spinal cord compression.[9] However, the risk to the spinal cord increases with the severity of the fracture.

Patients who sustain a hangman's fracture typically present with acute neck pain after a traumatic incident. Most patients do not have neurologic symptoms; however, neurologic symptoms can occur and depend on which part of the spinal cord is affected. Patients may also have delayed stroke if there has been damage to the vertebral artery.

Other fractures of the cervical spine that are important to recognize are odontoid fractures, Jefferson fracture, extension teardrop fractures, hyperextension dislocation fractures, flexion teardrop fractures, and clay shoveler's fractures.

There are three classifications of **odontoid fractures**.[10] A type 1 fracture is an infrequent, stable fracture of the tip of the odontoid process. A type 2 fracture is an unstable fracture through the base of the odontoid process *(Fig. 37-4)*. A type 3 fracture is a stable fracture that passes through a portion of the superior body of C2 *(Fig. 37-5)*. Type 2 fractures are the most common, occurring in 31% to 65% of cases, and are complicated by nonunion in 26% to 36% of cases.[5] Odontoid fractures, being in an axial plane, are best visualized in the coronal or sagittal plane either directly with magnetic resonance (MR) imaging or with reformatted computed tomography (CT) imaging, but can be visualized with plain radiographs as well. MRI can be used to evaluate the chronicity of the

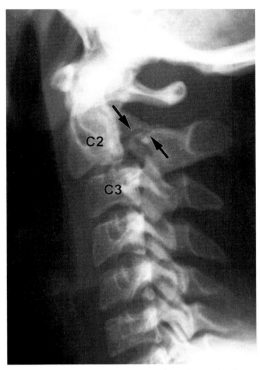

Figure 37-1 ▶ Hangman's Fracture, Lateral Radiograph. There is anterior subluxation of C2 with respect to C3. Note overlapping fracture lines (*black arrows*) of the C2 pedicles.

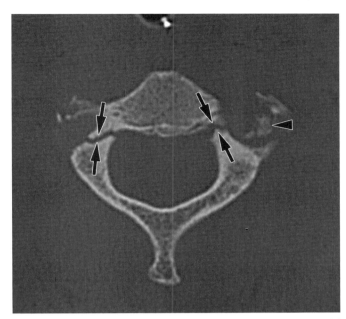

Figure 37-2 ▶ Hangman's Fracture, CT. Same patient as in Figure 37-1. Axial CT image confirms bilateral pedicle fractures (*between arrows*).

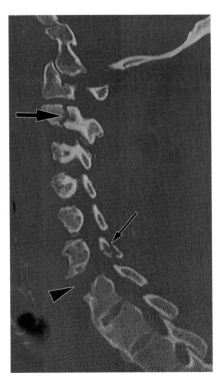

Figure 37-3 ▶ Hangman's Fracture. Off-midline sagittal CT image demonstrates a vertical fracture through the posterior body of C2 (*large arrow*). A concomitant hyperextension fracture at is seen C6-7 with distraction of the disc (*arrowhead*) and fracture through the C6 lamina (*small arrow*).

fracture. A recent fracture will demonstrate increased signal intensity on fat-saturated, T2-weighted or short tau inversion recovery (STIR) acquisitions and increased prevertebral soft tissue signal. A type 1 fracture can have an appearance similar to an os odontoideum (unfused ossification center cephalad to the dens). A type 1 fracture will have irregular noncorticated borders as opposed to the well-corticated periphery of an os odontoideum.

The **Jefferson fracture** is an axial loading compression fracture of the lateral masses of the atlas between the occipital condyles and articular facets of C2. The lateral masses are driven laterally away from C2 by the compressive force, which results in fractures of the anterior and posterior ring of C1. The fractures may be unilateral or bilateral and can consist of 2 to 4 fragments.[5] Jefferson fractures are typically stable with an intact transverse ligament.[11] The separation of the lateral masses can be seen with open-mouth plain radiographs of the craniocervical junction. The more definitive diagnosis is best identified with axial CT with coronal reformatted images demonstrating noncorticated fracture lines and prevertebral soft tissue edema *(Fig. 37-6)*. However, one should not mistake a fracture with a congenital developmental cleft, which has well-corticated margins and no associated soft tissue edema.

Extension teardrop fractures occur frequently and represent 19% of all fractures of C2.[5] This fracture is due to avulsion of the anterior longitudinal ligament with a triangular piece of bone from the anterior inferior vertebral body *(Fig. 37-7)*. One important characteristic of the fracture fragment is that its vertical height is either equal to or greater than its transverse dimension. This distinguishes an extension teardrop fracture from the similarly appearing hyperextension dislocation injury. Furthermore, patients with extension teardrop fractures typically do not have any neurologic symptoms, unlike those with hyperextension dislocation.[5]

A **hyperextension dislocation fracture** is an unstable fracture that is often the result of a high-velocity, abrupt deceleration motor

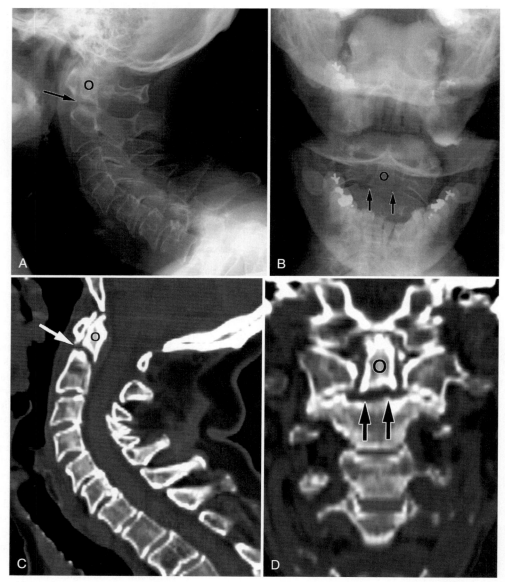

Figure 37-4 ▶ Odontoid Fracture, Type 2. Lateral (image **A**) and open-mouth frontal (image **B**) radiographs, sagittal (image **C**) and coronal (image **D**) reformatted CT of the cervical spine. Note fracture line (*arrows*) through the base of the odontoid process (*O*).

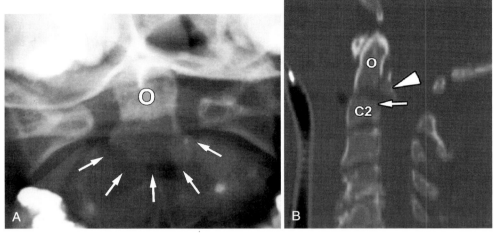

Figure 37-5 ▶ Odontoid Fracture, Type 3. Open-mouth frontal radiograph (image **A**) demonstrates a curvilinear fracture line (*arrows*) that extends more inferiorly into the body of C2. Sagittal reformatted CT (image **B**) shows separation of the odontoid process (*O*) from the C2 vertebral body and a posterior fracture fragment (*arrowhead*) that has avulsed a portion of the posterior superior body of C2 (*arrow*).

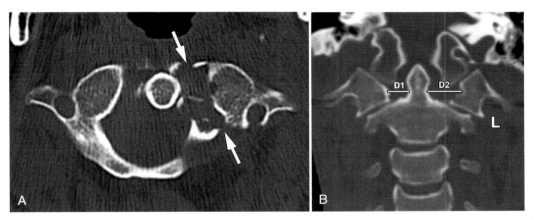

Figure 37-6 ▶ Jefferson Fracture. Axial CT, image **A**. Fracture through the left side of the ring of C1 (*arrows*). Coronal reformatted CT image **B** reveals asymmetry in the distance between the lateral aspect of the dens and the medial border of the C1 ring with greater separation on the left secondary to the complete ring fracture (*D2 > D1*).

vehicle accident, but can occur with any etiology that causes a significant, abrupt posteriorly directed force to the face.[12] There is rupture of the anterior longitudinal ligament and either avulsion of a fracture fragment with an appearance similar to an extension teardrop fracture (except that the diameter of the fracture fragment may be greater than its vertical height), a horizontal rupture through the intervertebral disc, and/or fracture(s) through the vertebral lamina (*Fig. 37-8*).[12] This type of fracture commonly involves the lower cervical vertebrae although it can occur anywhere throughout the cervical spine. Severe hyperextension causes posterior dislocation of the vertebra and is commonly associated with an acute cervical cord syndrome.[5] Fat-saturated, T2-weighted or STIR acquisitions can demonstrate abnormal increased signal intensity in the cervical cord, anterior longitudinal ligament,

retrospinal soft tissues, and intervertebral disc compatible with edema and/or hemorrhage.

A **flexion teardrop fracture** most commonly occurs at the C5-6 level. This also produces a triangular fracture from the anterior inferior corner of the vertebral body; however, there is significant ligamentous disruption with this type of injury. This type of injury presents with an acute anterior cervical cord syndrome.[5] This is an unstable fracture with a poor prognosis.

A **Clay shoveler's fracture** is a fracture of the spinous process of a lower cervical vertebral body, usually C7 (*Fig. 37-9*). The colloquialism *Clay shoveler's fracture* was used to describe the fracture seen in men digging drainage ditches in clay soil in southwestern Australia. As workers tossed their clay-filled shovel upward, some of the clay sometimes stuck to it, producing an unexpected

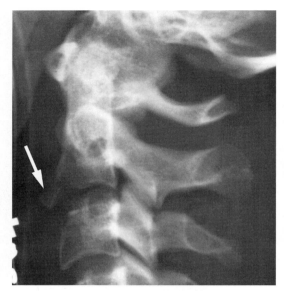

Figure 37-7 ▶ **Extension Teardrop Fracture.** Lateral radiograph. Note triangular fracture (*arrow*) of the anterior inferior C2 vertebral body at its attachment to the anterior longitudinal ligament.

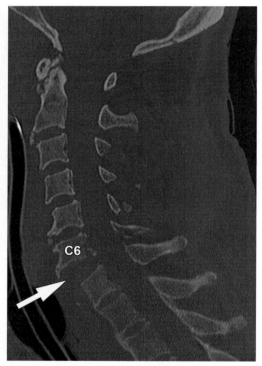

Figure 37-8 ▶ **Hyperextension Dislocation Fracture.** Sagittal reformatted CT image. Note distraction injury at C6-7 (*arrow*) with fracture extending through the disc and anterior subluxation of C6 with respect to C7.

opposite force on the workers' neck and back muscles. This would lead to fatigue of the spinous process, which could be heard occasionally as an audible crack accompanied by the immediate onset of pain from avulsion of the tip of the spinous process.[13] Today, such fractures occur as a result of motor vehicle accidents, sudden muscle contractions, or direct trauma.

With any of the fractures of the upper cervical spine, one should make a thorough evaluation for ligamentous injury. There are many published indirect signs of ligamentous injury described with plain film radiographs or CT, as well as more direct signs of ligamentous injury as seen with MR imaging. The most common measurements are those used for the diagnosis of atlanto-occipital dissociation or

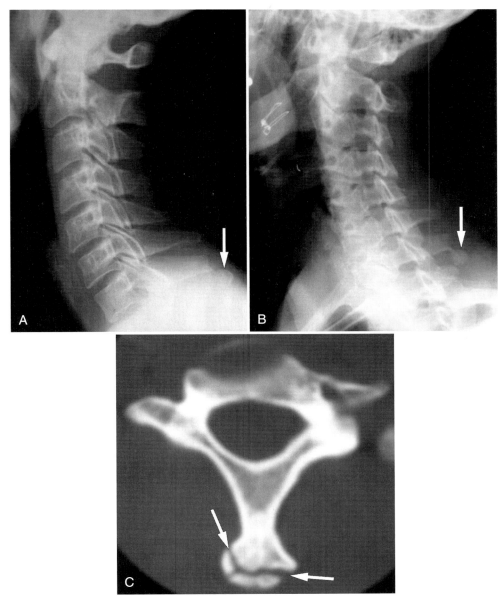

Figure 37-9 ▶ Clay Shoveler's Fracture. Lateral radiograph (image **A**), oblique radiograph (image **B**), and axial CT (image **C**) demonstrate the classic avulsion of the dorsal aspect of the C7 spinous process (*arrows*).

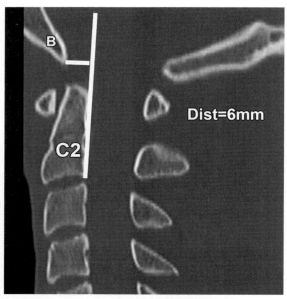

Figure 37-10 ▸ **Basion Axial Interval (BAI).** Midline sagittal CT. Normal patient. Measured by drawing a tangent along the posterior slope of the body of C2 in the midsagittal plane (*long white line*) and extending it cephalad past the basion (*B*). The distance between the basion and this line is the BAI. The normal BAT is considered to be less than 12 mm.

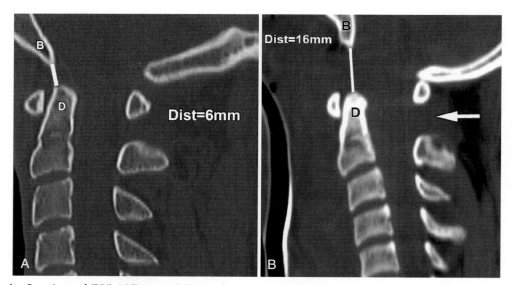

Figure 37-11 ▸ **Basion-Dens Interval (BDI).** Midline sagittal CT. Normal patient image **A**. Measured as the distance between the inferior most tip of the basion (*B*) to the closest point of the tip of the dens (*D*). A distance of 8.5 mm would be inclusive of greater than 95% of normal patients. Image **B** demonstrates an increase in the BDI in a patient with atlanto-occipital dissociation. Note also the widening of the space between the C1 and C2 spinous processes (*arrow*).

subluxation and include the basion-dens interval, basion-axial interval, the Powers ratio, the atlantodental interval, and atlanto-occipital interval.

The **basion axial interval (BAI)** is measured by drawing a tangent along the posterior slope of the body of C2 (midsagittal plane) and extending it cephalad past the basion *(Fig. 37-10)*. The distance between the basion and this line is the BAI. The normal BAI is considered to be less than 12 mm.[14]

The **basion-dens interval (BDI)** is measured as the distance between the inferior most tip of the basion (clivus) to the closest point of the tip of the dens *(Fig. 37-11, A, and B)*. Published norms of 12 mm on plain films are likely excessive. From CT measurements, a distance of 8.5 mm would be inclusive of greater than 95% of normal patients.[15]

The **Powers ratio** is a measurement of anterior atlanto-occipital dissociation or subluxation. It is measured by dividing the distance

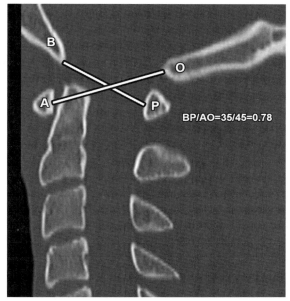

Figure 37-12 ▶ Powers Ratio. Midline sagittal CT. Normal patient. Measured by dividing the distance of a line connecting the tip of the basion (*B*) to the spinolamellar line of the posterior arch of the atlas (*P*) by the distance from the ventral edge of the opisthion (*O*) to the midposterior surface of the anterior arch of C1 (*A*). A ratio of less than 0.9 would include 95% of the normal population.

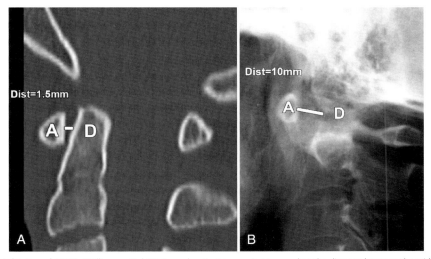

Figure 37-13 ▶ Atlantodental Interval (ADI). Midline sagittal CT. Normal patient image **A**. Measured as the distance between the midpoint of the posterior surface of the anterior arch of C1 (*A*) to the nearest point on the anterior surface of the dens (*D*). Published reports based on plain films state norms are 3 mm or less in men and 2.5 mm or less in women. CT measurements find no difference between men and women with a normal value of less than 2 mm. Lateral radiograph image **B** demonstrates widening of the ADI compatible with atlantoaxial subluxation.

of a line connecting the tip of the basion to the spinolamellar line of the posterior arch of the atlas by the distance from the ventral edge of the opisthion to the midposterior surface of the anterior arch of C1 (*Fig. 37-12*). A ratio of less than 0.9 would include 95% of the normal population.

The **atlantodental interval (ADI)** is used to evaluate the atlanto-axial relationship. It is measured as the distance between the midpoint of the posterior surface of the anterior arch of C1 to the nearest point on the anterior surface of the dens (*Fig. 37-13, A and B*). Published reports based on plain films state norms are 3 mm or less in men and 2.5 mm or less in women.[14] CT measurements find no difference between men and women with a normal value of less than 2 mm.[15]

The **atlanto-occipital interval (AOI)** is measured using an off-midline sagittal image at the level of the occipital condyles. The AOI is the distance of a line drawn perpendicular to the articular

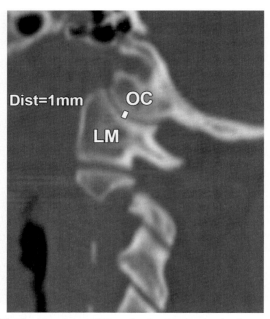

Figure 37-14 ▶ **Atlanto-Occipital Interval (AOI).** Off-midline sagittal CT. Normal patient. Measured as the distance of a line drawn perpendicular to the articular surfaces of the occipital condyle (*OC*) and lateral mass of C1 (*LM*). Normal measurements ranged between 0.6 and 1.4 mm with an average of 1 mm.

surfaces of the occipital condyle and lateral mass of C1 (*Fig. 37-14*). Normal measurements ranged between 0.6 and 1.4 mm with an average of 1 mm.

Other findings that suggest ligamentous injury is widening of the distance between the spinous processes, particularly at the spinolaminar line (*Fig. 37-15*). It is often stated that this distance can be evaluated at the level of the spinous processes; however, spinous processes can have various curvatures or can be bifid making an objective evaluation of widening difficult. Perched or locked facet joints are compatible with ligamentous disruption (*Figs. 37-16 and 37-17*). A significant kyphotic deformity may reflect injury to the posterior ligamentous complex. A spondylolisthesis can be caused by ligamentous injury, but can also be caused by ligamentous laxity. As with other ligamentous injuries, a direct evaluation of the ligaments cannot be made with plain films or CT, but rather inferred. MR imaging will demonstrate abnormal increased T2 or STIR signal intensity in regions of ligamentous injury (*Fig. 37-18*).

IMAGING FEATURES

Hangman's fractures can be identified with several different imaging modalities. The typical patient is imaged with plain radiographs. This will typically demonstrate anterior subluxation of C2 with respect to C3 and a lucency in the region of the C2 pedicles (see Fig. 37-1). Prevertebral soft tissue swelling can be appreciated, which is not seen with a similarly appearing pseudosubluxation of C2 on C3. The spinolamellar line is usually intact.

CT is often the next imaging modality obtained to evaluate any additional fractures and to determine the relationship of fracture fragments to the spinal canal, neural foramen, and vertebral artery foramen (see Fig. 37-2). Prevertebral soft tissue edema can be appreciated. The dens is usually spared. A fracture may extend through the C2 vertebral body. Fractures through the C2 vertebral

pedicles are readily identified. If the fracture line extends through the vertebral artery foramen or if a fracture fragment lies within the vertebral artery foramen, then one should raise the question of vertebral artery damage. Vertebral artery damage could be further evaluated with CT angiography, MR angiography, or conventional angiography.

MR imaging is used to identify abnormalities related to the cervical spinal cord and to provide a more direct evaluation of ligamentous stability. T2-weighted acquisitions using fat-saturation technique or STIR images can identify regions of increased cord signal intensity if there is cord edema/ischemia. This same acquisition will demonstrate increased signal intensity in the marrow adjacent to the fracture lines compatible with marrow edema, increased signal intensity in the prevertebral soft tissues from soft tissue edema, and increased signal intensity in the interspinous regions, which may reflect partial or complete ligamentous disruption.

DIFFERENTIAL DIAGNOSIS

1. **Pseudosubluxation of C2 on C3**: This can be a normal finding in children because of ligamentous laxity. There is no associated soft tissue swelling. The spinolamellar line remains intact.
2. **C2 spondylolysis**: This can look similar to a hangman's fracture; however, there is no associated soft tissue swelling and the edges of the spondylolysis are usually well corticated.

TREATMENT

1. **External cervical immobilization**: Most patients that survive the initial injury have good results after cervical immobilization. Initially, most patients are treated with external bracing.

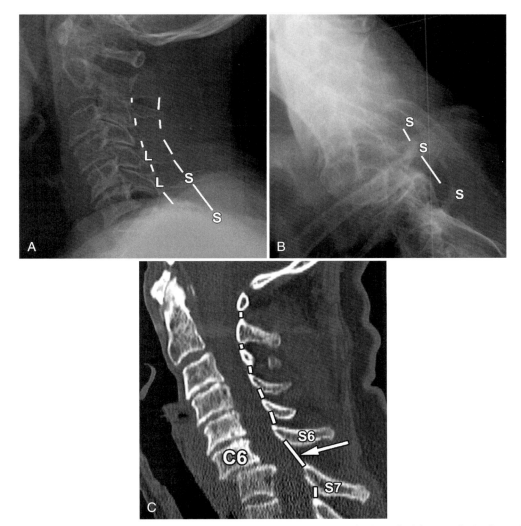

Figure 37-15 ► **Ligamentous Injury Suggested by Widening of the Interspinous Distance.** Lateral radiograph of the cervical spine (image **A**) suggests widening of the interspinous process distance (*L*, lamina, *S*, spinous process); however, the C7 spinous process is difficult to visualize because of the patient's shoulders. A lateral swimmer's view (image **B**) shows more clearly the abnormal separation between the C6 and C7 spinous processes (*S*). Sagittal reformatted CT of the same patient confirms abnormal separation (*arrow*) of the C6 (*S6*) and C7 (*S7*) spinous processes at the level of the spinolaminar line (*short lines*) compatible with injury to the interspinous ligament and anterior subluxation of C6 with respect to C7. This patient may also have sustained injury to the anterior and posterior longitudinal ligaments.

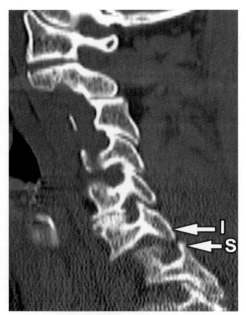

Figure 37-16 ▶ Perched Cervical Facet. Inferior articular process (*I*) is perched superior to the superior articular process (*S*) of the adjacent inferior level.

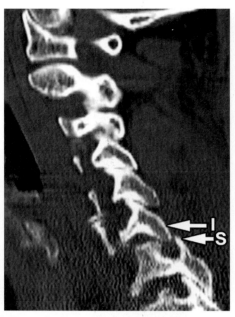

Figure 37-17 ▶ Locked Cervical Facet. The inferior articular process (*I*) has jumped over the superior articular process (*S*) of the adjacent inferior level and has settled so that the inferior tip of the inferior articular process is unable to move posteriorly because of the superior aspect of the superior articular process blocking its motion.

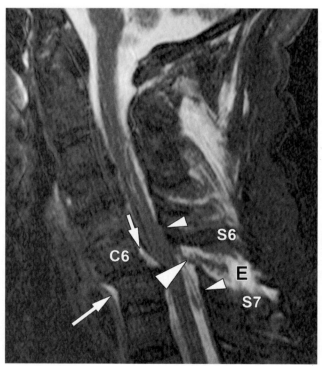

Figure 37-18 ▶ Ligamentous Injury. Same patient as in Figure 37-15. Sagittal fat-saturated, midline T2-weighted image. Increased signal intensity is seen throughout the widened space between the C6 (*S6*) and C7 (*S7*) spinous processes compatible with edema (*E*) and a complete tear of the interspinous ligament. The anterior aspect of the interspinous ligament is depicted by *small arrowheads*. There is discontinuity of the anterior interspinous ligament at C6-7 (*large arrowhead*). Fluid signal posterior to the C6 vertebral body (*short arrow*) and anterior to C7 (*long arrow*) suggests disruption of the posterior and anterior longitudinal ligaments.

2. **Surgical stabilization**: It has been recommended that surgical stabilization should be considered in cases where there is severe angulation of C2 with respect to C3, disruption of the C2-3 intervertebral disc, or failure of external bracing.[4]

References

1. Wood-Jones F. The ideal lesion produced by judicial hanging. *Lancet.* 1913;1:53.
2. Garber J. Abnormalities of the atlas and axis vertebrae: Congenital and traumatic. *J Bone Joing Surg Am.* 1964;46:1782-1791.
3. Schneider RC, Livingston KE, Cave AJ, Hamilton G. "Hangman's fracture" of the cervical spine. *J Neurosurg.* 1965;22:141-154.
4. Isolated fractures of the axis in adults. *Neurosurgery.* 2002;50:S125-S139.
5. Pratt H, Davies E, King L. Traumatic injuries of the C1/C2 complex: Computed tomographic imaging appearances. *Curr Prob Diag Radiol.* 2008;37:26-38.
6. Effendi B, Roy D, Cornish B, et al. Fractures of the ring of the axis: A classification based on the analysis of 131 cases. *J Bone Joint Surg Br.* 1981;63:319-327.
7. Levine AM, Edwards CC. The management of traumatic spondylolisthesis of the axis. *J Bone Joint Surg Am.* 1985;67:217-226.
8. Greene KA, Dickman CA, Marciano FF, et al. Acute axis fractures: Analysis of management and outcome in 340 consecutive cases. *Spine.* 1997;22:1843-1852.
9. Mollan RA, Watt PC. Hangman's fracture. *Injury.* 1982;14:265-267.
10. Anderson LD, D'Alonzo RT. Fractures of the odontoid process of the axis. *J Bone Joint Surg Am.* 1974;56:1663-1674.
11. Jefferson G. Fracture of the atlas vertebra. *Br J Surg.* 1920;407-421.
12. Edeiken-Monroe B, Wagner LK, Harris JH. Hyperextension dislocation of the cervical spine. *AJR Am J Roentgenol.* 1986;146:803-808.
13. Lee P, Hunter TB, Taljanovic M. Musculoskeletal colloquialisms: How did we come up with these names? *Radiographics.* 2004;24:1009-1027.
14. Harris JH, Carson GC, Wagner LK. Radiologic diagnosis of traumatic occipitovertebral dissociation: 1. Normal occipitovertebral relationships on lateral radiographs of supine subjects. *AJR Am J Roentgenol.* 1994;162:881-886.
15. Rojas CA, Bertozzi JC, Martinez CR, Whitlow J. Reassessment of the craniocervical junction: Normal values on CT. *AJNR Am J Neuroradiol.* 2007;28:1819-1823.

INFLAMMATORY POLYNEUROPATHY OF THE CAUDA EQUINA

Leo F. Czervionke, M.D.

CLINICAL PRESENTATION

The patient is a 16-year-old male who presented with history of a "cold and sore throat that lasted a month" followed by progressive acute lower extremity weakness. This was followed by numbness in the toes and fingers and later dizziness. On physical examination, he had absent lower extremity reflexes and reduced strength in the feet, toes, hip flexors, deltoid, and finger flexors. He was observed to be ataxic and had a mild upper extremity tremor. A magnetic resonance (MR) scan of the lumbar spine was ordered. Nerve conduction studies revealed findings consistent with a demyelinating polyradiculomyelopathy. The protein level in the cerebrospinal fluid (CSF) was elevated (115 mg/dL). A diagnosis of Guillain-Barré syndrome was made. He was treated with intravenous immunoglobulin (IVIg), and symptoms improved but did not resolve completely after several months of follow-up.

IMAGING PRESENTATION

MR imaging of the lumbar spine obtained at time of presentation revealed diffuse thickening and enhancement of the nerve rootlets of the cauda equina and nerve roots consistent with diffuse inflammatory polyneuritis in keeping with the clinical diagnosis (*Figs. 38-1 to 38-4*).

DISCUSSION

Diffuse inflammatory polyneuropathies of the cauda equina, spinal nerve roots, and peripheral nerves represent a diverse group of disorders with many similarities in terms of pathogenesis, clinical presentation, biochemical properties, and histologic origins and in terms of similarities seen on imaging studies. Acute polyneuropathy or polyradiculoneuropathy is usually classified under the general category of **Guillain-Barré syndrome (GBS)**. GBS is the most common cause of acute muscle weakness in patients under age 40, and its incidence is 1 to 2 per 100,000 people.[1-3] GBS most commonly occurs in children and young adults.[4] Chronic inflammatory polyradiculoneuropathy (CIPD) is a condition that usually has a different presentation and clinical course. However, GBS may progress to CIDP or resemble CIDP clinically in the later stages of the disease.[5]

There are at least six clinical subtypes of Guillain-Barré syndrome: (1) Acute inflammatory demyelinating polyradiculo-neuropathy (AIDP) is often used synonymously with GBS because AIDP is by far the most common subtype of GBS. AIDP is a post-infectious or post-vaccination, immune-mediated process that attacks the Schwann cells, causing neural inflammation and demyelination that may involve the cauda equina, nerve roots, peripheral nerves, and/or cranial nerves. AIDP classically manifests as an *ascending paralysis* beginning in the distal lower extremities and extending cephalad to a varying degree in thethorax, cervical region, and sometimes into the brainstem. (2) Acute motor axonal neuropathy (AMAN), also called *Chinese paralytic syndrome*, attacks motor nerves at the nodes of Ranvier, which are gaps in the myelin sheath between adjacent Schwann cells. AMAN is prevalent in China and Mexico.[6] (3) Acute motor sensory axonal neuropathy (AMSAN) is similar to AMAN with motor dysfunction, but also causes severe axonal dysfunction of sensory nerves.[7] (4) Miller-Fisher syndrome (MFS) is a rare form of GBS with patients presenting initially with opthalmoplegia, ataxia, and areflexia. A *descending pattern of paralysis* occurs in MFS. (5) Bickerstaff's brainstem encephalitis (BBE) is believed to be a variant of GBS characterized by acute onset of opthalmoplegia, ataxia, disturbance of consciousness, hyperreflexia, and a positive Babinski sign.[8,9] (6) Acute panautonomic neuropathy (APAN) is the rarest form of GBS, which manifests as diffuse autonomic nervous system dysfunction.[10] Patients present with sympathetic and parasympathetic nervous system dysfunction, cardiac dysrhythmias, orthostatic hypotension, and sometimes encephalopathy. APAN has a high mortality rate.

GBS is an acute motor and sensory axonal neuropathy. Symptoms usually develop after a viral illness or after vaccination. Patients present with lower extremity flaccid paralysis or distal lower extremity paresthesias (numbness and tingling), hyporeflexia, or areflexia. This is followed by *ascending paralysis*. Eventually the paralysis may involve the brainstem, which causes respiratory paralysis requiring ventilator support. Autonomic nerve dysfunction is common. Cranial nerve palsies may occur in up to one half of patients, facial nerve paralysis being the most common.[3]

Neuropathic pain is not considered a common primary feature of GBS but does develop in many patients, and the pain can be severe.[11,12] However, many types of pain can occur in patients with GBS.[13] In one series of 55 GBS patients, nearly one half of the patients presented with moderate to severe pain.[14] The back and leg pain usually resolves by 8 weeks after onset, but dysesthetic pain in the extremities may persist.[14] GBS must always be considered in the differential diagnosis of children presenting with back or leg pain.[4] The extremity pain associated with GBS is often worse

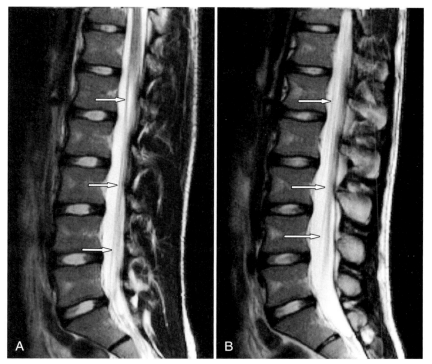

Figure 38-1 ▶ Guillain-Barré Syndrome (GBS). 16-year-old male. In midline sagittal T2-weighted lumbar MR image **A** and T2-weighted paramidline image **B**, the nerve roots of the cauda equina (*arrows*) are thickened.

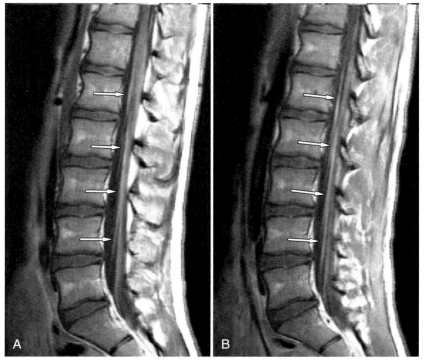

Figure 38-2 ▶ Guillain-Barré Syndrome. Same patient as in Figure 38-1. Corresponding sagittal contrast enhanced midline T1-weighted image **A** and parasagittal image **B**, the nerve roots of the cauda equina (*arrows*) appear diffusely thickened without nodularity and enhance uniformly.

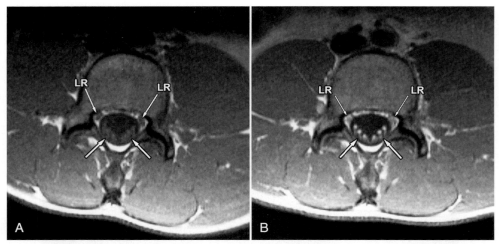

Figure 38-3 ▸ Guillain-Barré Syndrome, L2 Level. Same patient as in Figures 38-I and 38-2. In unenhanced axial T1-weighted image **A**, cauda equina nerve roots (*arrows*) are slightly enlarged and enhance on contrast enhanced axial T1-weighted image **B**. The ventral nerve rootlets of the cauda equina are larger and enhance to a greater degree than the dorsal rootlets (*arrows*). The nerve roots in the lateral recesses (*LR*) also enhance bilaterally.

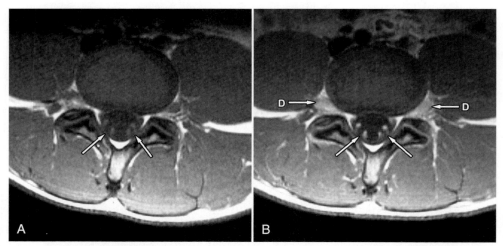

Figure 38-4 ▸ Guillain-Barré Syndrome, L3-4 level. Same patient as in Figures 38-1 to 38-3. On unenhanced axial T1-weighted image **A**, the cauda equina nerve roots (*arrows*) are slightly enlarged. In contrast enhanced image **B**, the nerve roots (*arrows*) enhance, although ventral nerve rootlets are larger and enhance to a greater degree than the dorsal rootlets (*arrows*). The dorsal root ganglia (*D*) are slightly enlarged and also enhance to a greater degree than normal.

at night and can be a deep muscular aching pain or spasmodic pain, described commonly as a *charley horse*. Painful dysesthesia may also occur similar to that commonly seen with diabetic neuropathy.[15] Patients with GBS may also experience abdominal pain.[3,16] Muscle weakness and fatigue may be prominent features in more chronic cases of GBS.[11] Patients with GBS typically have elevated protein in the CSF. The majority of patients with GBS show improvement in 2 to 3 months, but up to 50% have persistent symptoms at 1 year follow-up. Permanent deficits remain in up to 10% of cases. Up to 8% of AIDP cases can be fatal. GBS may evolve into a condition that is clinically similar to or indistinguishable from CIDP. The diagnosis of CIDP should be considered if a patient with GBS deteriorates after 9 weeks from onset of symptoms or when the patient's condition deteriorates three times or more.[5]

GBS is believed to be an immune-mediated process that causes inflammatory demyelinating lesions in the cauda equina, nerve roots, peripheral nerves, or cranial nerves. Antibodies to ganglioside GM1 (anti-GM1 antibodies) are elevated in the serum and CSF of patients with GBS and AMAN.[17,18] Anti-GM1 antibodies have also been implicated in the pathogenesis of amyotrophic lateral sclerosis (ALS).[19] The GM1 epitope is present in motor neurons and their axons, in the dorsal root ganglia, and in sensory axons. The precise role of anti-GM1 antibodies in the pathogenesis of GBS is still not fully known.[17] There is some evidence that patients with GBS who have anti-GM1 antibodies more often experience a rapidly progressive and more severe neuropathy with predominantly distal distribution of weakness.[18] Other autoantibodies may also be involved in the pathogenesis of GBS. For example, patients with acute polyneuropathies may have elevated titers of IgG autoantibodies against disialosyl epitopes.[20] Histologically, patients have focal segmental demyelination, perivascular and endoneural lymphocytic infiltrates, and macrophage infiltrates; axonal degeneration may eventually occur.

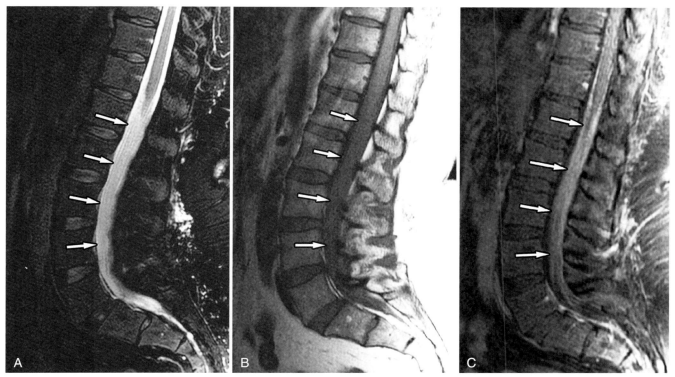

Figure 38-5 ▶ Chronic Inflammatory Demyelinating Polyradiculoneuropathy (CIDP). Post-liver transplantation patient receiving tacrolimus who developed a cytomegalovirus infection. On sagittal T2-weighted image **A** and T1-weighted image **B**, the cauda equina nerve roots (*arrows*) are indistinct and individual nerve roots cannot be seen. On contrast-enhanced fat-saturated T1-weighted MR image **C**, the cauda equina nerve roots (*arrows*) are thickened and enhance diffusely. The pial surface of the conus medullaris and lower thoracic spinal cord also enhance diffusely.

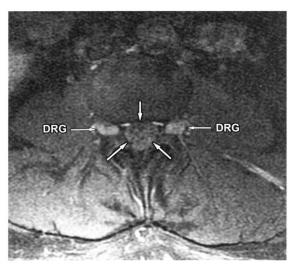

Figure 38-6 ▶ Chronic Inflammatory Demyelinating Polyradiculoneuropathy (CIDP). Same patient as in Figure 38-5. Axial contrast enhanced T1-weighted image shows diffuse ill-defined enhancement of the diffusely enlarged nerve roots of the cauda equina which fill the thecal sac. The dorsal root ganglia (*D*) also enhance intensely.

A *Campylobacter jejuni* infection can trigger GBS. Patients with *C. jejuni* infection more commonly experience severe pure motor deficits. In one study, patients with *C. jejuni* infections responded better to intravenous immunoglobulin (IVIg) therapy than to plasma exchange.[18]

Chronic inflammatory demyelinating polyradiculoneuropathy (CIDP) is an acquired immune-mediated demyelinating disorder involving spinal nerve roots, cauda equina (*Figs. 38-5 to 38-10*), lumbar plexus, brachial plexus, or peripheral nerve roots. The prevalence of CIDP is probably grossly underestimated.[21] The pathogenesis of CIDP is unknown but is believed to be related to both abnormal humoral and cellular immune responses to some nerve antigen or antigens. Activated T cells are involved in the generation of inflammatory lesions in the nervous system in general and are also involved in CIDP.[22] The CD4 and CD8 T-cell subgroups have both been implicated in this process.[23,24] The same type of invariant T-cell found in patients with multiple sclerosis is also present in the majority of patients with CIDP.[24] Regardless of the precise immunologic mechanism, T-lymphocytes, monocytes, and macrophages infiltrate the nerves and adjacent tissue and cause release of enzymes that cause inflammation in the nerves. Soluble cytokines and chemokines also contribute to the pathogenesis of CIDP, and concentrations of these substances are elevated in the CSF in patients with CIDP.[25]

Histologically, the nerves in patients with CIDP show segmental demyelination and remyelination and thinning of myelin sheaths, and the nerves often have an *onion bulb* appearance,[26,27] features present in many of the chronic polyneuropathies. Mononuclear cell infiltrates may be present in the endoneurium. There may be a preferential involvement of the motor nerves, which may account for negative sural nerve biopsies in some patients.[21]

Most cases of CIDP are idiopathic, but it can be associated with a variety of disorders including diabetes, HIV infection, celiac disease (gluten-sensitive enteropathy), melanoma, Sjögren's

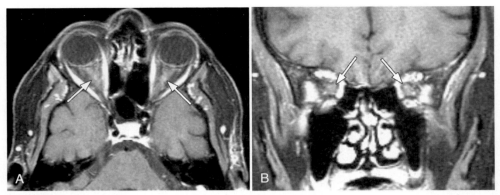

Figure 38-7 ► **Chronic Inflammatory Demyelinating Polyradiculoneuropathy (CIDP).** Same patient as in Figures 38-5 and 38-6. The patient also had bilateral optic neuritis attributed to cytomegalovirus infection. Axial contrast enhanced fat-saturated T1-weighted images of the orbits shows diffuse enhancement and enlargement of both optic nerves (*arrows*) on axial image **A** and coronal image **B**.

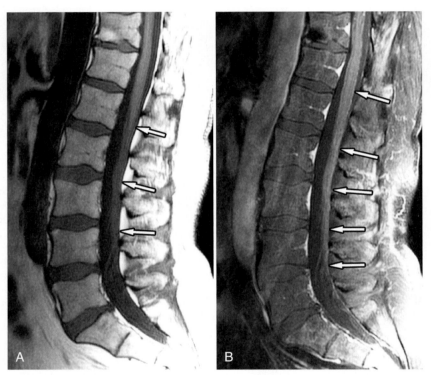

Figure 38-8 ► **Chronic Inflammatory Demyelinating Polyradiculoneuropathy (CIDP).** Unenhanced sagittal image **A** and contrast-enhanced fat-saturated T1-weighted MR image **B**. The nerve roots of the cauda equina (*arrows*) appear thickened and enhance diffusely.

syndrome, lymphoma, IgM gammopathy (polyclonal or monoclonal), or with hepatitis.[23,28] Patients with chronic polyneuropathies often have elevated antiganglioside and/or antisulfatide IgM antibodies.[20] The peripheral nerves are most commonly involved in patients with CIDP. Biopsy of the sural nerve may help confirm the diagnosis.[22] In the spine, CIDP affects the cauda equina and lumbar nerve roots more commonly than the cervical nerve roots. The thoracic nerve roots and cranial nerves may also be affected but are less commonly involved than in AIDP (see Fig. 38-7).

Patients with CIDP classically present with a history of a chronic, progressive, or relapsing disorder with muscle weakness and often sensory loss. Patients with sensory neuropathy have predominant involvement of large-fiber nerves.[21] This is usually a polyradicular condition with symmetric or asymmetric involvement of proximal and distal muscles in the lower extremity.[21] Neurogenic pain is not a common initial manifestation of CIDP, but pain may occur as the disease evolves.[29] Rarely, neurogenic pain is the initial manifestation of CIDP.[30] Neuropathic pain is very common in patients with small-fiber peripheral neuropathies, such as patients with diabetic neuropathy or amyloidosis-related neuropathy.[15,30,31] Patients may present with symptoms similar to multiple sclerosis.

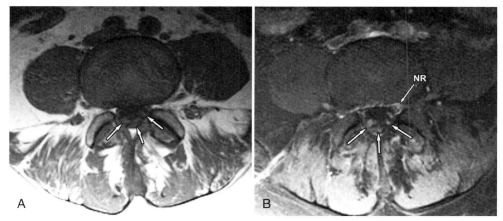

Figure 38-9 ► **Chronic Inflammatory Demyelinating Polyradiculoneuropathy (CIDP).** Same patient as in Figure 38-8. Axial unenhanced T1-weighted image **A** and contrast-enhanced fat-saturated T1-weighted MR image **B** reveals asymmetric enlargement and enhancement of the nerve roots of the cauda equina (*arrows*) at the L3 level and enhancement of the left L3 nerve root (*NR*) in the left lateral recess.

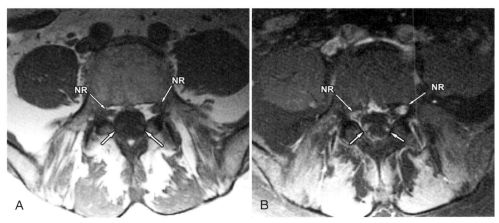

Figure 38-10 ► **Chronic Inflammatory Demyelinating Polyradiculoneuropathy (CIDP).** Same patient as in Figures 38-8 and 38-9. L5 level. Axial unenhanced T1-weighted image **A** and contrast-enhanced fat-saturated T1-weighted image **B**. All nerve roots of the cauda equina (*arrows*) enhance but are asymmetrically enlarged. The L5 nerve roots (*NR*) enhance within the lateral recess of L5 bilaterally.

Classically, GBS symptoms progress within the first few weeks and are maximal at 4 weeks from onset of the disease, and thereafter the disorder is usually monophasic. In CIDP, symptoms usually progress for at least 2 months, and thereafter the disorder may be monophasic, relapsing-remitting, or steadily progressive.[5] In practice, however, it may be difficult clinically to differentiate CIDP from progressive GBS, especially in the early stages of the disease.[5] The major electromyographic (EMG) finding in CIDP is slow nerve conduction similar to that seen with demyelinating disorders in general. A more detailed summary of the EMG findings of CIDP can be found elsewhere.[21] Patients with mild cases of CIDP tend to recover with complete or near complete regaining of function. Severe cases have a chronic, progressive, relapsing-remitting illness. Rarely, CIDP can be fatal.

Sensory ganglioneuropathies, which involve the dorsal root ganglia, represent a subgroup of polyneuropathies that may occur with paraneoplastic subacute sensory neuronopathy (SSN), Sjögren's syndrome, Miller-Fisher syndrome, Bickerstaff's brainstem encephalitis, inherited ganglioneuropathies (Friedreich's ataxia and other inherited cerebellar ataxias), and with certain drugs (pyridoxine, vincristine, taxane, and cisplatin).[20,32] There is a predisposition to developing chemotherapy-induced neuropathy in patients who are diabetic, chronic alcoholics, and in patients with inherited neuropathies.[32]

Paraneoplastic neuropathy (PPN) is rarely encountered in routine practice but may produce clinical manifestations and an MR imaging appearance identical to GBS or CIDP. Indeed, PPN may be considered to be a subtype of CIDP.[33] There are other paraneoplastic syndromes that affect the nervous system, including paraneoplastic encephalomyelitis, paraneoplastic cerebellar degeneration, cancer-associated retinopathy, and paraneoplastic opsoclonus-myoclonus-ataxia syndrome.[33] Paraneoplastic neuropathy commonly involves the dorsal root ganglia, but the spinal cauda equina, nerve roots, and peripheral nerves may be involved as well (*Fig. 38-11*).[33]

Paraneoplastic syndromes in the nervous system are believed to be the result of an immune response to proteins normally present in the nervous system. When these same proteins are expressed by tumors, these proteins are called *onconeural antigens*.[34-36] Autoantibodies to these antigens are detected in up to 30% of patients with PPN.[35,37] In the majority of patients with paraneoplastic polyneuropathy, nonprotein molecules act as onconeural antigens.[34] Gangliosides, normally found in plasma cell membranes and concentrated in the nervous system, often act as

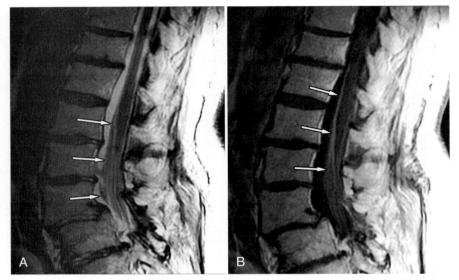

Figure 38-11 ▶ Paraneoplastic Polyneuropathy of the Cauda Equina. On T2-weighted image **A**, the nerve roots of the cauda equina (*arrows*) are thickened and appear matted together. On sagittal contrast enhanced T1-weighted image **B**, the cauda equina roots (*arrows*) are thickened and enhance diffusely, relative to the nonenhancing spinal cord. The pial surfaces of the conus medullaris also enhance (*upper arrows in image* **B**).

onconeural antigens in paraneoplastic neuropathy, and antigan-glioside antibodies (anti-GM1 antibodies) are often found in patients with paraneoplastic polyneuropath.[34] Onconeural antigens on tumor cells may also trigger IgG autoantibody formation and production of cytotoxic T-lymphocytes.[34,38] Other antineural antibodies may be present in the serum and CSF of patients with paraneoplastic disorders including anti-Hu, anti-Yo, and anti-P/Q type voltage-gated calcium channel (VGCC) antibodies.[33,39]

The CSF in patients with PPN contains lymphocytes (pleocytosis) in the early stages of this condition and elevated IgG, and oligoclonal bands are present in the CSF weeks to months later. Organ-specific antineuronal antibodies may be present in the CSF or serum in these patients.[40] Whole body fluorodeoxyglucose positron emission tomography (FDG-PET) scanning may be helpful in patients with paraneoplastic syndrome to identify the source of the malignancy. Small cell lung carcinoma is the most common malignancy associated with PPN,[40] and FDG-PET is highly sensitive for the detection and staging of lung carcinoma.[41,42]

POEMS Syndrome

Polyneuropathy is one component of POEMS (*p*olyneuropathy, *o*rganomegaly, *e*ndocrinopathy, *M* protein, *s*kin changes) syndrome. POEMS syndrome is a rare multisystemic paraneoplastic syndrome caused by an underlying plasma cell dyscrasia. More than 95% of patients with POEMS syndrome have a characteristic monoclonal lambda osteosclerotic plasmacytoma or bone marrow infiltration.[43]

Inherited Sensory and Motor Neuropathies

The inherited sensory and motor neuropathies (ISMN) represent a group of disorders that may manifest with motor weakness, sensory disturbance, diminished nerve conduction velocities on EMG, and polyneuropathy. The most widely known conditions in this category are Charcot-Marie-Tooth disease and Dejerine-Sottas

disease.[44-48] A mutation in chromosome *17p11* has been found in some patients with Charcot-Marie-Tooth disease type 1A (CMT1A).[49,50] Interestingly, a mutation in the same gene has been reported in a patient with GBS.[49,50] The peripheral nerves are commonly involved in these conditions, but the spinal nerve roots, cauda equina, and cranial nerves may also be involved, the nerves appearing diffusely enlarged, sometimes clumped, and enhancing on MR images.[44,51]

IMAGING FEATURES

Inflammatory polyneuropathy involving the cauda equina is best demonstrated with MR imaging. However, the activity or clinical severity of the disease often does not correlate well with the MR appearance.[52] Furthermore, contrast enhancement of the nerves or cauda equina does not indicate that the affected nerves are necessarily associated with pain.

In GBS or CIDP, the cauda equina nerve roots may be involved, more commonly in GBS (see Figs. 38-1 to 38-4). The enhancement of the surface of the conus medullaris and cauda equina can be extensive and intense.[4,53,54] Patients with CIDP may have relatively more extraforaminal involvement than cauda equina involvement.[52] Nerve root enlargement, if present, can be seen on T2-weighted or T1-weighted MR images (see Figs. 38-1 and 38-2), on myelographic images or on post-myelogram CT scans.[52-57] The nerve roots of the cauda equina on sagittal images appear either thickened (see Figs. 38-1 and 38-2) or difficult to differentiate, sometimes appearing as a single cord of tissue within the lumbar spinal canal (see Figs. 38-5 and 38-8). The pial surfaces of the inflamed conus medullaris and cauda equina nerve roots enhance uniformly and symmetrically after IV contrast enhancement (see Figs. 38-5 and 38-8).[4,55] Usually the nerves are diffusely involved without nodularity, but occasionally the nerve roots of the cauda equina are asymmetrically enlarged in CIDP (see Figs. 38-9 and 38-10). The enlargement and contrast enhancement of the nerve roots are often diffuse but can be asymmetrically involved (see Figs. 38-9 and 38-10).

The presence of ventral nerve root enhancement strongly suggests GBS (see Figs. 38-3 and 38-4).[58] However, motor manifestations in GBS occur in only 3% of patients, so more commonly, diffuse enhancement of the cauda equina is expected in GBS.[59] The pial margins of the conus medullaris often enhance in GBS or CIDP, but the conus medullaris is usually not enlarged.

Enlargement and enhancement of the dorsal root ganglia within the neural foramina are often present at multiple levels throughout the spine (see Figs. 38-4, 38-6, and 38-10). Cranial nerve enlargement and enhancement may also be visible (see Fig. 38-7).[55,60,61] In patients with sensory ganglioneuropathies, the dorsal root ganglia are often enlarged at multiple levels and enhance to a greater degree than normal. The appearance is similar to that seen in neurofibromatosis patients with nerve root involvement. Cranial nerve involvement may occur in GBS or CIDP but is more common in GBS.

DIFFERENTIAL DIAGNOSIS

Many conditions can cause enlargement and enhancement of the cauda equina rootlets, nerve roots, and peripheral nerves similar to GBS or CIDP.

1. **Leptomeningeal metastasis (LM) (leptomeningeal carcinomatosis):** LM is the most common cause of diffuse enhancement of the cauda equina and pial surface of the conus medullaris. Metastatic involvement of the pial surface of the conus and cauda equina tends to be multinodular, but occasionally a diffuse pattern of enhancement is seen, so called *zuckerguss* (sugarcoated) pattern occurs with LM metastases. The patient with LM metastases usually has a known malignancy.

2. **Paraneoplastic polyneuropathy:** May simulate the appearance of leptomeningeal metastasis, CIDP, or GBS. Elevated paraneoplastic antibody titers are typically present in the CSF and serum (see Fig. 38-11).[33]

3. **Infectious polyneuropathy secondary to cytomegalovirus (CMV)** (see Figs. 38-5 to 38-7), **Lyme disease** (Borrelia infection), or **neurosyphilis** (*Treponema pallidum*)[55] or **tuberculosis**.[62]

4. **Tacrolimus (FK506):** An immunosuppressive agent that inhibits cytokine synthesis and blocks T-cell development. It may be used in patients after liver transplantation. Tacrolimus may be neurotoxic to the central nervous system (CNS) causing CNS symptoms in up to 26% of patients. In 4% of patients, it affects the peripheral neuromuscular system, usually causing myopathy or a peripheral mononeuropathy. In a minority of patients, it can cause an acute or chronic polyneuropathy, similar to Guillain-Barré syndrome or CIDP (see Figs. 38-5 to 38-7).[63,64]

5. **Neurofibromatosis and CIDP:** Neurofibromatosis and CIDP may have a similar imaging appearance if multifocal nerve root enlargement is present.[65] Clinical manifestations and presentation are different allowing differentiation between these conditions.

6. **Inherited polyneuropathies:** Polyneuropathies such as Charcot-Marie-Tooth disease or Dejerine-Sottas disease may be difficult to differentiate from GBS or CIDP with imaging alone. Diagnosis relies on family history and genetic testing.[44,46,51]

7. **Nitrous oxide inhalation:** Whippet-induced myeloneuropathy may produce clinical manifestations identical to GBS.[66]

8. **Subacute combined degeneration (SCD):** SCD caused by vitamin B_{12} deficiency may manifest with clinical findings similar to GBS. However, patients with SCD do not have imaging evidence of cauda equina polyneuropathy. On MR imaging, patients with SCD have a characteristic linear band of T2 hyperintensity in the dorsal aspect of the cervical spinal cord (in the dorsal funiculus) that usually extends over several levels *(Fig. 38-12)*. A similar MR appearance and clinical presentation can be seen in patients with vitamin B_6 (pyridoxine) toxicity.

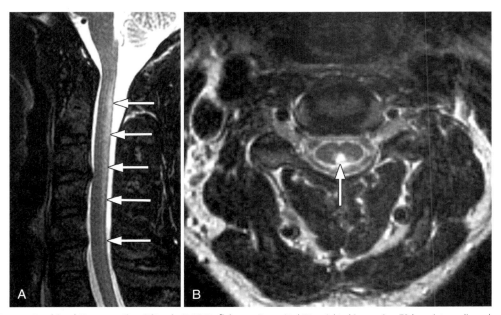

Figure 38-12 ▶ **Subacute Combined Degeneration, Vitamin B-12 Deficiency.** On sagittal T2-weighted image **A**, a T2 hyperintense linear band is seen in the dorsal aspect of the spinal cord (*arrows*). On axial T2-weighted image **B**, the hyperintense signal (*arrow*) is located in the dorsal funiculus.

TREATMENT

A discussion of the detailed therapeutic approach for GBS and CIDP is beyond the scope of this book, but a detailed discussion of the therapeutic approach to these disorders can be found elsewhere.[2,67-68] In general immunomodulation or immunosuppressive therapies are used to treat these conditions. A brief summary of the therapeutic options follows.

GBS

1. **Plasma exchange in combination with IV immunoglobulin (IVIg) therapy:** Effective in many but not all patients. Early treatment with plasma exchange can lead to more rapid and complete recovery.[2,3]
2. **Corticosteroid therapy:** Used alone for the treatment of patients with AIDP, corticosteroid therapy is probably not beneficial, but combined corticosteroid and IVIg therapy may have a minor positive synergistic effect.[1,2,69]
3. **Respiratory support with a ventilator:** Required if brainstem involvement results in respiratory compromise.

CIDP

The following therapeutic options are used alone or in combination.

1. **Plasma exchange**
2. **Intravenous immunoglobulin (IVIg)**
3. **Corticosteroid therapy**
4. **Immunosuppressive or cytotoxic drugs**: Drugs such as methotrexate, azathioprine, cyclosporin-A, etanercept, and mycophenolate have been used for the treatment of CIDP.[2] Interferons are naturally occurring cytokines that have also been used with some success for treatment of patients with multiple sclerosis, but a therapeutic benefit of using interferon for treating patients with CIDP has not been proved.[70]

Neuropathic Pain Treatment

Mediations are often prescribed for treatment of neuropathic pain associated with the inflammatory polyneuropathies. Some drugs that have been used to treat neuropathic pain include gabapentin, pregabalin, topiramate, and amitryptyline.[71,72] Persistent dysesthetic pain may be treated with conventional analgesics.[14]

References

1. Van Koningsveld R, Van Doorn PA, Schmitz PI, et al. Mild forms of Guillain-Barré syndrome in an epidemiologic survey in The Netherlands. *Neurology*. 2000;54(3):620-625.
2. van Doorn PA. Treatment of Guillain-Barré syndrome and CIDP. *J Peripher Nerv Syst*. 2005;10(2):113-127.
3. Wong PS, Fothergill NJ, Touquet R. Abdominal pain as a presenting symptom of the Guillain-Barré syndrome. *Arch Emerg Med*. 1988;5(4):242-245.
4. Wilmshurst JM, Thomas NH, Robinson RO, et al. Lower limb and back pain in Guillain-Barré syndrome and associated contrast enhancement in MRI of the cauda equina. *Acta Paediatr*. 2001;90(6):691-694.
5. Ruts L, van Koningsveld R, van Doorn PA. Distinguishing acute-onset CIDP from Guillain-Barré syndrome with treatment related fluctuations. *Neurology*. 2005;65(1):138-140.
6. McKhann GM, Cornblath DR, Ho T, et al. Clinical and electrophysiological aspects of acute paralytic disease of children and young adults in northern China. *Lancet*. 1991;338(8767):593-597.
7. Griffin JW, Li CY, Ho TW, et al. Guillain-Barré syndrome in northern China: The spectrum of neuropathological changes in clinically defined cases. *Brain*. 1995;118(Pt 3):577-595.
8. Al-Din AN, Anderson M, Bickerstaff ER, Harvey I. Brainstem encephalitis and the syndrome of Miller Fisher: A clinical study. *Brain*. 1982;105(Pt 3):481-495.
9. Bickerstaff ER. Brain-stem encephalitis; Further observations on a grave syndrome with benign prognosis. *Br Med J*. 1957;1(5032):1384-1387.
10. Suarez GA, Fealey RD, Camilleri M, Low PA. Idiopathic autonomic neuropathy: Clinical, neurophysiologic, and follow-up studies on 27 patients. *Neurology*. 1994;44(9):1675-1682.
11. Rekand T, Gramstad A, Vedeler CA. Fatigue, pain and muscle weakness are frequent after Guillain-Barré syndrome and poliomyelitis. *J Neurol*. 2009;256(3):349-354.
12. Ruts L, Rico R, van Koningsveld R, et al. Pain accompanies pure motor Guillain-Barré syndrome. *J Peripher Nerv Syst*. 2008;13(4):305-306.
13. Pentland B, Donald SM. Pain in the Guillain-Barré syndrome: A clinical review. *Pain*. 1994;59(2):159-164.
14. Moulin DE, Hagen N, Feasby TE, Amireh R, Hahn A. Pain in Guillain-Barré syndrome. *Neurology*. 1997;48(2):328-331.
15. Otto M, Bak S, Bach FW, Jensen TS, Sindrup SH. Pain phenomena and possible mechanisms in patients with painful polyneuropathy. *Pain*. 2003;101(1-2):187-192.
16. Lyons R. Elusive belly pain and Guillain-Barré syndrome. *J Pediatr Health Care*. 2008;22(5):310-314.
17. Kaji R, Kimura J. Facts and fallacies on anti-GM1 antibodies: Physiology of motor neuropathies. *Brain*. 1999;122 (Pt 5):797-798.
18. Jacobs BC, van Doorn PA, Schmitz PI, et al. *Campylobacter jejuni* infections and anti-GM1 antibodies in Guillain-Barré syndrome. *Ann Neurol*. 1996;40(2):181-187.
19. Annunziata P, Maimone D, Guazzi GC. Association of polyclonal anti-GM1 IgM and anti-neurofilament antibodies with CSF oligoclonal bands in a young with amyotrophic lateral sclerosis. *Acta Neurol Scand*. 1995;92(5):387-393.
20. Kuntzer T, Antoine JC, Steck AJ. Clinical features and pathophysiological basis of sensory neuronopathies (ganglionopathies). *Muscle Nerve*. 2004;30(3):255-268.
21. Latov N. Diagnosis of CIDP. *Neurology*. 2002;59(12 Suppl 6):S2-S6.
22. Koller H, Schroeter M, Kieseier BC, Hartung HP. Chronic inflammatory demyelinating polyneuropathy—update on pathogenesis, diagnostic criteria and therapy. *Curr Opin Neurol*. 2005;18(3):273-278.
23. Koller H, Kieseier BC, Jander S, Hartung HP. Chronic inflammatory demyelinating polyneuropathy. *N Engl J Med*. 2005;352(13):1343-1356.
24. Illes Z, Shimamura M, Newcombe J, et al. Accumulation of Valpha7.2-Jalpha33 invariant T cells in human autoimmune inflammatory lesions in the nervous system. *Int Immunol*. 2004;16(2):223-230.
25. Kieseier BC, Kiefer R, Gold R, et al. Advances in understanding and treatment of immune-mediated disorders of the peripheral nervous system. *Muscle Nerve*. 2004;30(2):131-156.
26. Bouchard C, Lacroix C, Plante V, et al. Clinicopathologic findings and prognosis of chronic inflammatory demyelinating polyneuropathy. *Neurology*. 1999;52(3):498-503.
27. Vital C, Vital A, Lagueny A, et al. Chronic inflammatory demyelinating polyneuropathy: Immunopathological and ultrastructural study of peripheral nerve biopsy in 42 cases. *Ultrastruct Pathol*. 2000;24(6):363-369.
28. Rajabally Y, Vital A, Ferrer X, et al. Chronic inflammatory demyelinating polyneuropathy caused by HIV infection in a patient with asymptomatic CMT 1A. *J Peripher Nerv Syst*. 2000;5(3):158-162.
29. Di Guglielmo G, Di Muzio A, Torrieri F, et al. Low back pain due to hypertrophic roots as presenting symptom of CIDP. *Ital J Neurol Sci*. 1997;18(5):297-299.
30. Boukhris S, Magy L, Khalil M, et al. Pain as the presenting symptom of chronic inflammatory demyelinating polyradiculoneuropathy (CIDP). *J Neurol Sci*. 2007;254(1-2):33-38.
31. Stewart JD, McKelvey R, Durcan L, et al. Chronic inflammatory demyelinating polyneuropathy (CIDP) in diabetics. *J Neurol Sci*. 1996;142(1-2):59-64.
32. Quasthoff S, Hartung HP. Chemotherapy-induced peripheral neuropathy. *J Neurol*. 2002;249(1):9-17.
33. Nath U, Grant R. Neurological paraneoplastic syndromes. *J Clin Pathol*. 1997;50(12):975-980.
34. De Toni L, Marconi S, Nardelli E, et al. Gangliosides act as onconeural antigens in paraneoplastic neuropathies. *J Neuroimmunol*. 2004;156(1-2):178-187.
35. Sutton I. Paraneoplastic neurological syndromes. *Curr Opin Neurol*. 2002;15(6):685-690.
36. Giometto B, Scaravilli F. Paraneoplastic syndromes. *Brain Pathol*. 1999;9(2):247-250.
37. Antoine JC, Mosnier JF, Absi L, et al. Carcinoma associated paraneoplastic peripheral neuropathies in patients with and without anti-onconeural antibodies. *J Neurol Neurosurg Psychiatry*. 1999;67(1):7-14.
38. Albert ML, Darnell JC, Bender A, et al. Tumor-specific killer cells in paraneoplastic cerebellar degeneration. *Nat Med*. 1998;4(11):1321-1324.

39. Giometto B, Taraloto B, Graus F. Autoimmunity in paraneoplastic neurological syndromes. *Brain Pathol.* 1999;9(2):261-273.

40. Giannopoulou C. Navigating the paraneoplastic neurological syndromes. *Eur J Nucl Med Mol Imaging.* 2003;30(3):333-338.

41. Chin R, Jr, McCain TW, Miller AA, et al. Whole body FDG-PET for the evaluation and staging of small cell lung cancer: A preliminary study. *Lung Cancer.* 2002;37(1):1-6.

42. Gould MK, Maclean CC, Kuschner WG, et al. Accuracy of positron emission tomography for diagnosis of pulmonary nodules and mass lesions: A meta-analysis. *JAMA.* 2001;285(7):914-924.

43. Dispenzieri A, Gertz MA. Treatment of POEMS syndrome. *Curr Treat Options Oncol.* 2004;5(3):249-257.

44. Aho TR, Wallace RC, Pitt AM, Sivakumar K. Charcot-Marie-Tooth disease: Extensive cranial nerve involvement on CT and MR imaging. *AJNR Am J Neuroradiol.* 2004;25(3):494-497.

45. Ouvrier RA, McLeod JG, Conchin TE. The hypertrophic forms of hereditary motor and sensory neuropathy: A study of hypertrophic Charcot-Marie-Tooth disease (HMSN type I) and Dejerine-Sottas disease (HMSN type III) in childhood. *Brain.* 1987;110(Pt 1):121-148.

46. Satran R. Dejerine-Sottas disease revisited. *Arch Neurol.* 1980;37(2):67-68.

47. Rao CV, Fitz CR, Harwood-Nash DC. Dejerine-Sottas syndrome in children. (Hypertrophic interstitial polyneuritis). *Am J Roentgenol Radium Ther Nucl Med.* 1974;122(1):70-74.

48. Cox MJ. Progressive familial hypertrophic polyneuritis (Dejerine-Sottas syndrome, 1893). *Proc R Soc Med.* 1956;49(4):183-184.

49. Pareyson D, Scaioli V, Taroni F, et al. Phenotypic heterogeneity in hereditary neuropathy with liability to pressure palsies associated with chromosome 17p11.2-12 deletion. *Neurology.* 1996;46(4):1133-1137.

50. Upadhyaya M, Roberts SH, Farnham J, et al. Charcot-Marie-tooth disease 1A (CMT1A) associated with a maternal duplication of chromosome 17p11.2—>12. *Hum Genet.* 1993;91(4):392-394.

51. Maki DD, Yousem DM, Corcoran C, Galetta SL. MR imaging of Dejerine-Sottas disease. *AJNR Am J Neuroradiol.* 1999;20(3):378-380.

52. Midroni G, de Tilly LN, Gray B, Vajsar J. MRI of the cauda equina in CIDP: Clinical correlations. *J Neurol Sci.* 1999;170(1):36-44.

53. Iwata F, Utsumi Y. MR imaging in Guillain-Barré syndrome. *Pediatr Radiol.* 1997;27(1):36-38.

54. Georgy BA, Chong B, Chamberlain M, et al. MR of the spine in Guillain-Barré syndrome. *AJNR Am J Neuroradiol.* 1994;15(2):300-301.

55. Kale HA, Sklar E. Magnetic resonance imaging findings in chronic inflammatory demyelinating polyneuropathy with intracranial findings and enhancing, thickened cranial and spinal nerves. *Australas Radiol.* 2007;51(Spec No.):B21-B24.

56. Perry JR, Fung A, Poon P, Bayer N. Magnetic resonance imaging of nerve root inflammation in the Guillain-Barré syndrome. *Neuroradiology.* 1994;36(2):139-140.

57. Hvidsten K, Larsen JL, Nyland H. Myelography in Guillain-Barré syndrome (acute inflammatory polyradiculoneuropathy). *Neuroradiology.* 1978;14(5):235-239.

58. Byun WM, Park WK, Park BH, et al. Guillain-Barré syndrome: MR imaging findings of the spine in eight patients. *Radiology.* 1998;208(1):137-141.

59. Berciano J. MR imaging in Guillain-Barré syndrome. *Radiology.* 1999;211(1):290-291.

60. Fletcher GP, Roberts CC. AJR teaching file: progressive polyradiculopathy. *AJR Am J Roentgenol.* 2006;186(3 Suppl):S230-S232.

61. Duarte J, Martinez AC, Rodriguez F, et al. Hypertrophy of multiple cranial nerves and spinal roots in chronic inflammatory demyelinating neuropathy. *J Neurol Neurosurg Psychiatry.* 1999;67(5):685-687.

62. Chong VH, Joseph TP, Telisinghe PU, Jalihal A. Chronic inflammatory demyelinating polyneuropathy associated with intestinal tuberculosis. *J Microbiol Immunol Infect.* 2007;40(4):377-380.

63. De Weerdt A, Claeys KG, De Jonghe P, et al. Tacrolimus-related polyneuropathy: Case report and review of the literature. *Clin Neurol Neurosurg.* 2008;110(3):291-294.

64. Kaushik P, Cohen AJ, Zuckerman SJ, et al. Miller Fisher variant of Guillain-Barré syndrome requiring a cardiac pacemaker in a patient on tacrolimus after liver transplantation. *Ann Pharmacother.* 2005;39(6):1124-1127.

65. Pytel P, Rezania K, Soliven B, et al. Chronic inflammatory demyelinating polyradiculoneuropathy (CIDP) with hypertrophic spinal radiculopathy mimicking neurofibromatosis. *Acta Neuropathol.* 2003;105(2):185-188.

66. Tatum WO, Bui DD, Grant EG, Murtagh R. Pseudo-Guillain-Barré syndrome due to "whippet"-induced myeloneuropathy. *J Neuroimaging.* May 20, 2009. [E-pub ahead of print.]

67. Hadden RD, Hughes RA. Treatment of immune-mediated inflammatory neuropathies. *Curr Opin Neurol.* 1999;12(5):573-579.

68. Ropper AH. Current treatments for CIDP. *Neurology.* 2003;60(8 Suppl 3):S16-S22.

69. Hughes R, Bensa S, Willison H, et al. Randomized controlled trial of intravenous immunoglobulin versus oral prednisolone in chronic inflammatory demyelinating polyradiculoneuropathy. *Ann Neurol.* 2001;50(2):195-201.

70. Hadden RD, Sharrack B, Bensa S, et al. Randomized trial of interferon beta-1a in chronic inflammatory demyelinating polyradiculoneuropathy. *Neurology.* 1999;53(1):57-61.

71. Toth C, Au S. A prospective identification of neuropathic pain in specific chronic polyneuropathy syndromes and response to pharmacological therapy. *Pain.* 2008;138(3):657-666.

72. Pandey CK, Bose N, Garg G, et al. Gabapentin for the treatment of pain in Guillain-Barré syndrome: A double-blinded, placebo-controlled, crossover study. *Anesth Analg.* 2002;95(6):1719-1723, table of contents.

INTERSPINOUS BURSITIS (BAASTRUP'S DISEASE)

Leo F. Czervionke, M.D.

CLINICAL PRESENTATION

The patient is a 75-year-old male who presented with severe mid low back pain. He has difficulty walking distances but reports no lower extremity pain. Physical examination reveals some vague tenderness to deep palpation of the back. No lower extremity weakness. Normal sensory examination. Normal deep tendon reflexes.

IMAGING PRESENTATION

Multilevel spondylosis deformans, intervertebral disc degeneration, and generalized disc bulging are seen with imaging. Severe circumferential thecal sac narrowing is present at the L3-4 level as a result of disc bulging, thickened ligamentum flava, and bilateral facet hypertrophy. Abnormal T2 signal hyperintensity and contrast enhancement is demonstrated in the L3-4 interspinous ligaments and adjacent spinous processes, and contrast enhancement of the L3-4 facet capsules is shown bilaterally. Findings are consistent with severe central stenosis at the L3-4 level, active inflammatory facet arthropathy, and interspinous ligamentous inflammation (i.e., interspinous bursitis, also known as *Baastrup's disease*) (*Figs. 39-1 to 39-7*).

DISCUSSION

The space between adjacent lumbar spinous processes contains an interspinous ligament or ligaments and bilateral paraligamentous bursae. Small, short bilateral paired muscles, the interspinous lumborum muscles, are located on both sides of the interspinous ligament at a given lumbar level. These tissues can become inflamed and be a source of back pain. Interspinous ligamentous inflammation or bursitis (often referred to as *Baastrup's disease* or *Baastrup's sign*) most commonly occurs at the L4-5 level but can occur at any lumbar level.[1,2]

Normally, the spinous processes are covered by noncartilaginous connective tissue. As this disorder evolves, chronic active or episodic inflammation occurs in the interspinous ligaments, and over time the abutting surfaces of the involved spinous processes contact and eventually become flattened and sclerotic, with small cystic erosions or geodes occurring where the spinous processes contact (*Figs. 39-8 to 39-10*). This process may lead to interspinous adventitial bursal formation and eventually formation of a synovial-lined articulation between the spinous processes.[2,3] When interspinous bursal formation occurs, both calcium pyrophosphate dihydrate (CPPD) and hydroxyapatite crystal deposition may be present in the bursa.[2] When interspinous ligamentous inflammation occurs, the adjacent posterior paraspinal musculature and nearby facet capsules may also be inflamed (*Figs. 39-11 to 39-13*). Patients with interspinous ligamentous inflammation are usually symptomatic, reporting moderate to intense low back pain near the midline.

The etiology of this type of Baastrup's disease is not precisely known. Traditionally, the cause of this disorder has been attributed to translational movement or abutting of the posterior spinous processes during spine hyperextension or excessive lumbar lordosis. However, it is also possible that this represents a primary degenerative process of the interspinous ligaments.[1]

We have observed that interspinous inflammation or bursitis commonly occurs frequently in the setting of active inflammatory facet arthropathy (facet synovitis), and we suggest an alternate hypothesis: that Baastrup's disease may occur secondary to chronic active inflammatory facet arthropathy. Alternatively, it is possible that some cases of facet synovitis occur secondary to active interspinous bursitis. Supporting this hypothesis is the fact that the interspinous bursae may communicate with the nearby ipsilateral facet joint via a potential space along the dorsal surface of the ipsilateral lamina. This communication can be demonstrated in some patients by injecting contrast agent into the ipsilateral facet joint or into the interspinous ligaments at a given level (*Figs. 39-14 to 39-16*). In these cases, the contrast agent not only opacifies the facet joint but also is seen extending along the ipsilateral dorsal surface of the lamina and into the tissues adjacent to the interspinous ligament, which is believed to represent an interspinous bursa. A communication between the interspinous bursa and the facet joint has been demonstrated in some patients by injecting the interspinous bursa.[4] Occasionally, these bursae may also communicate with posterior epidural intraspinal cysts.[4]

Any spine structure or articulation innervated by afferent nociceptive nerve fibers is a potential pain generator.[5,6] The majority of back pain sensation is detected by nociceptors in the zygapophyseal (facet) joints, along the margins of the intervertebral discs or sacroiliac joints, or in paraspinal myofascial tissues. Nociceptors may also occur adjacent to developing vertebral osteophytes and adjacent to the paraspinous ligaments.[5,7]

The prevalence of symptomatic interspinous inflammation is unknown but is probably considerably greater than once believed, because active interspinous ligamentous inflammation cannot

Text continued on page 307

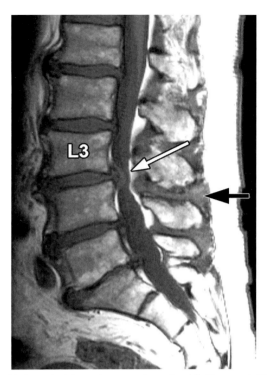

Figure 39-1 ▶ Spinal Stenosis, Interspinous Bursitis (Baastrup's Disease). Sagittal T1-weighted MRI reveals severe central canal stenosis at L3-4 level (*white arrow*) due to disc bulging and ligamentum flavum thickening. The L3-4 interspinous ligament is thickened (*black arrow*).

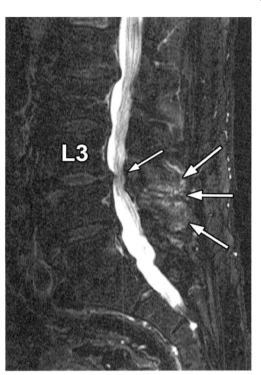

Figure 39-2 ▶ Spinal Stenosis, Interspinous Bursitis. Corresponding sagittal fat-saturated sagittal MRI in same patient as in Figure 39-1. T2 hyperintensity in L3-4 interspinous tissues and adjacent L3 and L4 spinous processes (*large white arrows*). Central canal stenosis indicated by *small white arrow.*

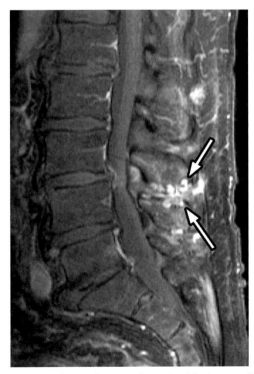

Figure 39-3 ▶ Spinal Stenosis, Interspinous Bursitis. Corresponding sagittal contrast-enhanced T1-weighted fat-saturated sagittal image in same patient as in Figures 39-1 and 39-2. There is narrowing of the interspinous space and enhancing tissue in the interspinous space associated with small erosions of the adjacent spinous processes (*arrows*).

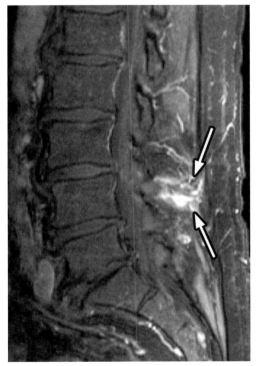

Figure 39-4 ▶ Spinal Stenosis, Interspinous Bursitis. Same patient as in Figures 39-1 to 39-3. Contrast-enhanced parasagittal T1-weighted fat-saturated sagittal MR image reveals enhancing tissue (*arrows*) in the interspinous and paraspinous regions consistent with inflammation of the interspinous ligaments and interspinous bursae.

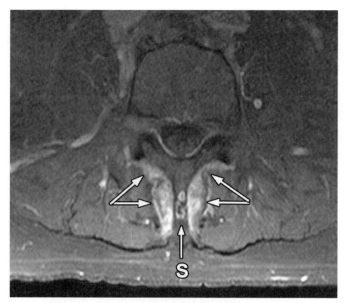

Figure 39-5 ▶ Spinal Stenosis, Interspinous Bursitis. Corresponding axial T1-weighted fat-saturated sagittal MRI in same patient as in Figures 39-1 to 39-4, at level of L3 spinous process. Enhancing tissue (*arrows*) is present on either side of the spinous process (*S*) is consistent with enhancement of paraspinous ligaments and/ or margins of interspinous bursae. There are 2 ovoid erosions within the spinous process (*S*) containing enhancing tissue.

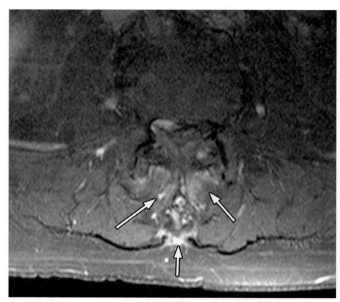

Figure 39-6 ▶ Spinal Stenosis, Interspinous Bursitis. Corresponding axial T1-weighted fat-saturated sagittal MR image in same patient as in Figures 39-1 to 39-5, at L3-4 intervertebral disc level. Heterogeneous enhancement of the interspinous ligaments and paraspinous tissues is demonstrated (*arrows*).

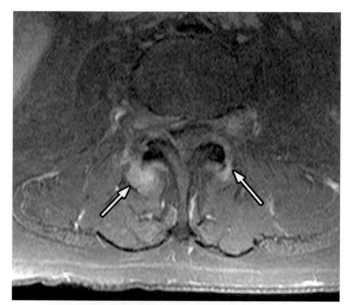

Figure 39-7 ▶ Spinal Stenosis, Interspinous Bursitis. Corresponding axial T1-weighted fat-saturated sagittal image in same patient as in Figures 39-1 to 39-6, at level of L4 spinous process. Enhancement of parafacetal soft tissues (*arrows*) is consistent with active inflammatory facet arthropathy (facet synovitis).

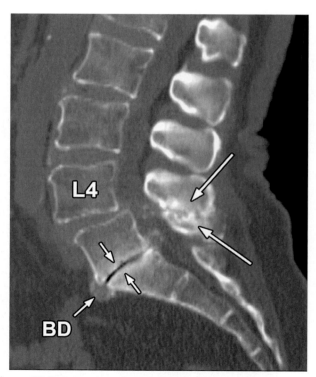

Figure 39-8 ▶ Interspinous Bursitis. 67-year-old female with chronic low back pain, intervertebral disc degeneration, and Baastrup's disease. Sagittal CT image showing large L5-S1 bulging disc (*BD*) and intervertebral disc narrowing associated with vacuum disc phenomenon (*small arrows*). The L5-S1 interspinous space markedly narrowed and there are bone erosions and sclerosis where the spinous processes contact each other (*arrows*).

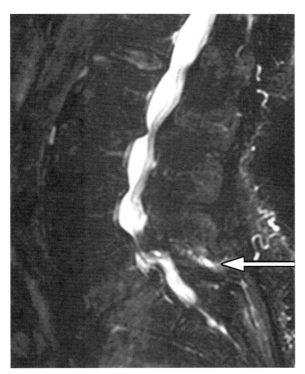

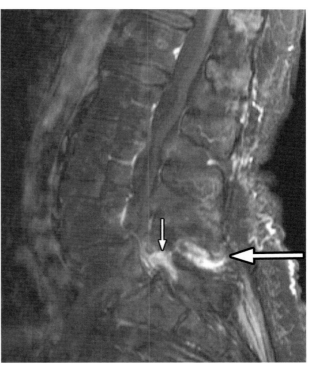

Figure 39-9 ▶ Interspinous Bursitis. Corresponding sagittal T2-weighted MRI in same patient as in Figure 39-8. T2 hyperintense tissue is demonstrated in the L4-5 interspinous tissues (*arrow*). Note multilevel central canal stenosis.

Figure 39-10 ▶ Interspinous Bursitis. Corresponding sagittal contrast-enhanced T1-weighted MRI in same patient as in Figures 39-8 and 39-9. The inflamed interspinous tissues (*long arrow*) and ligamentum flavum (*small arrow*) enhance intensely at the L4-5 level.

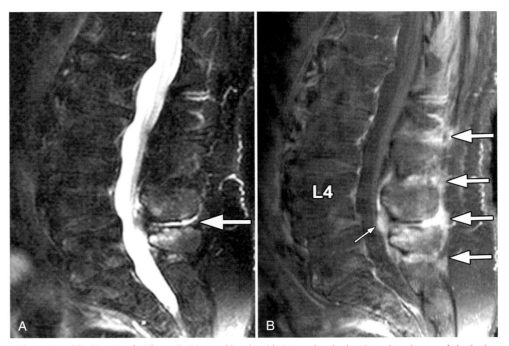

Figure 39-11 ▶ Interspinous Bursitis (Baastrup's Disease). 64-year-old male with intense low back pain and tenderness of the back to palpation. On sagittal T2-weighted MR image **A**, the interspinous tissues at L4-5 (*arrow*) are T2 hyperintense and subtle T2 hyperintensity is present in the adjacent L4 and L5 spinous processes. On sagittal contrast-enhanced fat-saturated T1-weighted MR image **B**, the L2-3 through L5-S1 interspinous ligaments enhance (*large arrows*) and the ligamentum flavum (*small arrow*) also enhances indicating a multilevel ligamentous inflammatory process.

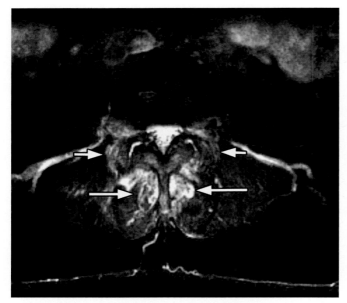

Figure 39-12 ▶ **Interspinous Bursitis (Baastrup's Disease).** Same patient as in Figure 39-11. Axial fat-saturated T2-weighted MRI obtained at L4-5 level. The paraspinous tissues (*long arrows*) and the parafacetal tissues (*short arrows*) are diffusely hyperintense, consistent with active edema or inflammation involving the interspinous ligament, interspinous bursae, and the facets bilaterally.

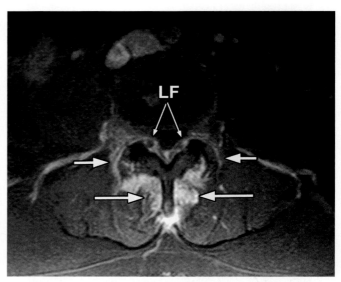

Figure 39-13 ▶ **Interspinous Bursitis.** Corresponding axial contrast-enhanced fat-saturated T1-weighted MR image to Figure 39-12. There is diffuse enhancement of the paraspinous ligaments (*long arrows*), parafacetal soft tissues (*short arrows*), and ligamentum flavum (LF) consistent with active inflammatory interspinous bursitis (Baastrup's disease) and inflammatory facet arthropathy (facet synovitis).

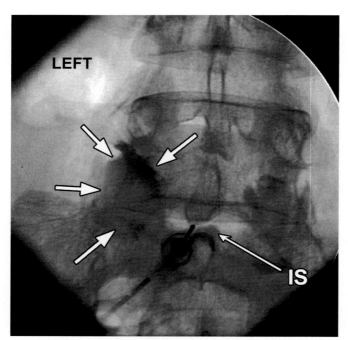

Figure 39-14 ▶ **Interspinous Bursa Injection.** PA radiograph obtained with patient prone. Injection of contrast agent into the L4-5 interspinous (*IS*) bursa results in opacification of the left L4-5 facet joint (*arrows*) indicating communication between the interspinous bursa and facet joint. The L5 vertebra is a partially sacralized transitional vertebral segment.

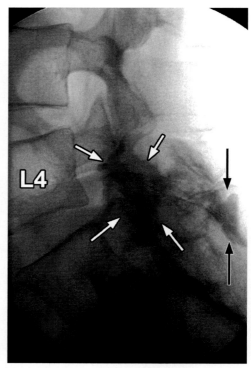

Figure 39-15 ▶ **Interspinous Bursa Injection.** Lateral radiograph obtained post injection of contrast agent into L4-5 interspinous bursa (*black arrows*) in same patient as in Figure 39-14. The contrast agent fills not only the interspinous bursa (*black arrows*) but also the left L4-5 facet joint (*white arrows*).

be diagnosed on radiographs or computed tomography (CT), and is not visible with magnetic resonance (MR) imaging unless fat-saturated images or short tau inversion recovery (STIR) images are obtained.

Not all patients with the radiographic appearance of Baastrup's disease are symptomatic. However, this condition can be acutely painful and should always be considered in patients with low back pain. Clinical manifestations include midline back pain, limited back motion, and paraspinal muscular spasm. Localized tenderness is often elicited upon palpation of the spinous processes or interspinous spaces, and the back pain is usually accentuated by hyperextension.[2]

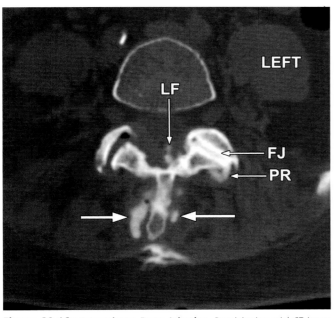

Figure 39-16 ▶ Interspinous Bursa Injection. Post injection axial CT image obtained at L4-5 level in patient described in Figures 39-14 and 39-15. The contrast agent is in the interspinous/paraspinous bursae (*long arrows*), in a small fluid collection in the left ligamentum flavum (*LF*), in the left facet joint (*FJ*), and in the posterior recess (*PR*) of left facet joint.

IMAGING FEATURES

On radiographs or CT, the involved spinous processes are typically in close proximity ("kissing spinous processes"), and the spinous processes are usually flattened and sclerotic (see Fig. 39-8). Small bone erosions or geodes are often seen where the spinous processes contact, which may be visible on CT or MR imaging (see Figs. 39-3, 39-5, and 39-8). Erosions and sclerosis of contacting spinous processes are usually seen in the late, advanced stages of Baastrup's disease, when the patient may or may not be symptomatic.

Special attention should be given to examining the interspinous ligaments on all patients with back pain. Interspinous ligamentous inflammation is the hallmark of active or ongoing, progressive Baastrup's disease. MR imaging evidence of interspinous ligamentous inflammation is usually present in symptomatic patients with Baastrup's disease. As in all spinal inflammatory conditions, interspinous ligamentous inflammation is best demonstrated with contrast-enhanced, fat-saturated, T1-weighted MR imaging, although it can be detected on T2-weighted, fat-saturated images or by using STIR imaging sequences (see Figs. 39-1 to 39-13). In some patients, the interspinous ligamentous inflammation is not visible on fat-saturated, T2-weighted or STIR images and is only visible on contrast-enhanced MR images (*Figs. 39-17 and 39-18*).

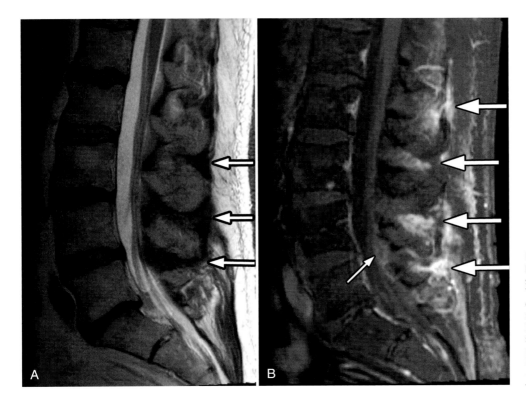

Figure 39-17 ▶ Multilevel Interspinous Bursitis. Patient with severe low back pain secondary to Baastrup's disease. Sagittal T2-weighted MR image **A** reveals thickening of the L2-3, L3-4, and L4-5 interspinous ligaments (*arrows*) but no hyperintensity of the ligaments. Sagittal contrast-enhanced fat-saturated T1-weighted MR image **B** reveals multilevel enhancement of the interspinous ligaments and ligamentum flavum (*small arrow*).

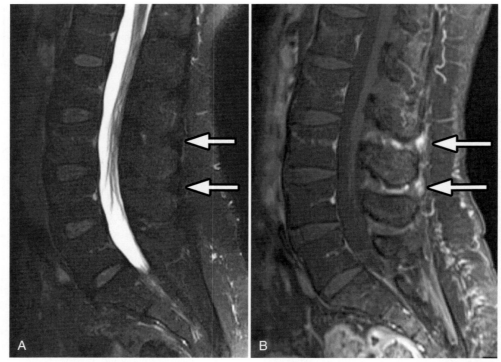

Figure 39-18 ► **Interspinous Bursitis (Baastrup's Disease) in Patient with Severe Low Back Pain.** The interspinous ligaments (*arrows*) at L2-3 and L3-4 levels have normal intensity sagittal T2-weighted MR image **A**, but enhance following IV contrast on sagittal contrast-enhanced fat-saturated T1-weighted MR image **B**.

Therefore, interspinous ligamentous inflammation may go undetected if contrast-enhanced, fat-saturated MR images are not obtained. The abnormal signal is most commonly seen at the L4-5 level followed by the L3-4 level. Often symptomatic patients have multilevel lumbar interspinous ligamentous involvement (see Fig. 39-17).

There may be associated inflammation visible in the adjacent paraspinal muscles or nearby facet capsules, especially when interspinous bursal formation has occurred (see Figs. 39-7, 39-12, and 39-13). T1 hypointense and T2 hyperintense cystic outpouchings may be seen along the margins of the interspinous ligaments secondary to active or chronic interspinous ligamentous inflammation *(Fig. 39-19)*. Inflamed bursae or bursal cysts may enhance along their margins *(Figs. 39-19 and 39-20)*. As mentioned above, these bursae may communicate with the adjacent facet joints or occasionally with posterior midline or paramidline epidural cystic fluid collections (see Figs. 39-14 to 39-16), which, if present, could cause compression of the thecal sac and contribute to spinal stenosis.[4,8]

F-18 fluorodeoxyglucose (FDG) uptake may also be observed in inflamed interspinous ligaments using positron emission tomography/computed tomography (PET-CT imaging) in patients with Baastrup's disease.[9,10]

Rarely, a fracture or stress fracture may develop in one of the involved spinous processes in patients with Baastrup's disease. Fractures are usually symptomatic and visible on technetium-99m methylene diphosphonate (Tc-99m MDP) radionuclide bone scan images, because of the reparative bone response to the fracture.[3]

DIFFERENTIAL DIAGNOSIS

1. **Proliferative hyperostosis of the spinous processes**: May be seen in diffuse idiopathic skeletal hyperostosis (DISH), fluorosis, acromegaly, and hypervitaminosis states.[2]
2. **Ankylosing spondylitis:** May cause erosions and resorption of the spinous processes. In longstanding ankylosing spondylitis, the interspinous ligaments may calcify and eventually ossify, resulting in fusion of the spinous processes.[2]
3. **Chronic juvenile arthritis:** May be associated with increased osteoclastic activity manifested as erosion of the spinous processes and development of interspinous bursae.[2]
4. **Cysts:** Posterior epidural cysts that communicate with interspinous bursa may be confused with intraspinal juxtafacet (ganglion) cysts or synovial cysts.[4] These communications can be confirmed by bursography.

TREATMENT

1. **Nonsteroidal anti-inflammatory drugs (NSAIDs):** Typically prescribed for this condition and may or may not be beneficial.
2. **Steroid dose pack:** Short-term administration of steroids may be effective therapy in many patients with Baastrup's disease, provided there is no contraindication to the use of steroids.
3. **Anesthetic-steroid mixture:** Direct injection of anesthetic-steroid mixture into the inflamed interspinous bursa and/or interspinous ligaments.[5] In patients with associated active

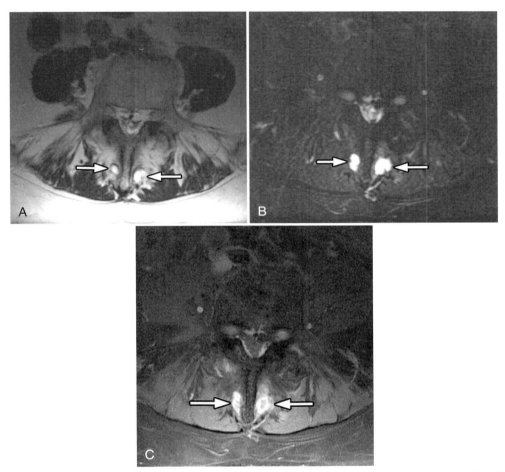

Figure 39-19 ▶ Baastrup's Disease, Interspinal Bursal Cyst Formation. L3-4 paraspinous bursal cysts (*arrows*) shown on axial T2-weighted MR image **A**, fat-saturated T2-weighted image **B**, and contrast-enhanced fat-saturated image **C**. The cysts are T2 hyperintense on images **A** and **B** and marginal enhancement of the bursal cysts is shown in image **C**.

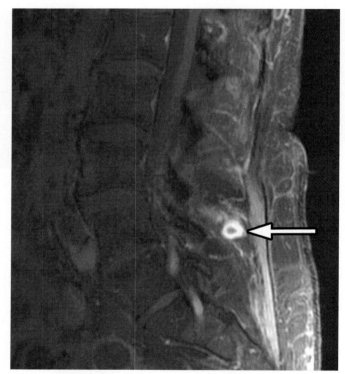

Figure 39-20 ▶ **Baastrup's Disease, Interspinal Bursal Cyst Formation.** Same patient as in Figure 39-19. Left parasagittal contrast-enhanced fat-saturated T1-weighted MR image. The inflamed left paraspinous bursal cyst has intense peripheral rim enhancement (*arrow*).

inflammatory facet arthropathy (facet synovitis), the facet joints should be injected initially, because the interspinous bursae may fill during facet injection and thus can be treated along with the inflamed facet joint. If the facet joint does not communicate with the nearby interspinous bursa, as verified by iodinated contrast injection, then a separate injection is made into the affected interspinous bursa or ligament.

4. **Surgery:** Surgery is not a first-line treatment of Baastrup's disease. However, if the patient fails to respond to the above more conservative therapies, surgical excision of the affected spinous processes is an option.[5] If there is associated vertebral instability at the involved level or levels, a surgical fusion procedure should be considered.

References

1. Maes R, Morrison WB, Parker L, et al. Lumbar interspinous bursitis (Baastrup disease) in a symptomatic population: Prevalence on magnetic resonance imaging. *Spine (Phila Pa 1976)*. 2008;33(7):E211-E215.

2. Sartoris DJ, Resnick D, Tyson R, Haghighi P. Age-related alterations in the vertebral spinous processes and intervening soft tissues: Radiologic-pathologic correlation. *AJR Am J Roentgenol*. 1985;145(5):1025-1030.

3. Pinto PS, Boutin RD, Resnick D. Spinous process fractures associated with Baastrup disease. *Clin Imaging*. 2004;28(3):219-222.

4. Chen CK, Yeh L, Resnick D, et al. Intraspinal posterior epidural cysts associated with Baastrup's disease: Report of 10 patients. *AJR Am J Roentgenol*. 2004;182(1):191-194.

5. Lamer TJ, Tiede JM, Fenton DS. Fluoroscopically-guided injections to treat "kissing spine" disease. *Pain Physician*. 2008;11(4):549-554.

6. Jonsson B, Stromqvist B, Egund N. Anomalous lumbosacral articulations and low-back pain: Evaluation and treatment. *Spine (Phila Pa 1976)*. 1989;14(8):831-834.

7. Lamer TJ. Lumbar spine pain originating from vertebral osteophytes. *Reg Anesth Pain Med*. 1999;24(4):347-351.

8. Hui C, Cox I. Two unusual presentations of Baastrup's disease. *Clin Radiol*. 2007;62(5):495-497.

9. Abul-Kasim K, Thurnher MM, McKeever P, Sundgren PC. Intradural spinal tumors: Current classification and MRI features. *Neuroradiology*. 2008;50(4):301-314.

10. Gorospe L, Jover R, Vicente-Bartulos A, et al. FDG-PET/CT demonstration of Baastrup disease ("Kissing" Spine). *Clin Nucl Med*. 2008;33(2):133-134.

CHAPTER 40

INTRATHECAL RADICULITIS

Leo F. Czervionke, M.D.

CLINICAL PRESENTATION

The patient is a 30-year-old female with severe low back pain and right lower extremity pain in the right S1 distribution. On physical examination, she has diffuse lower extremity weakness, right heel drop when she walks on her toes, and decreased right ankle jerk.

IMAGING PRESENTATION

Magnetic resonance (MR) imaging reveals a very large disc extrusion compressing the thecal sac on the right at the L5-S1 level. There is intense contrast enhancement surrounding the disc fragment and diffuse enhancement of the intrathecal right S1 nerve root above the level of the disc herniation, indicating S1 radiculitis (*Figs. 40-1 to 40-3*).

DISCUSSION

Intrathecal radiculitis is an important pain-producing condition that is frequently not recognized, which is supported by the fact that there exists a paucity of publications in the literature on this subject. Takata and colleagues[1] in 1988 described visible intrathecal nerve root swelling on post-myelogram computed tomography (CT) images in 60% of the patients in their series who had symptomatic lumbar disc herniations. The enlarged intrathecal nerve root is often caused by a disc herniation, central canal stenosis, or postoperative granulation tissue (*Figs. 40-1 to 40-11*). The affected nerve corresponds to the patient's radicular pain distribution.[1] Intrathecal nerve roots of the cauda equina may enhance on MR imaging after IV contrast enhancement if the blood nerve barrier that normally exists is disrupted. The blood-nerve barrier can break down as a result of mechanical factors, trauma, an autoimmune response, or ischemia.[2] Mechanical compression of the nerve root can result in neural edema and eventually ischemic compromise of the nerve root if the condition is prolonged.[3] Although the precise cause of the blood-nerve breakdown is not known, the nerve root enhancement likely reflects a low-grade inflammatory process involving one or more cauda equina nerve roots; hence, we refer to this condition as *intrathecal radiculitis.* Intrathecal radiculitis may occur preoperatively or postoperatively and may occur with or without nerve root enlargement (see Figs. 40-1 to 40-9).[2]

Contrast enhancement of intrathecal nerve roots occurs in 5% of patients undergoing spinal MR imaging in the unoperated spine.[4] Contrast enhancement occurs because of disruption in the normal blood-nerve barrier in these patients. This could be secondary to mechanical factors, trauma, or ischemic breakdown. Uncommonly, nerve roots of the cauda equina may become inflamed without associated demonstrable nerve root impingement and without any predisposing conditions for arachnoiditis.[2,4] In the unoperated spine, this most commonly occurs as a result of nerve root impingement secondary to a large disc herniation.[3] However, in some cases a small herniated disc or large bulging disc is responsible for the mechanical compression (see Figs. 40-1 to 40-4 and 40-10). Central canal stenosis or lateral recess stenosis can also be associated with intrathecal nerve root entrapment (see Figs. 40-4 to 40-6).[2,5] An entrapped root in the lateral recess may exhibit contrast enhancement.[2,3]

In the postoperative spine, one could consider this a form of localized arachnoiditis, usually affecting a solitary root, but sometimes a few nerve roots are involved. This likely represents postoperative inflammation of the root and is most commonly associated with the presence of postoperative granulation tissue often encasing the involved root.[2] However, postoperative radiculitis can occur secondary to residual or recurrent herniated disc, nonspecific postoperative inflammation, or infection, as a result of nerve root edema or ischemia.[2] Painful postoperative radiculitis may represent one of many causes of so called *failed back syndrome.*[6]

Isolated preoperative or postoperative radiculitis is usually a painful, yet self-limited condition that likely does not often progress to adhesive arachnoiditis.[3] Not all patients exhibiting nerve root enhancement on MR imaging will be symptomatic, but in our experience, these patients are the exception. Classically, the patient with MR imaging manifestations of intrathecal radiculitis describes radicular pain in the distribution of the enhancing nerve root if a solitary nerve root is involved. If multiple nerve roots are involved, the patient usually has polyradicular symptoms. In some cases, the radiculopathy does not precisely correlate with the number or level of the enhancing root or roots.[2] Some patients with a solitary enhancing root present with radicular pain in the distribution of more than one nerve root.[2] In rare cases, the enhancing (and symptomatic) nerve root will be located on the opposite side of a large herniated disc, for an unknown reason.[2]

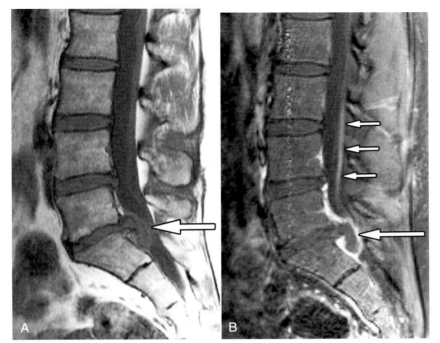

Figure 40-1 ▶ Disc Extrusion, Nerve Root Inflammation. Large L5-S1 herniated disc extrusion (*long arrow*) shown on unenhanced T1-weighted MR image **A** and contrast-enhanced T1-weighted MR image **B**. There are diffuse enlargement and enhancement of right S1 intrathecal nerve root (*short arrows in image* **B**). Note intense enhancement along the margin of the T1 hypointense disc fragment on image **B** representing inflammation.

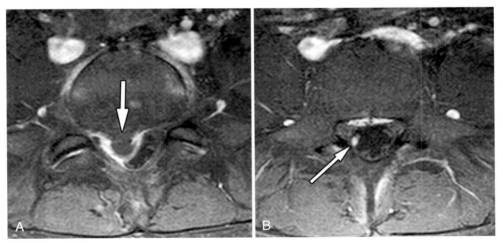

Figure 40-2 ▶ Disc Extrusion, Nerve Root Inflammation. Axial contiguous contrast-enhanced T1-weighted images at L5-S1 level. Same patient as in Figure 40-1. In axial image **A**, the herniated disc (*arrow*) is isointense relative to the intervertebral disc. Intense contrast-enhancement is demonstrated at margin of disc fragment. On axial image **B**, obtained just superior to the L5-S1 disc herniation at mid-L5 vertebral level, the intrathecal portion of the right S1 nerve root (*arrow*) is enlarged and enhances intensely compared with other nonenhancing intrathecal nerve roots.

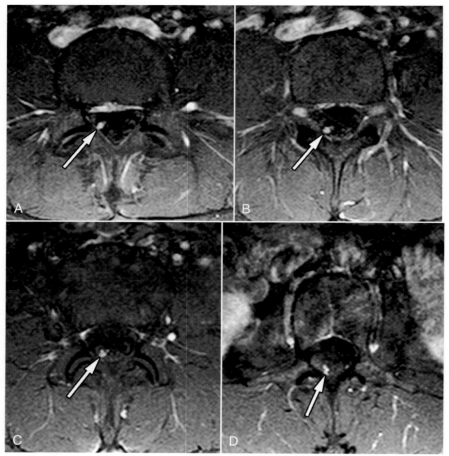

Figure 40-3 ▶ Disc Extrusion, Nerve Root Inflammation. Axial images in mid- and upper lumbar regions in same patient as in Figures 40-1 and 40-2. The right intrathecal S1 nerve root (*arrow in images* **A** *through* **D**) is enlarged and enhances intensely at all visible lumbar levels above the disc herniation.

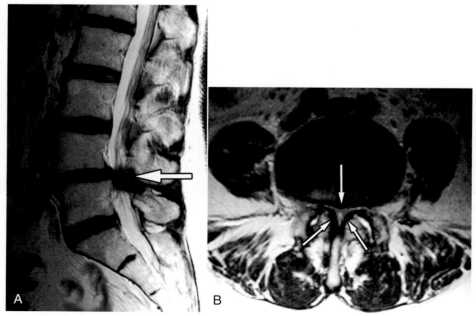

Figure 40-4 ▶ Central Canal Stenosis and Left S1 Radiculitis. Patient with severe L4-5 central canal stenosis and left S1 radiculitis with difficulty walking and left lower extremity pain. Severe central canal stenosis (*arrow*) is demonstrated at the L4-5 level shown on sagittal T2-weighted MR image **A**. On axial T2-weighted image **B**, the severe central canal stenosis (*arrows*) is shown to be secondary to disc bulging, ligamentum flavum thickening, and facet hypertrophy.

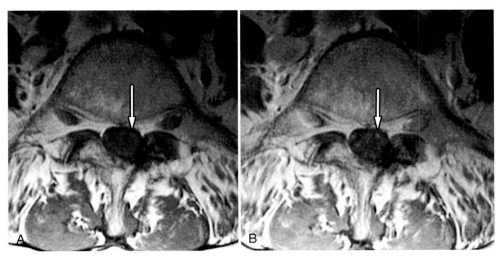

Figure 40-5 ▶ Central Canal Stenosis and Left S1 Radiculitis. Same patient as in Figure 40-4. Unenhanced T1-weighted MR image **A** and contrast-enhanced image **B** obtained at L4 level. The intrathecal left S1 nerve root (*arrow in* **A** *and* **B**) is not enlarged but enhances following IV contrast at the L4 level, relative to other intrathecal roots.

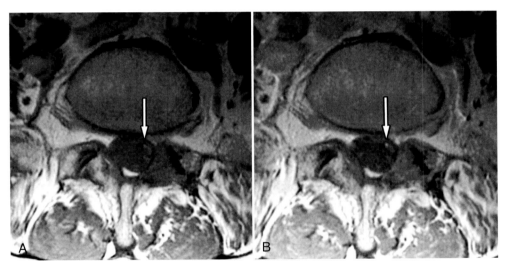

Figure 40-6 ▶ Central Canal Stenosis and Left S1 Radiculitis. Same patient as in Figures 40-4 and 40-5. Unenhanced T1-weighted MR image **A** and contrast-enhanced image **B** obtained at L3 level. The intrathecal left S1 nerve root (*arrow in* **A** *and* **B**) is not enlarged but enhances following IV contrast at the L3 level, relative to other intrathecal roots. The nerve root enhanced at every lumbar level above the L4-5 stenosis to the level of the conus medullaris (*not shown*).

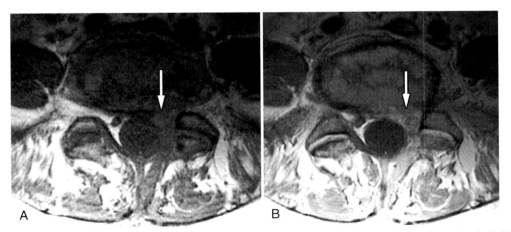

Figure 40-7 ▶ Postoperative Radiculitis. Postoperative left L5 and S1 radiculopathy secondary to L5 and S1 nerve root inflammation (radiculitis). Unenhanced axial T1-weighted MR image **A** and contrast-enhanced axial image **B**. Relatively T1 hypointense scar/granulation tissue (*arrow in image* **A**) located anterolateral to thecal sac at the L5-S1 level. The postoperative scar/granulation tissue (*arrow in image* **B**) enhances following IV contrast.

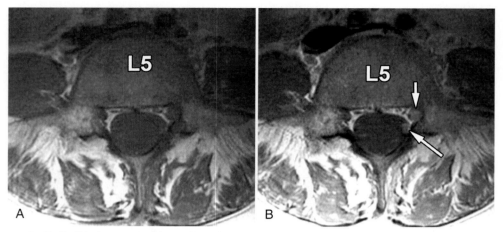

Figure 40-8 ▶ Postoperative Radiculitis. Postoperative left S1 and L5 radiculitis. Same patient as in Figure 40-7. L5 vertebral level. Intrathecal portions of the nerve roots are not well seen on axial unenhanced T1-weighted MR image **A**. On corresponding axial contrast-enhanced T1-weighted MR image **B**, the left S1 root (*long arrow*) is enlarged and enhances. Extrathecal portion of the L5 nerve root (*short arrow*), located in the left L5 lateral recess, is also enlarged and enhances to a greater degree compared to corresponding normal L5 nerve root on the right.

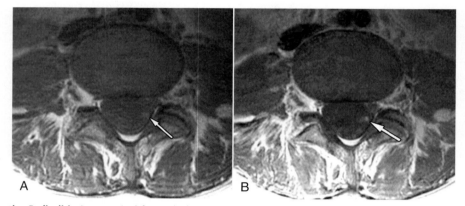

Figure 40-9 ▶ Postoperative Radiculitis. Postoperative left S1 radiculitis. Same patient as in Figures 40-7 and 40-8. L3-4 intervertebral disc level. The left intrathecal S1 nerve root is visible and enlarged (*arrow*) on unenhanced T1-weighted MR image **A**. On corresponding axial contrast-enhanced MR image **B**, the left S1 nerve root (*arrow*) enhances.

IMAGING FEATURES

Inflammation of an intrathecal nerve root is most easily recognized on contrast-enhanced MR imaging (see Figs. 40-1 to 40-3 and 40-5; *Fig. 40-12*). Radiculitis may go undiagnosed if preoperative and post contrast-enhanced axial images are not obtained and carefully scrutinized side by side by the study interpreter. Occasionally, radiculitis can be diagnosed on unenhanced MR imaging if an enlarged nerve root is visible within the thecal sac on contiguous images (see Fig. 40-10). The affected nerve root or roots enhance uniformly and may or may not be enlarged. Isolated preoperative or postoperative radiculitis is usually a painful but often a self-limited condition that probably does not result in adhesive arachnoiditis.[3,4,7] The S1 intrathecal nerve root is most commonly involved followed by L5. Rarely, radiculitis involves an upper lumbar nerve root *(Fig. 40-13)*.

In most cases, a single intrathecal nerve root is involved, and the enhancement extends above the level of the nerve root impingement cephalad to the level of the conus medullaris (see Figs. 40-1

to 40-3, 40-11, and 40-12). Manifestations of adhesive arachnoiditis usually are absent. Characteristically, nerve root clumping and thecal sac adhesions do not occur after resolution of isolated or localized intrathecal radiculitis.

DIFFERENTIAL DIAGNOSIS

1. **Intradural vessel simulating radiculitis** (*Figs. 40-14 to 40-16*): Such vessels are occasionally seen within the thecal sac on sagittal and axial contrast-enhanced MR images, and should be considered a normal variant. These intrathecal vessels are usually somewhat tortuous within the thecal sac and can be traced from the anterior surface of the spinal cord, where they appear to join the anterior spinal artery, and the vessel courses inferiorly along with an intrathecal nerve root, usually entering the S1 or occasionally the L5 nerve root sheath (see Fig. 40-15). These vessels characteristically are not

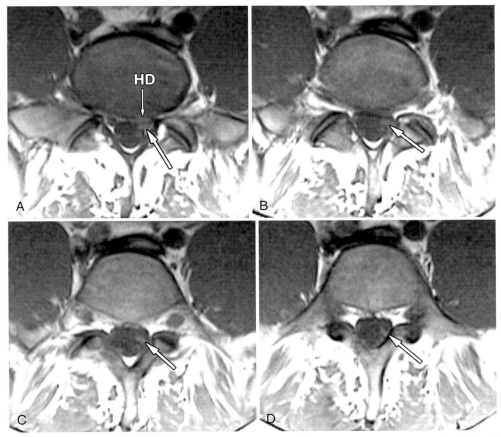

Figure 40-10 ► **Left S1 Radiculitis.** Left L5-S1 herniated disc produces left S1 radiculitis, visible on axial contiguous unenhanced axial T1-weighted images **A** through **D**. Small left paramidline herniated disc (*HD*) is slightly T1 hyperintense relative to intrathecal CSF on image **A**. The enlarged intrathecal S1 nerve root (*arrow in images* **A** *through* **D**) is slightly T1 hyperintense at and above the level of the herniated disc. No IV contrast agent given.

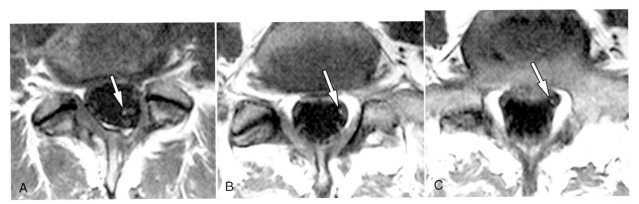

Figure 40-11 ► **Left S1 Radiculitis.** Patient with mild left leg pain and moderate weakness in left S1 distribution secondary to left S1 radiculitis. No associated herniated disc or spinal stenosis. Axial contrast-enhanced T1-weighted MR images **A** through **C** of the lower lumbar spine. Image **A**, obtained at the L4-5 level, reveals enhancement of the intrathecal left motor rootlet of S1 (*arrow*), which is located medial to nonenhancing left sensory rootlet of S1. On image **B**, located at the L5-S1 intervertebral disc level, the left L1 motor root (*arrow*) enhances relative to the more lateral nonenhancing left S1 sensory root. On image **C**, obtained at S1 level just below L5-S1 intervertebral disc level, the enhancing left S1 motor root (*arrow*) enters the axillary root pouch with the non-enhancing, normal sensory rootlet.

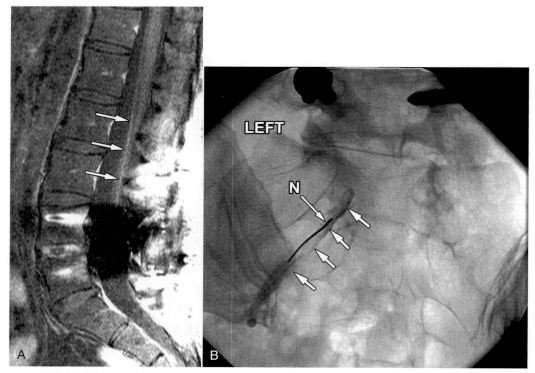

Figure 40-12 ▶ **Persistent Left S1 Radiculitis Following Surgery.** The patient described in Figure 40-11 underwent posterior pedicle screw fixation procedure at L4-5 with absolutely no relief of left leg pain or weakness. After a few weeks, a repeat MR study was obtained. On postoperative sagittal contrast-enhanced fat-saturated T1-weighted MR image **A**, the intrathecal portion of the left S1 nerve root (*arrows*), above the ferromagnetic artifact, is seen to enhance diffusely. A selective left S1 nerve root injection was subsequently performed (PA radiographic image **B**), resulting in complete and immediate relief of left leg pain, and delayed resolution of the leg weakness within a few days post injection.

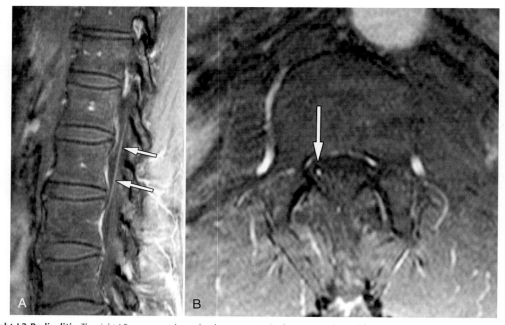

Figure 40-13 ▶ **Right L2 Radiculitis.** The right L2 nerve root (*arrow*) enhances on sagittal contrast-enhanced fat-saturated T1-weighted MR image **A** and axial image **B**.

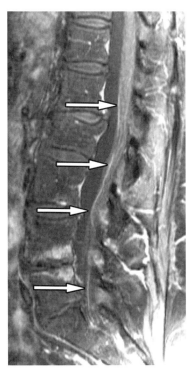

Figure 40-14 ▶ Intradural Vessel Simulating Radiculitis. The enhancing vessel (*arrows*) arises along the anterior spinal cord surface, likely communicating with the anterior spinal artery, and extends inferiorly to the S1 level.

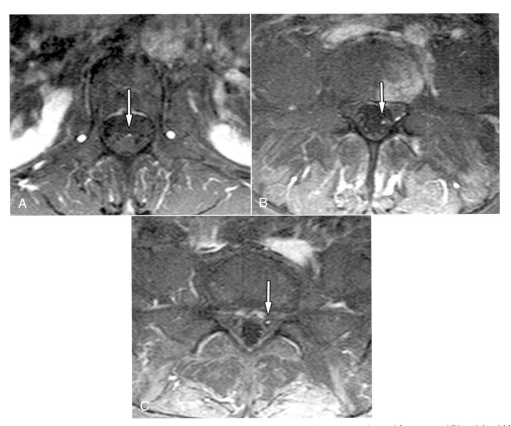

Figure 40-15 ▶ Intradural Vessel Simulating Radiculitis. Same patient as in Figure 40-14. Axial contrast-enhanced fat-saturated T1-weighted MR images obtained in upper lumbar (image **A**) region and in the lower lumbar region (images **B** and **C**). The tiny, well-defined, enhancing intradural vessel (*arrow in images* **A**, **B** and **C**) is located along the anterior surface of the conus medullaris (image **A**) and is positioned medial to the intrathecal portion of the left S1 nerve root at the L5 level (image **B**). The enhancing vessel (*arrow*) enters the left S1 nerve root pouch in image **C**, obtained at the L5-S1 levels.

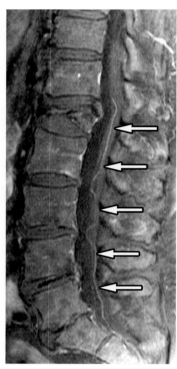

Figure 40-16 ▶ Normal Intradural Vessel Simulating Radiculitis. Tortuous "normal" intradural enhancing vessel (*arrows*) demonstrated on sagittal contrast-enhanced fat-saturated T1-weighted MR image in patient with nonspecific back pain but no leg pain or lower extremity weakness. Noted is L1 vertebral compression fracture and multilevel intervertebral disc degeneration.

associated with radicular symptoms, are slightly smaller than a normal intrathecal nerve root, and have very well defined margins. The vessel is nearly always located anterior or medial to the adjacent intrathecal nerve root (see Fig. 40-15). The vessel most commonly accompanies the S1 or less commonly the L5 nerve root, and the intrathecal course occasionally is quite tortuous (see Fig. 40-16). Rarely, an intradural vessel may be seen to accompany an upper lumbar nerve root.

Normal intradural vessels must be differentiated from intrathecal arterial feeders supplying dural atrioventricular fistulas (AVFs) near the conus medullaris. Such arterial feeders are usually larger in caliber and are associated with tortuous arterialized veins surrounding the lower thoracic spinal cord. In patients with type I dural AVF involving the lower spinal cord, there is typically a region of abnormal T2 hyperintensity in the lower thoracic spinal cord related to chronic ischemia secondary to the AVF.

2. **Arachnoiditis:** In the acute stage, the nerve roots and thecal sac may enhance, but this stage is rarely observed. It is conceivable, but not known, whether isolated intrathecal radiculitis can ultimately result in full-blown chronic arachnoiditis. Most commonly, patients with arachnoiditis present in the chronic stage with chronic intractable low back pain and polyradicular pain. MR or CT myelogram images in patients with chronic arachnoiditis reveal thickened, clumped nerve roots, adhesions between the nerve roots and thecal sac, and deformity of the thecal sac. Occasionally, an *empty thecal sac* sign is seen in patients with chronic arachnoiditis, after the chronically inflamed roots adhere to the thecal sac.

3. **Guillain-Barré syndrome (GBS):** An acute polyradiculitis that causes the acute inflammation of the nerve roots of the cauda equina. The anterior intrathecal nerve roots may be larger and enhance more intensely on contrast-enhanced MR images than the posterior roots. These patients classically present with ascending paraparesis and less commonly with pain and paresthesias (see Chapter 33 for further discussion of Guillain-Barré syndrome).

4. **Chronic inflammatory demyelinating polyradiculopathy (CIDP):** This is a chronic inflammatory condition usually involving all nerve roots of the cauda equina. The nerve roots of the cauda equina are smooth, slightly enlarged, and enhance diffusely. This condition causes a diffuse polyneuropathy, but pain is uncommonly reported in this condition upon presentation.

TREATMENT

Conservative therapy may be sufficient to treat intrathecal radiculitis because radiculitis may be a self-limited condition, especially if it occurs in the postoperative setting.

1. **Nonsteroidal anti-inflammatory agents:** Are of limited benefit in treating this condition.

2. **Short-term systemic steroid therapy:** May be helpful in some patients.

3. **Selective nerve root injection or transforaminal epidural injection of anesthetic-steroid agents:** Can be both diagnostic and therapeutic in patients with intrathecal preoperative or postoperative radiculitis by confirming whether the enhancing nerve root is indeed symptomatic if the patient's pain is relieved by the injection (see Fig. 40-12). In the situation in which a disc herniation is responsible for the radiculitis, selective nerve block may provide relief of pain by reducing inflammation in the nerve root until the herniated disc fragment

either involutes spontaneously or is removed surgically. In cases of spinal stenosis causing the nerve root impingement, a nerve root or transforaminal epidural injection may break the cycle of pain sufficiently to provide short-term and sometimes long-term relief of pain.

4. **Surgery:** If the above methods fail, surgery such as discectomy or decompression laminectomy may be required to alleviate the inciting cause of the radiculitis.

References

1. Takata K, Inoue S, Takahashi K, Ohtsuka Y. Swelling of the cauda equina in patients who have herniation of a lumbar disc: A possible pathogenesis of sciatica. *J Bone Joint Surg Am.* 1988;70(3):361-368.

2. Jinkins JR. Magnetic resonance imaging of benign nerve root enhancement in the unoperated and postoperative lumbosacral spine. *Neuroimaging Clin N Am.* 1993;3(3):525-541.

3. Itoh R, Murata K, Kamata M, et al. Lumbosacral nerve root enhancement with disk herniation on contrast-enhanced MR. *AJNR Am J Neuroradiol.* 1996;17(9):1619-1625.

4. Jinkins JR. MR of enhancing nerve roots in the unoperated lumbosacral spine. *AJNR Am J Neuroradiol.* 1993;14(1):193-202.

5. Lucantoni D, Galzio R, Zenobii M, et al. Involvement of lumbosacral roots caused by lateral recess stenosis. *J Neurosurg Sci.* 1984;28(2):93-96.

6. Jinkins JR. Enhanced MR clarifies cause of failed back surgery. *Diagn Imaging (San Franc).* 1993;15(11):108-112.

7. Jinkins JR. Acquired degenerative changes of the intervertebral segments at and suprajacent to the lumbosacral junction: A radioanatomic analysis of the nondiscal structures of the spinal column and perispinal soft tissues. *Eur J Radiol.* 2004;50(2):134-158.

LATERAL RECESS STENOSIS

Leo F. Czervionke, M.D.

CLINICAL PRESENTATION

The patient is a 57-year-old male with chronic low back pain, bilateral lower extremity pain, paresthesias, and difficulty walking. The pain is exacerbated by standing and walking even short distances. On physical examination, the patient has moderate weakness of the hip flexors bilaterally, increased tone in the lower extremities, bilateral hyperreflexia, and sustained clonus bilaterally. The patient has a cardiac defibrillator, so a computed tomography (CT) scan was ordered instead of a magnetic resonance (MR) scan.

IMAGING PRESENTATION

CT scan of the lumbar spine revealed severe central canal stenosis at the L4-5 level caused by generalized disc bulging, bilateral ligamentum flavum thickening, and facet hypertrophy. Bilateral lateral recess stenosis is present below the L4-5 intervertebral disc level (L4-5 subarticular zone) (*Figs. 41-1 and 41-2*).

DISCUSSION

The lateral recess is sometimes referred to as the *subarticular zone* or *subarticular groove* because it is anatomically located below the intervertebral disc level. There is controversy in the literature as to what actually constitutes the lateral recess. There are those who consider the intervertebral neural foramen as part of the lateral recess.[1,2] We consider the neural foramen (lateral intervertebral canal) and the lateral recess (subarticular zone) as distinct anatomic entities. Even with the advanced imaging techniques available today, the lateral recess remains a misunderstood anatomic concept, and unfortunately, stenosis of the lateral recess is still overlooked by some who evaluate CT and MR imaging studies.

Anatomically, the lumbar lateral recess is formed anteriorly by the posterolateral surface of the vertebral body and overlying posterior longitudinal ligament, posteriorly by the superior articular facet and overlying ligamentum flavum, and laterally by the pedicle (*Figs. 41-3 to 41-5*).[3-5] There are some who also consider the intervertebral disc margin as an anterior boundary of the lateral recess.[6,7] However, the disc margin is not anatomically part of the lateral recess or *subarticular zone*.[8] The nerve root that exits the thecal sac at a given disc level is positioned within the lateral recess. This nerve root, which has the same level name as the adjacent pedicle,

will course below the pedicle before exiting the spinal canal within the intervertebral neural foramen below. For example, the L4 nerve root exits the thecal sac at the L3-4 disc level, enters the lateral recess, which is a three- sided structure bound by the L4 pedicle medially, the L4 vertebral body anteriorly, and superior articular process of L4 posteriorly. The L4 nerve root courses inferiorly beneath the L4 pedicle to exit the spinal canal via the L4-5 neural foramen.

By far the most common level affected with lateral recess stenosis is L4-5 (see Figs. 41-1 and 41-3), which causes compression of the L5 nerve root.[7] The second most common level of lateral recess stenosis is L5-S1, which affects the S1 nerve root (Figs. 41-5 and *41-6*). The lateral recess may be congenitally narrowed, for example, in patients with developmentally "short" pedicles or in patients with achondroplasia. Acquired lateral recess stenosis is far more common than and is often associated with central canal stenosis secondary to vertebral spondylitic bony ridges and facet osteoarthritis resulting in overgrowth (hypertrophy) of the facets (see Figs. 41-1 and 41-3). The lateral recess tends to be most narrowed just below the level of the intervertebral disc, at the level of the superior margin of the vertebral endplate and medial to the pedicle (see Figs. 41-1, 41-2, and *41-7*). At this level, a nerve root that has exited the thecal sac becomes trapped between hypertrophic spondylitic ridges arising along the posterolateral vertebral endplate margin and the hypertrophic superior articular process (see Figs. 41-1 and *41-8*).[3,6,9] Central canal stenosis is often present in patients with bony lateral recess stenosis (see Figs. 41-4 and *41-9*). In patients with central canal stenosis, hypertrophic spondylitis ridges, facet hypertrophy, and ligamentum flavum are the common components that cause circumferential thecal sac narrowing at the intervertebral disc level. These same three components also cause bony lateral recess stenosis immediately below the disc level in the subarticular zone (see Figs. 41-1 to 41-9). In addition, herniated disc fragments or synovial cysts may occupy a normal-sized bony lateral recess and produce symptoms identical to lateral recess stenosis (*Figs. 41-10 to 41-13*). Therefore, it is imperative to carefully evaluate the lateral recess preoperatively in all patients undergoing discectomy or decompressive laminectomy.[10]

With spondylolisthesis, the bulging or protruding posterior disc margin tends to be drawn up or displaced (*uncovered*) superiorly and laterally, which tends to trap the exiting nerve root beneath the pedicle.[11] Spondylolisthesis therefore tends to compromise the medial portion of the neural foramen rather than the lateral recess.[11] Occasionally, the uncovered, superiorly displaced disc in patients with spondylolisthesis will extend more superiorly to compress

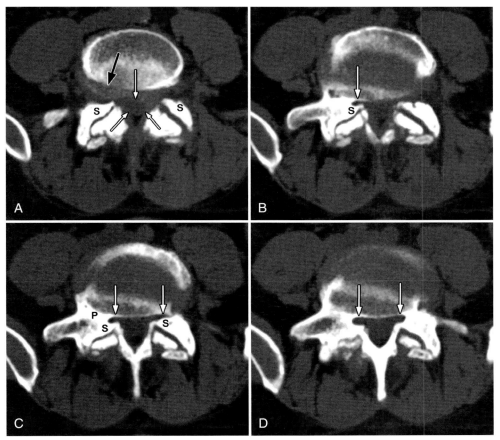

Figure 41-1 ▶ **L4-5 Level Central Canal Stenosis and Subarticular Lateral Recess Stenosis.** Axial CT image **A**, obtained at the L4-5 intervertebral disc level, reveals central canal stenosis (*white arrows*) secondary to disc bulging, facet hypertrophy, and ligamentum flavum thickening. A right posterolateral disc protrusion/herniation (*black arrow*) encroaches upon the right L4-5 neural foramen. S = superior articular processes of L5. Images **B**, **C**, and **D** are rostral to caudal axial CT sections obtained through the L4-5 subarticular zone showing bilateral lateral recess stenosis (*arrows*) bounded anteriorly by the L5 vertebral body margin, laterally by the pedicle (P), and posteriorly by the hypertrophic superior articular processes (*S*) of L5.

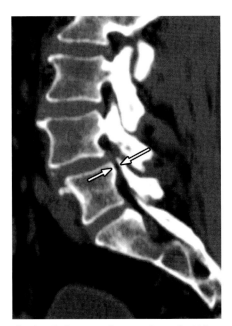

Figure 41-2 ▶ **L4-5 Level Central Canal Stenosis and Subarticular Lateral Recess Stenosis.** Right parasagittal CT image in same patient as in Figure 41-1. The narrowed right lateral recess (*arrows*) is bounded anteriorly by the posterior L5 vertebral body margin and posteriorly by the anterior surface of the superior articular process of L5. The lateral recess is more narrowed superiorly near the L5 superior endplate.

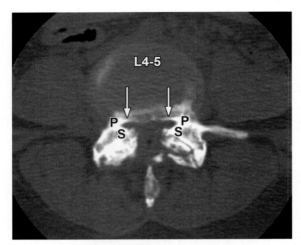

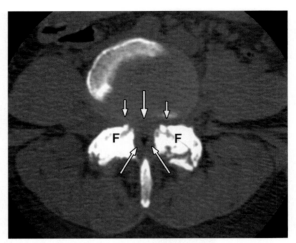

Figure 41-3 ▶ Lateral Recess Stenosis. 54-year-old female with coexistent severe L4-5 central canal stenosis. The lateral recess narrowed bilaterally (*arrows*) but more narrowed on the right. The lateral recesses are located medial to the respective pedicles (*P*) and are narrowed due to bilateral overgrowth of the superior articular processes (*S*) of L5.

Figure 41-4 ▶ Lateral Recess Stenosis. Axial CT scan, in same patient as in Figure 41-3, showing classic CT appearance of circumferential thecal sac narrowing (central stenosis) secondary to bulging disc (*midline long arrow*), ligamentum flavum thickening (*paramidline long arrows*) and bilateral articular process hypertrophy/facet hypertrophy (*F*). *Short arrows* indicate location of bilateral "medial foraminal stenosis" secondary to disc bulging and bilateral facet hypertrophy.

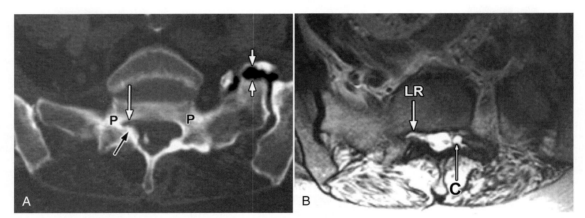

Figure 41-5 ▶ Lateral Recess Stenosis. Patient with severe right L5-S1 bony lateral recess stenosis (*long white arrow*), due primarily to hypertrophy of the right superior articular process (*black arrow*) of transitional S1 vertebra shown on axial CT image **A**. P = pedicles of S1. Note gas filled degenerative pseudoarthrosis (*short white arrows*) on the left. On corresponding axial T2-weighted MR image **B**, the severe bony lateral recess stenosis (*LR*) on the right is visible. A synovial cyst (*C*) is shown encroaching upon the left lateral recess. This synovial cyst is not visible on CT image **A**.

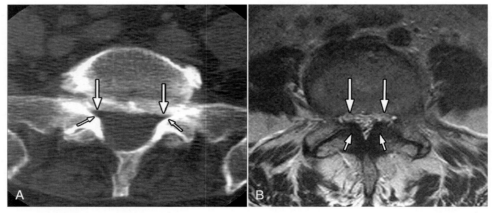

Figure 41-6 ▶ Bilateral Lateral Recess Stenosis At L5-S1. Axial CT image **A** and axial T2-weighted MR image **B**. The stenotic lateral recesses (*long arrows in images* **A** *and* **B**) are caused by bilateral superior articular facet hypertrophy (*short arrows image* **A**) and by thickened ligamentum flava (*short arrows in image* **B**).

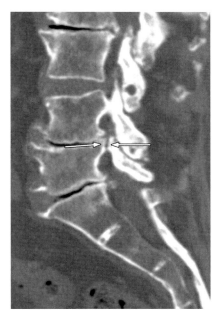

Figure 41-7 ▶ Right Lateral Recess Stenosis. Severe right lateral recess stenosis (*arrows*) at L4-5 as demonstrated on parasagittal CT image obtained just medial to the right pedicle of L5. Typically, lateral recess stenosis is most severe superiorly near the superior endplate of L5 due to hypertrophic vertebral spondylitic ridge anteriorly and superior L5 articular process and facet hypertrophy.

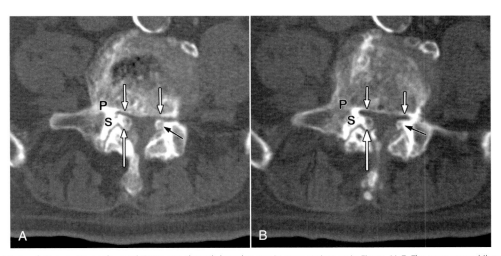

Figure 41-8 ▶ Right Lateral Recess Stenosis. Axial CT images through lateral recess in same patient as in Figure 41-7. The most severe bilateral recess stenosis is at level of the L5 superior vertebral endplate (*short white arrows*) shown in axial CT image **A**. On the right, a large L5 superior articular process spur (*long white arrow*) encroaches on the right lateral recess and a smaller L5 superior articular process spur (*black arrow*) narrows the left lateral recess. On contiguous more inferior axial CT image **B**, the bilateral superior facet spurs are still visible and the lateral recesses (*short white arrows*) are still narrowed but are slightly larger than demonstrated in more rostral image **A**. P = right pedicle of L5. S = right superior articular process of L5.

the exiting nerve root within the inferior portion of the lateral recess.

Bulging discs coexist with marginal vertebral endplate spondylitic ridging (spondylosis deformans), and therefore some consider the bulging disc at a given disc level to contribute to lateral recess stenosis.[6] We consider the true lateral recess to exist only at the level of the pedicle, and therefore *lateral recess,* as we use the term, is not found at a given lumbar intervertebral disc level, because the neural foramen (which is not a blind recess) is located at the lumbar disc level. A bulging or posterolateral protruding disc,

along with facet hypertrophy and overlying ligamentum flavum thickening, will indeed narrow the axillary root pouch of the thecal sac at the medial entry zone of the neural foramen (see Figs. 41-1, 41-4, and 41-9) . When this occurs, we refer to this as *medial foraminal stenosis* rather than lateral recess stenosis, which occurs just below a given disc level. Medial foraminal stenosis can also be a clinically significant condition that may coexist with disc herniation or central stenosis, and therefore the medial portion of the neural foramen must be carefully assessed before discectomy or decompressive laminectomy.

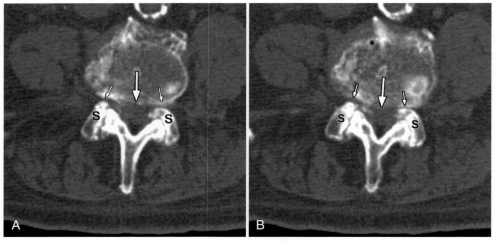

Figure 41-9 ▶ Severe Central Canal Stenosis and Bilateral Neural Foraminal Stenosis at L4-5 Level. Same patient as in Figures 41-7 and 41-8. Axial CT image **A** and more caudal image **B** are contiguous images through the L4-5 intervertebral disc at the inferior most level of the L4-5 neural foramina. No lateral recess exists at this level. Bilateral medial foraminal stenosis (*short arrows*) and central canal stenosis (*long arrow*) are demonstrated. S = superior articular processes of L5.

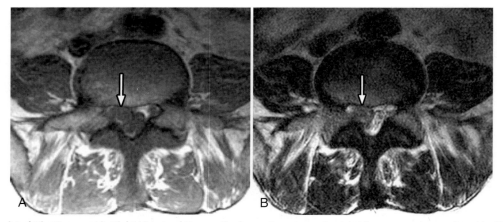

Figure 41-10 ▶ Herniated Disc Fragment in Right L5 Lateral Recess. Disc fragment compresses the right L5 nerve root, obscures the epidural fat in the lateral recess, and deforms the right anterolateral margin of the thecal sac. On axial T1-weighted MR image **A**, the disc fragment (*arrow*) is nearly isointense relative to the CSF. On axial T2-weighted image **B**, the disc fragment (*arrow*) is T2 hypointense relative to intrathecal CSF.

Lateral recess stenosis causes leg pain and paresthesias. The leg pain is made worse by standing and walking. The pain with lateral recess stenosis is typically relieved by squatting or sitting.[7] Leg pain caused by herniated discs is usually made worse by sitting.[12] Most patients with lateral recess stenosis or a herniated disc in the lateral recess experience intense radicular leg pain when a Laségue maneuver is performed (positive straight leg–raising sign).[9,10,13] Deep tendon reflexes are usually diminished or abolished, although they can be brisk if there is acute nerve root entrapment such as a herniated disc encroaching upon the lateral recess.[9,10] Patients with lateral recess compromise often have motor disturbances as well, including weakness of the ipsilateral anterior tibial muscle and the extensor hallucis longus muscle. Muscle weakness and a positive straight leg–raising sign are more likely to occur when a disc herniation contributes to the lateral recess stenosis.[10]

IMAGING FEATURES

Myelography alone tends to underestimate the degree of lateral recess stenosis.[7] If myelography is performed, it is important to obtain CT scans after every myelogram. However, plain CT scans are sufficient for diagnosing bony lateral recess stenosis (see Figs. 41-1 and 41-8). Lateral recess stenosis is diagnosed when the distance between the posterior vertebral body margin and superior articular process is 3 mm or less, as measured on axial CT images.[5,7] Lateral recess stenosis is usually most severe just below a given disc level, where posterolateral osteophytic ridges from the superior vertebral body margin and the adjacent hypertrophic superior articular facet cause the greatest degree of lateral recess narrowing (see Fig. 41-8).

Special attention should be given to the lateral recess when evaluating lumbar MR scans. Lateral recess stenosis is certainly

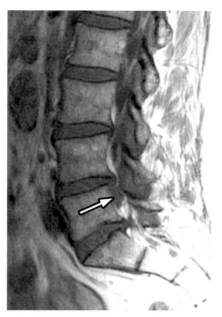

Figure 41-11 ▶ Herniated Disc Fragment in Right L5 Lateral Recess. Right parasagittal T1-weighted MR image **A**, in same patient as in Figure 41-10. The disc fragment (*arrow*) is positioned in the lateral recess below the L4-5 intervertebral disc level.

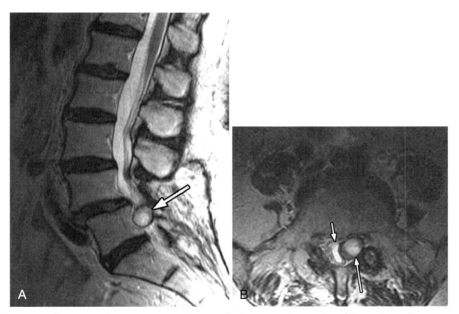

Figure 41-12 ▶ Synovial Cyst in Left L5 Lateral Recess. On sagittal T2-weighted image **A**, the cyst (*arrow*) has a thin T2 hypointense margin and T2 hyperintense fluid-filled center. On axial T2-weighted image **B**, the cyst (*long arrow*) compresses and displaces the thecal sac (*short arrow*) to the right of midline.

visible using current MR imaging techniques (see Figs. 41-5 and 41-6), but there is a tendency to overlook the lateral recess when evaluating the lumbar spine with MR. The degree of nerve root compression by lateral recess stenosis may be underestimated with MR.[6]

CT and MR are valuable for evaluating not only the lateral recess but also diagnosing associated disc herniation (see Fig.

41-10). A posterolateral disc herniation that extends slightly below the disc level can cause radiculopathy by encroaching upon the nerve within the lateral recess.[3,10] Synovial cysts may also occupy the lateral recesses and are T2 hypointense and T2 hyperintense on MR imaging. Synovial cysts usually have a faint hyperdense rim on unenhanced CT images, probably because of the presence of calcification in the cyst wall (see Fig. 41-13).

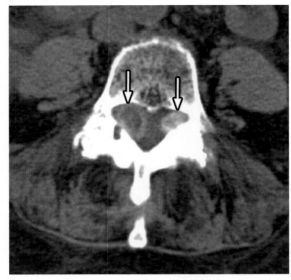

Figure 41-13 ▶ **Synovial Cysts Causing Lateral Recess Stenosis.** Bilateral L4-5 synovial cysts encroach upon the L4-5 subarticular zones (*lateral recesses*) adjacent to the L5 pedicles. Axial CT image. The synovial cysts (*arrows*) are relatively hyperdense peripherally and hypodense centrally.

The nerve root in the stenotic lateral recess may enhance after IV contrast administration indicating disruption in the blood-nerve barrier, which can be secondary to any insult to the nerve root including trauma, inflammation, demyelination, ischemia, or axonal degeneration.[14,15] Nerve roots that enhance in this manner are nearly always symptomatic to some degree.

DIFFERENTIAL DIAGNOSIS

Lateral recess stenosis is one of the three types of spinal stenosis, the others being vertebral canal stenosis (central canal stenosis) and neural foraminal stenosis (lateral canal stenosis). Lateral recess stenosis has a classic imaging appearance. Narrowing of the medial portion of the neural foramen is sometimes erroneously referred to as *lateral recess stenosis*.

TREATMENT

1. **Surgical decompression** is the definitive therapy for lateral recess stenosis. The standard surgical treatment of lateral recess stenosis is laminectomy along with partial facetectomy, removing the hypertrophied superior articular process.[7,9] Endoscopic decompression of the lateral recess has been suggested as an alternative to extensive laminectomy.[16] When a partial facetectomy is performed, there is the possibility of rotational instability developing.[7] For this reason, it may be necessary to perform a posterolateral fusion procedure in addition to the laminectomy and facetectomy. Furthermore, disc herniation and bony lateral recess stenosis may coexist.[10] If surgery is performed to remove a herniated disc at a given disc level, it is important to decompress coexistent adjacent bony lateral recess stenosis if present.[10]

2. **Selective nerve root injection or transforaminal epidural injection** with anesthetic-steroid agents can be a very valuable provocative test to confirm the diagnosis of symptomatic lateral recess stenosis and also to provide temporary relief of symptoms. The selective nerve root block or transforaminal injection should be performed by introducing the needle into the neural foramen below the level of the stenotic lateral recess. In some patients, a single injection or repeated injections may provide long-term relief of pain in patients with significant lateral recess stenosis, sometimes obviating the need for surgery. Patients with persistent or recurrent leg pain or those patients with developing leg weakness should be treated surgically.

References

1. Furman MB, Puttlitz KM, Pannullo R, Simon J. Spinal stenosis and neurogenic claudication. WebMD; 2009 [cited 2009]; Available from: http://emedicine.medscape.com/article/310528-overview.
2. Amundsen T, Weber H, Lilleas F, et al. Lumbar spinal stenosis: Clinical and radiologic features. *Spine.* 1995;20(10):1178-1186.
3. Demondion X, Manelfe C, Prere J, Francke J. [Lumbar lateral recess and intervertebral foramen: Radio-anatomical study]. *J Radiol.* 2000;81(6 Suppl):734-745.
4. Matozzi F, Moreau JJ, Jiddane M, et al. Correlative anatomic and CT study of the lumbar lateral recess. *AJNR Am J Neuroradiol.* 1983;4(3):650-652.
5. Mikhael MA, Ciric I, Tarkington JA, Vick NA. Neuroradiological evaluation of lateral recess syndrome. *Radiology.* 1981;140(1):97-107.
6. Bartynski WS, Lin L. Lumbar root compression in the lateral recess: MR imaging, conventional myelography, and CT myelography comparison with surgical confirmation. *AJNR Am J Neuroradiol.* 2003;24(3):348-360.
7. Ciric I, Mikhael MA, Tarkington JA, Vick NA. The lateral recess syndrome: A variant of spinal stenosis. *J Neurosurg.* 1980;53(4):433-443.
8. Wiltse LL, Berger PE, McCulloch JA. A system for reporting the size and location of lesions in the spine. *Spine.* 1997;22(13):1534-1537.
9. Lucantoni D, Galzio R, Zenobii M, et al. Involvement of lumbosacral roots caused by lateral recess stenosis. *J Neurosurg Sci.* 1984;28(2):93-96.
10. Kanamiya T, Kida H, Seki M, et al. Effect of lumbar disc herniation on clinical symptoms in lateral recess syndrome. *Clin Orthop Relat Res.* 2002;(398):131-135.
11. MacMahon PJ, Taylor DH, Duke D, et al. Disc displacement patterns in lumbar anterior spondylolisthesis: Contribution to foraminal stenosis. *Eur J Radiol.* 2009;70(1):149-154.
12. Major NM, Helms CA. Central and foraminal stenosis of the lumbar spine. *Neuroimaging Clin N Am.* 1993;3(3):564-565.

13. Epstein JA, Epstein BS, Rosenthal AD, et al. Sciatica caused by nerve root entrapment in the lateral recess: The superior facet syndrome. *J Neurosurg.* 1972;36(5):584-589.

14. Xiong L, Jinkins JR. Sterile, benign radiculitis associated with lumbosacral lateral recess spinal canal stenosis: Evaluation with enhanced magnetic resonance imaging. *J Spinal Disord.* 2001;14(1):73-75.

15. Jinkins JR. MR of enhancing nerve roots in the unoperated lumbosacral spine. *AJNR Am J Neuroradiol.* 1993;14(1):193-202.

16. Ruetten S, Komp M, Merk H, Godolias G. Surgical treatment for lumbar lateral recess stenosis with the full-endoscopic interlaminar approach versus conventional microsurgical technique: A prospective, randomized, controlled study. *J Neurosurg Spine.* 2009;10(5):476-485.

CHAPTER
42

LEPTOMENINGEAL METASTASIS

Leo F. Czervionke, M.D.

CLINICAL PRESENTATION

The patient is a 45-year-old female who presented in the emergency department with nausea, vomiting, severe headache, dizziness, neck pain and stiffness, severe low back pain, and lower extremity weakness. The patient was diagnosed 9 months previously with right upper lobe small cell lung carcinoma, stage IIIB, which has been treated with chemotherapy.

IMAGING PRESENTATION

Magnetic resonance (MR) imaging of the brain and entire spinal axis was obtained. The patient has leptomeningeal contrast enhancement on the surfaces of the temporal lobes posteriorly, along the pial surfaces of the cerebellar hemispheres, along the margins of the brainstem and the cisternal segment of cranial nerve V bilaterally, and involvement of the cisternal and intracanalicular portions of cranial nerve VIII bilaterally. Diffuse leptomeningeal enhancement of the entire spinal cord and cauda equina was also apparent (*Figs. 42-1 to 42-3*). MR imaging findings are consistent with intracranial and spinal leptomeningeal carcinomatosis.

DISCUSSION

Leptomeningeal metastases, also known as *leptomeningeal carcinomatosis* or *carcinomatous meningitis*, is a neoplastic condition, whereby tumor disseminates throughout the central nervous system. In the spinal canal, the tumor deposits along the surface of the spinal cord attaching to the leptomeninges. The leptomeninges anatomically includes the arachnoid and pia mater. This may occur due to tumor originating outside or inside the central nervous system (CNS).

Tumors that arise outside the CNS most commonly cause leptomeningeal metastases, and these are most commonly from primary neoplasms of the lung and breast (*Figs. 42-1 to 42-5*), but also may occur secondary to extra-CNS melanoma, lymphoma, and leukemia.[1,2] Leptomeningeal spread of tumor rarely occurs with tumors of the gastrointestinal (GI) tract, genitourinary (GU) tract, prostate cancer,[3] mesothelioma,[4] and myeloma.[5] Leptomeningeal involvement by melanoma is most often from metastatic melanoma, but rarely primary leptomeningeal melanoma can occur.[6]

In patients with extra-CNS lymphoma, leptomeningeal spread rarely occurs in patients with Hodgkin's disease and commonly occurs in patients with AIDS-related non-Hodgkin's lymphoma, immunoblastic lymphoma, and Burkitt's lymphoma.[1,7] In patients with myeloid malignancies, the presence of specific cytogenetic abnormalities are strongly associated with the development of leptomeningeal tumor, including translocation of chromosome 8-21, translocation of chromosome 9-11, deletion of chromosome 11q23, and inversion or deletion of chromosome 16.[1]

Leptomeningeal spread of tumor may occur secondary to tumors originating inside the CNS, although this occurs in less than 2% of patients with primary CNS tumors overall. Primitive neuroectodermal tumors (PNET, such as medulloblastoma), primary CNS lymphoma, and glioneuronal tumors[8] have a much higher incidence of leptomeningeal spread.[1,9]

Other intracranial tumors can seed the leptomeninges producing so called *drop metastases*, tumors that deposit along the cord surface or in the cauda equina. Drop metastases most commonly occur with intracranial ependymomas and less commonly astrocytomas. Intradural ependymomas arising in the lumbosacral spinal canal may also cause leptomeningeal dissemination superiorly to involve the thoracic, cervical, or intracranial leptomeninges. Intracranial germ cell tumors, such as pineal germinomas, are also known to spread along cerebrospinal fluid (CSF) pathways and may involve the intracranial or spinal leptomeninges (*Figs. 42-6 and 42-7*).

Glioblastoma multiforme and rarely oligodendroglioma may spread along the leptomeninges.[10] Hemangioblastomotosis, a histologically benign yet highly aggressive and devastating condition, has the same imaging appearance as leptomeningeal carcinomatosis.[11,12] The clear cell subtype of meningioma has an aggressive nature and has a propensity to spread along the leptomeninges.[13]

Leptomeningeal tumors in general carry a dire prognosis, usually leading to the demise of the patient within weeks to months.[1,14] Untreated patients with leptomeningeal cancer usually die within a month. The median survival is only 4 to 5 months with treatment.[15]

Hematogenous spread via arachnoidal vessels is believed to be the most common mechanism of spread to the leptomeninges.[1,16] Direct extension may also occur from tumors located along the ependymal or meningeal surfaces.[1] Another proposed mechanism of leptomeningeal dissemination is iatrogenic spread at the time of surgical removal of a parenchymal brain tumor, which is believed to occur more commonly after resection of a brain metastasis, especially when the metastasis is located in the posterior fossa.[17,18]

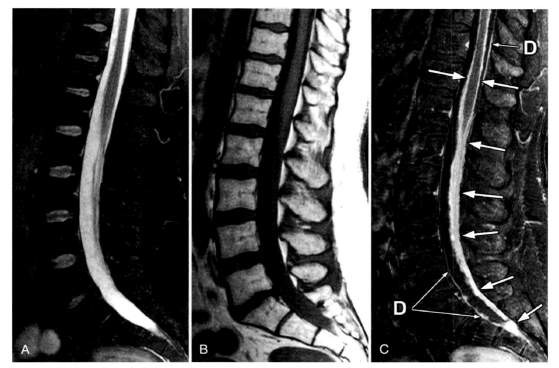

Figure 42-1 ▶ **Leptomeningeal Carcinomatosis Secondary to Small Cell Lung Carcinoma.** No definite abnormality is visible on sagittal T2-weighted MR image **A** or T1-weighted image **B**. On sagittal contrast enhanced image **C**, diffuse leptomeningeal enhancing tumor envelops the spinal cord and nerve roots of the cauda equina (*arrows*). The thecal sac dura (*D*) also enhances uniformly due to diffuse infiltration by tumor.

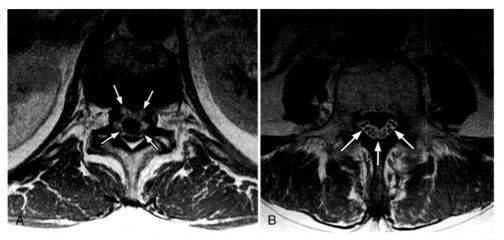

Figure 42-2 ▶ **Leptomeningeal Carcinomatosis Secondary to Small Cell Lung Carcinoma.** Corresponding contrast enhanced axial T1-weighted MR image **A** through conus medullaris and image **B** through cauda equina reveal diffuse enhancing tissue enveloping the conus medullaris and nerve rootlets (*arrows*) in image **A** and cauda equina nerve roots (*arrows*) in image **B**.

There is almost always a history of known malignant neoplasm in patients with leptomeningeal metastasis. Patients with this condition typically present with severe back pain and weakness. They may have polyradicular symptoms and bladder or bowel dysfunction.[19] Nuchal rigidity may exist, similar to patients with meningitis. Absent deep tendon reflexes and sensory loss may be present.[1]

A lumbar puncture is usually performed in these patients to obtain CSF for chemical analysis, cell count, and cytology and to aid in excluding meningitis, which may have a similar clinical presentation. Ideally, the lumbar puncture should be performed after brain computed tomography (CT) or magnetic resonance (MR) imaging to exclude a space-occupying intracranial mass. In leptomeningeal carcinomatosis, CSF protein is usually elevated, CSF glucose may be low, lymphocytic pleocytosis may be present, and the opening pressure is often elevated.[1,20,21] The absence of positive cytology does not exclude leptomeningeal metastasis. Malignant cells are usually detected in the CSF, but negative CSF cytology

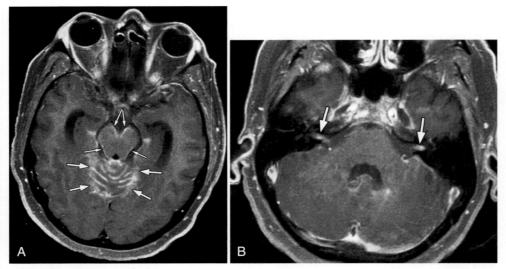

Figure 42-3 ▶ **Leptomeningeal Carcinomatosis.** Same patient as in Figures 42-1 and 42-2. Intracranial leptomeningeal enhancement "coats" the surface of the midbrain (*small arrows*) and cerebellar vermis (*long arrows*) in contrast enhanced T1-weighted MR image **A**. The intracanalicular portion of cranial nerve VIII enhances bilaterally (*arrows*) in contrast enhanced image **B** due to metastatic infiltration by tumor, simulating bilateral CN VIII schwannomas.

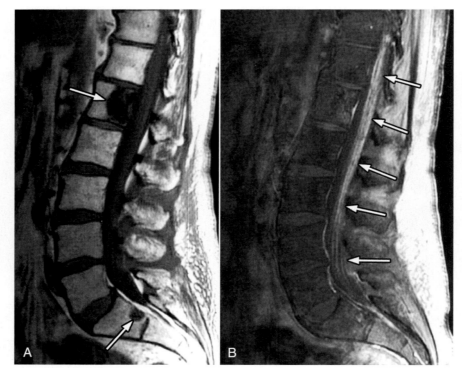

Figure 42-4 ▶ **Osteoblastic Metastases, Leptomeningeal Carcinomatosis.** 59-year-old female patient who has been treated for breast cancer developed severe low back and lower extremity weakness. Unenhanced sagittal T1-weighted MR image **A** reveals T1 hypointense lesions in the L1 and S1 vertebral bodies (*arrows*) representing osteoblastic bone metastases. No abnormality visible in spinal canal. On sagittal contrast enhanced T1-weighted MR image **B**, there is diffuse micronodular enhancement of the cauda equina nerve roots and surface of the conus medullaris representing diffuse leptomeningeal carcinomatosis.

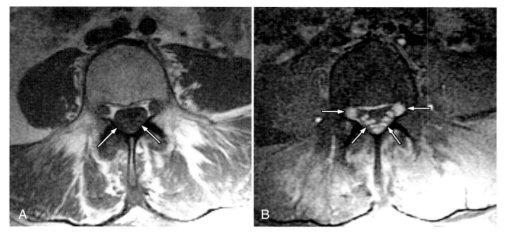

Figure 42-5 ▶ Leptomeningeal Carcinomatosis. Axial unenhanced T1-weighted image **A** and contrast enhanced image **B** in same patient as in Figure 42-4, obtained through cauda equina at L3 level. There is diffuse enhancement and slight enlargement of all visible nerve roots (*arrows*) at this level.

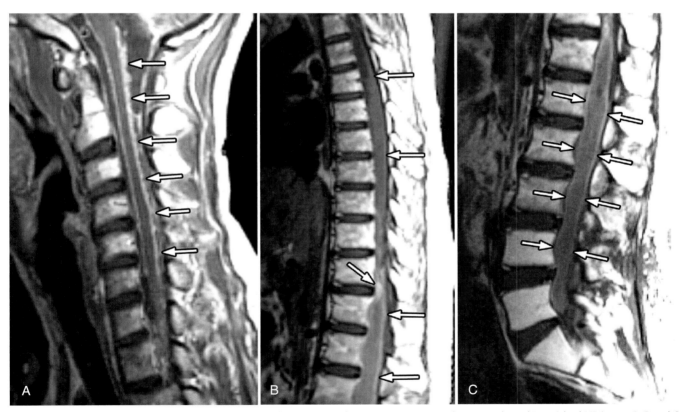

Figure 42-6 ▶ Pineal Germinoma With Dissemination Throughout the Spinal Leptomeninges. Sagittal contrast enhanced T1-weighted MR images **A**, **B**, and **C** of the cervical, thoracic and lumbar spine. The pial surface of the entire spinal cord and thecal sac enhance diffusely (*arrows*) due to diffuse infiltration of the spinal meninges by tumor.

does not exclude the presence of leptomeningeal metastasis, because cytology may be negative in 10% to 15% of patients even after repeated lumbar punctures.[22,23] In a patient with known malignancy and in the appropriate clinical setting with the characteristic MR imaging appearance of leptomeningeal disease, positive CSF cytology is not required to make the diagnosis.[1,24]

IMAGING FEATURES

If leptomeningeal carcinomatosis is suspected, contrast-enhanced MR imaging of the entire spinal axis and brain should be obtained.[1] Contrast-enhanced MR imaging is far more sensitive than contrast-enhanced CT[25,26] or CT myelography.[27] Leptomeningeal spread of

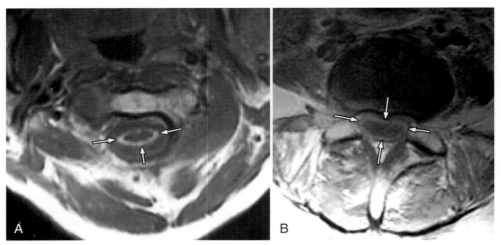

Figure 42-7 ▶ **Pineal Germinoma.** Same patient as in Figure 42-6. Axial contrast enhanced T1-weighted MR image **A** at the C2 level reveals diffuse circumferential enhancement of the pial surface of the spinal cord (*arrows*). On axial contrast enhanced T1-weighted image **B** at the L4-5 level, diffuse enhancement of the dura (*arrows*) is demonstrated. The cauda equina nerve roots within the thecal sac are not seen. The cauda equina roots may be matted together but do not enhance.

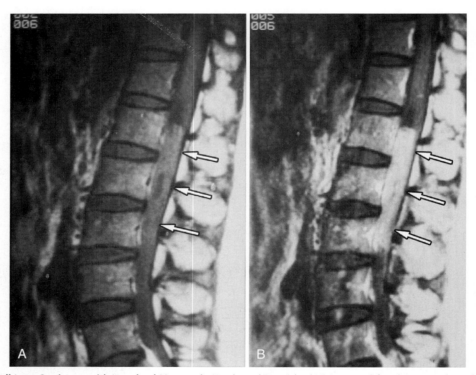

Figure 42-8 ▶ **Small Cell Lung Carcinoma with Intradural Metastasis.** Unenhanced T1-weighted MR image on left and contrast enhanced image on right. Intradural leptomeningeal tumor (*arrows*) fills the entire spinal canal from the L1 to L3 level involving the conus medullaris and cauda equina.

tumor may manifest as a solitary nodule or a mass lesion along the surface of the spinal cord, cauda equina, or in the caudal aspect of the thecal sac (*Fig. 42-8*). More commonly, multiple small nodular tumors arise along the cord surface or cauda equina,[2] which are visible on post-myelogram CT images, but better demonstrated on contrast-enhanced MR images (see Figs. 42-1 to 42-5). Diffuse leptomeningeal tumor often manifests as

a fine multinodular pattern or uniform sheet-like pattern of tumor enveloping the spinal cord and nerve rootlets of the cauda equina, but this may not easily be seen on myelographic or post-myelogram CT images. Larger nodular tumor deposits may be visible as filling defects within the intrathecal contrast column on the cord surface on myelographic radiographs or on post-myelogram CT images.

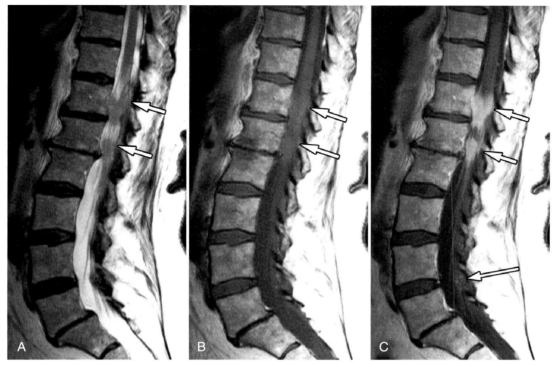

Figure 42-9 ▶ Leptomeningeal Lymphoma. Tumor (*arrows*) encases the conus medullaris and upper cauda equina nerve roots on sagittal T2-weighted MR image **A** and T1-weighted image **B**. The tumor is T2 hypointense relative to the CSF on image **A** and isointense relative to the spinal cord on image **B**. The tumor (*arrows*) enhances with a "melted wax" appearance on contrast enhanced T1-weighted sagittal image **C**. There is a small amount of tumor involving the cauda equina at the L5 level as well.

MR imaging is the modality of choice for detection and evaluating the extent of leptomeningeal neoplasia. Nodular metastatic deposits are readily visible on contrast-enhanced images and also on unenhanced, T2-weighted MR images. These tumor nodules are usually T1 isointense and therefore may be difficult to visualize on unenhanced, T1-weighted images (see Figs. 42-1, 42-4, and 42-5). Diffuse, sheet-like leptomeningeal carcinomatosis may not be visible on unenhanced, T1- or T2-weighted images along the cord surface, but typically the cauda equina nerve rootlets appear thickened or indistinct on unenhanced T1- or T2-weighted images in these cases. If a leptomeningeal tumor is discovered, it is important to scan the entire neuroaxis for other possible tumors.

Contrast-enhanced, T1-weighted MR imaging is the technique of choice for evaluating patients with suspected spinal leptomeningeal carcinomatosis.[23,25,28] The leptomeningeal tumor is most conspicuous on fat-saturated, contrast-enhanced, T1-weighted images (see Fig. 42-1). A diffuse multifocal nodular pattern of enhancement or diffuse sheet-like leptomeningeal enhancement may be seen on MR imaging along the surface of the spinal cord or involving the cauda equina nerve roots. When the enhancing neoplasm completely envelopes the spinal cord and nerve roots of the cauda equina, this is commonly referred to as the *zuckerguss* (sugar icing) pattern (see Figs. 42-1, 42-2, and 42-4).

Another pattern that may be seen with leptomeningeal carcinomatosis is a large, dominant mass enveloping the conus medullaris and cauda equina (see Fig. 42-8). Leptomeningeal lymphoma may also produce a similar appearance (*Fig. 42-9*).

Rarely, multiple myeloma will invade the central nervous system and disseminate along CSF pathways, producing leptomeningeal myelomatosis.[5,14,29] The imaging appearance of leptomeningeal myelomatosis is identical to leptomeningeal carcinomatosis, causing diffuse or micronodular enhancement of the leptomeninges of the brain, spinal cord, and/or cauda equina (*Fig. 42-10*). Occasionally, the intracranial dura is also involved by the myelomatous process, which can simulate the appearance of a subdural hematoma.[5]

Fluorine-18 fluorodeoxyglucose positron emission tomography (FDG-PET) scanning has been shown to be valuable for detection and evaluating the extent of leptomeningeal carcinomatosis,[30] but has not been widely used for evaluating leptomeningeal tumors to date. It is likely that PET scanning will prove to be an essential imaging tool for evaluating leptomeningeal tumors. If a leptomeningeal tumor is detected by MR, it is recommended that a whole body PET scan be obtained. This is especially important if the patient has no known primary tumor.

DIFFERENTIAL DIAGNOSIS

1. **Multiple schwannomas:** Numerous tiny intradural schwannomas can have an appearance similar to leptomeningeal carcinomatosis. The tiny schwannomas can be attached to the pial surface of the spinal cord or nerve roots of the cauda equina (*Fig. 42-11*).

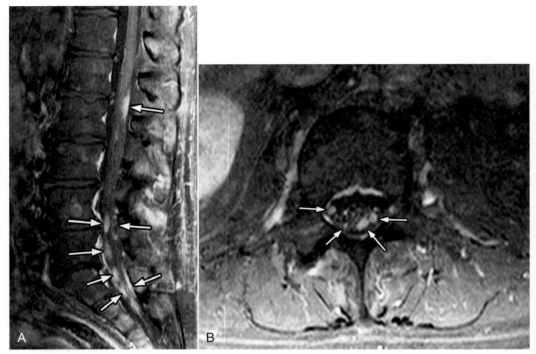

Figure 42-10 ▶ Leptomeningeal Myelomatosis. Contrast enhanced sagittal fat saturated MR image **A** and axial image **B**. Multiple nodular and fusiform enhancing lesions (*arrows in* **A** *and* **B**) involve the nerve roots of the cauda equina asymmetrically. This condition cannot be differentiated from leptomeningeal carcinomatosis by MR imaging.

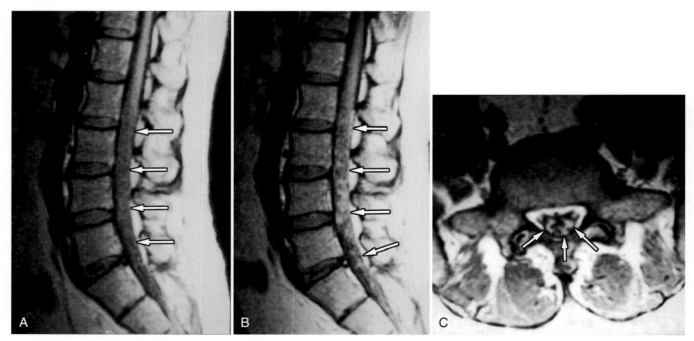

Figure 42-11 ▶ Leptomeningeal Schwannomatosis Simulating Leptomeningeal Carcinomatosis. On sagittal T1-weighted MR image **A**, multiple ill-defined tiny nodular lesions (*arrows*) are demonstrated within the thecal sac. The numerous tiny schwannomas (*arrows*) enhance intensely on contrast enhanced sagittal T1-weighted image **B**.

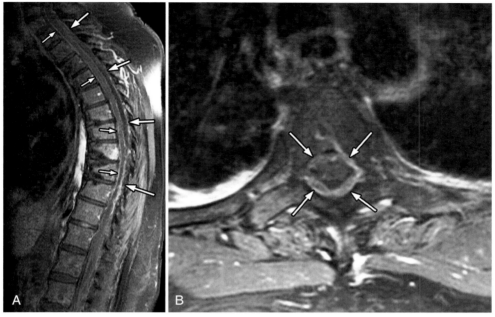

Figure 42-12 ▶ **Pneumococcal Meningitis.** On sagittal fat saturated contrast enhanced T1-weighted image **A**, there is enhancement of the dura (*long arrows*) and pial surface of the thoracic spinal cord (*short arrows*). Thick meningeal enhancement (*arrows*) surrounds the spinal cord on fat saturated axial contrast enhanced image **B**. Also noted is bilateral pleural thickening and pleural contrast enhancement.

2. **Meningitis secondary to bacterial or granulomatous infection:** This can cause lesions in or along the surface of the spinal cord or thickening of the cauda equina (*Fig. 42-12*).[2] AIDS-related leptomeningitis, tuberculous leptomeningitis, and West Nile virus leptomeningitis[31] may have an imaging appearance similar to diffuse leptomeningeal metastasis. Clinical presentation (history, fever, elevated white blood cell count, etc.) and CSF analysis are used to differentiate leptomeningeal infection from neoplasm.

3. **Primary intramedullary or intradural tumors:** Tumors such as ependymoma, lymphoma, or hemangioblastoma, may spread along the CSF pathways and can have the same appearance as leptomeningeal metastases (*Fig. 42-13*).

4. **Aggressive hemangioblastomatosis:** After removal of a cerebellar or spinal hemangioblastoma, which is a histologically benign tumor, multicentric hemangioblastomas may occur along the leptomeninges. Rarely, a diffuse form of this disease, *aggressive hemangioblastomatosis* can occur, manifesting as diffuse tumor infiltration along the basilar leptomeninges and surface of the spinal cord mimicking leptomeningeal carcinomatosis (*Fig. 42-14*).[11,12]

5. **Paraneoplastic syndrome:** One of many possible manifestations of a paraneoplastic syndrome is diffuse enhancement of the conus medullaris and cauda equina simulating the appearance of leptomeningeal metastasis (*Fig. 42-15*). Patients with paraneoplastic syndrome often have cerebellar symptomatology unrelated to neoplasia and have elevated paraneoplastic antibodies in the serum and CSF.[19]

6. **Inflammatory polyradiculopathy:** A variety of acute and chronic non-neoplastic disorders can cause thickening and enhancement of the nerve rootlets of the cauda equina and margins of the spinal cord that may simulate the MR appearance of leptomeningeal metastasis. These polyradiculopathies can be congenital (Charcot-Marie Tooth disease or Dejerine-Sottas disease) or acquired (Guillain-Barré syndrome, post-chemotherapy leptomeningitis). A variable degree of contrast enhancement is seen along the margins of the spinal cord and cauda equina on MR imaging in these conditions. The contrast enhancement pattern of the cauda equina and cord surface tends to be smooth and uniform rather than nodular in these conditions (*Fig. 42-16*). Back pain is common in patients with Guillain-Barré syndrome, although ascending paralysis is the most common clinical presentation. Patients with chronic polyradiculopathy usually present with flaccid paralysis and sensory disturbances. Back pain may occur in these chronic conditions but is usually a less common secondary finding.

7. **Arachnoiditis:** Arachnoiditis secondary to the presence of intrathecal blood from prior surgery or a percutaneous interventional procedure can cause thickening and adhesions involving the cauda equina. There may be enhancement of the involved nerve roots early in the disease, but the enhancement tends to be minimal and usually resolves. Most patients with chronic arachnoiditis have no discernable nerve rootlet enhancement.

TREATMENT

The prognosis in patients with leptomeningeal metastasis is extremely poor and any treatment is considered palliative. Because current treatments are not considered to be curative, therapy is given with the primary goal of improving quality of remaining life. The clinical status of the patient and risk versus benefit of the

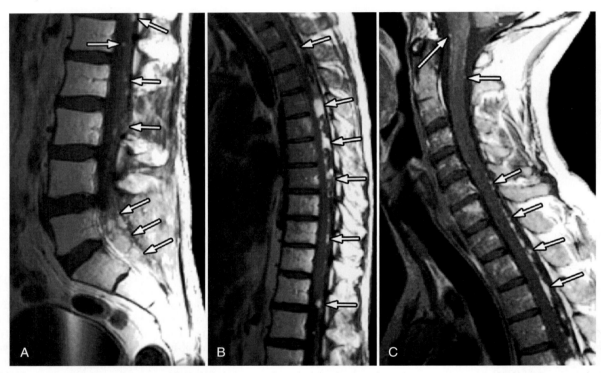

Figure 42-13 ► **Lumbosacral Ependymoma with Cephalad Leptomeningeal Dissemination.** The primary tumor was an intradural ependymoma at the L5-S1 level (*lower 3 arrows on sagittal contrast enhanced T1-weighted image* **A**).Tiny upper lumbar leptomeningeal tumors are indicated by upper lumbar arrows on image **A**. Multiple small nodular and coalescent enhancing leptomeningeal ependymomas (*arrows*) are demonstrated in the thoracic region and cervical region on contrast enhanced sagittal images **B** and **C**.

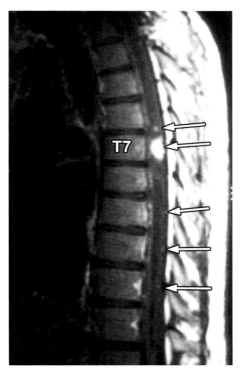

Figure 42-14 ▶ Multiple Hemangioblastomas. Sagittal contrast enhanced T1-weighted MR image. Relatively large intramedullary lesion at the T7 level and tiny enhancing lesions above and below are visible along the cord surface (*arrows*). Note T1 hypointense spinal cord syrinx above and below the T7 level.

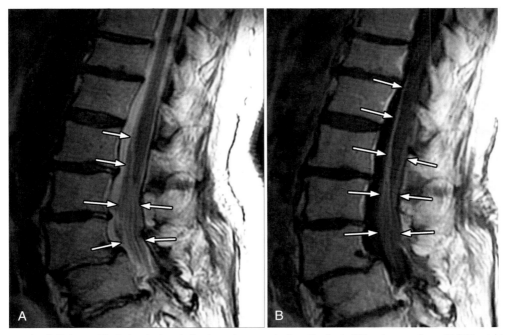

Figure 42-15 ▶ Paraneoplastic Polyneuritis. Patient had markedly elevated paraneoplastic antibodies in CSF and serum. On sagittal T2-weighted image **A**, the cauda equina roots (*arrows*) are thickened. On sagittal T1-weighted image **B**, the cauda equina nerve roots and pial surface of the lower spinal cord enhance uniformly (*arrows*).

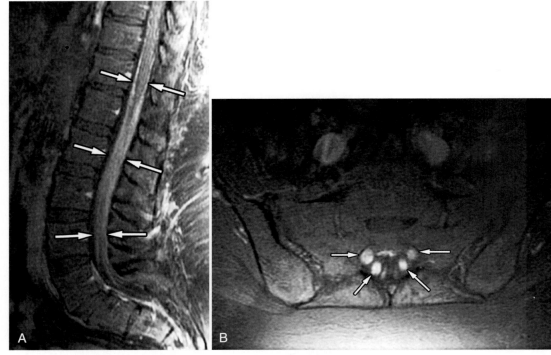

Figure 42-16 ▶ Chronic Inflammatory Demyelinating Polyradiculoneuropathy (CIDP). Diffuse enhancement (*arrows*) is seen along the pial surface of the spinal cord and cauda equina nerve roots on contrast enhanced sagittal T1-weighted image **A**. On axial image **B**, obtained through the S1 level, the nerve roots (*arrows*) enhance uniformly and symmetrically.

therapy must always be taken into consideration in planning the therapeutic approach.

1. **Conservative, supportive care:** Analgesics, steroids, and anticonvulsants are administered when judged to be appropriate.
2. **Intrathecal chemotherapy:** Often administered if the tumor is chemosensitive (e.g., small cell lung carcinoma or lymphoma). The agent can be given via repeated lumbar punctures or through a ventriculostomy catheter (e.g., Ommayo reservoir). Obtaining a radionuclide flow study with indium-111 diethylenetriaminepentaacetic acid (DTPA) is recommended before instituting intrathecal chemotherapy to determine whether a normal CSF flow pattern exists.[1] If an abnormal CSF flow pattern is present, the chemotherapeutic agent may not reach its intended target, and other therapeutic approaches, such as radiotherapy, should be considered. Complications such as aseptic meningitis or leukoencephalopathy may develop in a minority of patients after intrathecal chemotherapy.
3. **Radiotherapy**: May be administered alone or with chemotherapy. The radiotherapy is given to the whole brain, entire spinal axis, or focused to symptomatic sites, depending on the location and extent of the leptomeningeal tumor.[1]
4. **Surgery:** Surgical biopsy is rarely performed to confirm presence of leptomeningeal tumor. A ventriculostomy catheter may be inserted for chemotherapy instillation or ventriculo-peritoneal (VP) shunt if hydrocephalus develops in the patient.
5. **Investigational therapies:** Including intrathecal immunotherapy (e.g., with cytokines or monoclonal antibodies) and intrathecal radioimmunotherapy (e.g., radioisotopes

conjugated with monoclonal antibodies) have been used in some patients.[32,33]

References

1. O'Meara WP, Borkar SA, Stambuk HE, Lymberis SC. Leptomeningeal metastasis. *Curr Probl Cancer.* 2007;31(6):367-424.
2. Yousem DM, Patrone PM, Grossman RI. Leptomeningeal metastases: MR evaluation. *J Comput Assist Tomogr.* 1990;14(2):255-261.
3. Deinsberger R, Regatschnig R, Kaiser B, Bankl HC. Spinal leptomeningeal metastases from prostate cancer. *Acta Neurochir (Wien).* 2006;148(4):467-471.
4. Petrovic BD, Kozic DB, Semnic RR, et al. Leptomeningeal metastasis from malignant pleural mesothelioma. *AJNR Am J Neuroradiol.* 2004;25(7):1223-1224.
5. Schluterman KO, Fassas AB, Van Hemert RL, Harik SI. Multiple myeloma invasion of the central nervous system. *Arch Neurol.* 2004;61(9):1423-1429.
6. Schneider F, Putzier M. Primary leptomeningeal melanoma. *Spine.* 2002;27(24):E545-E547.
7. Davies CL, Chinn R, Nelson M, et al. Outcome in AIDS-related systemic non-Hodgkin lymphoma and leptomeningeal disease is not predicted by a CT brain scan. *AJNR Am J Neuroradiol.* 2007;28(10):1988-1990.
8. Gardiman MP, Fassan M, Orvieto E, et al. Diffuse leptomeningeal glioneuronal tumors: A new entity? *Brain Pathol.* 2010;20(2):361-366. Epub 2009, May 22.
9. Kesari S, Batchelor TT. Leptomeningeal metastases. *Neurol Clin.* 2003;21(1):25-66.
10. Armao DM, Stone J, Castillo M, et al. Diffuse leptomeningeal oligodendrogliomatosis: Radiologic/pathologic correlation. *AJNR Am J Neuroradiol.* 2000;21(6):1122-1226.
11. Courcoutsakis NA, Prassopoulos PK, Patronas NJ. Aggressive leptomeningeal hemangioblastomatosis of the central nervous system in a patient with von Hippel-Lindau disease. *AJNR Am J Neuroradiol.* 2009;30(4):758-760.
12. Bakshi R, Mechtler LL, Patel MJ, et al. Spinal leptomeningeal hemangioblastomatosis in von Hippel-Lindau disease: Magnetic resonance and pathological findings. *J Neuroimaging.* 1997;7(4):242-244.

13. Lee W, Chang KH, Choe G, et al. MR imaging features of clear-cell meningioma with diffuse leptomeningeal seeding. *AJNR Am J Neuroradiol.* 2000;21(1):130-132.
14. Shalay KM, Parikh JR. Meningeal myelomatosis. *Can Assoc Radiol J.* 1994;45(6):460-462.
15. Herrlinger U, Forschler H, Kuker W, et al. Leptomeningeal metastasis: Survival and prognostic factors in 155 patients. *J Neurol Sci.* 2004;223(2):167-178.
16. Olson ME, Chernik NL, Posner JB. Infiltration of the leptomeninges by systemic cancer: A clinical and pathologic study. *Arch Neurol.* 1974;30(2):122-137.
17. van der Ree TC, Dippel DW, Avezaat CJ, et al. Leptomeningeal metastasis after surgical resection of brain metastases. *J Neurol Neurosurg Psychiatry.* 1999;66(2):225-227.
18. Norris LK, Grossman SA, Olivi A. Neoplastic meningitis following surgical resection of isolated cerebellar metastasis: A potentially preventable complication. *J Neurooncol.* 1997;32(3):215-223.
19. Connolly ES, Jr., Winfree CJ, McCormick PC, et al. Intramedullary spinal cord metastasis: Report of three cases and review of the literature. *Surg Neurol.* 1996;46(4):329-337; discussion 37-38.
20. Glass JP, Melamed M, Chernik NL, Posner JB. Malignant cells in cerebrospinal fluid (CSF): The meaning of a positive CSF cytology. *Neurology.* 1979;29(10):1369-1375.
21. Jaeckle KA. Assessment of tumor markers in cerebrospinal fluid. *Clin Lab Med.* 1985;5(2):303-315.
22. Wasserstrom WR, Glass JP, Posner JB. Diagnosis and treatment of leptomeningeal metastases from solid tumors: Experience with 90 patients. *Cancer.* 1982;49(4):759-772.
23. Sze G. Leptomeningeal tumor: The "plain vanilla" approach remains the best. *AJNR Am J Neuroradiol.* 2002;23(5):745-746.
24. Straathof CS, de Bruin HG, Dippel DW, Vecht CJ. The diagnostic accuracy of magnetic resonance imaging and cerebrospinal fluid cytology in leptomeningeal metastasis. *J Neurol.* 1999;246(9):810-814.
25. Collie DA, Brush JP, Lammie GA, et al. Imaging features of leptomeningeal metastases. *Clin Radiol.* 1999;54(11):765-771.
26. Chamberlain MC, Sandy AD, Press GA. Leptomeningeal metastasis: A comparison of gadolinium-enhanced MR and contrast-enhanced CT of the brain. *Neurology.* 1990;40(3 Pt 1):435-438.
27. Heinz R, Wiener D, Friedman H, Tien R. Detection of cerebrospinal fluid metastasis: CT myelography or MR? *AJNR Am J Neuroradiol.* 1995;16(5):1147-1151.
28. Singh SK, Leeds NE, Ginsberg LE. MR imaging of leptomeningeal metastases: comparison of three sequences. *AJNR Am J Neuroradiol.* 2002;23(5):817-821.
29. Leifer D, Grabowski T, Simonian N, Demirjian ZN. Leptomeningeal myelomatosis presenting with mental status changes and other neurologic findings. *Cancer.* 1992;70(7):1899-1904.
30. Komori T, Delbeke D. Leptomeningeal carcinomatosis and intramedullary spinal cord metastases from lung cancer: Detection with FDG positron emission tomography. *Clin Nucl Med.* 2001;26(11):905-907.
31. Olsan AD, Milburn JM, Baumgarten KL, Durham HL. Leptomeningeal enhancement in a patient with proven West Nile virus infection. *AJR Am J Roentgenol.* 2003;181(2):591-592.
32. Chamberlain MC. A phase II trial of intra-cerebrospinal fluid alpha interferon in the treatment of neoplastic meningitis. *Cancer.* 2002;94(10):2675-2680.
33. Coakham HB, Kemshead JT. Treatment of neoplastic meningitis by targeted radiation using (131)I-radiolabelled monoclonal antibodies: Results of responses and long term follow-up in 40 patients. *J Neurooncol.* 1998;38(2-3):225-232.

CHAPTER 43

LIPOMA

Douglas S. Fenton, M.D.

CLINICAL PRESENTATION

The patient is a 52-year-old female with symptoms of progressive decrease in strength in both legs and urinary incontinence. There is no history of antecedent trauma. No recent infection or vaccinations. She had a similar bout of leg weakness and urinary incontinence, although much less severe, 25 years ago when she was pregnant. These symptoms went away approximately 3 months postpartum. On physical examination, the patient has a decrease in sensation from approximately T2 inferiorly. Her gait is slightly broad-based and there is symmetric, mild lower extremity weakness.

IMAGING PRESENTATION

Sagittal T1- and fat-saturated, T2-weighted magnetic resonance (MR) images reveal an oblong intraspinal mass with increased T1 signal intensity and low signal intensity on the fat-saturated acquisition. A nonfat-saturated, T2-weighted sequence (not pictured) revealed the mass to be of increased signal intensity. The mass has the imaging characteristics of fat and represents an intradural lipoma (*Fig. 43-1*).

DISCUSSION

Intradural lipomas of the spinal canal are rare and comprise less than 1% of all primary tumors of the spine.[1] Vertebral, dermal, and renal abnormalities are not a feature of intradural lipomas because they, along with other fatty neoplasms, are associated with spinal dysraphism.[2] Of all fatty neoplasms of the spinal canal, intradural lipomas account for 4% of the tumors, lipomyelomeningoceles for 84%, and lipomas of the filum terminale for 12%.[3] Intradural spinal lipomas have nearly equal gender preference with a very slight female predominance.[1,4] They most commonly manifest in the second and third decades of life (55%), and to a lesser extent in the first year of life (24%) and fifth decade of life (16%).[4] The thoracic region is most commonly involved in adults (32%), followed by the cervicothoracic region (24%), and cervical region (13%).[4] Intradural spinal lipomas are usually posterior (67%) or posterolateral (23%) to the spinal cord.[5] The cervical region is most commonly involved in children.[6]

There is debate as to the embryology of intradural spinal lipomas. It is thought that lipomas develop when there is premature dysjunction of the cutaneous ectoderm from the forming neural tube. The surrounding mesenchyme migrates underneath the ectoderm into the neural tube and adheres to the primitive ependyma, which induces it to dedifferentiate into fat. Normally, the mesenchyme migrates into the space between the neural tube and superficial ectoderm and differentiates into the vasculature for the spinal cord, meninges, and vertebral column.[7-9] Histologically, intradural spinal lipomas consist of mature fat cells separated by connective tissue strands and are partially to fully encapsulated.[7,10] The lipoma is admixed with nerve bundles that are often located at the periphery, which suggests secondary entrapment of adjacent nerve roots.[11] Although these lipomas are not considered neoplastic, they can demonstrate autonomous, slow growth. The fat of these lipomas is metabolically active like fat in the rest of the body. Growth of these lipomas can be seen with an increase in body fat and are associated with the metabolic changes of pregnancy.[4,10,12]

The clinical course of patients with intradural spinal lipomas is one of slow progression of myelopathic symptoms.[4] Fifty-five to sixty-eight percent of patients become symptomatic in the first three decades of life.[4,13] Patients often present with a long history of disabilities that rapidly progress prior to them seeking medical attention. Symptoms include spinal pain, sensory changes, loss of positional sense, gait disturbance, weakness, hypotonia, and incontinence.[11,14] Early gait disturbance is caused by dorsal column dysfunction (secondary to the posterior location of most lipomas) rather than weakness in the legs.[4,15] The most frequently reported symptoms are numbness or spastic weakness in the extremities.[4] Radicular pain is uncommon.[4]

IMAGING FEATURES

Magnetic resonance imaging (MRI) is the imaging modality of choice. The mass is readily identified, as are its location and effect on the spinal cord, other nervous tissue, and vasculature. Intradural lipomas often appear as round or lobulated masses that display signal characteristics of normal fat. The spinal canal may demonstrate widening in the region of the mass because of chronic pressure erosion. The mass is of increased signal intensity on T1- and T2-weighted acquisitions, and displays low signal intensity on both sequences when a fat-saturation technique or short tau inversion recovery (STIR) technique is applied (see Fig. 43-1). Lipomas do not demonstrate contrast enhancement. If the fatty mass demonstrates a region of contrast enhancement, then a more ominous

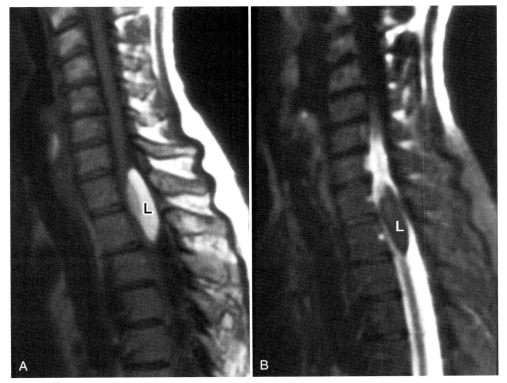

Figure 43-1 ▶ Intradural Lipoma. Ovoid intradural mass (*L*) in the upper thoracic spine of primarily increased T1 signal intensity on image **A** and of uniformly low signal intensity on sagittal fat-saturated, T2-weighted image **B** compatible with a fatty mass/lipoma.

etiology such as liposarcoma should be entertained. The adjacent spinal cord may be compressed or appear stretched. There may be increased T2 signal in the intrinsic cord compatible with cord ischemic change or myelomalacia. Computerized tomography (CT) demonstrates spinal lipomas as a lobulated/ovoid hypodense (fat density Hounsfield unit) mass (*Fig. 43-2*). CT does not identify the relationship of the mass to the spinal cord and nerve roots as well as MRI. Myelography does not identify the mass but demonstrates the effect of the mass on the dural sac and spinal cord. When viewed in a plane parallel to the mass and spinal cord, an intradural extramedullary mass will appear as a negative defect in the spinal column with widening of the contrast-filled space immediately cephalad and caudad to the mass, between the dural sac and the negative defect from the spinal cord (*Fig. 43-3*). The addition of CT to myelography gives only marginally more benefit than CT alone. Ultrasound can be used in infants suspected of having a spinal lipoma. Ultrasound, unlike CT, does not use ionizing radiation, and it is unnecessary to sedate an infant for an ultrasound examination, unlike MRI. A lipoma will appear as an echogenic mass.

DIFFERENTIAL DIAGNOSIS

1. **Dermoid cysts** arise from misplaced ectodermal elements in early gestation. They can contain hair follicles, sebaceous glands, and sweat glands. The oil from sebaceous glands can have similar imaging characteristics to fat; however, dermoids are typically of mixed density/signal intensity (*Fig. 43-4*).

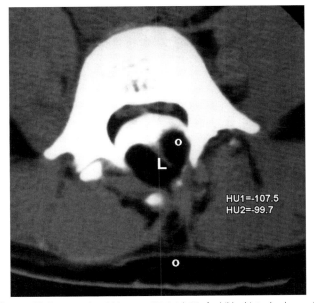

HU1=-107.5
HU2=-99.7

Figure 43-2 ▶ Intradural Lipoma, CT. Axial CT of a bibbed intradural mass (*L*) in the lower lumbar spine with a very low Hounsfield measurement (HU = −107.5) similar to the Hounsfield measurement of subcutaneous fat (HU = −99.7).

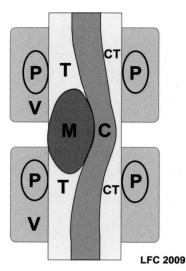

LFC 2009

Figure 43-3 ► **Intradural, Extramedullary Mass.** Coronal view. Intradural mass (*M*) displaces the spinal cord (*C*) laterally. There is widening of the CSF-filled space (*T*) both immediately cephalad and caudad to the mass with acute angles between the mass and the spinal cord and between the mass and the wall of the thecal sac. The thecal sac contralateral to the side of the mass (*CT*) is narrowed both cephalad and caudad to the level of the mass. *P* = vertebral pedicle; *V* = vertebral body. (Image courtesy of Leo F. Czervionke, M.D.)

2. **Lipoma of the filum terminale** can be found in the filum terminale anywhere from the lower thoracic spine through the sacrum. It can be associated with spinal dysraphism and tethered cord (*Fig. 43-5*).
3. **Lipomyelomeningoceles** are spinal dysraphisms where the intraspinal fat is connected through the dysraphism with subcutaneous fat (*Fig. 43-6*). There are often cutaneous stigmata associated with lipomyelomeningoceles.

TREATMENT

1. **Subtotal surgical excision** is the treatment of choice for symptomatic intradural spinal lipoma. Complete excision cannot be obtained because of frequent entrapment of the spinal nerve roots and the close adherence of the tumor to the spinal cord. Complete excision is associated with higher rates of neurologic damage. Surgeons may use sensory evoked potential (SEP) monitoring intraoperatively to minimize neurologic injury. The goal of surgical treatment is to halt progression of neurologic deficits. Because patients do not typically normalize postoperatively, there are those who believe that surgery should be performed in asymptomatic patients when a lipoma is discovered.
2. **Weight reduction** has been attempted to reduce the size of the lipoma; however, this has been questioned by the observation of rapid growth of a lipoma despite severe diet control.[12,16]

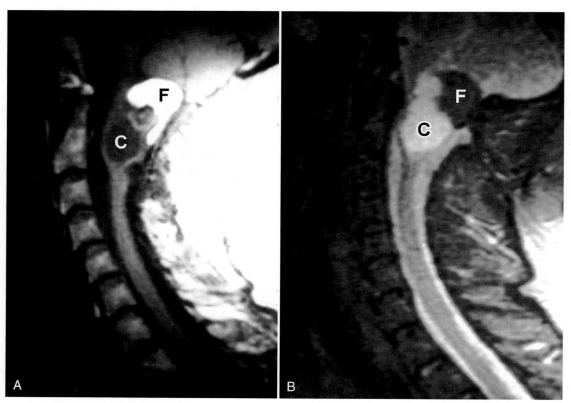

Figure 43-4 ► **Dermoid Cyst.** This mass is typically of mixed signal intensity having fatty and cystic components. Sagittal T1 image **A** and sagittal gradient recall image **B** demonstrate a large mixed signal intensity upper cervical mass with fat signal intensity (increased T1, decreased gradient) superiorly (*F*) and fluid-like signal intensity (decreased T1, increased gradient) inferiorly (*C*).

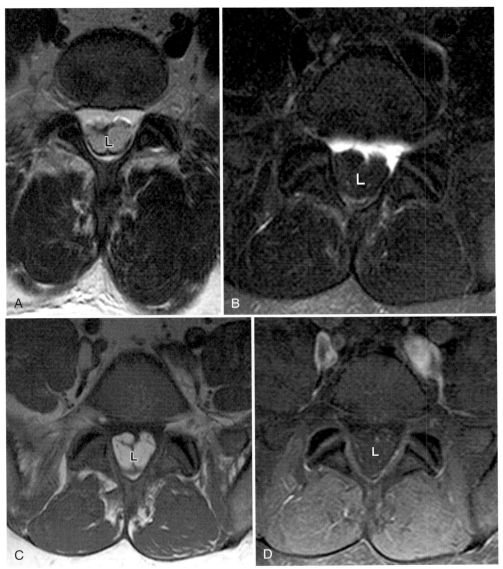

Figure 43-5 ▶ **Lipoma of Filum Terminale.** Bilobed fatty mass (lipoma of the filum terminale (*L*) in the lower lumbar spine. Axial T2 (**A**), axial T2 fat-saturated (**B**), axial T1 (**C**), axial T1 post-contrast, fat-saturated (**D**). Typical MR appearance of fat is of increased T1 (**C**) and T2 signal (**B**). Fat-saturated technique will cause uniform decrease in signal of a fatty mass (**B** and **D**). Furthermore, a purely fatty mass does not enhance (**D**).

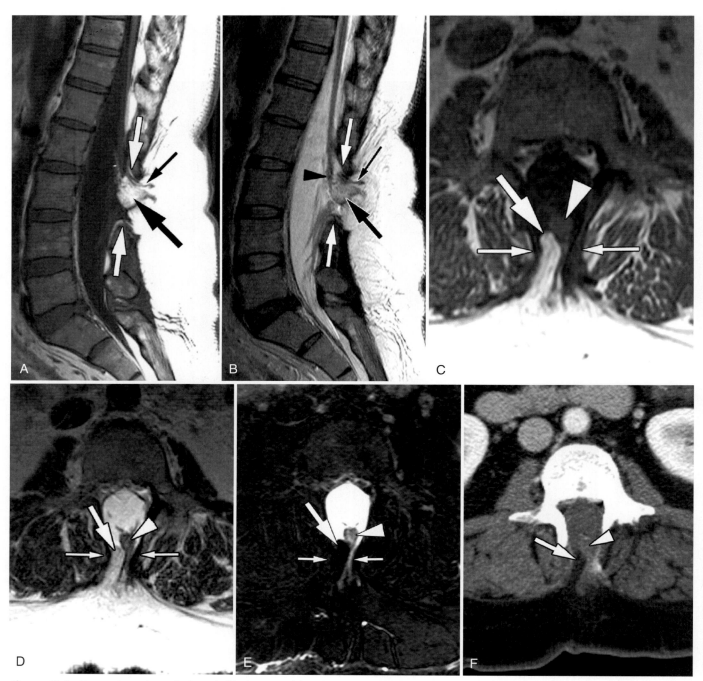

Figure 43-6 ▶ Lipomyelomeningocele. Intraspinal fat is connected through a dysraphism with subcutaneous fat. Sagittal T1-weighted image **A** and sagittal T2-weighted image **B** show a low-lying spinal cord (*arrowhead*, **B**) tethered to intraspinal fat (*large black arrow*) with neural elements (*small black arrow*, **A** and **B**) entering through a spinal dysraphism (*between white arrows*, **A** and **B**). Axial T1 image **C**, axial T2 image **D**, and axial T2 fat-saturated image **E** demonstrate the intraspinal fat (*large white arrow*) connected to the subcutaneous fat through a spinal dysraphism (*between small white arrows*). The low-lying terminus of the spinal cord (*white arrowhead*) is adjacent to the intraspinal fat and within the spinal dysraphism. Axial CT image **F** of same patient shows the characteristic low density of the intraspinal fat (*arrow*) adjacent to the spinal cord terminus (*arrowhead*) within the dysraphism.

References

1. Ehni G, Love JG. Intraspinal lipomas: Report of cases; review of the literature, and clinical and pathologic study. *Arch Neurol Psychiatry.* 1945;53: 1-28.
2. Johnson RE, Roberson GH. Subpial lipoma of the spinal cord. *Radiology.* 1974;111:121-125.
3. Bulsara KR, Zomorodi AR, Villavicencio AT, et al. Clinical outcome differences for lipomyelomeningoceles, intraspinal lipomas, and lipomas of the filum terminale. *Neurosurg Rev.* 2001;24:192-194.
4. Giuffre R. Intradural spinal lipomas: Review of the literature (99 cases) and report of an additional case. *Acta Neurochir (Wien).* 1966;14:69-95.
5. Fan CJ, Veerapen RJ, Tan CT. Case report: Subdural spinal lipoma with posterior fossa extension. *Clin Radiol.* 1989;40:91-94.
6. Blount JP, Elton S. Spinal lipomas. *Neurosurg Focus.* 2001;10(1):e3.
7. Naidich TP, Zimmerman RA, McLone DG, et al. Congenital anomalies of the spine and spinal cord. In: Atlas SW, ed. *Magnetic resonance imaging of the brain and spine.* 2nd ed. Philadelphia: Lippincott-Raven; 1996:1265-1337.
8. Bhatoe HS, Singh P, Chaturvedi A, et al. Nondysraphic intramedullary spinal cord lipomas: A review. *Neurosurg Focus.* 2005;18:ECP1.
9. Muthusubramanian V, Pande A, Vasudevan MC, Ramamurthi R. Concomitant cervical and lumbar intradural intramedullary lipoma. *Surg Neurol.* 2008;69:314-317.
10. Klekamp J, Fusco M, Samii M. Thoracic intradural extramedullary lipomas: Report of three cases and review of the literature. *Acta Neurochir (Wien).* 2001;143:767-774.
11. Ammerman BJ, Henry JM, DeGirolami U, Earle KM. Intradural lipomas of the spinal cord: A clinicopathological correlation. *J Neurosurg.* 1976;44: 331-336.
12. Giudicelli Y, Pierre-Khan A, Bourdeaux AM, et al. Are the metabolic characteristics of congenital intraspinal lipoma cells identical to, or different from normal adipocytes? *Childs Nerv Syst.* 1986;2:290-296.
13. Heary RF, Bhandari Y. Intradural cervical lipoma in a neurologically intact patient: Case report. *Neurosurgery.* 1991;29:468-472.
14. Wood BP, Harwood-Nash, DC, Berger P, Goske M. Intradural spinal lipoma of the cervical cord. *AJR Am J Radiol.* 1985;145:174-176.
15. Lantos G, Epstein FE, Kory LA. Magnetic resonance imaging of intradural spinal lipoma. *Neurosurgery.* 1987;20:469-472.
16. Aoki N. Rapid growth of intraspinal lipoma demonstrated by magnetic resonance imaging. *Surg Neurol.* 1990;34:107-110.

LONGUS COLLI TENDINITIS

Douglas S. Fenton, M.D.

CLINICAL PRESENTATION

The patient is a 50-year-old female who presented with acute neck and shoulder pain. Over the last 2 weeks, she has noticed progressive, constant pain in the anterior midline aspect of her upper neck. She characterizes the pain as a dull ache. She has been having episodes of sharp neck pain that can be brought on by turning her head toward the right or the left or looking up. She notes intermittent, mild radiation of the pain into both of her shoulders. She describes some pain with swallowing. She does not confirm any weakness, numbness, or tingling in her arms, hands, or lower extremities. She has had no fever, chills, night sweats, weight loss, nausea, vomiting, diarrhea, changes in vision, syncope, or near syncope.

IMAGING PRESENTATION

Sagittal and axial computed tomography (CT) images of the upper cervical spine reveal a small amorphic calcific density ventral to the dens and inferior to the anterior arch of C1. There is associated very mild prevertebral soft tissue swelling. These imaging characteristics and the location of this finding are pathognomonic of longus colli tendinitis (*Fig. 44-1*).

DISCUSSION

Acute calcific tendinitis is an inflammatory condition caused by deposition of calcium hydroxyapatite crystals in the longus colli muscle. Acute calcific tendinitis, also known as *retropharyngeal calcific tendinitis, acute calcific prevertebral tendinitis*, or *longus colli tendinitis*, is a fairly uncommon condition. It is an under-recognized cause of acute cervical pain produced by inflammation of the longus colli muscle.[1] Patient may present with neck pain, dysphagia, or odynophagia and low grade fever. Laboratory evaluation may demonstrate a mildly elevated white blood cell count and a mildly elevated sedimentation rate.

Acute calcific tendinitis was first described by Hartley[2] in 1964. The etiology of calcium hydroxyapatite crystal deposition is unknown; however, some postulate that repetitive trauma, recent injury, tissue necrosis, or ischemia may play a factor.[3] It is thought that the crystals, once deposited within the longus colli muscle, start a foreign body–like inflammatory reaction.[4]

The primary differential diagnosis to exclude is retropharyngeal abscess. A retropharyngeal abscess is most likely to occur in infants, although it can occur in adults with the main cause being pharyngitis, tonsillitis, or a foreign body in the pharynx.[1] Other distinguishing features of acute calcific tendinitis are the lack of ring enhancement of the effusion, the lack of associated adenopathy, and the symmetric expansion of the prevertebral/retropharyngeal space by the effusion. The pathognomonic finding of acute calcific tendinitis is the amorphic calcification anterior to C1-2 in the superior oblique muscle where the longus colli tendon inserts.

IMAGING FEATURES

The principle radiographic findings of acute calcific tendinitis are prevertebral soft tissue swelling, typically extending from C1-C4, and a focus of amorphic calcification anterior to C1-2. The soft tissue swelling can be due either to an effusion or edema. Acute calcific tendinitis must be distinguished from a retropharyngeal abscess because they both can manifest similarly—swelling of the retropharyngeal wall, cervical pain, neck stiffness, sore throat, and fever—but they have very different treatments. The lack of enhancement surrounding the effusion is helpful because enhancement is not seen around the effusion in acute calcific tendinitis and is seen with abscess. The effusion also usually causes uniform expansion of the retropharyngeal space and may dissect through the fascia in a coronal plane. Retropharyngeal lymphadenopathy is associated with abscess and not with acute calcific tendonitis.[5] The amorphic calcification anterior to C1-2, where the superior oblique muscle of the longus colli tendon inserts, is pathognomonic for acute calcific tendinitis. Plain film radiography can demonstrate the amorphic calcification. Computed tomography (CT) with its superior spatial resolution demonstrates the amorphic calcification definitively as well as the effusion and/or edema and is the procedure of choice (see Fig. 44-1). Intravenous contrast should be given if there is clinical concern of abscess. Magnetic resonance (MR) imaging is usually not necessary to make the diagnosis, but can sometimes demonstrate increased T2 or short tau inversion recovery (STIR) signal intensity in the adjacent vertebra secondary to marrow reactive change as well as increased T2/STIR signal in the prevertebral soft tissues from soft tissue edema (*Fig. 44-2*).[6]

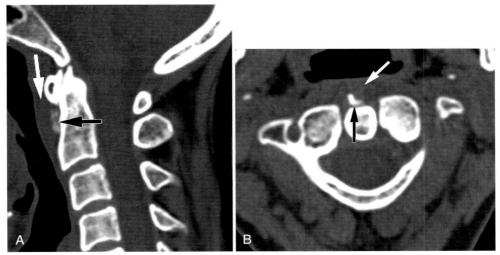

Figure 44-1 ► **Longus Colli Tendinitis.** Sagittal CT image **A** and axial CT image **B** demonstrate a small amorphic region of calcification in the midline just anterior to the dens (*black arrow*) with mild edematous changes in the prevertebral soft tissues (*white arrow*) with very slight mass effect on the posterior oral airway.

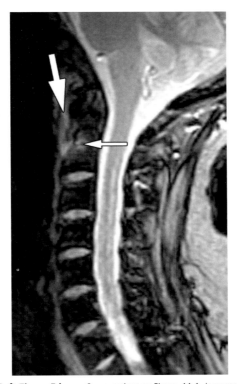

Figure 44-2 ► **Vertebral Marrow Reaction and Soft Tissue Edema.** Same patient as Figure 44-1. Increased signal intensity seen in the ventral dens (*small arrow*). Increased signal intensity also seen in the prevertebral soft tissues anterior to C1-C2 compatible with edema and/or effusion (*large arrow*).

DIFFERENTIAL DIAGNOSIS

1. **Retropharyngeal abscess:** Often retropharyngeal abscess has an associated rounded fluid collection with rim enhancement. The effusion of calcific tendonitis does not enhance (*Fig. 44-3*).

2. **Infectious/inflammatory spondylitis**: The inflammation is often centered on the intervertebral disc. There may be increased T2 signal intensity in the disc as well as enhancement of the prevertebral soft tissues (*Fig. 44-4*).

3. **Traumatic injury:** This can be ruled out with patient history and imaging.

4. **Foreign body aspiration:** This will be evident at patient history, direct visualization, or imaging.

5. **Retropharyngeal effusion/edema:** This can be caused by jugular vein thrombosis, radiation therapy, or retropharyngeal adenitis.

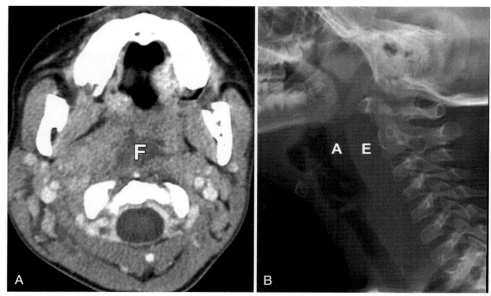

Figure 44-3 ▶ **Retropharyngeal Abscess.** Axial CT, image **A**. Midline retropharyngeal fluid collection with obliteration of the normal soft tissue/fat planes. Lateral radiograph image **B** shows significant widening of the prevertebral soft tissues (*E*) compatible with edema causing ventral bowing of the posterior wall of the airway (*A*).

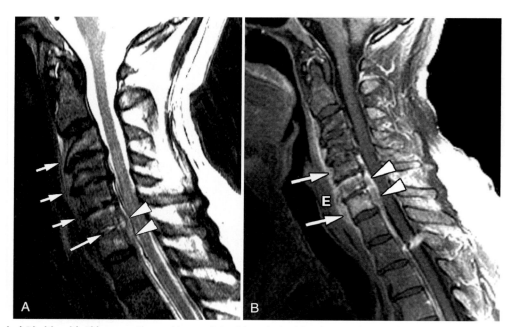

Figure 44-4 ▶ **Cervical Discitis with Phlegmon.** Abnormal increased signal intensity involving the C6 and C7 vertebral bodies on sagittal fat-saturated ,T2-weighted image **A**. There is also increased signal intensity within the C6-7 disc (*large arrow*) and ventral epidural soft tissue (*arrowheads*). Prevertebral increased T2 signal intensity (*small arrows*). Post-contrast, fat-saturated, T1-weighted image **B** shows diffuse enhancement of the C6 and C7 vertebral bodies consistent with discitis/osteomyelitis. There is enhancement of the ventral epidural soft tissue (*arrowheads*) and the prevertebral soft tissue (*arrows*) compatible with phlegmon. Nonenhancing soft tissue (*E*) is seen posterior to the airway compatible with retropharyngeal edema.

TREATMENT

Nonoperative management: Acute calcific tendinitis is a self-limited condition and spontaneously resolves within 1 to 2 weeks.[7] Conservative treatment includes nonsteroidal anti-inflammatory medications and avoiding painful neck movements.

References

1. Kusunoki T, Muramoto D, Murata K. A case of calcific retropharyngeal tendinitis suspected to be a retropharyngeal abscess upon the first medical examination. *Auris Nasus Larynx*. 2006;33:329-331.
2. Hartley J. Acute cervical pain associated with retropharyngeal calcium deposit: A case report. *J Bone Joint Surg Am*. 1964;46:1753-1754.
3. DeMaeseneer M, Vregde S, Laureys S, et al. Calcific tendinitis of the longus colli muscle. *Head Neck*. 1997;19:545-548.
4. Ring D, Vaccaro AR, Scuderi G, et al. Acute calcific retropharyngeal tendinitis: Clinical presentation and pathological characterization. *J Bone Joint Surg Am*. 1994;76:1636-1642.
5. Eastwood JD, Hudgins PA, Malone D. Retropharyngeal effusion in acute calcific prevertebral tendinitis: Diagnosis with CT and MR imaging. *AJNR Am J Neuroradiol*. 1998;19:1789-1792.
6. Mihmanli I, Karaarslan E, Kanberoglu K. Inflammation of vertebral bone associated with acute calcific tendinitis of the longus colli muscle. *Neurorad*. 2001;32:1098-1101.
7. Chung T, Rebello R, Gooden EA. Retropharyngeal calcific tendinitis: Case report and review of literature. *Emerg Radiol*. 2005;11:375-380.

LYMPHADENOPATHY

Douglas S. Fenton, M.D.

CLINICAL PRESENTATION

The patient is a 65-year-old male who presented with low back pain (visual analog scale [VAS] = 6/10) and report of mild bilateral knee pain for the last 6 months. There are no radicular symptoms. Patient states that his pain decreases when he is standing and flexing forward at the waist. Pain is worse at night or any time he is recumbent. There are no constitutional symptoms. Complete blood count (CBC) is normal. Patient has no history of cancer.

IMAGING PRESENTATION

Imaging demonstrates a large soft tissue mass in the retroperitoneal space, anterior to the L2 and L3 vertebral bodies, which displaces the inferior vena cava anteriorly and laterally and encircles a portion of the aorta. There is no evidence of adjacent bone destruction. The findings represent a conglomerate of lymph nodes (*Fig. 45-1*).

DISCUSSION

Lymph node evaluation is often performed with computed tomography (CT) or magnetic resonance imaging (MRI). Solitary retroperitoneal lymph nodes greater than 1.0 cm in long axis diameter or greater than 8 mm in short axis diameter are likely to be pathologic.[1-3] If multiple lymph nodes between 0.8 and 1.0 cm in diameter are present, then adenopathy should be suspected.[3] Pathologically enlarged lymph nodes can be caused primarily by lymphoma or may be metastatic resulting from a primary neoplasm. Pelvic retroperitoneal lymphadenopathy may be seen from spread of cervical, prostate, and bladder cancers.[1] Testicular cancer can spread to the renal perihilar regions on the left and the paracaval region just inferior to the right renal vein.[1] Colon, pancreatic, renal, lung, breast cancers, and melanoma frequently metastasize to the retroperitoneal lymph nodes.[1] It can be difficult to differentiate metastatic lymphadenopathy from retroperitoneal lymphoma. The presence of lymph node necrosis favors metastatic disease.[4]

Retroperitoneal lymphadenopathy can be a cause of back pain and extremity pain. Woll and Rankin[5] demonstrated a series of patients who each suffered from severe back pain for several months that was interfering with their sleep. Lying flat was unbearable for these patients, and the only time the symptoms were lessened or relieved was when they were sitting forward. Retroperitoneal

adenopathy was found in these cases, and it was not until these patients began their anticancer treatment with shrinkage of the lymph nodes that their pain subsided. Accordingly, any young patient with severe, persistent back pain that is relieved by sitting forward and without a history of trauma should be evaluated for malignant retroperitoneal lymphadenopathy.[5] Smith and colleagues[6] have had a similar experience in that new abdominal lymphadenopathy was discovered after patients with small cell bronchogenic carcinoma complained of new-onset back pain.

The etiology of lymphadenopathy-induced back pain is uncertain; however, it has been hypothesized that it may be due to direct neural compression or vascular compromise. Retroperitoneal metastatic adenopathy and lymphoma can affect the lumbosacral plexus. The lumbar plexus is formed from the anterior rami of the T12-L5 nerve roots and the sacral plexus is formed by the lumbosacral trunk and the anterior rami of the S1-S5 nerve roots.[7] The lumbar plexus is formed within the psoas major muscle, anterior to the transverse processes of the L2-L5 vertebrae.[7] The lumbosacral plexus can be affected by enlarged lymph nodes by extrinsic compression of the plexus causing low back pain and monoradicular or polyradicular symptoms.[7]

IMAGING FEATURES

Ultrasound has been widely used in imaging lymph nodes; however, there are inherent limitations of the use of ultrasound secondary to the depth in evaluating retroperitoneal lymph nodes and therefore is not the imaging modality of choice. A normal lymph node is a somewhat oval-shaped, hypoechoic, usually hypovascular structure with varying amounts of hilar fat (*Fig. 45-2*). When a node is infiltrated with malignancy, the node becomes rounded and demonstrates peripheral or mixed vascularity (*Fig. 45-3*).[8] Using these criteria, the accuracy of differentiating benign from malignant nodes is in the range of 84% to 94%.[9]

CT and MRI can demonstrate lymph nodes; however, these modalities rely on size criteria rather than function and physiology. The normal lymph node is often less than 1 cm in diameter, has a smooth, well-defined border, and shows uniform, homogeneous density or signal intensity.[10] Most benign nodes have a central fatty hilum seen as decreased density on CT and increased T1 and T2 signal intensity on MRI.[10] However, the size approach to nodal pathology has many false negatives. A lymph node that is only partially infiltrated with metastatic disease may appear "normal" if a size criterion alone is used. Furthermore, an inflammatory lymph

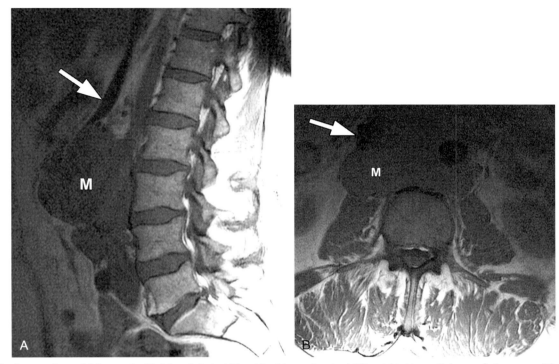

Figure 45-1 ▸ Retroperitoneal Adenopathy L2-3 Level. Sagittal T1-weighted image **A** and axial T1-weighted image **B**. Large soft tissue mass (*M*) ventral to the L2 and L3 vertebral bodies causes anterior displacement of the inferior vena cava (*arrow*).

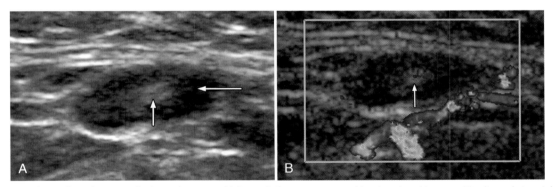

Figure 45-2 ▸ Normal Lymph Node. Longitudinal B-mode sonographic image **A** demonstrates normal lymph node architecture with a hypoechoic periphery (*long arrow*) and hyperechoic fatty central hilus (*short arrow*). Duplex sonogram image **B** demonstrates normal arterial (*red*) and venous (*blue*) flow in the central hilus (*short arrow*).

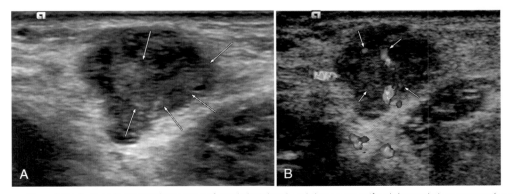

Figure 45-3 ▸ Abnormal Lymph Node. B-mode sonographic image **A** of a pathologic lymph node has a more uniformly hyperechoic appearance (*arrows*). Duplex sonogram image **B** shows increased vascularity (*arrows*).

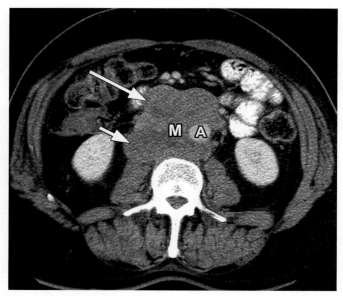

Figure 45-4 ▶ Malignant Lymphadenopathy. Axial CT through the lower lumbar region. Lobular mass of lymph nodes (*M*) surrounding and obliterating the inferior vena cava and encircling the aorta (*A*). The more posterior aspect of the mass (*short arrow*) is of lower density than the ventral portion (*long arrow*).

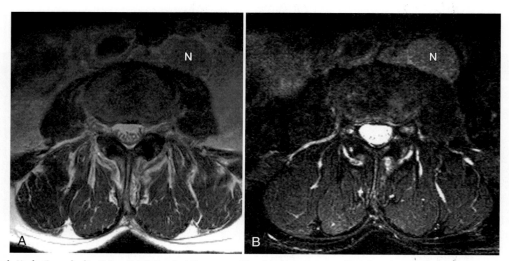

Figure 45-5 ▶ Lymph Node Conspicuity Using Fat-Saturated Sequence. T2-weighted appearance of lymph nodes is dependent on whether standard T2-weighting **A** or fat-saturated, T2-weighting **B** is performed. A lymph node (*N*) can be difficult to appreciate on standard T2-weighted images because it may blend with the adjacent intra-abdominal fat but becomes conspicuous when a fat-saturated pulse sequence is performed.

node can be enlarged and incorrectly classified as a malignant lymph node. Based on size criteria, MRI and CT are equally effective or ineffective in classifying lymph nodes.[11]

Malignant lymph nodes by CT may demonstrate intermediate to decreased density depending on whether there is necrosis *(Fig. 45-4)*. On MRI, lymph nodes are iso- to hypointense on T1-weighted images (see Fig. 45-1) and have variable T2 signal intensity dependent upon necrosis and whether a fat-saturated sequence was used *(Fig. 45-5)*. Lymph nodes demonstrate variable enhancement. Nuclear medicine positron emission tomography

(PET) imaging with ^{18}F-FDG (fluorodeoxyglucose) is of great importance in lymph node imaging. Malignant lymph nodes, with their increased rates of glycolysis, demonstrate avid uptake of FDG *(Fig. 45-6)*. Pieterman and colleagues[12] demonstrated a superior sensitivity and specificity of PET in comparison with CT in detecting lymph node involvement in the staging of lung cancer. However, the imaging resolution of PET alone is low. With the addition of fusion techniques of PET and CT, there has been improvement in the localization of areas of increased radiotracer uptake within lymph nodes.

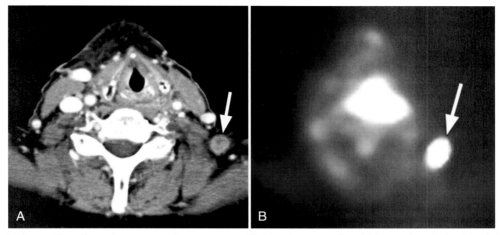

Figure 45-6 ▶ Pathologic Lymph Node. Axial CT image **A** demonstrates a mildly hyperdense, normal-sized left supraclavicular lymph node (*arrow*), which has avid radiotracer uptake on PET image **B**.

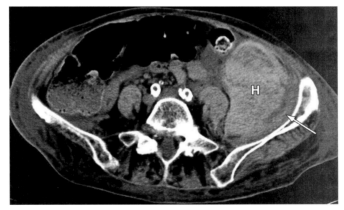

Figure 45-7 ▶ Retroperitoneal Hematoma. Axial noncontrast CT image. Large hyperdense retroperitoneal mass (*H*). The mass does not have discrete borders, as seen with adenopathy, and has an infiltrative appearance, blending borders with an enlarged left iliacus muscle (*arrow*).

DIFFERENTIAL DIAGNOSIS

1. **Retroperitoneal fibrosis** is typically of low T2-weighted signal with minimal enhancement.
2. **Retroperitoneal hematoma** has an infiltrative appearance, often with muscle enlargement (*Fig. 45-7*). It is hyperdense on CT. In its acute stage it is hypointense on both T1- and T2-weighted images and becomes hyperintense on T1-weighed images as it matures. One may see fluid-fluid levels if the patient is anticoagulated.
3. **Extramedullary hematopoiesis** is more paraspinal in location rather than retroperitoneal. It is often a well-defined mass that is iso- to hypointense on T1-weighed images, iso- to hyperintense on T2-weighted images, and can enhance. One should look for diffuse vertebral marrow signal intensity.
4. **Psoas abscess** is often associated with fever and potentially sepsis. The lesion is typically ill-defined, paraspinal, and enhancing and may have a fluid-like center. Gas can occasionally be seen within an abscess cavity (*Fig. 45-8*).
5. **Abdominal aortic aneurysm** typically has a smooth periphery. There may be calcification along the periphery. Contrast CT demonstrates a contrast-filled patent lumen coursing through the larger, rounded *mass* (*Fig. 45-9*). A reformatted sagittal or coronal image will demonstrate continuity of this

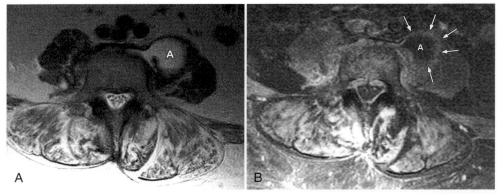

Figure 45-8 ▸ **Psoas Abscess.** Axial T2-weighted image **A** and fat-saturated, T1-weighted image **B** demonstrate a fluid signal intensity region (*A*) in the left psoas muscle with peripheral enhancement (*arrows*).

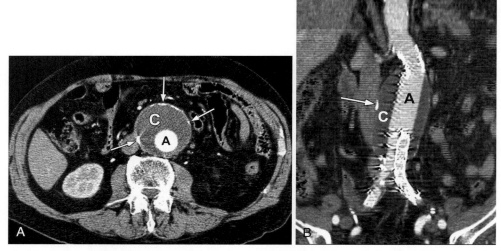

Figure 45-9 ▸ **Abdominal Aortic Aneurysm.** Axial post-contrast CT image **A** and coronal reformatted image **B**. Circumferential low density clot (C) around the contrast-enhanced aorta (*A*). An aortic aneurysm can be distinguished from lymphadenopathy in that the clot of an aneurysm typically surrounds the patent lumen and does not cause mass effect upon the patent aortic lumen. Coronal imaging is helpful with demonstrating the constant relationship of the clotted lumen to the patent lumen. Note the flecks of calcification in the aortic wall (*arrows*).

mass with the normal aorta above and aorta or iliac arteries below.

TREATMENT

The treatment of painful lymphadenopathy depends upon the cause of the lymphadenopathy.

1. **Systemic chemotherapy**
2. **Focused radiation therapy**

References

1. Barker CD, Brown JJ. MR imaging of the retroperitoneum. *Top Magn Reson Imaging*. 1995;7:102-111.
2. Vinnicombe S, Norman A, Husband J, et al. Normal pelvic lymph nodes: Documentation by CT scanning after bipedal lymphangiography. *Radiology*. 1995;194:349-355.
3. Einstein DM, Singer AA, Chilcote WA, Desai RK. Abdominal lymphadenopathy: Spectrum of CT findings. *Radiographics*. 1991;11:457-472.
4. Lee JK, Heiken JP, Ling D, et al. Magnetic resonance imaging of abdominal and pelvic lymphadenopathy. *Radiology*. 1984;153:181-188.
5. Woll PJ, Rankin EM. Persistent back pain due to malignant lymphadenopathy. *Ann Rheum Dis*. 1987;46:681-683.
6. Smith D, Johnson R, James RD, Thatcher N. Upper abdominal lymphadenopathy as first presentation of relapse, identified by ultrasonography in patients treated for small cell (oat cell) bronchogenic carcinoma. *Br J Dis Chest*. 1985;79:141-146.
7. Planner AC, Donaghy M, Moore NR. Causes of lumbosacral plexopathy. *Clin Radiol*. 2006;61:987-995.
8. Ahuja A, Ying M. Sonography of neck lymph nodes. Part II. Abnormal lymph nodes. *Clin Radiol*. 2003;58:359-366.

9. Griffith JF, Chan AC, Ahuja AT, et al. Neck ultrasound in staging squamous oesophageal carcinoma: A high yield technique. *Clin Radiol*. 2000;55: 696-701.

10. Torabi M, Aquino SL, Harisinghani MG. Current concepts in lymph node imaging. *J Nucl Med*. 2004;45:1509-1518.

11. Sohn KM, Lee JM, Lee SY, et al. Comparing MR imaging and CT in the staging of gastric carcinoma. *AJR Am J Roentgenol*. 2000;174:1551-1557.

12. Pieterman RM, van Putten JW, Meuzelaar JJ, et al. Preoperative staging of non-small-cell lung cancer with positron-emission tomography. *N Engl J Med*. 2000;343:254-261.

MALIGNANT (PATHOLOGIC) VERTEBRAL FRACTURE

Douglas S. Fenton, M.D.

CLINICAL PRESENTATION

The patient is a 63-year-old female with a history of thyroid cancer who presented with a recent 3-day history of neck pain, left arm weakness, and numbness of the left upper extremity. There are no symptoms involving the right upper extremity or lower extremities. She has no difficulty walking. There are no bowel or bladder symptoms.

IMAGING PRESENTATION

Sagittal T1-weighted and fat-saturated, T2-weighted images of the cervical spine show collapse of the C5 vertebral body with retropulsion of bone into the spinal canal causing compression and subtle increased T2 signal intensity within the cervical cord. The entire C5 vertebral body is replaced by abnormal decreased T1/increased T2 signal intensity compatible with metastatic disease in this patient with primary thyroid cancer. The increased cord signal intensity is consistent with spinal cord ischemia (*Fig. 46-1*).

DISCUSSION

Spinal fractures are common lesions and are a cause of significant back pain, which can lead to mechanical instability and neurologic deficits, ranging from radiculopathy to spinal cord compression and cauda equina syndrome. Differentiating between malignant and benign causes of a vertebral fracture is a problem that every radiologist faces. Referring physicians often press the radiologist to commit to a diagnosis although often a diagnosis is not obvious. Particularly difficult is the solitary fracture of a vertebral body in an elderly patient with a history of malignancy after minor or no trauma. The patient's advanced age puts him or her at a higher risk for a benign (osteoporotic) fracture; however, the history of malignancy increases the chance that the fracture is pathologic. The correct diagnosis is important with regard to clinical staging (if malignant), treatment, and prognosis.

Both malignant and benign vertebral fractures are just that, fractures, with imaging demonstrating varying degrees of loss of vertebral height. The most common cause of malignant vertebral collapse is metastatic disease from breast carcinoma, bronchogenic carcinoma, prostatic carcinoma, or renal carcinoma.[1,2] The spine is a common site for metastatic disease. Up to 39% of all bone metastases are in the spine.[3] Malignant collapse can also occur as a result of a primary bone neoplasm such as multiple myeloma, solitary plasmacytoma, or lymphoma.[1] Benign compression fractures are typically caused by osteoporosis. Other benign causes include trauma, eosinophilic granuloma, Paget's disease, and hemangioma.[4]

IMAGING FEATURES

Short of evaluating tissue for pathology via percutaneous or open biopsy, the radiologist can make a best guess as to the benignancy or malignancy of a vertebral lesion. Magnetic resonance (MR) imaging is the method of choice for evaluating a marrow infiltrative process such as a pathologic fracture although computed tomography (CT) can be used as well.

MR imaging findings that are suggestive of a malignant compression fracture include a convex bulging of the posterior cortex of the fractured vertebral body (found in 74% of metastatic fractures versus 20% of acute osteoporotic fractures), abnormal signal intensity extending into the pedicle (found in 85% of metastatic fractures versus 51% of acute osteoporotic fractures), or posterior elements (found in 59% of metastatic fractures versus 24% of acute osteoporotic fractures), an epidural mass (found in 74% of metastatic fractures versus 25% of acute osteoporotic fractures), and an associated paraspinal mass (found in 41% of metastatic fractures versus 7% of acute osteoporotic fractures).[5]

MR imaging findings that are suggestive of an acute osteoporotic compression fracture include a low signal intensity band on T1-weighted images that parallel the vertebral endplate (found in 93% of acute osteoporotic fractures versus 44% of metastatic fractures), a region of spared normal bone marrow signal intensity (found in 85% of acute osteoporotic fractures versus 19% of metastatic fractures), a retropulsed posterior bone fragment (found in 60% of acute osteoporotic fractures versus 11% of metastatic fractures), and multiple compression fractures (found in 58% of acute osteoporotic fractures versus 33% of metastatic fractures).[5] A new fracture in a patient with multiple chronic fractures with normal signal intensity makes the new fracture more likely to be an osteoporotic fracture; however, each new fracture must be individually evaluated, because malignant fractures and osteoporotic fractures can exist in the same patient.

CT can be useful for distinguishing between benign and malignant acute vertebral compression fractures. Cortical fractures without associated cortical destruction suggest a benign etiology. This is seen in nearly all acute osteoporotic compression

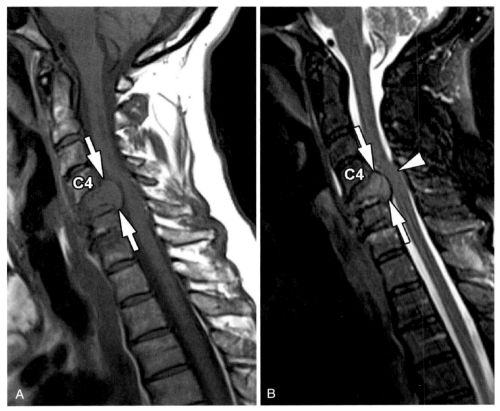

Figure 46-1 ► **Pathologic Fracture with Cord Compression.** Sagittal T1-weighted image **A** and sagittal T2-weighted image **B**. Complete replacement of the C5 vertebral body with pathologic signal (decreased T1, increased T2) and moderate loss of vertebral height. There is retropulsion of pathologic bone (*between arrows*) into the ventral epidural space with spinal cord compression. There is subtle increased T2 signal intensity (*arrowhead*, image **B**) in the cervical cord compatible with cord ischemia.

deformities and in only 9% of malignant compression deformities.[6] Fracture of the cortical bone of a vertebral body has a high diagnostic accuracy (95%) of an osteoporotic fracture, and cortical destruction has a high diagnostic accuracy (97%) for malignancy.[6] Retropulsion of a bone fragment into the spinal canal is seen in 35% of patients with benign compression fractures and in only 3% with malignant compression fractures. Retropulsion of a bone fragment must be distinguished from posterior convex bulging of the cortex seen with malignancy. Gas seen within the fractured vertebral body (gas cleft) is suggestive of a benign etiology, seen in 15% of osteoporotic acute compressions and rarely in malignant compressions.[6,7] Traditionally, it has been taught that a paraspinal soft tissue mass associated with a fracture is a sign of a malignant fracture. However, osteoporotic fractures can often be associated with small paraspinal soft tissues masses in their acute phase. The paraspinal mass with osteoporotic fractures generally surrounds the entire vertebral body, is less than 10 mm in thickness, and is of equal thickness all the way around or slightly more predominant anteriorly.[6] Malignant paraspinal masses are typically more eccentric in shape and involve only a portion of the periphery of the vertebral body.[6,8]

The CT findings more frequently found in malignant acute vertebral compression fractures are destruction of cortical and cancellous bone, destruction of a pedicle, an associated epidural mass, and an eccentric paraspinal mass. Destruction of cancellous bone

and the paraspinal mass have a lower specificity for malignancy than destruction of cortical bone, pedicle destruction, and epidural mass. Destruction of cancellous bone can be seen in up to 29% of patients with osteoporotic acute compression deformities.[6]

MR imaging is the preferred modality for evaluating acute vertebral compressions not only for diagnosing malignant versus benign causes, but also to identify the relationship of the fracture to the spinal cord and nerve roots. Acute malignant compressions demonstrate complete/near complete replacement of the vertebral body with low T1 signal intensity (Fig. 46-1, *A*, and *46-2*). Complete replacement is the rule because malignant fractures usually do not occur until the entire vertebral body is affected. T2 signal can be variable, depending on the type of cancer and whether the lesion is sclerotic, and also depends on whether a fat-suppression technique was used (see Fig. 46-1, *B*). There is often diffuse or patchy heterogeneous enhancement *(Fig. 46-3)*. Similar signal abnormality may be identified involving the pedicles *(Fig. 46-4)*. There may be an associated paraspinal soft tissue or epidural mass. With malignant fractures, the T1 signal intensity does not revert back to normal fatty marrow signal intensity as it does with osteoporotic fractures.

With MR imaging of acute osteoporotic fractures, the rule is that at least one area of normal T1 signal intensity remains in the vertebral body. The benign fracture often appears as a low T1 signal intensity band paralleling the fractured endplate *(Fig. 46-5, A)*.

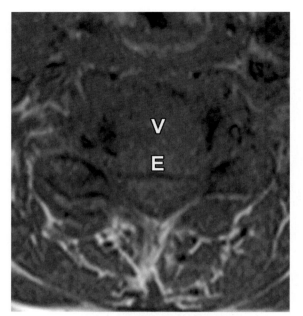

Figure 46-2 ► C5 Vertebral Body Replacement with Epidural Extension. Same patient as in Figure 46-1. Axial T1-weighted image. The vertebral body (*V*) is homogeneously replaced with low signal intensity with extension of pathologic tissue (*E*) into the ventral epidural space.

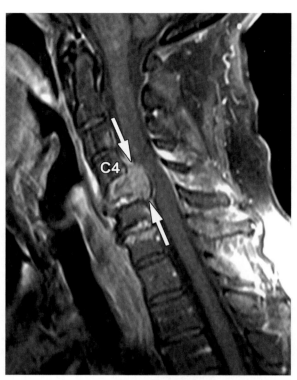

Figure 46-3 ► C5 Vertebral Body Replacement with Epidural Extension. Same patient as in Figures 46-1 and 46-2. Sagittal post-contrast, fat-saturated, T1-weighted image. Diffuse pathologic enhancement of the C5 vertebral body with similar abnormally enhancing soft tissue (*between arrows*) in the ventral epidural space.

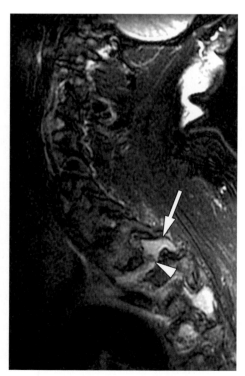

Figure 46-4 ► Pathologic Pedicle Involvement. Off-midline, sagittal, fat-saturated, T2-weighted image. Abnormal increased signal intensity involving the pedicle (*arrowhead*), superior articular process, and inferior articular process (*arrow*) of a single level.

T2-weighted images without fat saturation may appear normal because normal marrow and vertebral edema have similar signal characteristics, whereas the addition of a fat-saturation technique will demonstrate high signal intensity intravertebral edema, which can extend beyond the confines of the low T1 signal band (Fig. 46-5, *B*). Nonfat-saturated, post-contrast, T1-weighted images will demonstrate normalization of the endplate, bandlike signal intensity; however, with the addition of fat saturation, the abnormal bandlike area will enhance (Fig. 46-5, *C*). If there is a retropulsed bone fragment, it typically arises from the posterior superior endplate. One occasionally sees a *fluid sign* adjacent to the fractured endplate on fat-saturated, T2 acquisitions or on short tau inversion recovery (STIR) images. This is likely the same gas-containing structure that can be seen on CT in some fractures. The fluid sign depends on the length of time the patient is recumbent in the MR scanner. If he or she is recumbent for less than 10 minutes, the cleft will be of low T2 signal intensity. If he or she is recumbent for longer than 10 minutes, then the cleft may fill with fluid and appear bright on T2 (*Fig. 46-6*).[4,9] In the chronic phase of osteoporotic fractures, there is a return to normal signals on both T1- and T2-weighted images.

CT can be used in patients that have contraindications to MR imaging. Destruction of the vertebral cortex or pedicle from malignancy can readily be seen because of excellent soft tissue discrimination shown on CT (*Fig. 46-7*). Paraspinal and/or epidural abnormalities can be identified as intermediate density masses, although small epidural abnormalities may be difficult to appreciate.

Sagittal reconstructed CT images demonstrate the typical endplate compression and retropulsed fragment of an osteoporotic

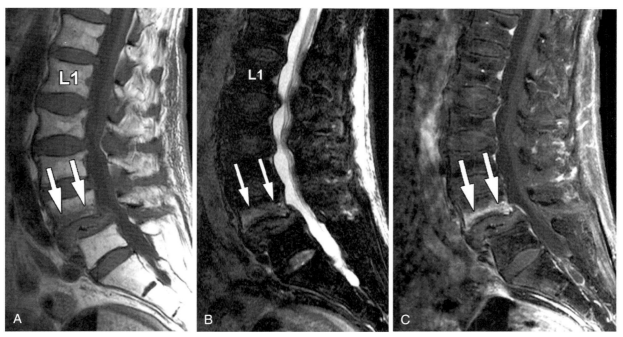

Figure 46-5 ▸ Recent Benign Compression Fracture. Sagittal T1-weighted image **A**, sagittal fat-saturated, T2-weighted image **B** and sagittal fat-saturated, post-contrast, T1-weighted image **C**. *Arrows* point to the band of signal abnormality and enhancement paralleling the mildly compressed inferior endplate. Note endplate deformities at several other levels, which demonstrate normal signal intensity and lack of enhancement compatible with chronic, healed compressions.

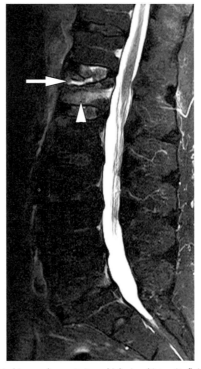

Figure 46-6 ▸ Fluid Sign. Sagittal fat-saturated, T2-weighted image demonstrates a high signal intensity fluid-filled cleft (*arrow*) in the anterior superior L1 vertebral body. Most of the remainder of the vertebral body demonstrates slightly less intense T2 signal intensity compatible with marrow edema (*arrowhead*).

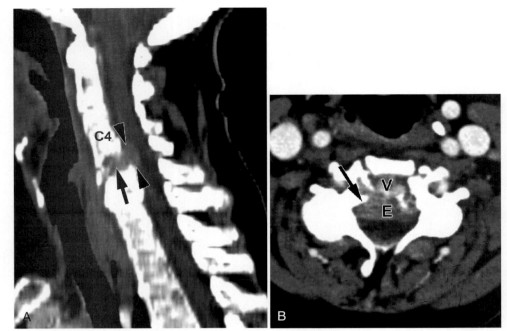

Figure 46-7 ▶ **Pathologic Replacement of Normal Bone.** Same patient as in Figures 46-1 to 46-3. Sagittal reformatted CT image **A** reveals replacement of normal high density bone with intermediate soft tissue (*arrow*). The soft tissue extends through the posterior cortex (between *arrowheads*) into the ventral epidural space. Axial image **B** shows destruction and replacement of the posterior vertebral body with soft tissue (*V*) with extension of pathologic soft tissue (*E*) into the epidural space. There is only a small spicule of remaining posterior cortex (*arrow*).

fracture. The compressed endplate may appear as a hyperdense band paralleling the endplate. There is typically no involvement of the vertebral pedicles (*Fig. 46-8*). At times, it is difficult to judge the age of a compression fracture by CT or plain radiographs. One can compare older studies with newer ones to formulate an impression as to the range of dates a compression has taken place and correlate it with physical examination and a nuclear medicine bone scan. A nuclear medicine bone scan will show intense increased radiotracer uptake in a recent fracture (*Fig. 46-9*). A combination of physical examination and fluoroscopy with palpation over the fractured vertebral body will elicit pain in a recent fracture.

In some equivocal cases, physicians are using combination positron emission tomography with CT (PET/CT) to assess malignant versus benign compressions. PET/CT has been shown to be both sensitive and specific for the detection of lytic and sclerotic lesions and can accurately differentiate between malignant and benign bone lesions with a sensitivity reaching 99%.[10] PET imaging will demonstrate increased radiotracer uptake in malignant fractures and not in osteoporotic fractures.

If a lesion remains equivocal, then the gold standard is to obtain tissue from the fracture from either a percutaneous or open biopsy.

DIFFERENTIAL DIAGNOSIS

1. **Osteoporotic compression deformity**: Cortical or pedicle destruction is not seen with osteoporotic compression deformities. Eccentric soft tissue masses or an epidural mass is not characteristic.

2. **Neuropathic joint**: This may be difficult to distinguish from a metastatic fracture. The pathology is typically centered on the intervertebral disc and facet joint. One may see flecks of bone within the neuropathic joint.

3. **Traumatic fracture**: Imaging findings can be similar to a metastatic fracture and there may be disruption of the vertebral cortex (*Fig. 46-10*). However, it is typically known that the patient has suffered a recent significant trauma. The difficulty may arise in a patient with known malignancy and minor trauma.

TREATMENT

Treatment depends on whether the fracture is malignant or benign, how significant the fracture is, and where it is located. One can adopt a wait-and-see attitude to define the etiology by reimaging the patient in 6 to 8 weeks. If the fracture was benign, signal intensity should revert toward normal. If it is malignant, the signal intensity should stay the same or worsen. This method is no longer acceptable, because patients with either osteoporotic or malignant fractures tend to do better with earlier treatment.

1. **Analgesic medication** is necessary to reduce pain. This could include nonsteroidal anti-inflammatory drugs (NSAIDs), a short course of steroids, or narcotic medication.

2. **Bracing** can be performed; however, it is best if the patient can be mobilized as soon as possible.

3. **Vertebral augmentation** with methymethacrylate is the accepted treatment for osteoporotic fracture pain relief and stabilization and can be performed in some patients with symptomatic metastatic compression deformities. Additional

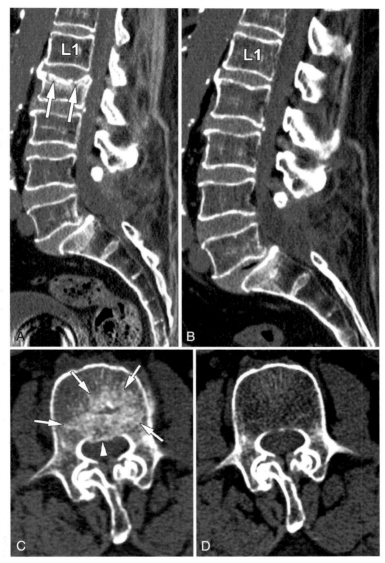

Figure 46-8 ▶ Fracture Age. Comparison images are important to grade the age of a fracture. Sagittal CT image **B** and axial CT image **D** were performed 1 month before similar images **A** and **C**. In the interim, there is new sclerotic density paralleling the superior endplate of L2 (*arrows*) and loss of vertebral height compatible with a probable benign fracture that has occurred since the prior examination. There is also a small retropulsed fragment (*arrow*).

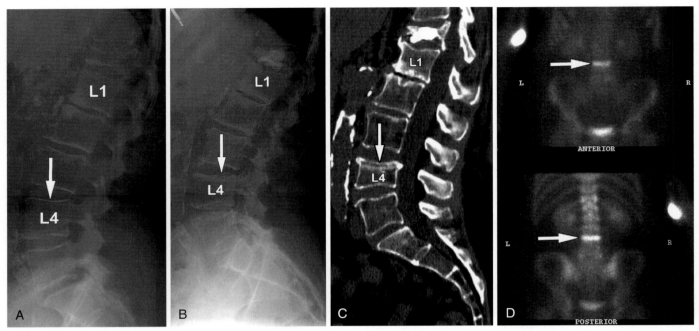

Figure 46-9 ► Fracture Age. Lateral plain radiographs **A** and **B** separated by 1 year (**B** most recent). Subtle loss of superior endplate height of the L4 vertebral body. Note evidence of an interim vertebral augmentation procedure of T12. Sagittal CT image **C** reveals the sclerotic band of compressed bone involving the superior endplate of L4 (*arrow*). Nuclear medicine bone scan demonstrates increased radiotracer uptake (*arrow*) on both the anterior and posterior projections compatible with osteoblastic activity.

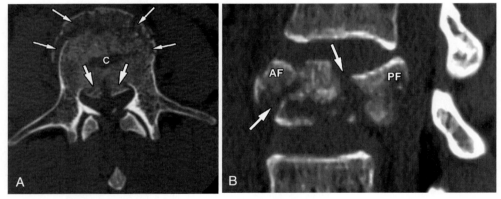

Figure 46-10 ► Traumatic Fracture. Axial image **A** and sagittal image **B** demonstrate a burst fracture with fragmentation of the vertebral body. Axial image shows a cleft (*C*) in the center of the body with fracture fragments both anteriorly (*small arrows*) and posteriorly (*large arrows*). Sagittal image shows the separation of the vertebra into prominent anterior (*AF*) and posterior (*PF*) fragments by large clefts (*arrows*). Note the posterior fragment is causing central spinal canal stenosis.

care must be taken in treating traumatic fractures with vertebral augmentation because one can cause an acute posterior displacement of a fracture fragment into the spinal canal causing cord compression or a cauda equina syndrome.

4. **Radiation therapy** may be needed to treat associated paraspinal or epidural masses with malignant compressions. This can be performed before or after vertebral augmentation.
5. **Open surgical curettage** with methacrylate packing or corpectomy and instrumented fusion may be necessary with some malignant compressions.

References

1. Cuénod CA, Laredo JD, Chevret S, et al. Acute vertebral collapse due to osteoporosis or malignancy: Appearance on unenhanced and gadolinium-enhanced MR images. *Radiology.* 1996;199:541-549.
2. An HS, Andreshak TG, Nguyen C, et al. Can we distinguish between benign versus malignant compression fractures of the spine by magnetic resonance imaging? *Spine.* 1995;20:1776-1782.
3. Yuh WT, Zachar CK, Barloon TJ, et al. Vertebral compression fractures: Distinction between benign and malignant causes with MR imaging. *Radiology.* 1989;172:215-218.
4. Uetani M, Hashmi R, Hayashi K. Malignant and benign compression fractures: Differentiation and diagnostic pitfalls on MRI. *Clin Radiol.* 2004;59:124-131.

5. Jung HS, Jee WH, McCauley TR, et al. Discrimination of metastatic from acute osteoporotic compression spinal fractures with MR imaging. *Radiographics.* 2003;23:179-187.

6. Laredo JD, Lakhdari K, Bellaïche L, et al. Acute vertebral collapse: CT findings in benign and malignant nontraumatic cases. *Radiology.* 1995;194: 41-48.

7. Maldague BE, Noel HM, Malghem JJ. The intervertebral vacuum cleft: A sign of ischemic vertebral collapse. *Radiology.* 1978;129:23-29.

8. Van Lom KJ, Kellerhouse LE, Pathria MN, et al. Infection versus tumor in the spine: Criteria for distinction with CT. *Radiology.* 1988;166:851-855.

9. Malghem J, Maldague B, Labaisse MA, et al. Intravertebral vacuum cleft: Changes in content after supine positioning. *Radiology.* 1993;187:483-487.

10. Even-Sapir E, Metser U, Flusser G, et al. Assessment of malignant skeletal disease: Initial experience with ^{18}F-Fluoride PET/CT and comparison between ^{18}F-Fluoride PET and ^{18}F-Fluoride PET/CT. *J Nucl Med.* 2004;45:272-278.

MENINGIOMA

Douglas S. Fenton, M.D.

CLINICAL PRESENTATION

The patient is an 85-year-old man who presented with numbness of the hands. He describes losing his balance 4 months ago and injuring his knee. He was told he had torn some ligaments in his knee; however, his balance problems have continued to progress. Over the last several weeks, he has developed a numb sensation in both hands, as if he were wearing cotton gloves. This particularly involves the fingers and includes the dorsal and palmer aspects of the hands and forearms. The numbness has leveled off and is no longer getting any worse. However, it has reached a point where he is no longer able to write or fasten his buttons. He does not have numbness in his feet. He must use a walker to maintain his balance or he will fall, particularly if he turns toward the left. There has been no incontinence. During neurologic examination, it was noted he has a severely ataxic, weaving, and lurching gait. He can barely stand independently. He needs assistance to reach the examination table and to walk. When he attempts to touch his nose with his left hand, he can barely get his finger to his face. There is prominent ataxia in the left hand and foot. There is weakness throughout the left upper extremity and also some weakness of the right hand and left foot. There is severe loss of proprioception in the left hand and left foot. There is a radicular band of absent pinprick sensation on the right following a C6 pattern.

IMAGING PRESENTATION

Sagittal T1 pre-contrast and post-contrast images of the cervical spine were obtained and reveal an ovoid intraspinal mass in the upper cervical region displaying intermediate T1 signal intensity and homogeneous enhancement. Axial imaging (not pictured) demonstrated the mass to be intradural and extramedullary and most compatible with a meningioma *(Fig. 47-1)*.

DISCUSSION

Spinal tumors are uncommon lesions. Spinal tumors can be classified as extradural, intradural/extramedullary, or intramedullary. Extradural lesions are most common, representing 60% of all spinal tumors, followed by intradural/extramedullary tumors (30%), and intramedullary tumors (10%).[1] The majority of extradural lesions arise from the vertebrae and are most frequently metastases. Nerve sheath tumors, meningiomas, and drop metastases are the most common intradural/extramedullary masses, with nerve sheath tumors and meningiomas comprising 90% of all intradural/extramedullary tumors.[1] Ependymomas and astrocytomas are the most common intramedullary neoplasms.

Meningiomas are the second most common intradural extramedullary neoplasm, second to nerve sheath tumors. Spinal meningiomas represent 12% of all meningiomas and 25% to 46% of primary spinal neoplasms.[2,3] The annual incidence of primary intraspinal neoplasms is about five per one million in females and three per one million in males.[2] Spinal meningiomas can affect people of all ages; however, they are most prevalent between the fifth and seventh decades of life.[4,5] Seventy percent of spinal meningiomas are found in females.[1] In women, spinal meningiomas are found with the highest frequency in the posterior, posterolateral (most common), or lateral thoracic region (80%), anterior cervical region (15%), and lumbosacral region (5%).[6,7] In men, the distribution of spinal meningiomas is 50% thoracic and 40% cervical.[1] Cervical meningiomas can be particularly problematic because they can adhere to the vertebral artery near its intradural entry and proximal intracranial course.

Embryologically, meningiomas arise from persistent arachnoid cap cells and not from the dura.[8] The arachnoid cap cells form the outer layer of the arachnoid mater and villi.[8] The most common histopathologic subtypes are psammomatous, meningothelial, fibrous, and transitional.[1] The psammomatous subtype is the most common histology of spinal meningioma, followed by meningothelial and transitional.[9] The psammomatous type contains numerous deposits of calcium. The etiology of meningiomas is uncertain; however, there are associations with exposure to ionizing radiation,[10] hormonal influences,[11] chemical exposure (lead),[12] viral infection,[13] and family history.[14]

Spinal meningiomas are usually benign, slow-growing tumors with lateral expansion into the subarachnoid space.[15,16] Patients often have a long clinical history prior to diagnosis because of the slow growth of the tumor. The mean duration of symptoms reported in the literature ranges from 12 to 24 months.[6,17,18] However, given the smaller space in the spinal canal, meningiomas can cause neurologic symptoms when they are quite small as opposed to intracranial meningiomas. Spinal meningiomas are typically well-circumscribed lesions that do not invade into normal tissue and generally do not seed other locations.[16] They are usually solitary; however, when multiple, raise the suspicion of neurofibromatosis type II. The incidence of multiple spinal meningiomas is 1% to 2%.[19] Malignant degeneration of a spinal meningioma is rare.[20]

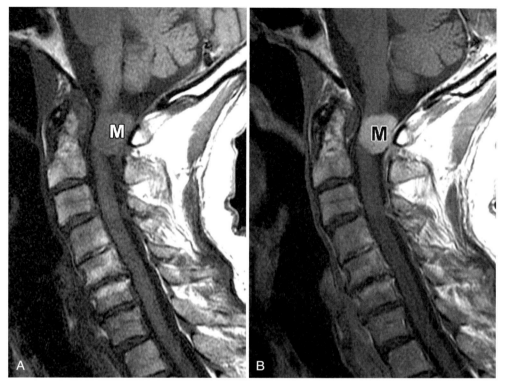

Figure 47-1 ► Meningioma. Sagittal T1 pre-contrast image **A** and post-contrast image **B**. Intraspinal mass (*M*) at the level of the dens demonstrating intermediate T1 signal intensity and homogeneous enhancement.

Focal pain is the most common manifesting symptom in patients with spinal meningiomas.[1,7] Radiating pain is less commonly seen. The pain is typically constant and described as burning or aching in quality.[16] Loss of strength, paresthesias, gait abnormalities, and bowel and bladder dysfunction can occur, although less frequently.[1] Although slow growing, spinal meningiomas can lead to chronic compressive myelopathy leading to spinal cord ischemia, either from direct compression or from alteration in blood supply. This can lead to permanent neurologic deficit even after successful surgery.[15,16]

IMAGING FEATURES

Magnetic resonance imaging (MRI) is the imaging modality of choice. The mass is readily identified, as well as its location and proximity to the spinal cord, other nervous tissue, and vasculature. The typical meningioma demonstrates iso- to hypointensity to the spinal cord on T1-weighted images and iso- to slight hyperintensity on T2-weighted acquisitions (*Fig. 47-2*). Calcifications in the mass are identified as regions of T1- and T2-weighted hypointensity (*Fig. 47-3*). Aside from regions of calcification, there is robust, homogeneous enhancement of meningiomas (see Fig. 47-2). One may see enhancement of the adjacent dura ("dural tail"), which is commonly seen as with intracranial meningiomas but is similarly not specific for meningioma.[21] Computed tomography (CT) demonstrates spinal meningiomas as an iso- to mildly hyperdense mass with homogeneous enhancement. Calcification can be readily identified on noncontrast CT as focal regions of hyperdensity (*Fig. 47-4*). Myelography does not identify the mass but demonstrates the effect of the mass on the dural sac and spinal cord. When viewed in a plane parallel to the mass and spinal cord, an intradural extramedullary mass will appear as a negative defect in the spinal column with widening of the contrast-filled space immediately cephalad and caudad to the mass, between the dural sac and the negative defect from the spinal cord (*Fig. 47-5*). The addition of CT to myelography gives only marginally more benefit than CT alone (*Fig. 47-6*).

DIFFERENTIAL DIAGNOSIS

1. **Schwannoma**: These tumors are more common than meningiomas in the intradural/extramedullary space. Schwannomas are often much more hyperintense on T2-weighted images, are not typically attached to the dura, and are less commonly dorsal to the spinal cord (*Fig. 47-7*).
2. **Intradural metastases**: Metastases are often multiple. Patients may also have a history of cancer.
3. **Epidermoid tumor**: These tumors have signal characteristics of cerebrospinal fluid on both T1- and T2-weighted acquisitions although debris in the cyst can alter the signal. Epidermoids are slow growing and often have undulating and insinuating margins.
4. **Dermoid cysts**: These have mixtures of hair follicles, sweat glands, sebaceous glands, and squamous epithelium. Signal characteristics are mixed on MR imaging secondary to its cystic and fatty features (*Fig. 47-8*).
5. **Lymphoma**: It is unusual for lymphoma to be intradural. When lymphoma mimics the appearance of meningioma, lymphoma is often in the epidural space.

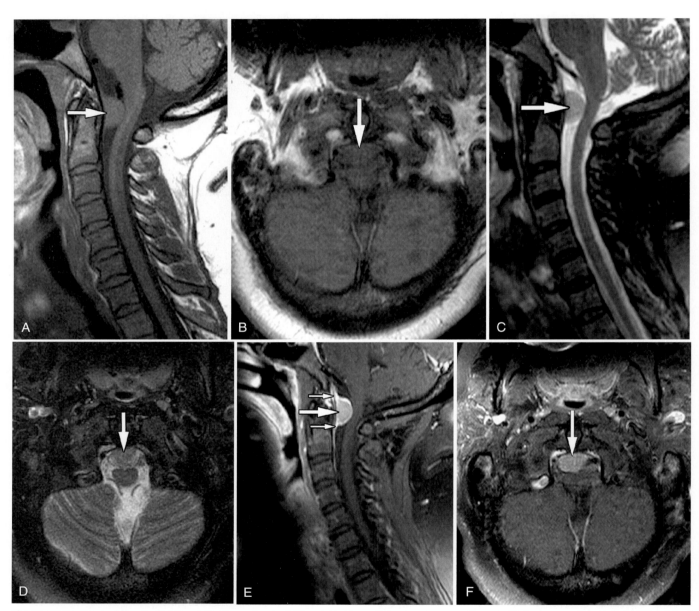

Figure 47-2 ▸ Meningioma. Sagittal T1-weighted image **A** and axial T1-weighted image **B** demonstrate a ventral intraspinal isointense mass (*arrow*). Sagittal T2-weighted image **C** and fat-saturated, T2-weighted image **D** reveal the mass (*arrow*) to be isointense to mildly hyperintense. There is robust enhancement of the meningioma (*large arrow*) on sagittal T1 post-contrast image **E** and axial post-contrast image **F**. Note the dural-based attachment with enhancing dural tails (*small arrows*, image **E**).

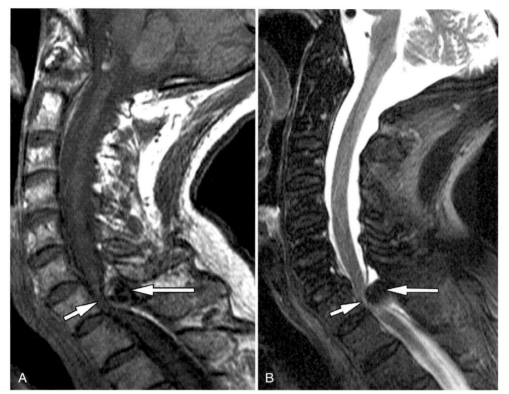

Figure 47-3 ► **Calcified Meningioma.** Sagittal T1-weighted image **A** and fat-saturated, sagittal, T2-weighted image **B**. Intraspinal mass posterior to the spinal cord at the level of C7 (*long arrow*) with very low T1 and T2 weighting. There is significant compression of the spinal cord at the C7 level (*short arrow*).

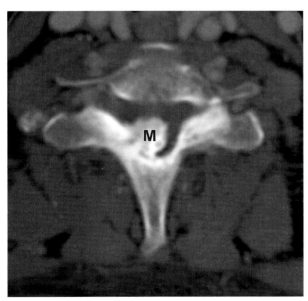

Figure 47-4 ► **Calcified Meningioma.** Same patient as in Figure 47-3. Axial CT image reveals dense calcification of a right posterior intraspinal meningioma (*M*), which occupies a large proportion of the spinal canal.

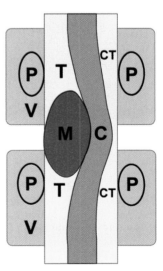

Figure 47-5 ► **Intradural, Extramedullary Mass.** Coronal view. Intradural mass (*M*) displaces the spinal cord (*C*) laterally. There is widening of the CSF-filled space (*T*) both immediately cephalad and caudad to the mass with acute angles between the mass and the spinal cord and between the mass and the wall of the thecal sac. The thecal sac contralateral to the side of the mass (*CT*) is narrowed both cephalad and caudad to the level of the mass. P = Vertebral pedicle; V = vertebral body. (Image courtesy of Leo F. Czervionke, M.D.)

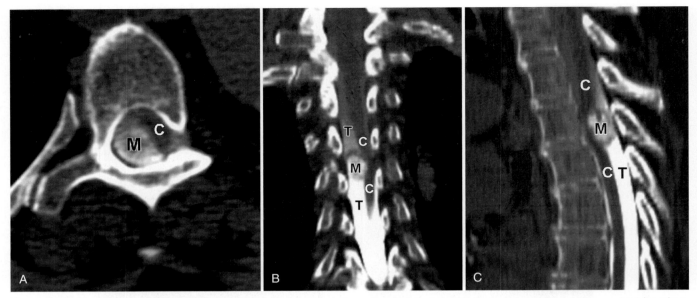

Figure 47-6 ▶ Meningioma, CT Myelogram. Axial image **A**, reformatted coronal image **B**, and reformatted sagittal image **C** post-myelogram CT images. Large hyperdense, intradural, extramedullary mass (*M*) causes ventral and left lateral displacement of the spinal cord (*C*) and causes severe narrowing of the spinal canal and cord. Typical contrast cap sign with widening of the thecal sac (*T*) ipsilateral to the side of the mass both above and below the mass with acute angles and narrowing of the thecal sac on the contralateral side (compare with Fig. 47-5).

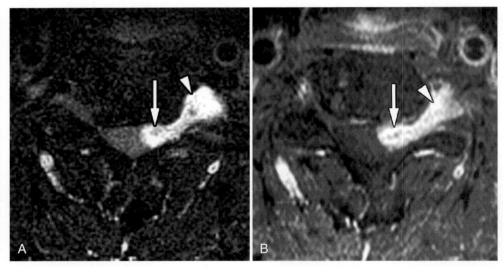

Figure 47-7 ▶ Schwannoma. Axial fat-saturated T2 image **A** and post-contrast, fat-saturated, T1-weighted image **B**. Note left intradural mass (*arrow*) that extends extradurally through the neural foramen (*arrowhead*).

TREATMENT

1. **Surgical resection and decompression** is the treatment of choice for spinal meningiomas. The most frequent approach is posteriorly via laminectomy.[15] Surgery is typically straightforward because there is often a well-defined plane between the meningioma and spinal cord. A literature review of surgical studies demonstrated uniform favorable outcomes with surgery.[15] Patients' functional outcome rate, defined as whether the patient remained neurologically intact or had improved since surgery, was in the range of 85% to 95%. The mean operative mortality rate ranged from 0% to 3.4%, most commonly caused by pulmonary embolism. Mean morbidity rate ranged from 0% to 24.1%, most commonly a result of cerebrospinal fluid leak. The mean recurrence rate ranged from 0% to 14.7%. Partial resection has been identified as an etiology of recurrence.[22] Spinal cord injury has been minimized through the use of somatosensory-evoked potential monitoring and nerve root stimulation.[16] Transcranial motor-evoked potential monitoring can be used to evaluate motor function from the cortex.[16]

2. **Radiation treatment** is controversial because meningiomas are such slow-growing neoplasms and surgical resection has such a high rate of success. Radiation may be used in recurrent and/or more aggressive neoplasms.

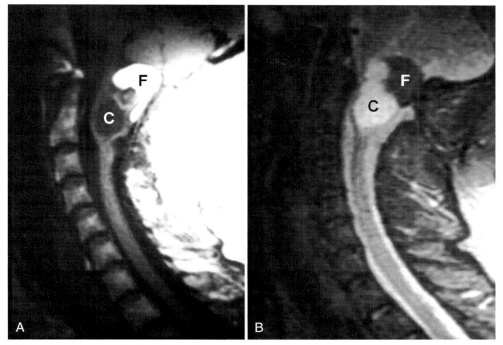

Figure 47-8 ▸ Dermoid Cyst. This mass is typically of mixed signal intensity having fatty and cystic components. Sagittal T1 image **A** and sagittal gradient recall image **B** demonstrate a large, mixed signal intensity, upper cervical mass with fat signal intensity (increased T1, decreased gradient signal) superiorly (*F*) and fluid-like signal intensity (decreased T1, increased gradient signal) inferiorly (*C*).

References

1. Van Goethem JWM, van den Hauwe L, Özsarlak Ö, et al. Spinal tumors. *Eur J Radiol*. 2004;50:159-176.
2. Helseth A, Mork SJ. Primary intra-spinal neoplasms in Norway, 1955 to 1986: A population-based survey of 467 patients. *J Neurosurg*. 1989;71: 842-845.
3. Levy W, Bay J, Dohn D. Spinal cord meningioma. *J Neurosurg*. 1982;57:804-812.
4. Traul DE, Shaffrey ME, Schiff D. Part I: spinal-cord neoplasms-intradural neoplasms. *Lancet Oncol*. 2007;8:35-45.
5. Albanese V, Platania N. Spinal intradural extramedullary tumors. *J Neurosurg Sci*. 2002;16:18-24.
6. Gottfried ON, Gluf W, Quinones-Hinojosa A, et al. Spinal meningiomas: Surgical management and outcome. *Neurosurg Focus*. 2003;14:E2.
7. McCormick PC, Post KD, Stein BM. Intradural extramedullary tumors in adults. *Neurosurg Clin N Am*. 1990;1:591-608.
8. Perry A, Gutmann DH, Reifenberger G. Molecular pathogenesis of meningiomas. *J Neurooncol*. 2004;70:183-202.
9. Sayagues JM, Tabernero MD, Maillo A, et al. Microarray-based analysis of spinal versus intracranial meningiomas: Different clinical, biological, and genetic characteristics associated with distinct patterns of gene expression. *J Neuropathol Exp Neurol*. 2006;65:445-454.
10. Shintani T, Hayakawa N, Hoshi M, et al. High incidence of meningiomas among Hiroshima atomic bomb survivors. *J Radiat Res*. 1999;40:49-57.
11. Lee E, Grutsch J, Persky V, et al. Association of meningiomas with reproductive factors. *Int J Cancer*. 2006;119:1152-1157.
12. Navas-Acién A, Pollán M, Gustavsson P, Plato N. Occupation, exposure to chemicals and risk of gliomas and meningiomas in Sweden. *Am J Ind Med*. 2002;42:214-227.
13. Altieri A, Castro F, Bermejo JL, Hemminki K. Association between number of siblings and nervous system tumors suggests an infectious etiology. *Neurology*. 2006;67:1979-1983.
14. Hemminki K, Li XJ, Collin VP. Parental cancer as a risk factor for brain tumors. *Cancer Causes Control*. 2001;12:195-199.
15. Setzer M, Vatter H, Marquardt G, et al. Management of spinal meningiomas: Surgical results and a review of the literature. *Neurosurg Focus*. 2007;23: E14.
16. Saraceni C, Harrop JS. Spinal meningiomas: Chronicles of contemporary neurosurgical diagnosis and management. *Clin Neurol Neurosurg*. 2009; 111:221-226.
17. King AT, Sharr M, Gullan RW, Bartlett LR. Spinal meningiomas: A 20-year review. *Br J Neurosurg*. 1998;12:521-526.
18. Klekamp J, Samii M. Surgical results for spinal meningiomas. *Surg Neurol*. 1999;52:552-562.
19. Chaparro MJ, Young RF, Smith M, et al. Multiple spinal meningiomas: A case of 47 distinct lesions in the absence of neurofibromatosis or identified chromosomal abnormality. *Neurosurgery*. 1993;32:298-301.
20. Beall DP, Googe DJ, Emery RL, et al. Extramedullary intradural spinal tumors: A pictorial review. *Curr Probl Diagn Radiol*. 2007;36:185-198.
21. Alorainy IA. Dural tail sign in spinal meningiomas. *Eur J Radiol*. 2006;60:387-391.
22. Gezen F, Bahaman S, Candace Z, Bedeck A. Review of 36 cases of spinal cord meningioma. *Spine*. 2000;25:727-731.

MULTIPLE MYELOMA

Douglas S. Fenton, M.D.

CLINICAL PRESENTATION

The patient is a 67-year-old male with a chief complaint of back pain and a history of prostate cancer. About 1 year ago, he began experiencing occasional chest pain. He would feel a "snapping-like" sensation in his chest. Six months ago he began feeling soreness in his hips and then developed back pain soon thereafter. Four months ago, he was ambulating on his own. Three months ago he was using a cane. Presently, he is wheelchair-bound. He feels the muscles in his back are tight and his legs are weak. He has also noticed some atrophy of his hand musculature.

IMAGING PRESENTATION

Sagittal T1-weighted and fat-saturated T2-weighted images of the cervical spine demonstrate several compressed vertebral bodies that display abnormal decreased T1/increased T2 signal intensity. There are also several other vertebral bodies of normal height but with rounded regions of abnormal signal intensity. Several spinous processes are also involved. There is retropulsion of pathologic bone from the T2 vertebral body that impresses the upper thoracic spinal cord *(Fig. 48-1)*.

DISCUSSION

Multiple myeloma (MM) is a neoplastic proliferation of monoclonal plasma cells within the bone marrow. It is the most common primary bone malignancy, with more than 50,000 active cases in the United States and 16,000 new cases diagnosed annually.[1] The median age at diagnosis is 70 years of age with a slight male predominance. The rate of MM is doubled in the black population as opposed to an age-matched white population. There is an increased risk of MM with exposure to ionizing radiation, farming pesticides, and possibly petrochemicals. There is also an increased risk of MM in people with rheumatoid arthritis or obesity.[2] Patients with monoclonal gammopathy of undetermined significance (MGUS) is found in 2% of people over 50 years of age, and the risk of this becoming MM is 1% each year.[3] Although most MM occurs de novo, it is thought that up to 20% progress from MGUS.[4] MM has a median survival rate of 3 to 5 years with chemotherapy and a 5% rate of complete remission.

In the normal person, plasma cells produce immunoglobulins to fight infection; however, in MM, the plasma cells proliferate and overproduce M protein, which can cause hyperviscosity. There may also be production of kappa and lambda light chain proteins that can cause end-organ damage, especially the kidneys. MM cells also produce cytokines that stimulate osteoclasts and suppress osteoblasts, which can lead to hypercalcemia and the typical lytic bone lesions without sclerosis and osteopenia. MM cells also produce angiogenesis factors that promote new blood vessel formation.[5]

Several staging systems have been developed for MM, the most widely used being those published by Durie and Salmon, dividing MM into three stages depending on overall tumor volume, blood hemoglobin, quantitative Bence-Jones protein, serum calcium levels, and number of bone lesions. Stage 1 has low tumor mass, greater hemoglobin, low Bence-Jones protein, normal serum calcium, and no more than a single bone lesion. Stage 3 has high tumor mass, lower hemoglobin, higher Bence-Jones protein, high serum calcium, and advanced lytic bone lesions. Stage 2 is intermediate between stages 1 and 3.[6] A more recent revision, called the *Durie/Salmon Plus staging system*, incorporates magnetic resonance imaging (MRI) and positron emission tomography (PET). From less severe to most, there is MGUS that has normal MRI and/or PET imaging, stage 1A (also known as *smoldering* or *indolent*) in which there can be a single plasmacytoma or very limited disease on imaging, stage 1B with less than 5 lesions, stages 2A or 2B (5-20 focal lesions), and stages 3A or 3B (greater than 20 focal lesions). Multiple myeloma is not diagnosed until stage 1B. An *A* designation is for those with a serum creatinine of less than 2 mg/dl and a *B* designation is for those above this level.[7]

The initial presentation of patients with MM is unexplained back pain or bone pain. The most commonly affected sites are the vertebrae (66% of cases), ribs (45% of cases), skull (40% of cases), and pelvis (30% of cases).[8] The long bones are also commonly affected; however, distal long bone disease is rare. Pathologic fracture is the manifesting symptom in up to one third of patients.[4] Other presentations include fatigue from anemia, weight loss, paresthesias, and fever.[4] If an older patient has bone or back pain lasting more than 2 to 4 weeks, despite symptomatic treatment, further evaluation is warranted to exclude MM.[5]

IMAGING FEATURES

A plain film skeletal survey of the skull, chest, pelvis, humera, and femora is easy to obtain, is of relatively low cost, and can cover a large area of the body. The skeletal survey can detect abnormalities

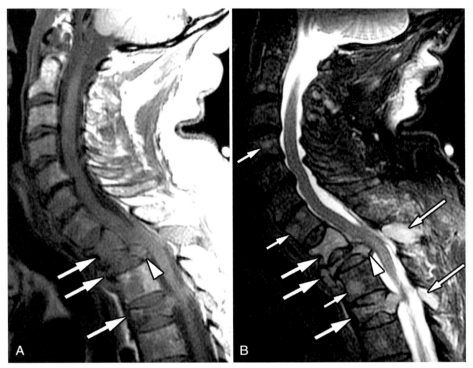

Figure 48-1 ► **Multiple Myleoma with Cord Compression.** Sagittal T1-weighted image **A** and fat-saturated, T2-weighted image **B**. Several compressed vertebral bodies with complete marrow replacement (*large arrows*) as well as several ovoid regions of marrow signal intensity (*small short arrows*). Posterior elements are also involved (*small, long arrows*, image **B**). Abnormal epidural soft tissue from collapsed vertebral body (*arrowhead*) compresses the spinal cord.

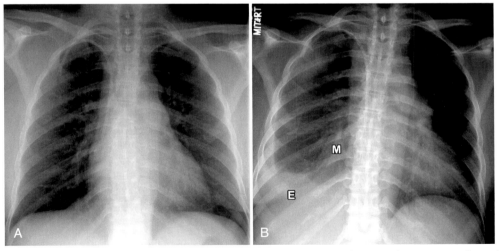

Figure 48-2 ► **Plasmacytoma.** Frontal radiographs **A** and **B** taken 1 year apart, **A** earlier. Image **A** is normal. Image **B** demonstrates an abnormal soft tissue density (*M*) along the right border of the cardiac silhouette, which was found to be a plasmacytoma and a large right pleural effusion (*E*).

in nearly 80% of patients diagnosed with MM.[8] However, the disadvantage of plain film radiography is sensitivity. Plain films rely on bone loss of 30% to 75% of the cancellous bone to be detected, which can be problematic for early diagnosis.[9] Despite this drawback, most centers believe plain film radiography surveys are the first imaging choice for routine diagnosis and staging of MM. If there has been sufficient bone loss, plain films can demonstrate the osteopenia of MM and/or the well-defined punched-out lytic

lesions of MM. The typical lesion is lytic with endosteal scalloping without evidence of marginal sclerosis. Plain films can also demonstrate plasmacytomas, which are often large and expansile, sometimes with septations (*Fig. 48-2*). Plain films can also demonstrate the complications of MM such as vertebral fracture.

Computed tomography (CT) is much more sensitive than plain films in detecting small or early lesions as well as fractures; however, a greater amount of ionizing radiation is used and

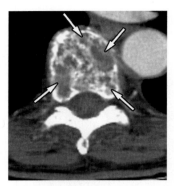

Figure 48-3 ► **Multiple Myeloma, Lytic Lesions.** Axial CT image. Multiple nonsclerotic lytic vertebral body lesions (*arrows*).

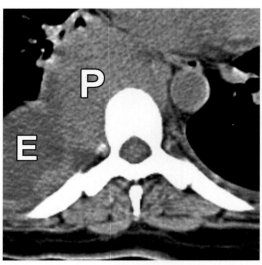

Figure 48-4 ► **Plasmacytoma.** Same patient as in Figure 48-2. Axial CT image. Large soft tissue mass (*P*) along the ventral and right lateral vertebral body plus pleural effusion (*E*).

therefore is often used as an adjunct to plain film radiography. CT well demonstrates the lytic lesion(s) of MM without evidence of sclerosis (*Fig. 48-3*). CT can also demonstrate extraosseous soft tissue abnormalities, including plasmacytomas, and their relationship to adjacent structures (*Fig. 48-4*). In addition, CT demonstrates the relationship of fractured bone to the spinal canal.

MR, including the use of fat-suppression techniques, is the most sensitive examination for bone marrow abnormalities; however, it is not specific for myeloma. In one study, disease was found in 19% of patients with a "normal" plain film survey, whereas 6% had a false-positive plain film survey.[10] The typical appearance of myeloma are vertebral lesions that are of decreased T1 signal intensity, increased T2 signal intensity, and enhancement (*Fig. 48-5*). These are the same imaging findings as with metastatic disease.

Given the costs associated with MRI and the greater access to radiography, the plain film survey remains the imaging of choice to diagnose and stage MM. However, MRI becomes the imaging of choice for the patient with a solitary plasmacytoma (*Fig. 48-6*) or when a patient has symptoms suggestive of cord compression (*Fig. 48-7*) because radiography is quite insensitive to soft tissue abnormalities and MRI (and CT) can be used for radiation and/or surgical planning. Nuclear medicine bone scans are often normal, even in the setting of severe MM, because of the lack of osteoblastic response. PET imaging with CT has been shown to be useful in the diagnosis and staging of MM with sensitivity being near that of MRI.[11] PET imaging will demonstrate regions of increased radiotracer activity that can be correlated with the associated CT scan.

DIFFERENTIAL DIAGNOSIS

1. **Metastatic disease** can have a similar appearance to multiple myeloma. Urinalysis does not demonstrate Bence-Jones proteinuria. Involvement of the vertebral pedicles is seen earlier with metastatic disease (*Fig. 48-8*).
2. **Osteoporosis** can have a patchy appearance on MR imaging; however, no discrete lesions are identified.
3. **Marrow hyperplasia**, as with osteoporosis, may have a patchy MR imaging appearance without discrete lesions. Marrow hyperplasia does not typically enhance.

TREATMENT

MM is considered incurable, but may have long periods of inactivity. Relapses occur in most cases, with death usually resulting from bacterial infection, renal insufficiency, or thromboembolism.[12]

1. **No treatment**: Patients with MGUS or smoldering myeloma do not require treatment because earlier treatment does not have any effect on mortality and may increase the risk of acute leukemia.[13,14] These patients should have follow-up examinations every 3 to 4 months including laboratory tests.
2. **Autologous stem cell transplantation (ASCT):** Treatment for patients with symptomatic MM who are younger than 65 years of age or older patients that can tolerate the treatment can receive ASCT. Patients who receive this treatment along with chemotherapy have a median survival of 68 months.[15]
3. **Melphalan and prednisolone:** Patients that are not candidates for ASCT can receive melphalan and prednisolone with or without thalidomide.[16]
4. **Treatment of MM complications:** The complications of MM can be treated as needed. Vertebroplasty or kyphoplasty can be performed on pathologic fractures for pain relief. Bisphosphonates have been shown to decrease vertebral fractures and pain in those with symptomatic disease.[17] Single-fraction radiotherapy is effective in relieving bone pain.[18] Spinal cord compression can be treated with radiotherapy as well, although surgical decompression should be performed if there is a fractured bone fragment causing spinal stenosis or cauda equina syndrome or to treat instability. Hypercalcemia can be treated with hydration with intravenous normal saline and steroids.[16] Plasmapheresis can be performed to treat myeloma protein–related hyperviscosity with arterial or venous thrombosis, and symptomatic anemia can be treated with transfusions with erythropoietin therapy and transfusions.[19] Infection is a frequent and potentially life-threatening complication, particularly in the first 3 months of chemotherapy, during relapse, and after bone marrow transplantation and should be treated expediently.[7]

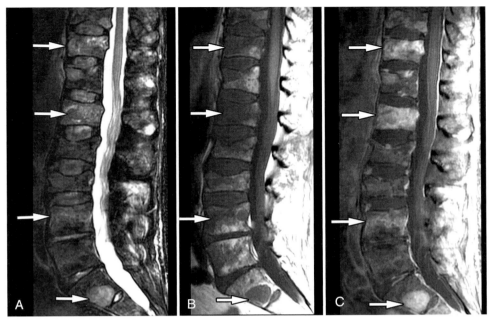

Figure 48-5 ▶ Multiple Myeloma. Sagittal fat-saturated, T2-weighted image **A**, sagittal T1-weighted image **B**, and sagittal fat-saturated, T1 post-contrast image **C**. Typical appearance of myeloma is similar to metastatic disease displaying increased T2 signal, decreased T1 signal, and enhancement (*arrows*). Notice the fairly characteristic round lesion in the S1 vertebral segment.

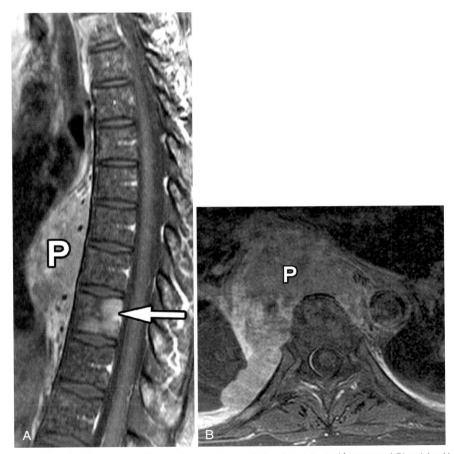

Figure 48-6 ▶ Plasmacytoma and Vertebral Body Lesion. Same patient as in Figures 48-2 and 48-4. Sagittal fat-saturated, T1-weighted image **A** and axial fatsaturated, T1-weighted image **B**. Large enhancing soft tissue mass (*P*) along the ventral and right lateral vertebral body. Enhancing vertebral body lesion seen on image **A** (*arrow*).

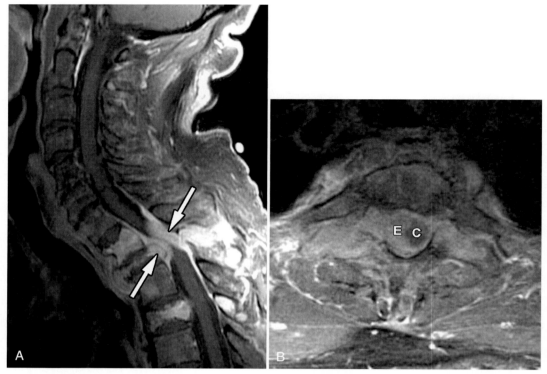

Figure 48-7 ▶ Multiple Myeloma with Cord Compression. Sagittal (**A**) and axial (**B**) T1-weighted, post-contrast, fat-saturated images. Enhancing epidural tumor (*arrows* image **A**, *E* image **B**). Mass effect from the epidural tumor displaces and compresses the spinal cord (*C*).

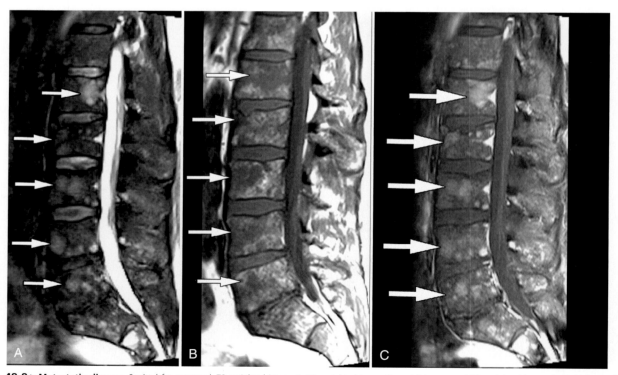

Figure 48-8 ▶ Metastatic disease. Sagittal fat-saturated, T2-weighted image **A**, T1-weighted image **B**, and fat-saturated, T1-weighted image **C**. Multiple small foci of decreased T1 signal, increased T2 signal and enhancement within all vertebral bodies (*arrows*) compatible with metastatic disease.

References

1. National Cancer Institute. SEER cancer statistics review, 1975-2003. Available at http://seer.cancer.gov/csr/1975_2003. Accessed May 11, 2009.
2. Sirohi B, Powles R. Epidemiology and outcomes research for MGUS, myeloma and amyloidosis. *Eur J Cancer.* 2006;42(11):1671-1683.
3. Kyle RA, Therneau TM, Rejkumar SV, et al. A long-term study of prognosis in monoclonal gammopathy of undetermined significance. *N Engl J Med.* 2002;346(8):564-569.
4. Kyle RA, Therneau TM, Rajkumar SV, et al. Review of 1027 patients with newly diagnosed multiple myeloma. *Mayo Clin Proc.* 2003;78(1):21-33.
5. Nau KC, Lewis WD. Multiple myeloma: Diagnosis and treatment. *Am Fam Physician.* 2008;78:853-859.
6. Durie BGM, Salmon SE. A clinical staging for multiple myeloma: Correlation of measured myeloma cell mass with presenting clinical features, response to treatment, and survival. *Cancer.* 1975:36:842-854.
7. Durie BG, Kyle RA, Belch A, et al. Scientific Advisors of the International Myeloma Foundation. Myeloma management guidelines: A consensus report from the scientific advisors of the international myeloma foundation. *Hematol J.* 2003;4:379-398.
8. Collins CD. Review multiple myeloma. *Cancer Imaging.* 2004;4:S47-S53.
9. Angtuaco EJ, Fassas AB, Walker R, et al. Multiple myeloma: Clinical review and diagnostic imaging. *Radiology.* 2004;231:11-23.
10. Ghanem N, Lohrmann C, Engelhardt M, et al. Whole-body MRI in the detection of bone marrow infiltration in patients with plasma cell neoplasms in comparison to the radiological skeletal survey. *Eur Radiol.* 2006;16:1005-1014.
11. Fonti R. Salvatore B Quarantelli M, et al. 18F-FDG PET/CT, 99mTc-MIBI, and MRI in evaluation of patients with multiple myeloma. *J Nuclear Med.* 2008;49:195-200.
12. Bredella MA, Steinbach L, Caputo G, et al. Value of FDG PET in the assessment of patients with multiple myeloma. *AJR Am J Roentgenol.* 2005;184:1199-1204.
13. Kyle RA, Remstein ED, Therneau TM, et al. Clinical course and prognosis of smoldering (asymptomatic) multiple myeloma. *N Engl J Ned.* 2007;356:2582-2590.
14. He Y, Wheatley K, Clark O, et al. Early versus deferred treatment for early stage multiple myeloma. *Cochrane Database Syst Rev.* 2003;(1):CD004023.
15. Sirohi B, Powles R, Mehta J, et al. An elective single autograft with high-dose melphalan: Single-center study of 451 patients. *Bone Marrow Transplant.* 2005;36(1):19-24.
16. Rajkumar SV, Kyle RA. Multiple myeloma: Diagnosis and treatment. *Mayo Clin Proc.* 2005;80:1371-1382.
17. Djulbegovic B, Wheatley K, Ross J, et al. Bisphosphonates in multiple myeloma. *Cochrane Database Syst Rev.* 2002;(3):CD003188.
18. Sze WM, Shelley M, Held I, Mason M. Palliation of metastatic bone pain:single fraction versus multifraction radiotherapy: A systematic review of the randomised trials. *Cochrane Database Syst Rev.* 2004;(2):CD004721.
19. Osterborg A, Brandberg Y, Molostova V, et al. Epoetin Beta Hematology Study Group. Randomized, double-blind, placebo-controlled trial of recombinant human erythropoietin, epoetin Beta, in hematologic malignancies. *J Clin Oncol.* 2002;20:2486-2494.

MYELITIS

Douglas S. Fenton, M.D.

CLINICAL PRESENTATION

The patient is a 33-year-old female with a 13-year history of recurrent events involving the nervous system. Initially, she noticed that her feet were painful on first arising in the morning. She had difficulty walking because of the intense discomfort that largely involved the soles of her feet. These symptoms abated spontaneously. Her next neurologic event occurred 4 years later, when she experienced an acute onset of weakness with difficulty in walking. Steroid therapy was introduced and these symptoms abated. On one occasion, she experienced transient double vision and has more recently noticed the onset of blurred vision in the left eye. The motor symptoms have involved all extremities. The most recent event occurred earlier this year. This was characterized by the acute onset of discomfort in the right upper extremity. Her arm became sensitive to sensory stimuli, and she has since been troubled by a feeling of burning, largely involving the right arm and also, to some extent, the lower limbs. Bladder function has deteriorated to the point where she is subject to marked urgency and frequency of micturition and is often incontinent of urine.

IMAGING PRESENTATION

Sagittal T2 and post-contrast, T1-weighted images reveal a long segment of patchy increased T2 signal intensity and enhancement in an enlarged cervical spinal cord from C2-C6 (*Fig. 49-1*).

DISCUSSION

Neuromyelitis optica (NMO), also known as *Devic's disease*, is an inflammatory disease of the central nervous system that mainly affects, as the name implies, the spinal cord and the optic nerves. NMO has frequently been thought of as a variant of multiple sclerosis (MS); however, clinical, radiologic, laboratory, and pathologic features and treatment have demonstrated that NMO is a distinct entity.[1] NMO can be monophasic or relapsing. Clinically, patients with relapsing NMO are similar to those with MS. However, patients with NMO have more severe attacks than those with MS. Radiologically, spinal cord lesions of NMO are located centrally within the spinal cord and extend over three or more vertebral segments. Atrophy and central cavitation can be seen in later stages of the disease. Patients with MS have more discrete lesions in the dorsolateral aspect of the spinal cord that are usually no longer than a single vertebral segment. Patients with NMO are seropositive for NMO-immunoglobulin G (NMO-IgG), which is rarely seen with MS.[2]

NMO affects young adults, but has been reported from infancy through the ninth decade.[3] The mean age at onset is 29 years (range 1-54 years) for the monophasic type and 39 years (range 6-72 years) for the relapsing type.[3] The ratio of women to men ranges from 1.4 to 1.8:1.[3] NMO appears to be more common in African-Americans, Japanese, and other Pacific Islanders. Demyelinating disease in Asia and India is typically NMO.

Clinically, a viral prodrome precedes the onset of NMO in 30% to 50% of cases.[3] This prodrome may consist of headache, fever, fatigue, respiratory, and gastrointestinal complaints. This may suggest that, at least in some cases, NMO is caused or triggered by an infectious agent. Spinal cord symptoms of NMO worsen over several hours to days and involve motor, sensory, and sphincter function.[3] This may be associated with deep or radicular pain, lower extremity paresthesias and/or weakness.[3] This weakness can progress to complete loss of sensation caudal to the spinal cord lesion. Myelitis in the cervical spine could lead to respiratory failure and death.[3] Optic neuritis in NMO may be uni- or bilateral and can be associated with retro-orbital pain. During a patient's first episode of NMO, 40% of eyes affected by optic neuritis become completely blind.[3] Most patients have some improvement in vision over time.

Newly proposed diagnostic criteria for NMO require the presence of optic neuritis and acute myelitis along with at least two of three supporting criteria: (1) a region of abnormal T2 signal intensity within the spinal cord extending over three or more vertebral segments, (2) brain magnetic resonance (MR) imaging not having the typical appearance of MS, and (3) NMO-IgG seropositivity.[4] It has been suggested to further subdivide NMO into partial or complete. A complete NMO would have involvement of the optic nerves and spinal cord either simultaneously or consecutively and positive NMO-IgG. A partial NMO would have involvement of either the optic nerves or spinal cord and positive NMO-IgG.[5]

NMO is only one of many etiologies that affect the spinal cord and cause myelopathy. Myelopathy is defined as a neurologic deficit related to the spinal cord. Myelopathy is most commonly caused by compression of the spinal cord either from an osteophyte or disc herniation in the cervical spine and less commonly in the thoracic spine.[6] Extrinsic compression of the spinal cord from trauma, metastatic disease, and primary neoplasm is the next most common cause of myelopathy. Other disease processes such as inflammatory, infectious, autoimmune, idiopathic, neoplastic,

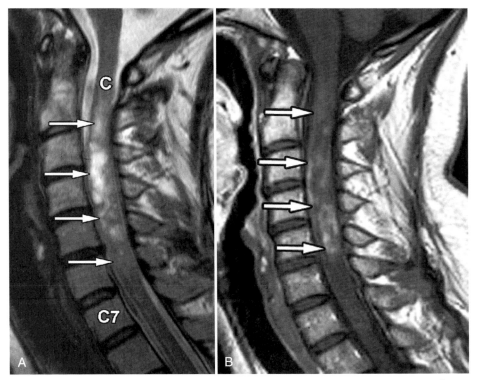

Figure 49-1 ▶ Neuromyelitis Optica. Sagittal T2-weighted image **A** and post-contrast, T1-weighted image **B**. Long segment expansile region of abnormal increased T2 signal intensity and patchy enhancement (*arrows*) in the cervical cord (*C*).

vascular, and nutritional disorders can effect the spinal cord directly, although they are more rare.

It is usually not a diagnostic dilemma in identifying causes of myelopathy extrinsic to the spinal cord versus intrinsic to the spinal cord. Computed tomography (CT) or, more preferred, magnetic resonance (MR) imaging readily demonstrates pathologic processes related to the vertebra or intervertebral discs and their relationship to the spinal cord. A history of recent trauma is also important information when evaluating an abnormality of the spinal cord. What is more challenging is narrowing the differential diagnosis of a patient presenting with myelopathic symptoms and an MR image demonstrating nonspecific increased T2 signal intensity in the spinal cord.

Clinically, myelopathy can be subdivided into their methods of presentation. When a patient presents with myelopathy associated with radicular pain, degenerative spondylosis from osteophyte and/or disc herniation, tumor and infection should be suspected. When myelopathy progresses in a stepwise fashion or has a sudden onset, then vascular processes such as vascular malformations, spinal cord infarction. and epidural hematoma should be considered.[6] If myelopathy is painless and slowly progressive, differential considerations should include neoplasm, demyelinating disease, degenerative disease, and nutritional deficiency.

IMAGING FEATURES

During an acute event of NMO, there is often a region of increased T2 signal intensity in the central spinal cord that extends over a length of at least three vertebral segments. There may be nodular, patchy, or diffuse enhancement of the spinal cord, sometimes

having a mass-like appearance (see Fig. 49-1). In the more chronic stages, the spinal cord may demonstrate atrophy and/or cavitation *(Fig. 49-2).* Increased T2 signal intensity lesions can be seen within one or both optic nerves. Regions of increased T2 signal intensity can be seen within the brain, most of which are not in the typical periventricular location or have the typical punched-out or flame-shaped configuration of MS lesions.

DIFFERENTIAL DIAGNOSIS

Magnetic resonance imaging is the only method of imaging able to evaluate abnormalities intrinsic to the spinal cord. Myelopathy related to an intrinsic spinal cord process has similar imaging characteristics of increased T2 signal intensity, variable enhancement, and/or cord swelling. The location of these signal abnormalities is important in narrowing the differential diagnosis. The spinal cord syndromes can be subdivided into broad categories of those that involve the whole cord, central cord, anterior cord, or posterior cord.[7] The major etiologies causing abnormal spinal cord T2 signal intensity are discussed separately below.

Whole Cross-Sectional Spinal Cord Abnormality

1. **Transverse myelitis** is the classic spinal abnormality that involves most or all of a portion of the spinal cord. Transverse myelitis is not a single process but rather a syndrome with multiple causes. Transverse myelitis is associated with viral

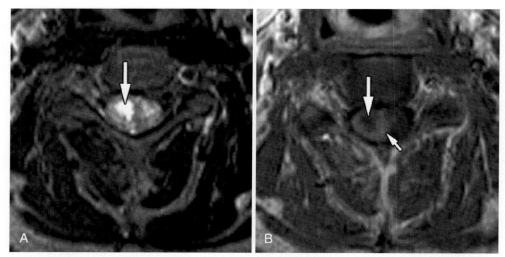

Figure 49-2 ▶ Neuromyelitis Optica. (Same patient as in Figure 49-1.) Axial T2-weighted image **A** and post-contrast, T1-weighted image **B**. Region of CSF signal intensity (*large arrow*) in the cervical cord compatible with cavitation. Peripheral rind of abnormal enhancement of the intramedullary lesion (*small arrow*).

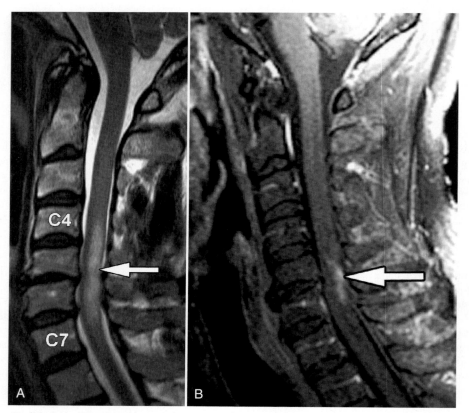

Figure 49-3 ▶ Transverse Myelitis. Sagittal T2-weighted image **A** demonstrates a long segment region of abnormal increased cord signal intensity (*arrow*) with a normal-sized spinal cord. There is patchy enhancement in the dorsal inferior aspect of this lesion on sagittal post-contrast, T1-weighted image **B** (*arrow*).

infections, vaccinations, autoimmune processes, and cancer, although most cases are idiopathic.[8,9] Transverse myelitis begins with back or radicular pain that quickly leads to bilateral leg paresthesias, an ascending sensory level, paraparesis, and paraplegia. It is most common in middle-aged adults. It is most frequently found in the thoracic spine. The characteristic imaging findings of transverse myelitis are normal size or segmental enlargement of the spinal cord, increased T2 signal

intensity involving more than two thirds of the cross-sectional area of the spinal cord, signal abnormality extending over three to four vertebral body levels, and either focal nodular enhancement or some enhancement at the periphery of the spinal cord *(Fig. 49-3)*.[8]

2. **Compressive lesions** from spondylosis, large disc herniation, and neoplasm can affect a segment of the entire spinal cord. The etiology of the myelopathy becomes obvious with imaging

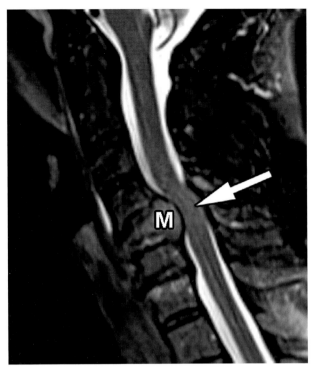

Figure 49-4 ▶ Pathologic Fracture with Cord Compression. Segmental subtle increased spinal cord T2 signal intensity (*arrow*) caused by compression from a pathologic fracture with retropulsion of pathologic bone (*M*).

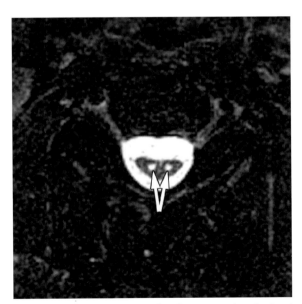

Figure 49-5 ▶ Myelomalacia from Chronic Compression. Focal regions of increased T2 signal intensity in the central gray matter of the spinal cord on both sides of midline (*arrows*) can be a late sequela of chronic cord compression with ensuing cord myelomalacia.

because MR readily demonstrates a large disc herniation, osteophyte, or primary bone abnormality compressing the spinal cord. Compression can cause increased T2 signal intensity throughout the affected segment of the spinal cord (*Fig. 49-4*), and in the subacute phase, may demonstrate some patchy enhancement. The signal abnormality is typically confined to the level of compression. Without decompressive treatment, there can be infarction of the spinal cord at the level of abnormality often seen as two foci of increased T2 signal intensity on either side of the spinal cord ("snake eyes") compatible with regions of myelomalacia (*Fig. 49-5*).

3. **Radiation myelopathy** causes injury to the white matter of the spinal cord. Patients usually present 9 to 15 months after the end of radiation.[10] Clinically, the patient can present early on with paresthesia (particularly with an inability to perceive pain and temperature). As it progresses, the patient can experience various symptoms including gait abnormalities and hemiplegia.[11] Several factors influence the development of radiation myelopathy including the total delivered dose of radiation, fractionation of the radiation dose (fractionation increases the latent period), the volume of the irradiated tissue (larger volumes decrease the latent period), the linear energy transfer (the greater the transfer the more likely myelopathy is going to occur), and the level of the spinal cord irradiated (posterior and lateral spinal cord involvement in the cervical/upper thoracic region; anterior and lateral spinal cord involvement in the lower thoracic/lumbar region).[11-13] Three criteria must be satisfied to diagnose radiation myelopathy: (1) the affected spinal cord must be within the radiation field, (2) the neurologic deficit must correspond to the affected spinal cord segment, and (3) metastases or other primary spinal cord lesions must have been excluded.[14] Radiation myelopathy is also best seen with MRI. In the acute phase of radiation myelopathy, the spinal cord is expanded and demonstrates decreased T1 signal and increased T2 signal. Contrast enhancement is variable and may be patchy or ringlike (*Fig. 49-6*). In the chronic phase of radiation myelopathy, the affected portions of the spinal cord (often the regions that enhanced) can become atrophic.

4. **Spinal cord neoplasms** typically cause T2 signal abnormality throughout the cross-sectional area of the spinal cord. The two most common spinal cord neoplasms are ependymoma and astrocytoma. These neoplasms often cause spinal cord expansion and may have associated hemorrhage and cysts. Because these are masses, there is a solid component that can be seen as decreased to intermediate T1 signal intensity that generally enhances. The nonenhancing T2 abnormality may represent cord edema or syrinx and extends over several vertebral segments (*Fig. 49-7*).

5. **Spinal cord abscesses** are uncommon and are often caused by pyogenic infections.[15] They can be of hematogenous origin, often from the respiratory tract, or from contiguous spread from an adjacent infection.[15] Spinal cord abscesses often demonstrate ill-defined decreased T1 signal intensity, increased T2 signal, and irregular enhancement. Short tau inversion recovery (STIR) images can sometimes separate the abscess from the associated edema, both of which are of increased T2 signal. A cord abscess may show positive diffusion, although absence of this does not exclude an abscess.

Central Spinal Cord Abnormality

1. The term **syrinx**, often is used to encompass both hydromyelia (ependymal-lined dilation of the central spinal canal) and syringomyelia (a gliotic-lined cystic spinal cord cavity not related to the central canal). Hydromyelia is a common imaging finding and most are asymptomatic. They are

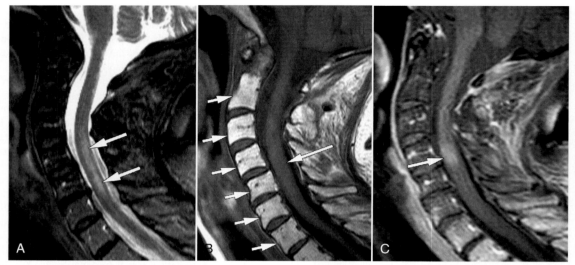

Figure 49-6 ▶ Radiation Myelopathy. Sagittal T2-weighted image **A** demonstrates a long segment region of central spinal cord T2 hyperintensity (*arrows*) with mild cord expansion. This abnormality is less well seen on sagittal T1-weighted image **B** (*long arrow*); however, note that there is diffuse increase in T1 signal intensity involving the cervical vertebrae that were in the field of radiation (*short arrows*). There is a focal region of enhancement of the cervical cord at the C4 level (image **C**, *arrow*).

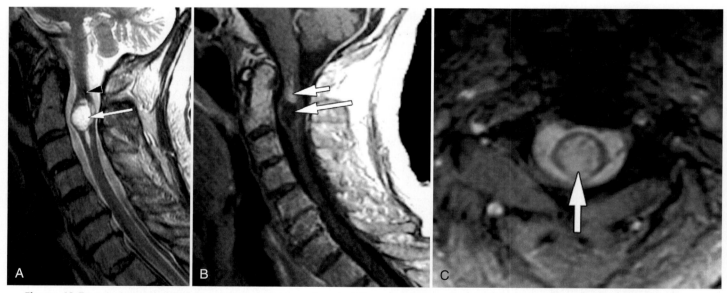

Figure 49-7 ▶ Spinal Cord Neoplasm. Sagittal T2-weighted image **A**, sagittal T1 post-contrast image **B**, and axial gradient recall image **C**. Intramedullary cystic lesion (*long arrow*) occupies nearly the entire cross-sectional area of the spinal cord. Hemosiderin staining (*arrowhead*, image **A**) and enhancement (*short arrow*, image **C**) cephalad to the cystic portion.

associated with Chiari malformations, spinal dysraphisms, scoliosis, and intramedullary tumors. Syrinx most commonly occurs in the cervical spine. When symptomatic, the classic clinical symptoms are loss of pain and temperature sensation with preservation of proprioception and light touch sensation, along a dermatome. A sensory loss in a cloaklike distribution over the neck, shoulders, and arms is common.[16] A syrinx is seen as a continuous or beaded, longitudinally oriented cerebrospinal fluid (CSF)-filled cavity within the center of the spinal cord. They follow CSF signal intensity on all pulse sequences (decreased T1 signal intensity, increased T2 signal intensity, no enhancement) (*Fig. 49-8*).

2. **Venous hypertension** can cause a myelopathy that demonstrates nonspecific central cord T2 signal changes. This is typically seen with dural arteriovenous fistulas or arteriovenous malformations of the spinal cord but has also been described with spinal epidural hematomas.[17] The hypothesis is that impaired venous drainage occurs because of a decrease in the arteriovenous pressure gradient. This leads to increased intramedullary pressure and congestion with spinal cord edema and a concomitant decrease in perfusion, resulting in ischemia and hypoxia.[18] Venous ischemia/infarction appears as increased T2 signal intensity in the central cord that progresses centripetally with variable enhancement (*Fig. 49-9*).

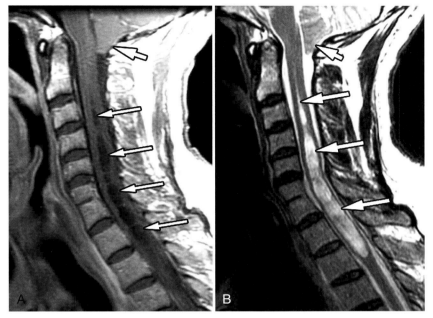

Figure 49-8 ▶ Syrinx. Sagittal Tl-weighted image **A** and T2-weighted image **B**. Cerebellar tonsil (*short white arrow*) is approximately 10 mm inferior to the foramen magnum. Long-segment region of CSF signal intensity within the spinal cord from C2-T2 (*long white arrows*). Findings compatible with Chiari 1 malformation with associated syringomyelia.

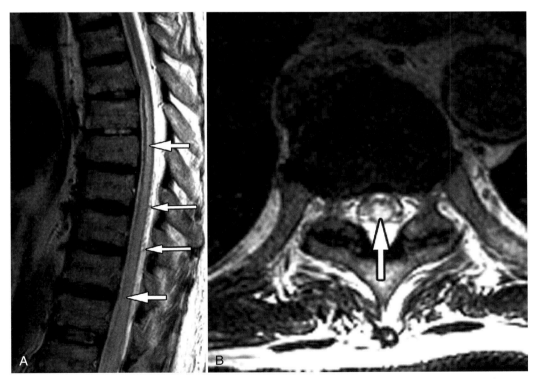

Figure 49-9 ▶ Venous Hypertension Secondary to Arteriovenous Fistula. Sagittal T2-weighted image **A** demonstrates increased signal intensity in the central spinal cord (*short arrows*). *Long arrows* point to abnormal vascularity on the posterior aspect of the thoracic spinal cord. Axial T2-weighted image **B** shows the central T2 abnormality in the spinal cord (*arrow*).

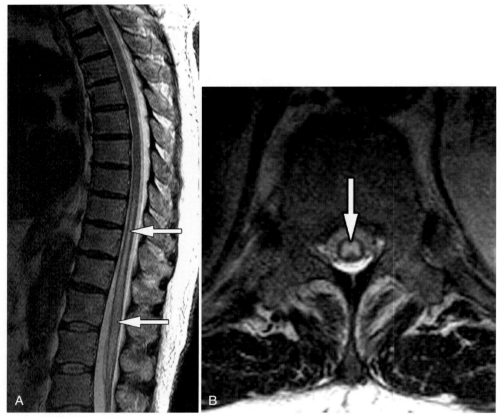

Figure 49-10 ▶ Spinal Cord Infarction. Early spinal cord infarction demonstrates increased T2 signal intensity in the central spinal cord gray matter on sagittal T2 image **A** and axial T2 image **B** (*arrows*).

Anterior Spinal Cord Abnormality

1. **Spinal cord infarction** most commonly involves the territory of the anterior spinal artery (ASA) in the thoracic region. The anterior spinal artery supplies the anterior two thirds of the spinal cord and the paired posterior spinal arteries supply the posterior one third. With bilateral involvement of the anterior horns, spinothalamic pathways, and lateral corticospinal tracts, one can see neurologic symptoms of para- or tetraparesis, bladder dysfunction, and bilateral dissociated sensation deficits with loss of temperature and pain sense inferior to the level of the infarction.[19] Causes of spinal cord ischemia or infarction include aortic aneurysms, vertebral artery dissection, spinal and aortic surgery, hypotension, cocaine abuse, and vasculitis.[7,19] MR imaging initially demonstrates abnormal T2 signal intensity involving the central gray matter (*Fig. 49-10*) and then extends to involve the anterior two thirds of a normal-sized spinal cord. With more severe cases, the entire cross-sectional area of the cord can be involved making it difficult to distinguish from other whole-cord syndromes. There may be patchy enhancement in the subacute phase. A helpful, albeit occasional, finding is one of increased T2 signal intensity in either the anterior aspect or near the endplate in the medullary portion of a vertebral body at the level of arterial occlusion compatible with vertebral infarction.

Posterior Spinal Cord Abnormality

1. **Multiple sclerosis (MS)** is a chronic, relapsing or slowly progressive disorder characterized by demyelinating plaques in the brain and/or spinal cord. The exact cause of MS is unknown, but many clinicians believe it is secondary to a viral or autoimmune process.[20] Although the number of plaques in the brain is positively correlated with the duration of the disease, spinal cord plaques correlate more with the degree of disability and not with disease duration.[21] Demyelinating plaques appear as well-defined ovoid T2 hyperintensities in the dorsolateral aspect of the spinal cord involving both gray and white matter (*Fig. 49-11*). The plaques may enhance in a nodular, arclike or ring fashion in the acute or subacute phase. Most demyelinating plaques involve a section of the spinal cord less than two vertebral segments in length and involving less than half of the cross-sectional area of the spinal cord. The cervical spine is more affected than the thoracic spine.[22] CSF examination may demonstrate oligoclonal bands.

2. **Acute disseminated encephalomyelitis (ADEM)** is a monophasic illness of children and young adults.[23] It has a rapid onset and can affect both the brain and the spine. Symptoms are often preceded by a viral illness. ADEM often involves the dorsal white matter of the spinal cord although it can involve the gray matter as well. The MR imaging findings of ADEM

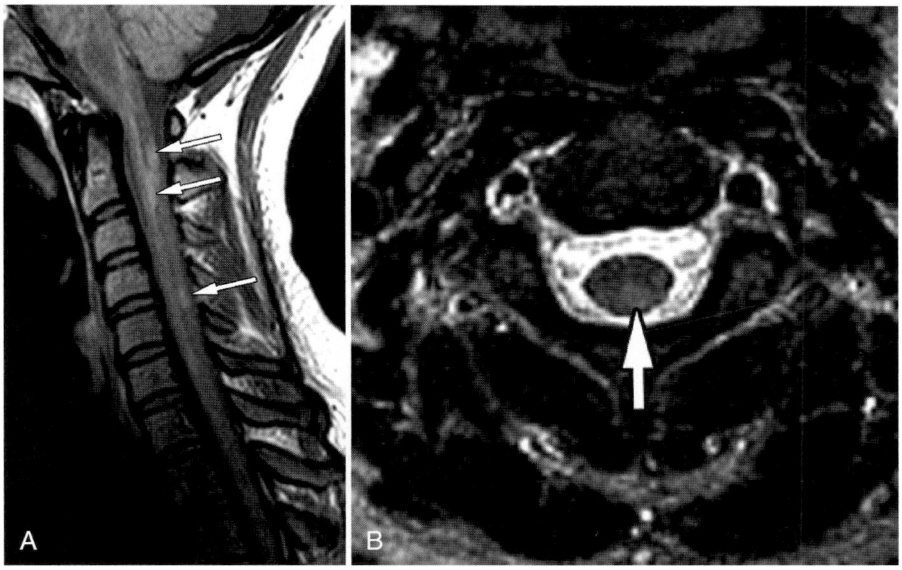

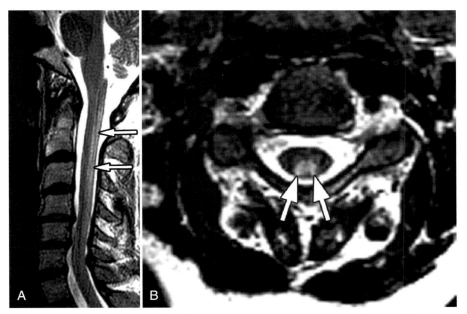

Figure 49-11 ▶ **Multiple Sclerosis.** Sagittal proton density image **A** reveals multiple short-segment hyperintensities primarily in the dorsal spinal cord (*arrows*). Axial T2-weighted image **B** shows a solitary demyelinating lesion of multiple sclerosis (*arrow*).

Figure 49-12 ▶ **Subacute Combined Degeneration.** Sagittal T2-weighted image demonstrates a long segment of increased T2 signal intensity in the dorsal spinal cord (*arrows*). Axial T2-weighted image shows the classic "inverted V" shape T2 abnormality involving the posterior columns (*arrows*).

can be indistinguishable from MS. There can be focal or diffuse regions of increased T2 signal intensity in the dorsal spinal cord. Focal, ring-shaped, or amorphic enhancement can occur in the acute phase. Differentiating ADEM and MS can be performed with CSF examination demonstrating high mononuclear cell titers and protein levels and absent oligoclonal bands.[24]

3. **Subacute combined degeneration (SCD)** can be caused by malabsorption (most common) or inadequate intake of vitamin B_{12}. SCD can manifest with numbness or tingling in the limbs, positional and vibratory sense disturbances, and spastic paraparesis or tetraparesis.[25] The disease predominantly involves the posterior columns followed by the anterolateral and anterior tracts.[26] The typical MR finding of SCD is T2 hyperintensity with occasional enhancement confined to the posterior columns with an "inverted V" appearance on axial T2-weighted images *(Fig. 49-12)*.[26] The signal abnormality usually resolves after appropriate vitamin B_{12} treatment.

4. **Human immunodeficiency virus (HIV) myelopathy** generally occurs late in the course of autoimmune immunodeficiency syndrome (AIDS).[27] Patients present with progressive spastic paraparesis, ataxia, bladder dysfunction, and sensory

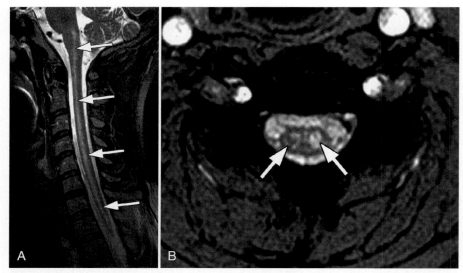

Figure 49-13 ▶ **HIV Myelopathy.** Off-midline sagittal T2-weighted image **A**. There is a long segment region of increased T2 signal intensity in the lateral aspect of the spinal cord (*arrows*). Axial T2-weighted image **B** shows the classic T2 abnormality involving the lateral columns (*arrows*).

loss.[28] There can be involvement of the posterior and/or lateral columns of the cervical and thoracic spinal cord. MRI signal characteristics can be identical to vitamin B_{12} deficiency. Patients will have a positive HIV test unlike vitamin B_{12} deficiency. The classic imaging presentation is increased T2 signal intensity bilaterally and symmetrically in the lateral columns of the spinal cord with occasional enhancement *(Fig. 49-13)* although posterior column or whole cord signal abnormality can occur. As the disease progresses, the affected spinal cord segments become atrophic.[27]

TREATMENT

1. **Immunosuppressive medications:** NMO is often first treated with immunosuppressive medications such as steroids and azathioprine.[29] If these treatments fail, then plasmapheresis may be effective.
2. **Intravenous steroids:** Transverse myelitis is often treated with intravenous steroids, although this treatment is debated in the literature.
3. **Surgical removal:** Compressive lesions are treated with surgical removal of the cause of compression.
4. **Hyperbaric oxygen:** Radiation myelopathy, unfortunately, tends to be progressive, without much improvement. There has been some success with hyperbaric oxygen in early cases.[30]
5. **Surgical resection with radiation and/or chemotherapy:** Spinal cord neoplasms are treated by surgical resection with possible radiation therapy and/or chemotherapy depending on tumor type.
6. **Surgical laminectomy, myotomy, and drainage:** Spinal cord abscess is treated with surgical laminectomy, myotomy and drainage. Abscess is cultured for appropriate antibiotic therapy.
7. **Treatment for syrinx:** Syrinx treatment depends on its etiology. If it is due to a tumor, then surgical resection of the tumor is performed. If it is due to trauma, then correcting any

traumatic deformities is performed. If the syrinx still causes symptoms, the syrinx can be directly drained or shunted.
8. **Treatment of venous hypertension:** Venous hypertension from an arteriovenous fistula or epidural hematoma has a better chance of fully resolving the earlier the cause is treated with either surgical or endovascular therapy.
9. **Treatment of spinal cord infarction:** Spinal cord infarction, in its acute stage, is often treated with steroids to minimize cord swelling. Blood pressure is kept slightly higher than normal to secure good perfusion. Anticoagulation medication can be given to minimize clotting. Patients will need physical therapy.
10. **Treatment for multiple sclerosis:** Multiple sclerosis is treated by many different medications including beta interferons, glatiramer, corticosteroids, and muscle relaxants. Plasma exchange can be used in patients with severe acute symptoms that do not respond to steroids. Patients should also get physical and occupational therapy and counseling to cope with emotional stress.[31]
11. **Treatment of ADEM:** ADEM is initially treated with corticosteroid therapy. If this fails to work, plasmapheresis, intravenous immunoglobulin therapy, or immunosuppressive therapy may be prescribed.
12. **Treatment of subacute combined degeneration:** Subacute combined degeneration is treated by first evaluating the underlying etiology, specifically whether it is due to malabsorption, and if so, treating that. Vitamin B_{12} administration is the mainstay of treatment.
13. **Treatment of HIV myelopathy:** HIV myelopathy has no known treatment to date. Patients have been treated with antiretroviral agents with mixed results.

References

1. Matiello M, Jacob A, Wingerchuk DM, Weinshenker BG. Neuromyelitis optica. *Curr Opin Neurol.* 2007;20:255-260.
2. Lennon VA, Wingerchuk DM, Kryzer TJ, et al. A serum autoantibody marker of neuromyelitis optica: Distinction from multiple sclerosis. *Lancet.* 2004;364:2106-2112.

3. Wingerchuk DM, Hogencamp WF, O'Brien PC, Weinshenker B. The clinical course of neuromyelitis optica (Devic's syndrome). *Neurology.* 1999;53:1107-1114.
4. Wingerchuk DM, Lennon VA, Pittock SJ, et al. Revised diagnostic criteria for neuromyelitis optica. *Neurology.* 2006;66:1485-1489.
5. Mandler RN. Neuromyelitis optica: Devic's syndrome, update. *Autoimmun Rev.* 2006;5:537-543.
6. Seidenwurm DJ. Myelopathy. *AJNR Am J Neuroradiol.* 2008;29:1032-1034.
7. Sheerin F, Collison K, Quaghebeur G. Magnetic resonance imaging of acute intramedullary myelopathy: Radiological differential diagnosis for the on-call radiologist. *Clin Radiol.* 2009;64:84-94.
8. Choi KH, Lee KS, Chung SO, et al. Idiopathic transverse myelitis: MR characteristics. *AJNR Am J Neuroradiol.* 1996;17:1151-1160.
9. Christensen PB, Wermuth L, Hinge HH, Bomers K. Clinical course and long-term prognosis of acute transverse myelopathy. *Acta Neurol Scand.* 1990;81:431-435.
10. Schultheiss TE, Higgins EM, El-Mahdi AM. The latent period in clinical radiation myelopathy. *Int J Radiat Oncol Biol Phys.* 1984;10:1109-1115.
11. Okada S, Okeda R. Pathology of radiation myelopathy. *Neuropathology.* 2001;21:247-265.
12. van der Kogel AJ. Radiation tolerance of the rat spinal cord: Time-dose relationships. *Radiology.* 1977;122:505-509.
13. Mastaglia FL, McDonald WI, Watson JV, Yogendran K. Effect of X-radiation on the spinal cord: An experimental study of the morphological changes in central nerve fibers. *Brain.* 1976;99:101-122.
14. Pallis CA, Louis S, Morgan RL. Radiation myelopathy. *Brain.* 1961;84:460-479.
15. Murphy KJ, Brunberg JA, Quint DJ, Kazanjian PH. Spinal cord infection: Myelitis and abscess formation. *AJNR Am J Neuroradiol.* 1998;19:341-348.
16. Poggi MM, Stockel J. Medical problems in patients with malignancy. *J Clin Oncol.* 2004;22:4019-4020.
17. Auler MA, Al-Okaili R, Rumboldt Z. Transient traumatic spinal venous hypertensive myelopathy. *AJNR Am J Neuroradiol.* 2005;26:1655-1658.
18. Kataoka H, Miyamoto S, Nagata I, et al. Venous congestion is a major cause of neurological deterioration in spinal arteriovenous malformations. *Neurosurgery.* 2001;48:1224-1229.
19. Weidauer S, Nichtweiss M, Lanfermann H, Zanella FE. Spinal cord infarction: MR imaging and clinical features in 16 cases. *Neuroradiology.* 2002;44:851-857.
20. Lampert PV. Autoimmune and virus induced demyelinating diseases. *Am J Pathol.* 1978;91:176-208.
21. Honig LS, Sheramata WA. Magnetic resonance imaging of spinal cord lesions in multiple sclerosis. *J Neurol Neurosurg Psychiatry.* 1989;52:459-466.
22. Ikuta F, Zimmerman HM. Distribution of plaques in seventy autopsy cases of multiple sclerosis in the United States. *Neurology.* 1976;26:26-28.
23. Atlas SW, Grossman RI, Goldberg HI, et al. MR diagnosis of acute disseminated encephalomyelitis. *J Comput Assist Tomogr.* 1986;10:798-801.
24. Honkaniemi J, Dastidar P, Kähärä V, Haapasalo H. Delayed MR imaging changes in acute disseminated encephalomyelitis. *AJNR Am J Neuroradiol.* 2001;22:1117-1124.
25. Hemmer B, Glocker FX, Schumacher M, et al. Subacute combined degeneration: Clinical, electrophysiological, and magnetic resonance imaging findings. *J Neurol Neurosurg Psychiatry.* 1998;65:822-827.
26. Pant SS, Asbury AK, Richardson EJ. The myelopathy of pernicious anemia: A neuropathological reappraisal. *Acta Neurol Scand.* 1968;5:1-36.
27. Chong J, Di Rocco A, Tagliati M, et al. MR findings in AIDS-associated myelopathy. *AJNR Am J Neuroradiol.* 1999;20:1412-1416.
28. Simpson DM, Tagliati M. Neurologic manifestations of HIV infection. *Ann Intern Med.* 1994;121:769-785.
29. Mandler RN, Ahmed W, Dencoff JE. Devic's neuromyelitis optica: A prospective study of seven patients treated with prednisone and azathioprine. *Neurology.* 1998;51:1219-1220.
30. Calabrò F, Jinkins JR. MRI of radiation myelitis: A report of a case treated with hyperbaric oxygen. *Eur Radiol.* 2000;10:1079-1084.
31. Mayo clinic staff: Multiple sclerosis. Available at http://www.mayoclinic.com/health/multiple-sclerosis/DS00188. Accessed July 19, 2009.

MYXOPAPILLARY EPENDYMOMA

Leo F. Czervionke, M.D.

CLINICAL AND IMAGING PRESENTATION

The patient is a 39-year-old man who initially presented with back pain and electric-like sensations that radiated down the backs of both legs. The pain was worse when he was lying down.

IMAGING PRESENTATION

Magnetic resonance (MR) image of the spine revealed a large enhancing intradural mass extending from the tip of the conus medullaris (mid T12) to the superior L2 level. A smaller intradural mass is located within the thecal sac at the L2-3 level (*Figs. 50-1 to 50-5*). The patient's symptoms eventually resolved and he delayed surgery until his symptoms returned 3 months later. Surgery consisted of L1-L5 decompressive laminectomy, intradural exploration, and gross total removal of the multilobulated tumor. Radiologic and pathologic diagnosis was myxopapillary ependymoma.

DISCUSSION

Of all intramedullary cord tumors, 95% are gliomas (astrocytomas or ependymomas); 65% of cord gliomas are ependymomas in adults.[1] Myxopapillary ependymomas comprise 30% of all ependymomas and 13% of spinal ependymomas. They represent the most common intradural tumor involving the conus medullaris and cauda equina.[1,2] Approximately 90% of tumors involving the conus medullaris/cauda equina junction are myxopapillary ependymomas.[3] They are histologically benign tumors, classified as World Health Organization (WHO) grade I, and although they may recur locally after surgery, rarely disseminate in the central nervous system (CNS).[4] They usually manifest in middle-aged adults, usually in the fourth decade of life,[5] with back pain, lower extremity weakness, and radiculopathy and may produce loss of bladder and bowel control.[1-3] The symptoms are usually slowly progressive because these tumors usually grow very slowly. Hemorrhage into the tumor can rarely cause rapid increase in tumor size, resulting in a cauda equina syndrome.[6] Myxopapillary ependymomas can rarely arise in the subcutaneous tissues posterior to the sacrococcygeal junction. Such tumors are believed to arise from the coccygeal medullary vestige or subcutaneous ependymal rests.[7,8]

IMAGING FEATURES

Typically, these lesions are relatively well circumscribed, lobulated masses that usually extend 1 or 2 vertebral levels,[2,9] but may be multiple or more extensive, filling the entire lumbar spinal canal.[3,10] They usually grow very slowly, so they may not be detected until they are quite large.[11] Plain radiographic (plain X-ray) findings are present in 60% of patients, more common with tumors occurring in the lumbar region.[12] They can produce expansion of the spinal canal and posterior vertebral body scalloping and also medial erosions/remodeling of the pedicles. MR imaging is the procedure of choice for evaluating spinal cord tumors.[13] On MRI, these masses are usually T1 isointense (see Fig. 50-1) but can be T1 hyperintense, because of the presence of intratumoral mucin.[5,12] Mucin is not usually present in cellular ependymomas of the cervical cord.[10] Myxopapillary ependymomas are predominantly T2 hyperintense with respect to the cord (see Fig. 50-2). They may contain small tumoral cysts or areas of necrosis and intratumoral hemorrhage (see Fig. 50-3) is common, as with cellular intramedullary ependymomas in the cervical region.[12] Myxopapillary ependymomas usually display intense heterogeneous enhancement (see Figs. 50-4 and 50-5). These tumors can produce subarachnoid hemorrhage, but this is rare.[14,15] The presence of superficial siderosis can be secondary to a myxopapillary ependymoma.[10] Myxopapillary ependymomas generally enhance intensely although somewhat heterogeneously after IV contrast (Figs. 50-5 and *50-6*). Myxopapillary ependymomas have an extremely low tendency to metastasize. However, ependymomas involving the conus or cauda equina may be secondary to ependymomas elsewhere in the CNS. Therefore, the entire spinal axis should be imaged if a spinal ependymoma is discovered, regardless of location. Calcifications rarely occur in spinal ependymomas.

DIFFERENTIAL DIAGNOSIS

1. **Schwannoma:** Occurring at the conus medullaris or in the cauda equina, a schwannoma may be difficult or impossible to differentiate from myxopapillary ependymoma. Schwannomas more commonly contain cystic areas, but some enhance homogeneously (see Fig. 50-6).
2. **Meningioma:** More common in the thoracic spine or in the cervical region near the foramen magnum level, these

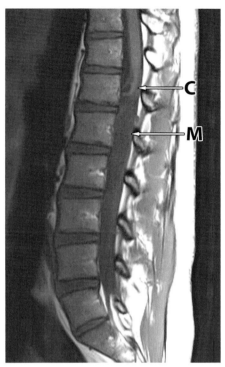

Figure 50-1 ▶ Myxopapillary Ependymoma. T1-weighted sagittal image shows distortion of the conus and upper cauda equina (*C*) by a vague mass (*M*), which is nearly isointense relative to CSF and therefore difficult to visualize.

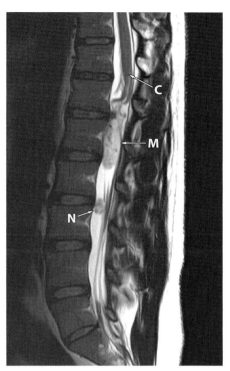

Figure 50-2 ▶ Myxopapillary Ependymoma. T2-weighted sagittal image shows distortion of the conus and upper cauda equina (*C*) by a heterogeneous mass (*M*), which contains focal areas of T2 hypointensity consistent with small areas of old hemorrhage, likely hemosiderin. *N*, T2 hypointense satellite nodule.

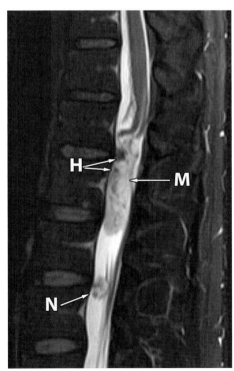

Figure 50-3 ▶ Myxopapillary Ependymoma. Fat-saturated, sagittal, T2-weighted image. T2 hypointense foci in mass (*M*) consistent with old hemorrhage (*H*). *N*, Satellite tumor nodule.

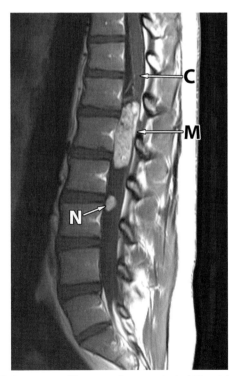

Figure 50-4 ▶ Myxopapillary Ependymoma. Sagittal T1-weighted, contrast-enhanced image. Distortion of conus medullaris (*C*) and upper cauda equina by heterogeneously enhancing intradural mass (*M*), which fills spinal canal at L1 level. Satellite intradural enhancing nodule (*N*) at L2-3 level.

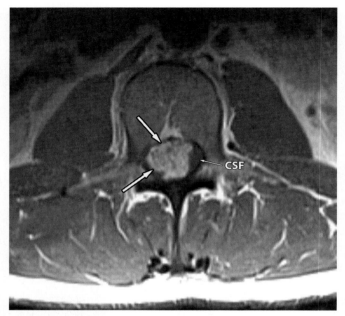

Figure 50-5 ▶ Myxopapillary Ependymoma. Axial T1-weighted, contrast-enhanced image at L1 level. The intensely enhancing, heterogeneous intradural mass fills the majority of the spinal canal except for a small amount of intrathecal CSF on the left.

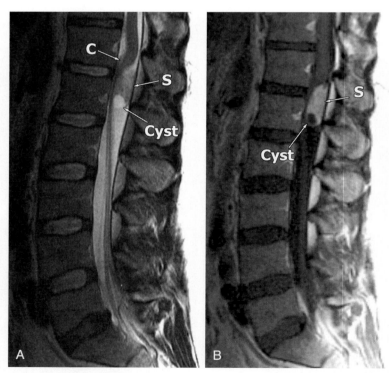

Figure 50-6 ▶ Intradural Schwannoma. In sagittal T2-weighted image **A**, the conus medullaris (*C*) and superior portion of the cauda equina are displaced anteriorly by the schwannoma (*S*). A cyst is located in the caudal pole of the tumor. In contrast-enhanced, T1-weighted image **B**, the solid portion of the schwannoma (*S*) enhances intensely and uniformly. The cyst does not enhance.

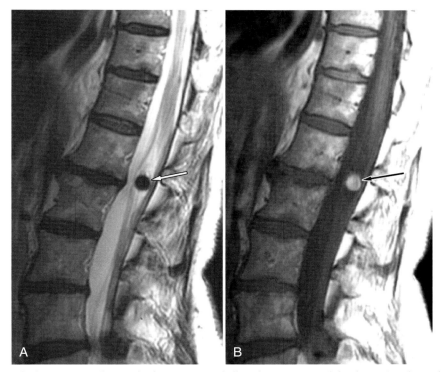

Figure 50-7 ▶ Intradural Meningioma. In sagittal T2-weighted image **A**, a markedly T2 hypointense round sharply marginated mass (*arrow*) arises within the cauda equina. In enhanced sagittal T1-weighted image **B**, the mass (*arrow*) enhances intensely and homogeneously. Conus level intradural meningiomas are far less common than intradural schwannomas.

tumors can arise in the conus/cauda equina region (*Fig. 50-7*). They are T1 isointense and T2 hyperintense relative to the spinal cord and enhance homogeneously after IV contrast.

3. **Metastasis involving the conus medullaris:** Lung and breast primary tumors are most common.[13] Look for leptomeningeal deposits elsewhere because metastases are often multiple. Enhancement may be homogenous or heterogeneous. Leptomeningeal metastases commonly involve the conus medullaris. See Chapter 37 for discussion of leptomeningeal metastasis.

4. **Lymphoma:** Can manifest as an intradural enhancing mass involving the conus medullaris, which resembles leptomeningeal metastasis (*Fig. 50-8*).

5. **Epidermoid:** Can usually be differentiated from ependymoma because epidermoids are T1 hypointense, T2 hyperintense masses that are classically hyperintense on diffusion-weighted images.

6. **Dermoid:** These lesions can involve the conus medullaris. They contain fat and a fluid-filled cyst (*Fig. 50-9*).

7. **Paraganglioma:** These are hypervascular tumors that rarely involve the conus/cauda equina. They tend to be more heterogeneous on MR imaging. Contrast enhancement pattern is variable.

TREATMENT

1. **En bloc surgical removal** is the procedure of choice[16] using microsurgical techniques.[17] Myxopapillary ependymomas may recur locally if not completely resected.

2. **Adjuvant radiotherapy** is given if the tumor cannot be completely resected or if there is tumor recurrence.[4,16]

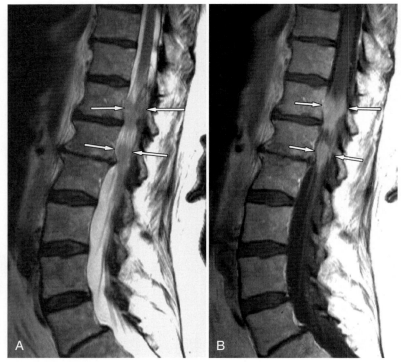

Figure 50-8 ▶ **Intradural Lymphoma Involving Conus Medullaris Region.** In sagittal T2-weighted image **A**, ill-defined T2 hypointense masses (*arrows*) involve the conus tip and upper cauda equina. In enhanced sagittal T1-weighted image. **B**, the masses (*arrows*) have a flame-shaped pattern of enhancement.

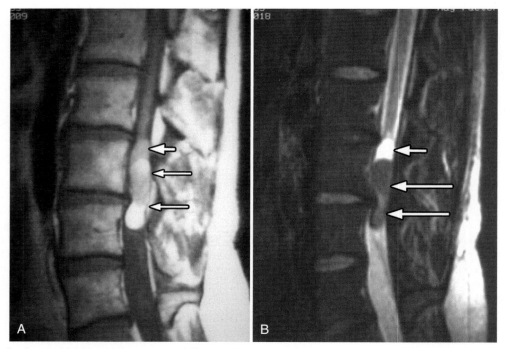

Figure 50-9 ▶ **Intradural Dermoid Arising at the Conus Medullaris Level.** Sagittal unenhanced T1-weighted MR image **A** and T2-weighted image **B**. Fat-containing portions of the dermoid are T1 hyperintense and T2 hypointense (*long arrows* in images **A** and **B**). The small rostral cyst in the dermoid is slightly T1 hyperintense and markedly T2 hyperintense (*short arrow* in images **A** and **B**) relative to the spinal cord.

References

1. Afshani E, Kuhn JP. Common causes of low back pain in children. *Radiographics.* 1991;11(2):269-291.
2. Koeller KK, Rosenblum RS, Morrison AL. Neoplasms of the spinal cord and filum terminale: Radiologic-pathologic correlation. *Radiographics.* 2000;20(6):1721-1749.
3. Friedman DP, Hollander MD. Neuroradiology case of the day. Myxopapillary ependymoma of the conus medullaris or filum terminale resulting in superficial siderosis and dissemination of tumor along CSF pathways. *Radiographics.* 1998;18(3):794-798.
4. Moynihan TJ. Ependymal tumors. *Curr Treat Options Oncol.* 2003;4(6):517-523.
5. Wagle WA, Jaufman B, Mincy JE. Intradural extramedullary ependymoma: MR-pathologic correlation. *J Comput Assist Tomogr.* 1988;12(4):705-707.
6. Tait MJ, Chelvarajah R, Garvan N, Bavetta S. Spontaneous hemorrhage of a spinal ependymoma: A rare cause of acute cauda equina syndrome: A case report. *Spine.* 2004;29(21):E502-E505.
7. Chung JY, Lee SK, Yang KH, Song MK. Subcutaneous sacrococcygeal myxopapillary ependymoma. *AJNR Am J Neuroradiol.* 1999;20(2):344-346.
8. Ma YT, Ramachandra P, Spooner D. Case report: Primary subcutaneous sacrococcygeal ependymoma: A case report and review of the literature. *Br J Radiol.* 2006;79(941):445-447.
9. Yamada CY, Whitman GJ, Chew FS. Myxopapillary ependymoma of the filum terminale. *AJR Am J Roentgenol.* 1997;168(2):366.
10. Wippold FJ, 2nd, Smirniotopoulos JG, Moran CJ, et al. MR imaging of myxopapillary ependymoma: Findings and value to determine extent of tumor and its relation to intraspinal structures. *AJR Am J Roentgenol.* 1995;165(5):1263-1267.
11. Baleriaux DL. Spinal cord tumors. *Eur Radiol.* 1999;9(7):1252-1258.
12. Kahan H, Sklar EM, Post MJ, Bruce JH. MR characteristics of histopathologic subtypes of spinal ependymoma. *AJNR Am J Neuroradiol.* 1996;17(1):143-150.
13. Lowe GM. Magnetic resonance imaging of intramedullary spinal cord tumors. *J Neurooncol.* 2000;47(3):195-210.
14. Argyropoulou PI, Argyropoulou MI, Tsampoulas C, et al. Myxopapillary ependymoma of the conus medullaris with subarachnoid haemorrhage: MRI in two cases. *Neuroradiology.* 2001;43(6):489-491.
15. Parmar H, Pang BC, Lim CC, et al. Spinal schwannoma with acute subarachnoid hemorrhage: A diagnostic challenge. *AJNR Am J Neuroradiol.* 2004;25(5):846-850.
16. Henson JW. Spinal cord gliomas. *Curr Opin Neurol.* 2001;14(6):679-682.
17. Asazuma T, Toyama Y, Suzuki N, et al. Ependymomas of the spinal cord and cauda equina: An analysis of 26 cases and a review of the literature. *Spinal Cord.* 1999;37(11):753-759.

NEUROFIBROMATOSIS

Douglas S. Fenton, M.D.

CLINICAL PRESENTATION

The patient is a 21-year-old man who has had neurologic symptoms for about 2 years. Initially, he had trouble holding a pen in the right hand. Over time, he has had more difficulty using his hands, especially the right hand. For the last 3 months, his symptoms have accelerated. He now has a spastic, unstable gait. The right leg is worse than the left. He has urinary hesitancy, but no incontinence. He has not experienced any falls. The patient has several café-au-lait spots and numerous subcutaneous soft tissue masses.

IMAGING PRESENTATION

Sagittal and coronal T2-weighted images reveal numerous hyperintense foraminal and paraspinal soft tissue masses. On the sagittal images, the neural foramina are enlarged by the soft tissue masses. The findings are compatible with multiple neurofibromas in this patient with neurofibromatosis type 1 (*Fig. 51-1*).

DISCUSSION

Neurofibromatosis (NF) is a subset of the phakomatoses. Phakomatoses, also known as *neurocutaneous syndromes,* consist of a group of disorders that tend to develop hamartomatous malformations and neoplastic growths affecting the skin, the nervous system, and other organs.[1] The most common phakomatoses are NF, tuberous sclerosis, von Hippel-Lindau syndrome, and Sturge-Weber disease. NF is the most common of the phakomatoses. NF is classically divided into two types: NF type 1 (NF-1), also known as *von Recklinghausen disease* or *peripheral neurofibromatosis,* and NF type 2 (NF-2) or central neurofibromatosis.

NF-1 is much more common than NF-2, accounting for greater than 90% of all cases of neurofibromatosis.[2] NF-1 occurs in 1 in 3500 live births.[3] It is an autosomal dominant disorder in 50% to 60% of cases and is localized to chromosome *17,* which encodes for neurofibromin. Neurofibromin is a tumor suppressor gene.[4] The remainder of the cases arise as spontaneous mutations. Diagnosic criteria that must be met for the diagnosis of NF-1 require the presence of two or more of the following: six or more café-au-lait spots, two or more neurofibromas, axillary or groin freckling, optic nerve glioma, two or more Lisch nodules (hamartomas of the iris), a distinctive bone lesion (such as hypoplasia of the sphenoid wing, pseudoarthrosis, severe kyphoscoliosis, or cortical thinning of a long bone), or a first-degree relative with NF-1.[5] Some patients may have a very mild disease, whereas others are profoundly affected. Some of the complications occur at different times of life, which can delay the actual diagnosis of NF-1. Café-au-lait spots and external plexiform neurofibromas are seen within the first year of life and are present in 95% of all patients.[6] Freckling and optic nerve gliomas are seen by 7 years of age. Cutaneous neurofibromas and Lisch nodules appear in teenage years or early adulthood. Malignancy and spinal plexiform neurofibromas are seen as adults.[6]

The many spinal manifestations of NF-1 can be divided into bone and soft tissue abnormalities. Scoliosis is the most common musculoskeletal manifestation of NF-1 with an incidence of 71%.[7] The scoliosis most often affects the thoracic spine.[8] The most common scoliosis is a nondystrophic curve with a Cobb angle of less than 10 degrees and a kyphosis between 20 and 45 degrees. Dystrophic curves have a Cobb angle of greater than 10 degrees and a kyphosis of greater than 45 degrees.[9] Primary bone involvement is known as *mesodermal dysplasia.*[10] Mesodermal dysplasia causes the bone to be weaker and susceptible to erosion and remodeling, which can lead to scoliosis, secondary vertebral scalloping from tumoral compression, and lateral meningoceles.[11] Soft tissue abnormalities include benign and malignant neurofibromas and schwannomas. Plexiform neurofibromas are present in 25% of cases of NF-1 and are considered pathognomonic for NF-1.[12] A neurofibroma is a fusiform tumor mass that is located along the path of a peripheral nerve. Most plexiform neurofibromas are slow growing and benign; however, some neurofibromas may undergo malignant degeneration and invade and/or erode adjacent bones. Malignant degeneration occurs in 3% of all patients with NF-1 and is greatest in patients between the ages of 15 and 40.[8]

There are no known predictive factors as to which tumors will undergo malignant degeneration. Most neurofibromas are asymptomatic. However, neurofibromas can affect large nerves, plexi, and spinal roots. The sacral plexus can be involved by tumor with compression of the ureters, rectum, and uterus.[6] Plexiform neurofibromas involving spinal roots can cause pain from neural foraminal narrowing and cause spinal stenosis and/or cord compression/myelopathy depending on the level of abnormality.[6] Other soft tissue involvement includes dural ectasias, which arise secondary to the pathologic (mesodermal dysplasia) bone with erosions of the vertebral bodies and the potential for formation of a lateral meningocele (pulsatile diverticula).[8]

NF-2 is also an autosomal dominant disorder, which is located on chromosome *22* and encodes the 595-amino acid protein

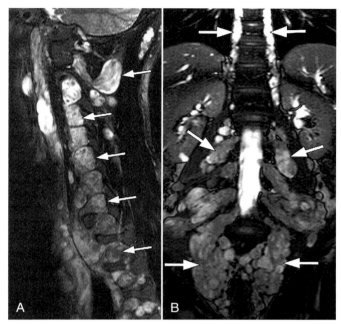

Figure 51-1 ► **Neurofibromatosis Type 1.** Off-midline sagittal T2-weighted image **A** and coronal T2-weighted image **B**. Innumerable large increased T2 signal intensity foraminal soft tissue masses (*arrows*), many of which are paravertebral. There is enlargement of all cervical neural foramina.

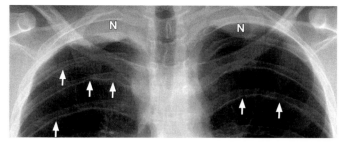

Figure 51-2 ► **Neurofibromatosis Type 1.** Frontal radiograph. Multiple regions of notching on the undersurface of several ribs (*arrows*). Note the soft tissue densities at both lung apices (*N*), which were discovered to be neurofibromas.

schwannomin (also known as *merlin* [moesin-ezin-radixin-like] protein), a tumor suppressor.[13] Like NF-1, 50% of the reported cases of NF-2 are spontaneous mutations. However, NF-2 is much more rare than NF-1, seen in 1 of 40,000 people.[14] There is no gender predilection. The term *neurofibromatosis 2* is a misnomer because neurofibromas are not seen with NF-2.

The most common type of spinal nerve sheath tumors associated with NF-2 are schwannomas and are present in more than 80% of patients.[14-16] In the spine of NF-2 patients, schwannomas and meningiomas have equal incidences and may occur simultaneously.[14] Spinal schwannomas are usually small and asymptomatic, although in some patients they can be large and cause compression of the spinal cord or adjacent neural structures with resulting myelopathy and radicular pain.[16] Peripheral schwannomas can arise from any nerve and can cause pain or impaired motor or sensory function.[16] The diagnosis of NF-2 can be made on the basis of a patient having either bilateral vestibular nerve masses (nearly one half of all patients present with hearing loss), a positive family history with either a unilateral vestibular mass or any two of meningiomas, gliomas, schwannomas, and congenital cataracts.[17] Because of the propensity of NF-2s for multiple intracranial and intraspinal neoplasms, NF-2 has also been called the *MISME (multiple inherited schwannomas, meningiomas, and ependymomas) syndrome*.

Comparing and contrasting NF-1 and NF-2, both entities are autosomal dominant.[4,13] NF-1 is 10 times more common than NF-2.[3,14] Both entities have intradural, extramedullary masses; however, these are seen more frequently with NF-2. Intramedullary masses are common with NF-2 and unusual with NF-1.[18] The neurofibromas of NF-1 have malignant potential, whereas the schwannomas of NF-2 have no malignant potential. Both entities have a similar incidence of bone abnormalities; however, these are usually secondary abnormalities such as neural foraminal widening/scalloping secondary to tumors.[18] Primary dysplastic

bone changes are only seen with NF-1. Scoliosis also appears to be much more frequent with NF-1.[18] Dural ectasias, although uncommon, are seen with NF-1 and not typical with NF-2.[18]

IMAGING FEATURES

Because neurofibromatosis types 1 and 2 are syndromes, the imaging characteristics depend upon which finding(s) the patient has. The imaging discussion below pertains only to findings in the spine.

Neurofibromatosis-1

Plain radiographs can demonstrate the scalloping of the vertebra seen with NF-1 and other bone changes such as kyphosis/scoliosis and dysplastic ("ribbon") or notched ribs (*Fig. 51-2*). The neurofibromas of NF-1 can be nodular or discrete or they can be plexiform neurofibromas that encase and enlarge the nerves. On computed tomography (CT), neurofibromas are hypodense with variable enhancement. There may be widening of the spinal canal and/or neural foramen secondary to dural ecstasia or the tumor itself (*Fig. 51-3*). On magnetic resonance imaging (MRI), neurofibromas are hypointense on T1-weighted sequences, hyperintense on T2-weighted sequences, and have a variable degree of enhancement (*Fig. 51-4*). Because neurofibromas and epidural/foraminal fat have similar signal intensity on T2-weighted sequences, it is best to perform fat-saturated, T2-weighted sequences. On T2 sequences imaged perpendicular to the axis, the neurofibroma appears like a target with a hyperintense rim and a low to intermediate signal intensity center (*Fig. 51-5*). The spinal neurofibromas often have a characteristic dumbbell shape with expansion of the neural foramen. There have been some studies that suggest that fluorodeoxyglucose positron emission tomography (FDG-PET) imaging may be useful in distinguishing benign from malignant neurofibromas.[18-20] These studies suggest that malignant neurofibromas have higher standard uptake values (SUV) than benign ones. Patients with NF-1 frequently have dural ectasias and lateral meningoceles (cerebrospinal fluid [CSF]-filled widenings of the spinal canal with or without extension through the neural foramen). They have imaging characteristics similar to water; hypodense on CT, increased T1/decreased T2 signal on MR, and no evidence of enhancement (*Fig. 51-6*).

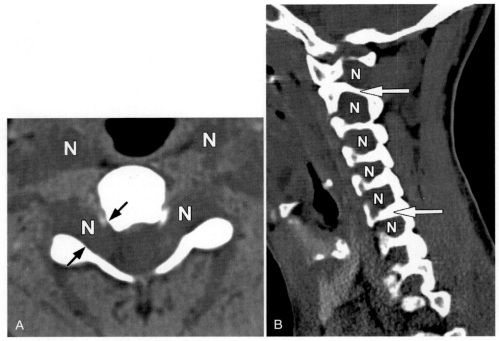

Figure 51-3 ▶ Multiple Neurofibromas, CT. Axial image **A** and off-midline sagittal image **B** CT images. Large hypodense neurofibromas (*N*) both in the neural foramen and in the soft tissues of the neck. The neural foramen are widened (*between arrows*, image **A**) and rounded (image **B**). The articular pillars have undergone chronic pressure erosion with thinning and stretching (*arrows*, image **B**) from the foraminal masses.

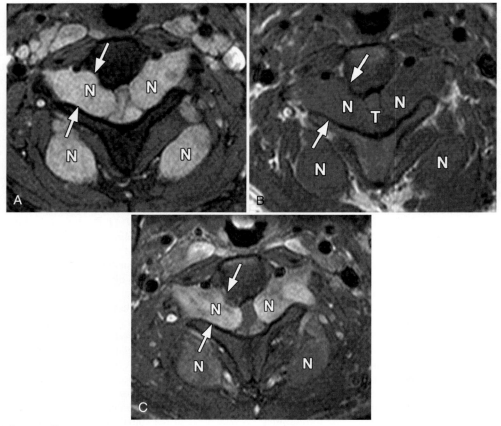

Figure 51-4 ▶ Multiple Neurofibromas, MRI. Axial fat-saturated, T2-weighted image **A**, T1-weighted image **B**, and fat-saturated, post-contrast, T1-weighted image **C**. Multiple soft tissue masses (*N*) displaying decreased T1 signal, increased T2 signal and enhancement both within the neural foramen and in the soft tissues. The neural foramina are widened (*between arrows*) and the foraminal masses cause significant narrowing of the thecal sac (*T*).

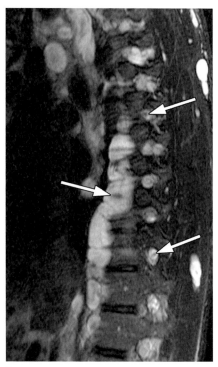

Figure 51-5 ▶ **Neurofibromas, Target Appearance.** Off-midline sagittal T2-weighted image. Imaging perpendicular to a neurofibroma demonstrates a target-like appearance with a low signal intensity center surrounded by a rim of higher signal intensity (*arrows*).

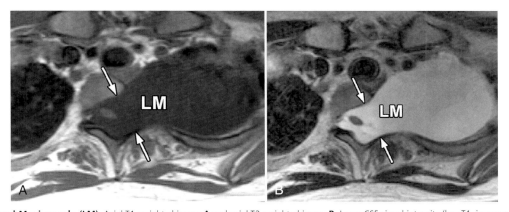

Figure 51-6 ▶ **Lateral Meningocele (LM).** Axial T1-weighted image **A** and axial T2-weighted image **B**. Large CSF signal intensity (low T1, increased T2) lateral extension of the thecal sac through a widened neural foramen (*between arrows*) into the upper left thoracic cavity.

Neurofibromatosis-2

Schwannomas of NF-2 can be primarily in the spinal canal or can be large, dumbbell-shaped masses that expand the neural foramen. They are commonly intradural, extramedullary masses. On CT, they are low to intermediate density tumors that enhance *(Fig. 51-7)*. On MRI, schwannomas are of low to intermediate signal intensity on T1 sequences, typically increased signal intensity on T2 sequences, and demonstrate avid, homogeneous enhancement *(Fig. 51-8)*. Plain radiographs, as with NF-1, can demonstrate spinal canal and/or neural foraminal expansion secondary to the tumors.

Meningiomas may be slightly hyperdense on CT and be dural-based. On MRI, they are typically of intermediate signal intensity on T1- and T2-weighted sequences (unless calcified where they are of decreased T1 and T2 signal). There is avid contrast enhancement aside from the calcified portions *(Fig. 51-9)*.

Ependymomas typically manifest as centrally located intramedullary masses in the spine. Ependymomas exhibit intermediate T1 and increased T2 signal intensity. There may be cystic areas in the tumor. The tumor may demonstrate avid enhancement of the entire tumor or of only the noncystic portions *(Fig. 51-10)*.

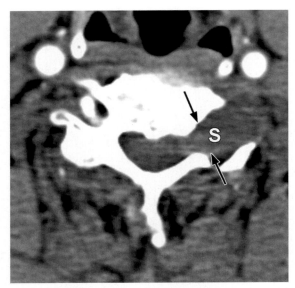

Figure 51-7 ▶ Schwannoma. Axial CT image. Soft tissue mass (*S*) extends from the left lateral epidural space into and through a widened neural foramen (*between arrows*).

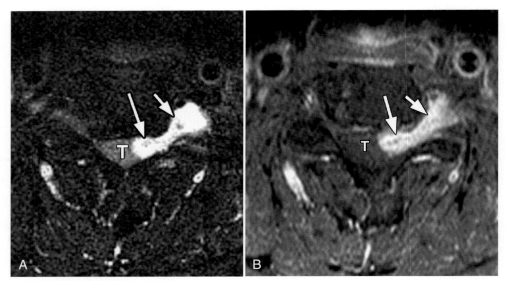

Figure 51-8 ▶ Schwannoma. Axial fat-saturated, T2-weighted image **A** and fat-saturated, post-contrast, T1-weighted image **B**. Dumbbell-shaped mass extending through the neural foramen having both intraspinal (*long arrow*) and extraforaminal (*short arrow*) components. The thecal sac (*T*) is compressed and displaced to the left.

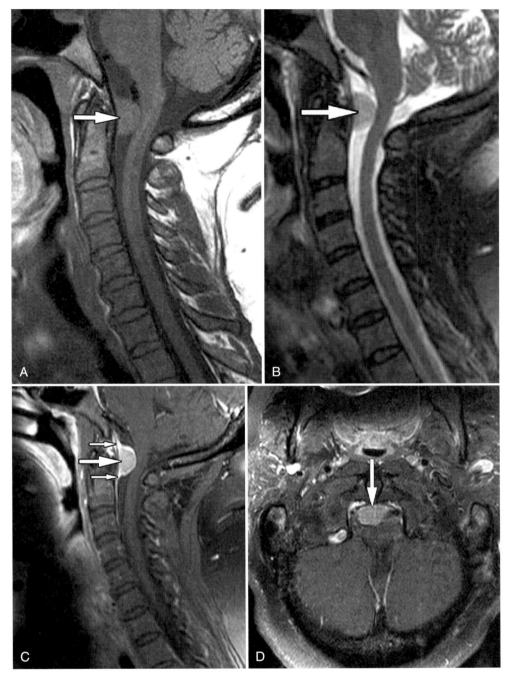

Figure 51-9 ▶ Meningioma. Sagittal T1-weighted image **A**, sagittal T2-weighted image **B**, sagittal fat-saturated, post-contrast, T1-weighted image **C,** and axial fat-saturated, post-contrast, T1-weighted image **D** demonstrate a ventral intradural mass (*arrow*) that is isointense on T1- and T2-weighted images and demonstrates robust enhancement (*arrow*). On sagittal post-contrast images there are small enhancing dural tails both cranial and caudal to the mass (*small arrows*).

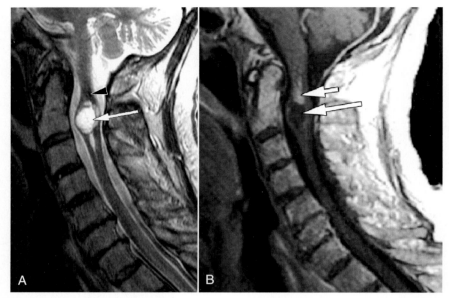

Figure 51-10 ▶ Ependymoma. Sagittal T2-weighted image **A** and post-contrast, T1-weighted image **B**. Large cystic intramedullary mass (*long arrow*) with enhancement on its cranial aspect (*short arrow*, image **B**) as well as hemosiderin deposition on its cranial aspect (*arrowhead*, image **A**).

DIFFERENTIAL DIAGNOSIS

Neurofibromatosis-1

1. **Neurofibromatosis-2:** The schwannomas of NF-2 can look identical to the neurofibromas of NF-1; however, one should evaluate for vestibular schwannomas, meningiomas, and/or ependymomas of NF-2. Spinal deformities are uncommon with NF-2.
2. **Chronic inflammatory demyelinating process (CIDP):** CIDP and NF-1 can have peripheral nerve root enlargement; however, there are no cutaneous stigmata with CIDP.
3. **Congenital hypertrophic polyradiculoneuropathies:** Entities such as Charcot-Marie-Tooth and Dejerine-Sottas disease can have enlarged peripheral nerve roots that appear radiographically like NF-1; however, there are no cutaneous stigmata.

Neurofibromatosis-2

1. **Solitary schwannomas, meningiomas, and ependymomas:** Each of these entities can exist as a separate process without belonging to a syndrome.
2. **Drop metastases:** These originate from the leptomeninges, not from the spinal roots.

TREATMENT

1. **Surgical excision:** There are no proved medical therapies for the schwannomas and neurofibromas of neurofibromatosis. Surgical excision of these tumors is the only treatment option despite there being significant risk of nerve injury, bleeding, and tumor recurrence.[6,21] Plexiform neurofibromas tend to infiltrate the adjacent nerve roots, whereas schwannomas displace them.[1] Therefore, patients with schwannomas tend to do better surgically because of their eccentric nature in relation to the nerve and it being encapsulated.[21] Surgery is usually only performed if there are significant symptoms or limitation of function.
2. **Cosmetic surgery:** Cosmetic surgery of the cutaneous lesions of NF-1 can be performed.[6,21] There are ongoing trials of drugs for the treatment of progressive plexiform neurofibromas.[21]
3. **Chemotherapy:** Chemotherapy is helpful with visual pathway tumors and higher grade astrocytomas.[6]
4. **Radiation therapy:** Radiation therapy should be avoided except with malignant tumors, because radiation can stimulate the growth of plexiform neurofibromas.[6]

References

1. Lin DDM, Barker PB. Neuroimaging of phakomatoses. *Semin Pediatr Neurol.* 2006;13:48-62.
2. Huson S. The different forms of neurofibromatosis. *Br Med J.* 1987;294:113-114.
3. Friedman JM. Epidemiology of neurofibromatosis type 1. *Am J Med Genet.* 1999;89:1-6.
4. Cichowski K, Jacks T. NF1 tumor suppressor gene function: Narrowing the GAP. *Cell.* 2001;104:593-604.
5. National Institutes of Health Consensus Development Conference. Neurofibromatosis: Conference statement. *Arch Neurol.* 1988;45:575-578.
6. Tonsgard JH. Clinical manifestations and management of neurofibromatosis type 1. *Semin Pediatr Neurol.* 2006;13:2-7.
7. Khong P, Goh WH, Wong VC, et al. MR imaging of spinal tumors in children with neurofibromatosis 1. *AJR.* 2003;180:413-417.
8. Rossi SE, Erasmus JJ, McAdams HP, Donnelly LF. Thoracic manifestations of neurofibromatosis-1. *AJR Am J Radiol.* 1999;173:1631-1638.
9. Ramachandran M, Tsirikos AI, Leww J, Saifuddin A. Whole-spine magnetic resonance imaging in patients with neurofibromatosis type 1 and spinal deformity. *J Spinal Disord Tech.* 2004;17:483-491.
10. Restrepo CS, Riascos RF, Hatta AA, Rojas R. Neurofibromatosis type 1: Spinal manifestations of a systemic disease. *J Comput Assist Tomogr.* 2005;29:532-539.

11. Tsirikos AI, Ramachandran M, Lee J, Saifuddin A. Assessment of vertebral scalloping in neurofibromatosis type 1 with plain radiography and MRI. *Clin Radiol.* 2004;59:1009-1017.
12. Poussaint TY, Jaramillo D, Chang Y, Korf B. Interobserver reproducibility of volumetric MR imaging measurements fo plexiform neurofibromas. *AJR Am J Radiol.* 2003;180:419-423.
13. Hovens CM, Kaye AH. The tumor suppressor protein NF2/merlin: The puzzle continues. *J Clin Neurosci.* 2001;8:4-7.
14. Malis L. Neurofibromatosis type 2 and central neurofibromatosis. *Neurosurg Focus.* 1998;4:e1.
15. Mautner VF, Lindenau M. The neuroimaging and clinical spectrum of neurofibromatosis 2. *Neurosurgery.* 1996;38:880-886.
16. Mautner VF. Spinal tumors in patients with neurofibromatosis type 2: MR imaging study of frequency, multiplicity and variety. *AJR Am J Roentgenol.* 1996;166:1231.
17. National Institutes of Health Consensus Development Conference Statement on Acoustic Neuroma, December 11-13, 1991. The Consensus Development Panel. *Arch Neurol.* 1994;51:201-207.
18. Egelhoff JC, Bates DJ, Ross JS, et al. Spinal MR finding in neurofibromatosis types 1 and 2. *AJNR Am J Neuroradiol.* 1992;13:1071-1077.
19. Ferner RE, Lucas JD, O'Doherty MJ, et al. Evaluation of (18)fluorodeoxy-glucose positron emission tomography ([18]FDG-PET) in the detection of malignant peripheral nerve sheath tumours arising from within plexiform neurofibromas in neurofibromatosis 1. *J Neurol Neurosurg Psychiatry.* 2000;68:353-357.
20. Solomon SB, Semih Dogan A, Nicol TL, et al. Positron emission tomography in the detection and management of sarcomatous transformation in neurofibromatosis. *Clin Nucl Med.* 2001;26:525-528.
21. Yohay K. Neurofibromatosis types 1 and 2. *Neurologist.* 2006;12:86-93.

OS ODONTOIDEUM

Leo F. Czervionke, M.D.

CLINICAL PRESENTATION

The patient is a 46-year-old female with dwarfism who suffers from chronic degenerative joint disease involving the large joints. The patient recently had high cervical myelopathic symptoms including neck pain, bilateral hand numbness associated with neck flexion, and weakness of the upper and lower extremities. She describes having recent episodes of intense tingling sensation that radiates down the spine (positive L'Hermitte's sign). On physical examination, neck motion is limited in all directions. She has mild distal upper extremity weakness bilaterally and moderate bilateral lower extremity weakness, mainly involving the hip flexors. Plantar flexion ability is diminished. There is a weak positive bilateral Babinski sign. Deep tendon reflexes are normal. No bladder or bowel dysfunction is present.

IMAGING PRESENTATION

Cervical spine computed tomography (CT) reveals an ossicle superior to a hypoplastic dens consistent with os odontoideum. The anterior arch of C1 is hypertrophic, whereas the posterior arch of C1 is diminutive. Both the anterior and posterior C1 arches contain a midline cleft (*Figs. 52-1 to 52-3*). Magnetic resonance (MR) imaging further reveals thickening of the cruciform ligament, which impinges upon the ventral cord surface at the C1-2 level. The anteroposterior (AP) diameter of the central canal is markedly narrowed (5 mm) with the neck in neutral position. Abnormal T2 signal hyperintensity is demonstrated in the spinal cord at the C1-2 level secondary to either cord edema or myelomalacia from cord compression (*Fig. 52-4*).

DISCUSSION

Os odontoideum is a term first used by Giacomini in 1886 to describe a potentially unstable condition, whereby the odontoid process is separated from the body of C2.[1] Os odontoideum is an uncommonly encountered condition in routine practice, but when present, is often discovered as an incidental finding on CT or MR scans of the cervical spine. Patients with os odontoideum may or may not have symptoms referable to the upper cervical region. Symptomatic cases of os odontoideum have upper neck pain, stiffness, or neurologic dysfunction secondary to atlantoaxial instability with cord compression.

Embryologically, the odontoid process develops from the fourth occipital sclerotome and the first cervical sclerotome. The C2 vertebral body is formed from the second cervical sclerotome.[2] The normal odontoid process (dens) develops from three ossification centers: a tiny terminal ossification center, the ossiculum terminale, and two larger, columnar-shaped ossification centers that form the majority of the odontoid process including its base. The ossiculum terminale develops from either mesenchyme from the fourth occipital sclerotome or proatlas (or both) and is not ossified at birth.[3] The normal ossiculum terminale appears at age 3 and fuses to the remainder of the dens by age 12.[2,3] The base of the odontoid process forms the superior portion of the C2 vertebral body centrally. The two basal columnar-shaped ossification centers of the dens begin to fuse in the sixth fetal month. The inferior portion of the dens begins to ossify in the seventh fetal month and ossification progresses from caudal to cephalad.[2] At birth, the cephalad portion of the odontoid is usually not ossified. By 3 to 4 years of age, the odontoid process is completely ossified, and by age 6 it is fused to the C2 vertebral body in most people.[4] Some unossified cartilage may persist into adult life in the center portion of the dens[5] and in the dental synchondrosis (sometimes called the *C1-2 disc anlage*), located at the junction of the C2 body and odontoid base.

Although relatively uncommon, os odontoideum is said to be the most common anomaly of the odontoid process (*Figs. 52-1 to 52-5*).[3] Other anomalies of the dens also occur. The dens may be developmentally hypoplastic, appearing as a small stump at the superior portion of the C2 body. Rarely, the odontoid process is aplastic.[5] However, true aplasia of the odontoid process would mean that there is complete absence of the dens including its base[3] and therefore some doubt that true odontoid aplasia even exists.[6] In patients with atlanto-occipital assimilation, the atlas is incorporated into or partially fused with the skull base; the dens is usually enlarged and elongated in this condition (*Fig. 52-6*). Atlantoaxial instability may be present with any anomaly of the C1-2 articulation.

The etiology of the condition we refer to as *os odontoideum* has been the subject of debate for decades, and this issue still remains unresolved.[4-7] There are three theories of os odontoideum development. The **first theory** maintains that os odontoideum occurs as a result of failure of the terminal ossification center at the tip of the odontoid process (dens) to fuse with the two basal columnar-shaped ossification centers of the dens.[4] This condition is referred to as *persistent terminal ossification center of the dens* or *persistent ossiculum terminale (POT)*. There is no doubt that POT occurs in

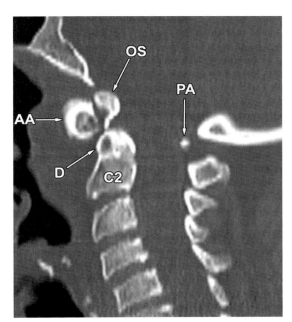

Figure 52-1 ▶ Os Odontoideum. Sagittal reformatted CT image. A separate ossicle, the os odontoideum (*OS*), is located between the hypoplastic dens (*D*) and the tip of the clivus (basion). The os odontoideum is centered slightly superior to the hypertrophic anterior arch (*AA*) of C1. The C1 posterior arch (*PA*) is smaller than normal in size. C2 = C2 vertebral body.

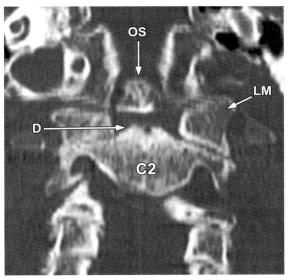

Figure 52-2 ▶ Os Odontoideum. Coronal reformatted CT image, same patient as in Figure 52-1. There is a gap between the os odontoideum (*OS*) and the hypoplastic dens (*D*). The os odontoideum is centered above the level of the lateral mass (*LM*) of C1. C2 = C2 vertebral body.

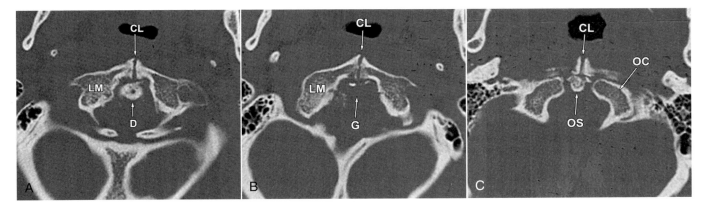

Figure 52-3 ▶ Os Odontoideum. Same patient as in Figures 52-1 and 52-2. Axial CT image **A** located at level of hypoplastic dens (*D*). Midline cleft (*CL*) in anterior arch of C1. Axial CT image **B** located at level of gap (*G*) between hypoplastic dens and os odontoideum (neither are visible on this image). Midline cleft (*CL*) in anterior arch of C1. LM = right apteral mass of C1 on image **A** and **B**. On axial CT image **C**, the os odontoideum (*OS*) is visible at the level of the occipital condyle (*OC*). The midline C1 cleft in the anterior arch of C1 is still visible at this level.

some patients. However, it is highly unlikely that POT is the same entity as os odontoideum.[8] The POT is a tiny ossification center, much smaller than os odontoideum, and is located above the level of the transverse atlantal ligament. Therefore, atlantoaxial instability is usually not associated with the presence of POT, and these patients are rarely symptomatic. Cases of symptomatic POT are probably misdiagnosed cases of os odontoideum.[9]

The **second theory** of os odontoideum formation is a traumatic theory of evolution, which is the most widely held theory.[9] In patients with a normally developing atlas, a fracture occurring through the odontoid process through the basal ossification centers of the dens could result in shearing of the upper portion of the odontoid process, resulting in a separate fragment, comprised of

three cartilaginous components: the upper portion of both basal dental ossification centers and the ossiculum terminale. Later these three fragments would ossify to become the os odontoideum.[8] This theory proposes that a weakness exists in the developing dens between the lower, ossified portions of the basal dental ossification centers and the upper, as yet unossified, cartilaginous portions of the basal dental ossification. Furthermore, this theory assumes that this interface between the ossified and cartilaginous basal portions of the basal dental ossifications is susceptible to fracture by traumatic shearing forces from an intact or disrupted transverse dental ligament.[8] This theory is definitely plausible and explains the imaging appearance of os odontoideum and the seemingly hypoplastic appearance of the base of the dens, which is attached to the

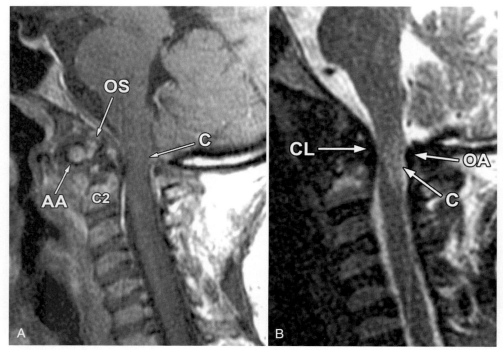

Figure 52-4 ▶ Os Odontoideum. Same patient as in Figures 52-1 to 52-3. On midline sagittal T1-weighted MR image **A**, the os odontoideum (*OS*) is located below the clival tip (basion) and centered slightly above the hypertrophic anterior arch of C1. C2 = C2 body. On midline sagittal T2-weighted MR image **B**, The spinal cord is compressed between the tectorial membrane/cruciform ligament (*CL*) anteriorly and the occipitoatlantal (*AO*) membrane posteriorly. T2 signal hyperintensity is present in the spinal cord (*C*) representing either cord edema or myelomalacia.

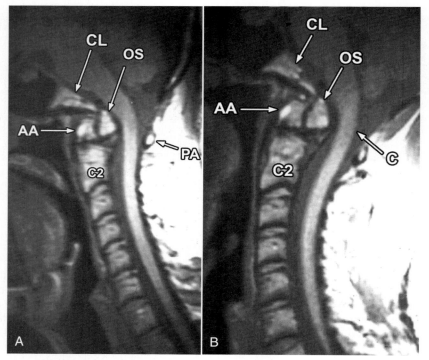

Figure 52-5 ▶ Os Odontoideum in Patient with Platybasia. On midline sagittal T1-weighted MR image **A**, obtained with the neck in flexion, the upper margin of the os odontoideum (*OS*) is positioned behind the tip of the clivus (*CL*), i.e., the basion. The inferior portion of the os odontoideum is located posterior to the hypertrophic anterior arch (*AA*) of C1. The C1 anterior arch is positioned beneath the clivus. The cruciform ligament and tectorial membrane, located posterior to the os odontoideum impinges upon the ventral cord surface with the neck in flexion. The posterior arch (*PA*) of C1 is relatively normal in size. C2 = C2 vertebral body. On midline sagittal T1-weighted MR image **B**, obtained with neck in relative extension, there is less impingement on the ventral cord surface by the os odontoideum (*OS*) and adjacent cruciform ligament/tectorial membrane. The relative position of the os odontoideum, anterior arch (*AA*) of C1 and clivus (*CL*) remain unchanged with the neck positioned in extension.

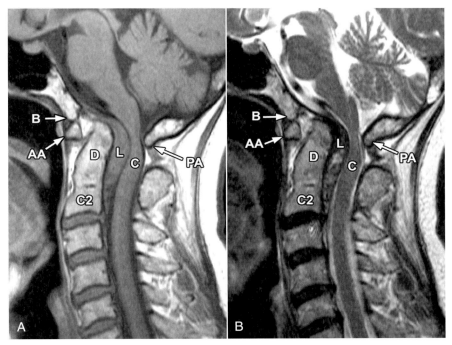

Figure 52-6 ▶ Atlantal-Occipital Assimilation. On midline sagittal T1-weighted image **A** and sagittal T2-weighted image **B**. The anterior arch (*AA*) of C1 contacts the undersurface of the basion (*B*), but is not fused to the basion. The body of C2 is normal in size but the dens (*D*) is elongated. The spinal cord (*C*) is severely compressed between the markedly enlarged cruciform ligament (*L*) and the posterior arch (*PA*) of C1, which is fused to the posterior margin of the foramen magnum (opisthion).

body of C2 in this condition. The fracture in this situation would likely have to occur in infancy or early childhood before the basal ossification centers of the dens are completely ossified, which is before the age of 5.[8-10] A fracture through the base of the odontoid at the dental synchondrosis is almost certainly not the cause of this anomaly because it does not explain the appearance of the atlas (with attached odontoid base) below the os odontoideum.[4,6]

A history of trauma is present in many patients with symptomatic os odontoideum, and therefore many cases of os odontoideum are almost certainly related to trauma in some way.[3,8,11,12] Further supporting the post-traumatic theory is the fact that some patients with os odontoideum have been reported to have a normal appearing odontoid process prior to a traumatic event.[3,6,8] However, trauma alone does not explain the imaging features of os odontoideum with the characteristic hypoplastic appearance of the dens and the hypertrophic anterior arch of C1.[9]

The **third theory** proposes that os odontoideum is a primary congenital or developmental anomaly that is detected incidentally or after a traumatic episode. This theory also has merit and seems to account for some, but not all, patients with os odontoideum. It is possible that the os odontoideum is a persistent, hypertrophied remnant of the proatlas. The proatlas is a small bone that normally exists in reptiles. In humans, a remnant of the proatlas and/or mesenchymal tissue from the fourth occipital sclerotome go on to form the ossiculum terminale of the dens. A tiny persistent proatlas ossicle may rarely be seen in humans between the tip of the odontoid and the basion.[4] A minority of patients with os odontoideum have no history of antecedent trauma.[3,7] Furthermore, os odontoideum may be associated with other congenital anomalies that seem to favor a congenital etiology of os odontoideum in these cases. These other congenital abnormalities or disorders include bipartite atlas, aplasia of the anterior C1 arch, Klippel-Feil malformation, Down syndrome, Morquio's disease, pseudochondrodysplasia, opsismodysplasia, and multiple epiphyseal dysplasia.[3,11,13-15] The anterior arch of C1 is often hypertrophic in patients with os odontoideum.[16] Supporting a congenital etiology of os odontoideum is the fact that familial cases of os odontoideum have been reported.[17-19] Os odontoideum may also occur in patients with Laron syndrome, because of an inborn genetic or metabolic pathway abnormality that causes resistance to growth hormone.[20] Patients with Laron syndrome often have a small oropharyngeal cross-sectional diameter and may develop significant degeneration of the C1-2 articulations with severe spinal stenosis and subsequent spinal cord myelomalacia.

The information presented above suggests that both congenital abnormalities and traumatic events play a role in the resulting condition referred to as *os odontoideum*. Because of this, some investigators believe that os odontoideum occurs when a pre-existing anomalous C2 vertebra is subjected to trauma in infancy or early childhood.[3,7,9,11]

CLINICAL FINDINGS

Many patients with os odontoideum are asymptomatic. Symptoms occur when there is spinal instability and/or cord compression. Symptomatic patients often have neck pain or discomfort ranging from mild to severe. Torticollis, light-headedness, and occipital headaches may be present. Approximately one third of patients in a large series of patients with os odontoideum had neurologic deficits although pain was more common.[3] Most neurologic deficits occur secondary to trauma and are related to atlantoaxial instability,[9] which in turn, may cause cord compression, cord swelling, edema, and resultant myelopathy.[21] Patients with cord compression may experience electric shocklike sensations in the extremities or trunk (L'Hermitte's sign).[11] Patients with os odontoideum with atlantoaxial instability who experience major or even minor trauma are at future risk for developing severe cord compression that can lead to quadraparesis or rarely to death.[6,22] Death can also occur after decompression of the cord following atlantoaxial dislocation, which may be secondary to development of hematomyelia.[22,23]

IMAGING FEATURES

Os odontoideum may go undetected on routine plain radiographs of the cervical spine because the ossicle may project over the lateral ring of C1 or be mistaken for the anterior arch of C1. On radiographs, CT or MR images, the os odontoideum is typically seen as a well-corticated, ovoid bone density superior to and separate from the C2 body. This ossicle may be in the expected location of the odontoid tip or close to the base of the occiput (just below the basion) (see Figs. 52-1 to 52-4).[12] An os odontoideum that moves with the anterior arch of C1 is most common and is said to be *dystopic*, whereas an os odontoideum that moves with the C2 body is much less common and said to be *orthotopic*.[9] In a minority of cases the os odontoideum is located within the foramen magnum posterior to the clivus.[9]

In os odontoideum, the superior margin of the C2 body may have one of three configurations as viewed on anteroposterior (AP) radiographs, tomograms, or coronal CT, as classified by Matsui:[24] type 1, a round, convex superior margin; type 2, a cone-shaped superior margin; or type 3, a tooth-like superior projection. The configuration of the upper C2 vertebral body margin has clinical implications. Myelopathy is more likely with type 1, followed by type 2. Myelopathy is usually not encountered in type 3.[24]

The anterior arch of C1 may appear hypertrophied relative to the posterior arch of C1 (see Figs. 52-1, 52-4, and 52-5).[25] It is uncertain whether the anterior C1 arch hypertrophy represents a congenital anomaly or is secondary to chronic stress on C1 because of atlantoaxial instability. A bipartite atlas or aplasia of the anterior arch of C1 may be associated with os odontoideum.[13,14]

Atlantoaxial instability is manifested by a widened space between the os odontoideum and the anterior arch of C1. Radiographs of the cervical spine in flexion and extension should be obtained in all patients with suspected atlantoaxial instability.[26] Atlantoaxial instability can also be diagnosed with flexion and extension MR imaging, which is helpful to assess the degree of cord impingement by the os odontoideum and cruciform ligament (see Fig. 52-5). In patients with os odontoideum, atlantoaxial instability usually occurs in the anterosuperior direction, but rotary subluxation may also be present in these patients.[21] A variety of measurements can be performed to assess the "space available for the cord" in patients with atlantoaxial subluxation.[26] Significant atlantoaxial instability is likely present if the distance between the posterior C2 vertebral body margin and the posterior arch of C1 is 13 mm or less with the neck flexed.[16,27] Watanabe and colleagues[21] recommend assessing atlantoaxial instability by calculating an *instability index* and *sagittal plane rotation angle*, based on differences in atlantoaxial subluxation and rotation with neck flexion and extension. Watanabe and colleagues[21] found that patients with an instability index of greater than 40% or a sagittal plane rotation angle greater than 20 degrees were far more likely to have myelopathy.

Vertebral artery compression and subsequent cerebellar infarction may occur from atlantoaxial instability secondary to os odontoideum.[10,28,29] The association of os odontoideum with a C1-2 synovial cyst has been reported that caused compression of the ventral epidural sac and spinal cord.[30]

Disruption of the nuchal ligament (nuchal cord) may occur with traumatic atlantoaxial dislocation with or without presence of os odontoideum, which is visible on MR imaging.[12]

DIFFERENTIAL DIAGNOSIS

1. **Persistent terminal ossification center of the dens** is a tiny ossicle that occurs at the tip of the dens and may be mistaken for a fracture.
2. **Odontoid hypoplasia** is usually not confused with os odontoideum. In this condition there is no ossicle above the hypoplastic dens.
3. **Atlanto-occipital fusion** (assimilation) is a congenital anomaly that is often associated with enlargement and cephalocaudal elongation of the dens. This may be associated with severe cord compression at the foramen magnum level (Fig. 52-6).

TREATMENT

1. **Cervical immobilization/traction or C1-2 fusion:** Asymptomatic patients with no atlantoaxial instability may be treated conservatively or not at all. Patients who have minimal atlantoaxial instability are sometimes treated conservatively with cervical immobilization or traction.[9,16] However, even patients with minor atlantoaxial subluxation are at risk for future neurologic deterioration, and therefore C1-2 fusion should be considered even in patients with relatively minimal atlantoaxial subluxation.[31]
2. **Decompressive laminectomy and fusion:** Patients with os odontoideum and atlantoaxial instability are usually treated by some form of posterior C1-2 fusion.[3,7,9,32] Unfortunately, C1-2 fusion results in 50% reduction of normal neck rotation. The posterior fusion may need to be extended to involve the occiput in some patients.[9] If the cord is compressed, a decompressive laminectomy and fusion may be performed, but decompressive laminectomy alone is not sufficient.[16] Some advocate internal screw fixation and posterior C1-2 bone graft/wiring for patients with os odontoideum.[31] A transoral transpalatopharyngeal approach has been used to decompress ventral epidural compression at the cervicomedullary junction that is irreducible by other means.[33]

References

1. Giacomini C. Sull' esistenza' dell' "os odontoideum" vomo. *Accad Med Torino*. 1886;49:24-28.
2. Choit RL, Jamieson DH, Reilly CW. Os odontoideum: A significant radiographic finding. *Pediatr Radiol*. 2005;35(8):803-807.
3. Fielding JW, Hensinger RN, Hawkins RJ. Os odontoideum. *J Bone Joint Surg Am*. 1980;62(3):376-383.
4. Wollin DG. The os odontoideum: Separate odontoid process. *J Bone Joint Surg Am*. 1963;45:1459-1471.
5. Flemming C, Hodson CJ. Os odontoideum; A congenital abnormality of the axis; case report. *J Bone Joint Surg Br*. 1955;37-B(4):622-623.
6. Fielding JW, Griffin PP. Os odontoideum: An acquired lesion. *J Bone Joint Surg Am*. 1974;56(1):187-190.

7. Sankar WN, Wills BP, Dormans JP, Drummond DS. Os odontoideum revisited: The case for a multifactorial etiology. *Spine.* 2006;31(9):979-984.

8. Hukuda S, Ota H, Okabe N, Tazima K. Traumatic atlantoaxial dislocation causing os odontoideum in infants. *Spine (Phila Pa 1976).* 1980;5(3):207-210.

9. Menezes AH. Pathogenesis, dynamics, and management of os odontoideum. *Neurosurg Focus.* 1999;6(6):e2.

10. Menezes AH. Craniocervical developmental anatomy and its implications. *Childs Nerv Syst.* 2008;24(10):1109-1122.

11. Brecknell JE, Malham GM. Os odontoideum: Report of three cases. *J Clin Neurosci.* 2008;15(3):295-301.

12. Kuhns LR, Loder RT, Farley FA, Hensinger RN. Nuchal cord changes in children with os odontoideum: Evidence for associated trauma. *J Pediatr Orthop.* 1998;18(6):815-819.

13. Osti M, Philipp H, Meusburger B, Benedetto KP. Os odontoideum with bipartite atlas and segmental instability: A case report. *Eur Spine J.* 2006;15(Suppl 5):564-567.

14. Garg A, Gaikwad SB, Gupta V, et al. Bipartite atlas with os odontoideum: Case report. *Spine (Phila Pa 1976).* 2004;29(2):E35-E38.

15. Al Kaissi A, Chehida FB, Ghachem MB, et al. Atlanto-axial segmentation defects and os odontoideum in two male siblings with opsismodysplasia. *Skeletal Radiol.* 2009;38(3):293-296.

16. Spierings EL, Braakman R. The management of os odontoideum: Analysis of 37 cases. *J Bone Joint Surg Br.* 1982;64(4):422-428.

17. Morgan MK, Onofrio BM, Bender CE. Familial os odontoideum: Case report. *J Neurosurg.* 1989;70(4):636-639.

18. Kirlew KA, Hathout GM, Reiter SD, Gold RH. Os odontoideum in identical twins: perspectives on etiology. *Skeletal Radiol.* 1993;22(7):525-527.

19. Saltzman CL, Hensinger RN, Blane CE, Phillips WA. Familial cervical dysplasia. *J Bone Joint Surg Am.* 1991;73(2):163-171.

20. Kornreich L, Horev G, Schwarz M, et al. Laron syndrome abnormalities: Spinal stenosis, os odontoideum, degenerative changes of the atlanto-odontoid joint, and small oropharynx. *AJNR Am J Neuroradiol.* 2002;23(4):625-631.

21. Watanabe M, Toyama Y, Fujimura Y. Atlantoaxial instability in os odontoideum with myelopathy. *Spine.* 1996;21(12):1435-1439.

22. Dastur DK, Wadia NH, Desai AD, Sinh G. Medullospinal compression due to atlanto-axial dislocation and sudden haematomyelia during decompression: Pathology, pathogenesis and clinical correlations. *Brain.* 1965;88(5):897-924.

23. Wadia NH. Myelopathy complicating congenital atlanto-axial dislocation: A study of 28 cases. *Brain.* 1967;90(2):449-472.

24. Matsui H, Imada K, Tsuji H. Radiographic classification of os odontoideum and its clinical significance. *Spine.* 1997;22(15):1706-1709.

25. Holt RG, Helms CA, Munk PL, Gillespy T, 3rd. Hypertrophy of C-1 anterior arch: useful sign to distinguish os odontoideum from acute dens fracture. *Radiology.* 1989;173(1):207-209.

26. Truumees E. Os Odontoideum. emedicine. 2008. Available at http://emedicine.medscape.com/article/1265065-overview. Accessed November 29, 2009, and November 6, 2010.

27. Greenberg AD. Atlanto-axial dislocations. *Brain.* 1968;91(4):655-684.

28. Takakuwa T, Hiroi S, Hasegawa H, et al. Os odontoideum with vertebral artery occlusion. *Spine.* 1994;19(4):460-462.

29. Fukuda M, Aiba T, Akiyama K, et al. Cerebellar infarction secondary to os odontoideum. *J Clin Neurosci.* 2003;10(5):625-626.

30. Aksoy FG, Gomori JM. Symptomatic cervical synovial cyst associated with an os odontoideum diagnosed by magnetic resonance imaging: Case report and review of the literature. *Spine.* 2000;25(10):1300-1302.

31. Klimo P Jr, Kan P, Rao G, et al. Os odontoideum: Presentation, diagnosis, and treatment in a series of 78 patients. *J Neurosurg Spine.* 2008;9(4):332-342.

32. Visocchi M, Fernandez E, Ciampini A, Di Rocco C. Reducible and irreducible os odontoideum in childhood treated with posterior wiring, instrumentation and fusion: Past or present? *Acta Neurochir (Wien).* 2009;151(10):1265-1274. Epub 2009 Apr 30.

33. Menezes AH. Surgical approaches: Postoperative care and complications "transoral-transpalatopharyngeal approach to the craniocervical junction." *Childs Nerv Syst.* 2008;24(10):1187-1193.

OSSIFICATION OF THE POSTERIOR LONGITUDINAL LIGAMENT

Douglas S. Fenton, M.D.

CLINICAL PRESENTATION

The patient is a 69-year-old female with a several-year history of progressive gait difficulty. She presently uses a wheelchair for longer distances outside the home and also a single point cane. She tends to lean on objects when she is walking because of her unsteadiness. Her gait problems have been evolving over the last 5 to 7 years. She reports acute hemiparesis involving the left face and upper and lower limbs. She says that she was diagnosed as having had a stroke and that similar recurrent spells have happened since then, lasting up to 2 hours. She has a continuing sense of tightness involving the right lower extremity that began in the distal leg and foot and now extends up to the knee with intermittent pins-and-needles sensation in the right lower limb. Sensory symptoms do not occur in the left lower extremity. She also feels that the right lower extremity is weak and that, in general, the lower extremity weakness bilaterally has gradually worsened.

IMAGING PRESENTATION

Sagittal T1- and T2-weighted images demonstrate flowing intermediate T1/decreased, T2 signal intensity along the posterior aspect of the vertebral bodies from C3-C7 causing moderate narrowing of the central spinal canal in the midline (*Fig. 53-1*).

DISCUSSION

Ossification of the posterior longitudinal ligament (OPLL) is a condition in which there is pathologic ossification of this ligament in the cervical and/or thoracic spine. If this ossification occupies enough of the spinal canal, then this condition can result in myelopathy and/or radiculopathy secondary to chronic pressure on the spinal cord and nerve roots.[1]

The posterior longitudinal ligament (PLL) is a band of collagen and elastin fibers that extends along a line along the posterior margins of the vertebral bodies from the atlas to the sacrum. The PLL is narrower and weaker than the anterior longitudinal ligament (ALL), which extends along the anterior margins of the vertebral bodies, also from the atlas to the sacrum. The fibers of both of these ligaments are firmly attached to the annulus of the intervertebral discs and the corner of the vertebral bodies.[2] The ligament is widest at the disc spaces and narrowest at the mid-vertebral

levels. The ligament is also thicker centrally and progressively thins out laterally.

With OPLL, there is initial hypertrophy of the ligament secondary to fibroblastic hyperplasia, which is followed by an increase in collagen deposition. Progressive mineralization and cartilaginous ingrowth form ossification centers that eventually result in formation of haversian canals.[3]

OPLL usually occurs in patients over 40 years of age and is very rare until the third decade. OPLL has been well studied in East Asian countries with an incidence of 2% to 4%.[4] The prevalence of OPLL in other countries has not been well studied. OPLL has been estimated to have a prevalence of 0.12%[5] in a radiology review. One quarter of North Americans and Japanese patients with cervical myelopathy exhibit OPLL.[6] Most often, OPLL is found in the upper cervical spine (70%, C2-C4) and less often in the upper thoracic spine (15%, T1-T4). Cervical OPLL occurs twice as often in males as in females.[7]

OPLL can be divided into four different patterns: (1) focal ossification at the posterior margin of the vertebral body; (2) segmental ossification, where each ossification does not extend beyond the adjacent disc level; (3) continuous or flowing ossification across several levels; and (4) mixed ossification, where there is a combination of segmental and continuous OPLL.[8]

Most patients with OPLL are asymptomatic. Matsunaga and colleagues[10] followed 359 patients with documented OPLL for 10 years. Of those, 323 patients at the onset of the study had no myelopathic symptoms and the remaining 36 did. Seventeen percent of those without myelopathy were treated conservatively and developed myelopathy during the follow-up period. Sixty-four percent of the patients who began with a myelopathy and declined surgery worsened. The authors concluded that if a patient was discovered to have OPLL without myelopathy, that prophylactic surgery was not necessary because of the slow progression of OPLL.

IMAGING FEATURES

Plain radiographs can demonstrate the ossification of OPLL behind the vertebral bodies; however, it can easily be overlooked and/or masked by the superimposed facet joint complex on the lateral radiograph (*Fig. 53-2*). Advanced imaging (computed tomography [CT], magnetic resonance [MR] imaging) is necessary to depict the degree of spinal canal stenosis and the effect of OPLL on the spinal cord. CT scanning with sagittal reformats

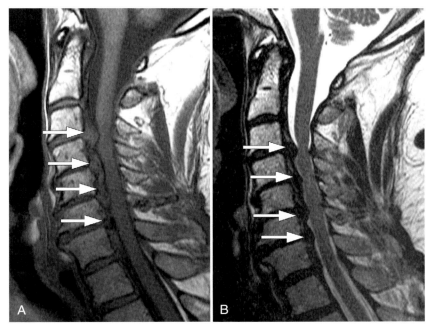

Figure 53-1 ▶ Ossification of the Posterior Longitudinal Ligament. Sagittal T1-weighted image **A** and sagittal T2-weighted image **B**. Flowing intermediate T1, decreased T2 signal intensity thickened soft tissue posterior to the vertebral bodies from mid C3 to C6-7 (*arrows*) causing varying degrees of narrowing of the central spinal canal in the anteroposterior dimension.

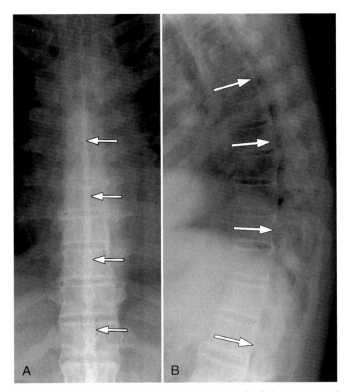

Figure 53-2 ▶ Ossification of the Posterior Longitudinal Ligament. Frontal (image **A**) and lateral (image **B**) radiographs of the thoracic spine. Dense contiguous high density ossification in the central midline along the posterior vertebral bodies (*arrows*) compatible with ossification of the posterior longitudinal ligament.

demonstrates the dense cortical bone of OPLL *(Fig. 53-3)*. A lower density marrow cavity may also be evident. On axial imaging, the ossification may have a "bow-tie" or "upside down T" appearance *(Fig. 53-4)*. Although CT can depict the degree of central canal narrowing, MR is necessary to demonstrate the effect of OPLL on the spinal cord if there are any signal changes in the spinal cord to suggest cord compromise *(Fig. 53-5)*. CT is often performed in conjunction with MR if surgery is contemplated because MR can overestimate the actual degree of spinal canal compromise. MR can demonstrate the flowing ossification of OPLL on sagittal images as well as the "bow-tie" or "upside down T" appearance. The dense cortical bone of mature OPLL is of decreased T1 and T2 signal intensity. However, increased T1 and T2 signal intensity will be seen where OPLL has acquired a marrow cavity. Furthermore, there may be increased signal intensity on T2-weighted acquisitions within the spinal cord secondary to spinal cord edema, ischemia, or infarction.

DIFFERENTIAL DIAGNOSIS

1. **Spondylosis/osteophyte:** Often spondylosis/osteophyte is centered at the disc level and rarely over several levels.
2. **Calcified disc herniation:** Usually calcified disc herniation is centered and connected to an intervertebral disc and does not extend over several levels *(Fig. 53-6)*.
3. **Meningioma:** Non-calcified portions of a meningioma will demonstrate avid enhancement.

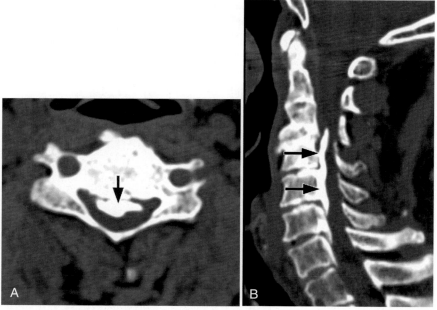

Figure 53-3 ► **Ossification of the Posterior Longitudinal Ligament, CT.** Axial CT image **A** and reformatted sagittal image **B**. Thick bone density posterior to the vertebral body extending from C3-C6 (*arrows*) causing moderate to severe narrowing of the central spinal canal.

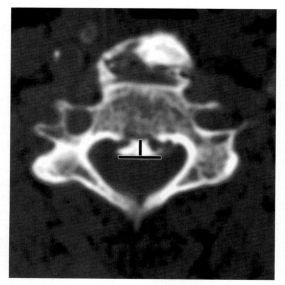

Figure 53-4 ► **"Upside-down T" Appearance of OPLL.** Axial CT image. Classic inverted T-shape ossification of the posterior longitudinal ligament.

TREATMENT

1. **Observation:** If OPLL is discovered as an incidental finding in an asymptomatic patient, then careful observation is warranted.
2. **Nonoperative management:** If the patient has minimal symptoms, then a trial of nonoperative management including injection therapy can be provided.
3. **Surgical management:** The indication for surgery is progressive myelopathy manifested by numbness, weakness of the

upper extremities, and a spastic gait.[8] There has been extensive debate as to the surgical treatment for OPLL; however, the direct removal of the ossified posterior longitudinal ligament via an anterior approach is considered to be the best option with good outcomes, low morbidity, and minimal trauma to the prevertebral soft tissues,[9] especially with the segmental form of OPLL. If OPLL is extensive and affects more than three levels, then a posterior approach with open-door laminoplasty is used. The open-door laminoplasty is an osteotomy of the posterior elements with reconstruction of the spinal canal.

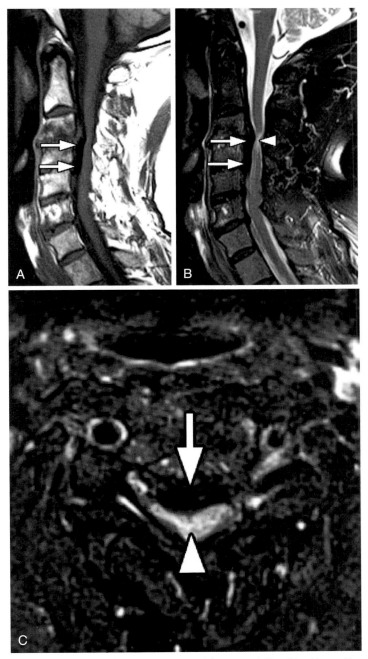

Figure 53-5 ▶ OPLL with Cord Compression. Sagittal T1-weighted image **A**, sagittal fat-saturated, T2-weighted image **B**, and axial fat-saturated, T2-weighted image **C** demonstrate the very low T1 and T2 signal intensity of mature OPLL (*arrows*). There is severe central spinal canal stenosis at the C3-4 level with increased spinal cord T2 signal intensity compatible with cord ischemia and/or myelomalacia (*arrowhead*).

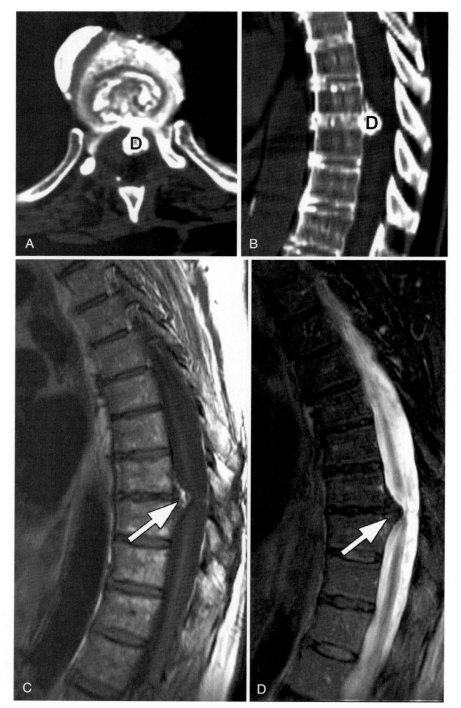

Figure 53-6 ▶ Calcified Disc Herniation. Axial, **A**, and sagittal, **B**, CT images demonstrate a focal, left paracentral calcified "mass" (*D*) centered on the intervertebral disc. Differential would include a calcified disc herniation or meningioma. Sagittal T1-weighted image **C** and T2-weighted image **D** from the same patient demonstrate contiguity with the disc (arrow) making the likely diagnosis a calcified disc herniation. Note that the periphery of this disc herniation is of increased T1 signal intensity, consistent with ossification of that portion of the disc and gaining a marrow cavity.

References

1. Schmidt MH, Quinones-Hinojosa A, Rosenberg WS. Cervical myelopathy associated with degenerative spine disease and ossification of the posterior longitudinal ligament. *Semin Neurol*. 2002;212:143-148.
2. Ehara S, Shimamura T, Nakamura R, Yamazaki K. Paravertebral ligamentous ossification: DISH, OPLL and OLF. *Eur J Radiol*. 1998;27:196-205.
3. Epstein N. Ossification of the cervical posterior longitudinal ligament: A review. *Neurosurg Focus*. 2002;13:ECP1.
4. Matsunga S, Yamaguchi M, Hayashi K, Sakou T. Genetic analysis of ossification fo the posterior longitudinal ligament. *Spine*. 1999;24:937-939.
5. Resnick D. *Diagnosis of Bone and Joint Disorders*. London: Saunders; 1994:1496-1507.
6. Epstein NE. The surgical management of ossification of the posterior longitudinal ligament in 43 North Americans. *Spine*. 1994;19:664-672.
7. Epstein NE. Ossification of the posterior longitudinal ligament: Diagnosis and surgical management. *Neurosurg Quart*. 1992;2:223-241.
8. Mizuno J, Nakagawa H. Ossified posterior longitudinal ligament: Management strategies and outcomes. *Spine J*. 2006;6:282S-288S.
9. Emery SE, Bolesta MJ, Banks MA, Jones PK. Robinson anterior cervical fusion: comparison of standard and modified techniques. *Spine*. 1994;19:660-663.
10. Matsunga S, Sakou T, Taketomi E, Komiya S. Clinical course of patients with ossification of the posterior longitudinal ligament: A minimum 10-year cohort study. *J Neurosurg*. 2004;100(3 Suppl Spine):245-248.

CHAPTER

54

OSTEOBLASTOMA

Douglas S. Fenton, M.D.

CLINICAL PRESENTATION

The patient is a 21-year-old male who presented with pain in the right lower lumbar spine. Over the past several weeks, the patient has noticed a sharp, focal pain in the right lower spine and hip. It is painful to the touch. The pain is worse at night and will occasionally awaken him from his sleep. His pain increases with activity. He notes that his pain goes away for several hours after he takes aspirin. A neurologic examination was normal.

IMAGING PRESENTATION

Axial and reformatted coronal computed tomography (CT) images reveal a large low-density mass containing calcification in the left posterolateral epidural space with irregularity and sclerosis of the left neural arch. The thecal sac is displaced anteriorly and to the left (*Fig. 54-1*). Surgical curettage revealed the mass to be an osteoblastoma.

DISCUSSION

Osteoid osteoma (OO) and osteoblastoma (OB) are benign osseous lesions of osteoblastic origin, consisting of a hypervascular nidus and surrounding sclerotic bone.[1] Osteoid osteoma was first described by Jaffe[2] in 1935. Osteoblastoma was later described by Licchtenstein[3] in 1956.

Both osteoid osteoma and osteoblastoma are most commonly found in the long bones.[4] The spine is the location of osteoid osteoma in 10% of cases and of osteoblastoma in 35% of cases.[4] Osteoid osteoma is usually seen in patients in their second decade of life, whereas osteoblastoma is seen in patients who are slightly older. Approximately 90% of osteoid osteomas and osteoblastomas occur before the age of 30. Both lesions are seen more commonly in males with ratios of 2 to 4:1.[4,5]

Histologically, osteoid osteoma and osteoblastoma are similar, consisting of an osteoid nidus surrounded by sclerotic bone.[4] Some clinicians believe that they are histologically indistinguishable and that their names should be changed to reflect that they are just different clinical expressions of the same process. They have remained distinct entities likely because of their different radiographic appearances and because they have different natural histories—osteoid osteoma tending to regress over time[6,7] and osteoblastoma having the ability to progress and even transform

into a malignancy.[8] Radiographically, osteoid osteomas are more sclerotic, nonexpansive, and painful earlier in their development as opposed to osteoblastoma that tends to be less sclerotic and more expansile.[4,9] McLeod and colleagues[9] used a cutoff of 1.5 cm to distinguish osteoid osteoma from osteoblastoma. A nidus of less than 1.5 cm in diameter is considered an osteoid osteoma, and those greater than 1.5 cm are osteoblastomas, a classification that has remained widely used. Osteoblastoma of the spine will frequently invade the epidural space, surround nerve roots, and possibly cause cord compression. The incidence of epidural invasion by osteoblastoma is approximately 50%.[10]

Osteoid osteomas and osteoblastomas have similar clinical symptomatology when they occur in the spine. The typical clinical symptoms are pain or varying intensity that increases with activity and often localizes at or near the site of the lesion.[11] The pain may be more apparent at night and may awaken the patient from sleep.[11] The pain is often reduced or may disappear altogether with the use of aspirin or other anti-inflammatory medications,[12] although aspirin therapy is less effective with osteoblastoma. Clinically, lesions in the spine can have radicular features; however, neurologic examination is often normal.[13] The incidence of neurologic deficits is significantly higher in patients with osteoblastoma than in those with osteoid osteoma.[5]

Osteoid osteoma is the most common cause of painful scoliosis in adolescents,[14] with all other causes of painful scoliosis being rare. One half of patients with osteoid osteoma in the cervical spine have scoliosis,[5] and over one half of patients with osteoblastoma anywhere in the spine have scoliosis.[14] It is important to consider the duration of a patient's osteoid osteoma or osteoblastoma-related scoliosis and also the patient's age because it appears that there is a critical amount of time that a patient with scoliosis related to osteoid osteoma or osteoblastoma has before it precludes resolution of the deformity. A study by Pettine and colleagues[15] suggests that 15 months is the critical duration of symptoms if antalgic scoliosis is to undergo spontaneous correction after excision of the tumor.[15] Patients with symptoms of less than 15 months duration had a decrease or complete correction of their scoliosis, and those with symptoms greater than 15 months did not. Furthermore, patients who were older when they had the onset of symptoms or those that were younger at the time of surgical excision had more spontaneous resolution of scoliosis.[15]

If complete resection of osteoid osteoma or osteoblastoma is not achieved, there is a significant potential for recurrence. Osteoblastoma has a recurrence rate of 10% to 15% with incomplete resection and has a potential for sarcomatous transformation

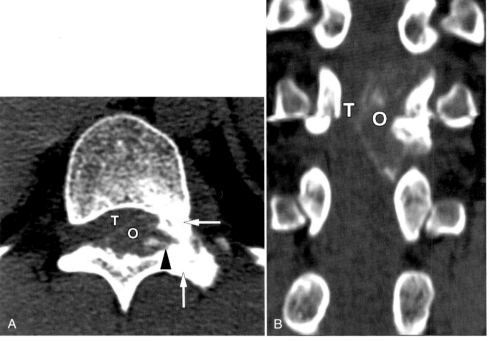

Figure 54-1 ► **Osteoblastoma.** Axial CT image **A** and coronal CT image **B**. Low-density soft tissue mass (*O*) in the left posterolateral epidural space causing right ventral displacement of the thecal sac (*T*). There is sclerosis of the adjacent left pedicle, transverse process, and lamina (*arrows*). The mass has caused some destruction of the right neural arch (*arrowshead*).

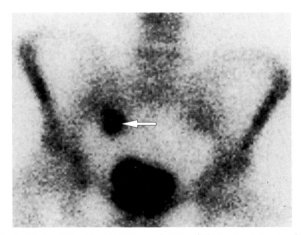

Figure 54-2 ► **Osteoid Osteoma, Nuclear Medicine Bone Scan.** Focal very hyperintense region of increased radiotracer uptake in the right inferior sacrum (*arrow*).

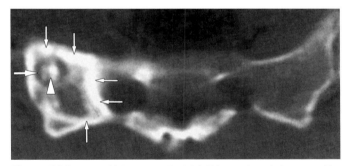

Figure 54-3 ► **Osteoid Osteoma, CT.** Axial CT image through the sacrum. The nidus of the osteoid osteoma is of low density (*large arrows*) with perinidal sclerosis (*small arrows*). There is frequently some central nidal mineralization (*arrowhead*).

and metastasizing.[4,16] Osteoid osteoma has a 4.5% recurrence rate[4] and no potential for malignant transformation.

IMAGING FEATURES

Osteoid Osteoma

The nidus of an osteoid osteoma is the most important part of the neoplasm to visualize. Plain radiography is not the imaging method of choice to evaluate for a radiolucent nidus because of the overlapping anatomy of the spine. Reactive sclerosis can be visualized; however, this is not specific for osteoid osteoma.

Technetium bone scans are very sensitive, but not specific for osteoid osteoma (*Fig. 54-2*).[15] These observations have been reported by Swee and colleagues[12] in which 75% of patients with osteoid osteoma on plain film radiographs had positive bone scans, and the 25% with radiographically negative/CT positive osteoid osteoma had positive bone scans. There have been no cases in the literature with a false-negative bone scan with proved osteoid osteoma. A nuclear medicine bone scan can be obtained to search for an intense focus of radiotracer uptake that would make one suspect osteoid osteoma; however, CT is regarded as the preferred imaging modality to localize the nidus for diagnosis, for presurgical evaluation for open procedures, and for localization purposes for percutaneous procedures. With CT, the nidus of an osteoid osteoma is usually of low attenuation with central mineralization and a varying degree of perinidal sclerosis (*Fig. 54-3*). The imaging

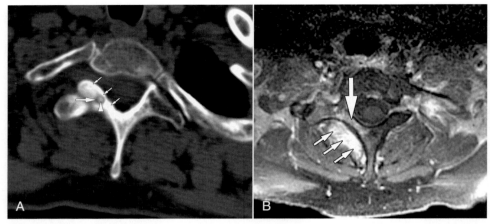

Figure 54-4 ▶ Osteoid Osteoma, CT vs. MRI. Axial CT image **A** and MR post-contrast, fat-saturated, T1 image **B** through the upper thoracic spine. CT image **A** demonstrates low density nidus (*large arrow*) with central mineralization (*arrowhead*) and perinidal sclerosis (*small arrows*). Fat-saturated, post-contrast, T1 MRI **B** reveals enhancement of the right lamina (*arrow*) and inflammatory enhancement in the adjacent soft tissues (*small arrows*).

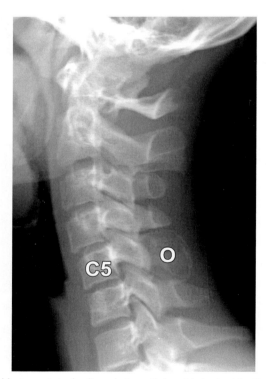

Figure 54-5 ▶ Osteoblastoma. Lateral radiograph. Expansile lucent lesion involving the C5 spinous process (*O*).

characteristics with magnetic resonance imaging (MRI) are variable. The typical nidus is of low to intermediate T1 signal intensity and variable T2 signal depending on the vascularity of the osteoma and/or presence of central mineralization. The nidus demonstrates rapid, avid contrast enhancement. The zone of sclerosis surrounding the nidus usually demonstrates increased T2 signal intensity and will enhance, although it enhances slower than the nidus. Inflammatory enhancement can be seen in the soft tissues adjacent to the osteoid ostoma *(Fig. 54-4)*. Dynamic contrast-enhanced MR is often used to separate nidus from the surrounding reactive zone.

Osteoblastoma

On plain radiography, an osteoblastoma appears as a lucent, expansile lesion with a varying degree of sclerosis, usually in the neural arch *(Fig. 54-5)*. CT better demonstrates the lesion as well as potential matrix mineralization or trabecula *(Fig. 54-6)*. CT can also demonstrate cortical breakthrough if the osteoblastoma is aggressive (see Fig. 54-1). On MRI, osteoblastomas have low to isointense T1 signal intensity and isointense to high T2 signal intensity, and they enhance *(Fig. 54-7)*. Occasionally, an osteoblastoma may have fluid-fluid levels; a characteristic of

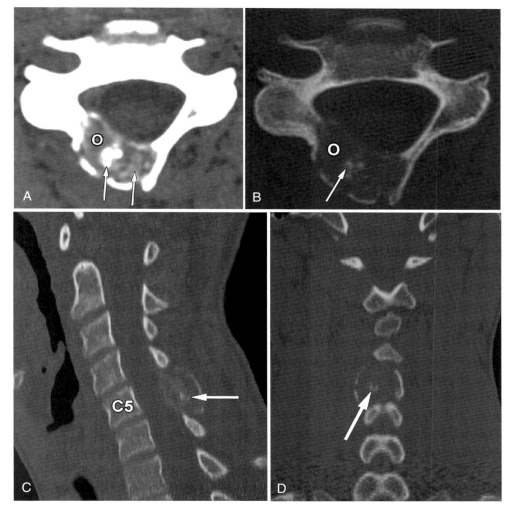

Figure 54-6 ▶ Osteoblastoma. Same patient as in Figure 54-5. Axial CT soft tissue window image **A**, axial bone window image **B**, sagittal image **C**, and coronal image **D**. Expansile low-density lesion (*O*) involving the right lamina and spinous process with areas of intrinsic mineralization (*arrow*).

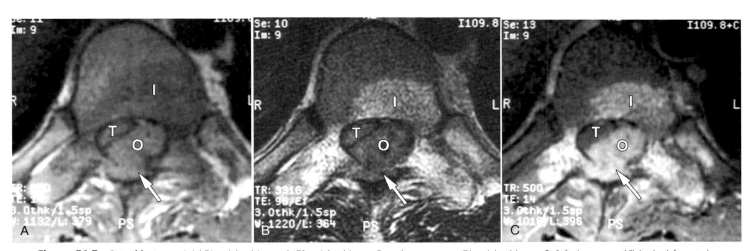

Figure 54-7 ▶ Osteoblastoma. Axial T1-weighted image **A**, T2-weighted image **B**, and post-contrast, T1-weighted image **C**. Soft tissue mass (*O*) in the left posterior epidural space displacing the thecal sac (*T*) anteriorly and to the right. The mass demonstrates intermediate to increased T1 signal intensity, intermediate to low T2 signal intensity, and intense enhancement. There is a break in the posterior cortex of the central spinal canal (*arrow*). Decreased T1 signal intensity, increased T2 signal intensity, and enhancement in the adjacent vertebral body, pedicles, lamina, and transverse processes represent edema and/or inflammation (*I*).

aneurysmal bone cysts. There may be extensive peritumoral edema/inflammation that is of low T1 signal intensity, high T2 signal intensity with variable enhancement. Bone scan demonstrates increased radiotracer uptake on all three phases.

DIFFERENTIAL DIAGNOSIS

Osteoid Osteoma

1. **Osteoblastoma**: By definition, the nidus of an osteoblastoma is greater than 1.5 cm in diameter and is an expansile lesion.
2. **Pedicle or lamina stress fracture**: The sclerosis around a fracture can have the identical appearance of osteoid osteoma–related sclerosis. A CT or MR scan may be necessary to evaluate for a fracture line. Pain associated with a fracture often improves at night during inactivity as opposed to osteoid osteoma, which classically is worse at night.
3. **Sclerotic metastasis**: The sclerosis of a sclerotic metastasis can look like the sclerosis of an osteoid osteoma. However, metastatic disease is usually in older patients. Metastases often involve the pedicle and may have an associated soft tissue mass.
4. **Osteomyelitis sequestrum**: A sequestrum usually involves the vertebral body, has an irregular shape, and is often associated with endplate irregularity.
5. **Unilateral spondylolysis**: The side contralateral to the spondylolysis may be sclerotic like an osteoid osteoma. Imaging is necessary to evaluate for a spondylotic defect.
6. **Unilateral absence of pedicle**: The side contralateral to the spondylolysis may be sclerotic like an osteoid osteoma. Imaging is necessary to evaluate for absence of the pedicle.

Osteoblastoma

1. **Osteoid osteoma**: By definition, the nidus of an osteoid osteoma is less than 1.5 cm in diameter.
2. **Metastasis**: Metastasis may have cortical destruction versus the cortical expansion seen with osteoblastoma. Metastasis is usually found in older patients.
3. **Aneurysmal bone cyst (ABC)**: ABC and osteoblastomas are both expansile lesions; however, ABC more typically has multiple blood-filled cavities with fluid-fluid levels. MRI is best able to demonstrate this finding.
4. **Infection**: Patients with infection are often sick and have elevated white blood cell counts and sedimentation rates. Imaging often demonstrates irregular endplates with infection.
5. **Osteogenic sarcoma**: Osteogenic sarcoma is an aggressive tumor with cortical destruction rather than the expansion seen with an osteoblastoma.

TREATMENT

Osteoid Osteoma

1. **Surgical resection**: Traditionally, surgical resection has been the recommended treatment for osteoid osteoma that causes disabling pain and/or deformity. As previously discussed, the earlier the surgical intervention, the better the chance for complete resolution of any scoliotic deformity. Scoliotic correction is unlikely to occur if symptoms have persisted for longer than 15 months.[15] Surgical excision has its complications and pitfalls. If the nidus is not completely resected, the lesion can recur. This may prompt a surgeon to remove more bone than necessary, which, in the spine, can lead to instability and may necessitate a fusion. There is also the possibility of nerve root or spinal cord injury.
2. **Nonsteroidal anti-inflammatory drugs**: If the patient's symptoms can be suppressed with nonsteroidal anti-inflammatory drugs (NSAIDs), then this may be the only treatment necessary and can be as effective as surgical excision. The patient may become pain free after several years, and the drug therapy then can be discontinued.[17]
3. **Percutaneous thermocoagulation**: In recent years, percutaneous thermocoagulation of the nidus has been used with success.[18] This procedure is performed using CT guidance with the patient under general anesthesia. The nidus location is confirmed with CT. A radiofrequency needle or other thermocoagulation device (laser) is placed into the center of the nidus. A bone drill may be necessary to gain access to the center of the nidus. The nidus is then thermocoagulated at 90° C for 6 minutes. It is important to measure the nidus size/diameter because if it is larger than the zone of thermocoagulation, then two adjacent needle pathways into the nidus separated by 1 cm may need to be used to thermocoagulate the entire lesion. There is concern for lesions in the spine and their proximity to nerve roots, dorsal root ganglia, and spinal cord. Some clinicians have used air injected into the adjacent epidural space prior to lesions to buffer nervous tissue structures from the heat.

Osteoblastoma

Surgical management: Osteoblastoma, by definition, is larger than an osteoid osteoma. Therefore, this lesion is most often not amenable to percutaneous thermocoagulation. Osteoblastoma is treated with surgical treatment that may include curettage and placement of bone graft or methylmethacrylate.

References

1. DePraeter MP, Dua GF, Seynaeve PC, et al. Occipital pain in osteoid osteoma of the atlas: A report of two cases. *Spine*. 1999;24:912-914.
2. Jaffe HL. "Osteoid-osteoma:" A benign osteoblastic tumor composed of osteoid and atypical bone. *Arch Surg*. 1935;31:709-728.
3. Lichtenstein L. Benign osteoblastoma: A category of osteoid-and bone forming tumors other than classical osteoid osteoma, which may be mistaken for giant-cell tumor or osteogenic sarcoma. *Cancer*. 1956;9:1044-1052.
4. Jackson RP, Reckling FW, Mants FA. Osteoid osteoma and osteoblastoma: Similar histologic lesions with different natural histories. *Clin Orthop Relat Res*. 1977;128:303-313.
5. MacLellan DI, Wilson FC. Osteoid osteoma of the spine: A review of the literature and report of six new cases. *J Bone and Joint Surg Am*. 1967;49:111-121.
6. Golding JSR. The natural history of osteoid osteoma with a report of twenty cases. *J Bone and Joint Surg*. 1954;36B:218.
7. Sabanas AO, Bickel WH, Moe JH. Natural history of osteoid osteoma of the spine: Review of the literature and report of three cases. *Am J Surg*. 1956;91:880.
8. Seki T, Fukuda H, Ishii Y, et al. Malignant transformation of benign osteoblastoma: A case report. *J Bone Joint Surg Am*. 1975;57:424.
9. McLeod RA, Dahlin DC, Beabout JW. The spectrum of osteoblastoma. *AJR Am J Radiol*. 1976;126:321-335.
10. Janin Y, Epstein JA, Carras R, Khan A. Osteoid osteomas and osteoblastomas of the spine. *Neurosurgery*. 1981;8:31-38.

11. Orlowski JP, Mercer RD. Osteoid osteoma in children and young adults. *Pediatrics.* 1977;59:526-532.

12. Swee RG, McLeod RA, Beabout JW. Osteoid osteoma: Detection, diagnosis, and localization. *Radiolgoy.* 1979;130:117-123.

13. Kirwan E, Hutton P, Pozo J, Ransford A. Osteoid osteoma and benign osteoblastoma of the spine: Clinical presentation and treatment. *J Bone and Joint Surg Br.* 1984;66:21-26.

14. Mehta MH. Pain provoked scoliosis: Observations on the evolution of the deformity. *Clin Orthop.* 1978;135:58-65.

15. Pettine KA, Klassen RA. Osteoid-osteoma and osteoblastoma of the spine. *J Bone and Joint Surg.* 1986;68A:354-361.

16. Mitchell ML, Ackerman LV. Metastatic and pseudomalignant osteoblastoma: A report of two unusual cases. *Skeletal Radiol.* 1986;15:213-218.

17. Kneisl J, Simon MA. Medical management compared with operative treatment for osteoid osteoma. *J Bone Joint Surg Am.* 1992;74:179-185.

18. Rosenthal DI, Alexander A, Rosenberg AE, Springfield D. Ablation of osteoid osteomas with a percutaneously placed electrode: A new procedure. *Radiology.* 1992;183:29-33.

OSTEOCHONDROMA

Douglas S. Fenton, M.D.

CLINICAL PRESENTATION

The patient is a 68-year-old woman who presented with instability and tinnitus. She has fallen several times but still ambulates without the use of a walker or cane. She states that she occasionally "loses control of her legs" for no reason, which causes her to fall. She feels that her instability has been occurring for at least 5 years and has progressed over the last year.

IMAGING PRESENTATION

Axial soft tissue and bone algorithm computed tomography (CT) images at the C2 level show bony densities along both the anterior and posterior aspect of the C2 vertebral body. The posterior bony density causes right ventrolateral impression upon the spinal cord. The posterior bony density has corticomedullary continuity with C2 (*Fig. 55-1*).

DISCUSSION

Osteochondromas are the most common benign tumors of the long bone.[1] They comprise 8.5% of all osseous tumors and 36% of all benign bone tumors.[2] Osteochondromas are actually considered hamartomas rather than true neoplasms. There are two presentations of osteochondroma: single and sporadic or multiple and hereditary. Multiple exostosis can occur sporadically (25% of cases) but usually results (75% of cases) from a hereditary autosomal dominant disorder known as *hereditary multiple exostosis, osteochondromatosis, Bessel-Hagel syndrome,* or *diaphyseal aclasis.*[2] The single and sporadic form affects the spine in 3% of cases, and the multiple form in 7% to 12% of cases.[2,3] Most spinal lesions are the solitary type, with spinal osteochondromas comprising 0.4% of all spinal tumors.[4] Approximately 10% to 15% of osteochondromas develop secondary to radiation exposure with an average latency of 8 years.[5] Osteochondromas are common in children who received radiation doses of greater than 25 Gy when they were younger than 2 years of age.[6] Osteochondroma is the only bone tumor that can be reproduced experimentally.[7] Solitary osteochondromas affect male patients more than females with a ratio of 2.5 : 1 and an average age at presentation of 30 years.[8] Patients with multiple exostoses present at an average age of 20 years.[8]

Approximately 50% of spinal osteochondromas occur in the cervical spine.[8] The most common level affected is C2, followed by C3 and C6. It has been postulated that microtrauma to the cervical vertebra resulting from its greater mobility might explain the higher incidence of osteochondroma in the cervical region.[8] The thoracic spine is the next most common site, typically affecting T8 followed by T4.[6] Spinal lesions most frequently occur in the posterior arch, usually arising from the tip of a spinous process or transverse process.[6]

Approximately 30% of solitary spinal osteochondromas cause spinal cord compression as opposed to 50% in the multiple form.[8] Clinical symptoms are often slow and progressive because of the slow nature of the growing neoplasm. However, some patients can have an acute presentation of symptoms after a sudden hyperextension or fall in the face of an already compromised spinal canal. Although rare, patients with a cervical osteochondroma can die suddenly from spinal cord compression.[9] Patients can exhibit symptoms of radicular pain, claudication, and/or myelopathy.

Malignant transformation of an osteochondroma to a chondrosarcoma is a well-known complication that is seen in 1% to 5% of patients with solitary osteochondromas and in 10% to 25% of those with the multiple hereditary form.[6] Malignant transformation should be suspected if the cartilaginous cap is greater than 2 cm in thickness,[10,11] if the lesion recurs after resection or grows after skeletal maturity, or if there is new onset of pain or a sudden increase in lesion size.[8,12]

IMAGING FEATURES

A mature osteochondroma consists of a stalk and body composed of mature bone, which is covered by a cartilaginous cap that never ossifies and is never seen on plain radiography.[12] Corticomedullary continuity of the osteochondroma with the parent bone is pathognomonic. On plain films, an osteochondroma appears as a pedunculated or sessile bony projection. At the point of attachment, the cortex of the bone or origin flares into the cortex of the osteochondroma (*Fig. 55-2*).[13] This is considered a pathognomonic finding. Due to multiple overlapping structures in the spine, plain films are often insufficient for diagnosis. Computerized tomography (CT) readily demonstrates the corticomedullary continuity of the osteochondroma with the parent bone where the cortex can be followed as a single line and the medullary cavities of the parent bone and osteochondroma are as one (*Fig. 55-3*).[6] Flocculent calcification or an "arcs and rings" matrix may be seen in the osteochondroma. Although CT can demonstrate the osseous component of an osteochondroma, it fails to demonstrate the cartilaginous cap in

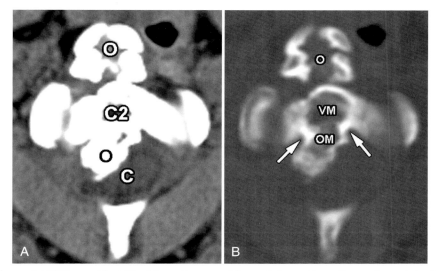

Figure 55-1 ▶ **Osteochondroma.** Axial CT image at the C2 level. Image **A** uses a soft tissue window and image **B** uses a bone window. There are large bony projections (*O*) from the anterior and posterior aspect of the C2 vertebral body. The posterior bony projection causes mass effect on the left ventral aspect of the spinal cord (*C*). The bone window image demonstrates continuity of the medullary cavity of the C2 vertebral body (*VM*) with the posterior bony projection medullary cavity (*OM*) and cortical continuity (*arrows*). The finding of corticomedullary continuity is consistent with an osteochondroma.

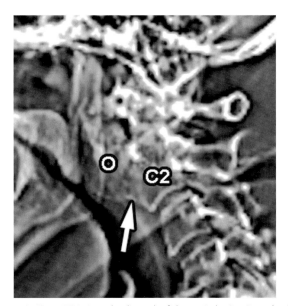

Figure 55-2 ▶ **Osteochondroma.** Same patient as in Figure 55-1. Lateral radiograph of the cervical spine. Bony density (*O*) projects from the ventral surface of the C2 vertebral body. The cortex of C2 appears to flare into the cortex of the bony density (*arrow*).

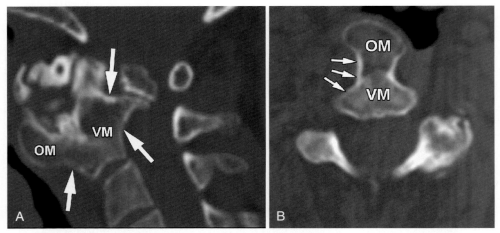

Figure 55-3 ▶ Osteochondroma, CT. Same patient as in Figures 55-1 and 55-2. Sagittal CT image **A** and axial CT image **B**. The medullary cavity of the ventral osteochondroma (*OM*) and the posterior osteochondroma are continuous with the C2 vertebral body medullary cavity (*VM*). The cortex of C2 flares into and is continuous with the cortex of the osteochondromas (*arrows*).

the majority of cases, and when it does, it often underestimates the size of the cartilaginous cap.[14] This makes it difficult to distinguish between an osteochondroma with a thick cartilaginous cap and a chondrosarcoma with a thin cartilaginous cap.

Magnetic resonance imaging (MRI) can demonstrate cartilaginous caps larger than 3 mm.[15] The cartilaginous cap can be seen in its entirety with MRI, which is important because caps greater than 2 cm in thickness should be suspect for malignant degeneration of the osteochondroma.[10,11] The cartilaginous cap appears isointense to hyperintense on T1-weighted images, hyperintense on T2-weighted images, and does not enhance. The cortex of the osteochondroma appears like normal bone cortex with decreased T1 and T2 signal intensity. The medullary cavity will appear hyperintense on T1-weighted images and iso- to hyperintense of T2-weighted images (*Fig. 55-4*). Occasionally, peripheral enhancement of osteochondromas is noted. MRI also better demonstrates the involvement of the surrounding tissues by the osteochondroma, particularly the spinal cord and nerve roots. A nuclear medicine bone scan may demonstrate increased radiotracer uptake when the osteochondroma is metabolically active and uptake is similar to normal bone when it is inactive.

DIFFERENTIAL DIAGNOSIS

1. **Chondrosarcoma:** A chondrosarcoma should be suspected if the cartilaginous cap is greater than 2 cm, if there has been

recurrence after excision, or there is an associated soft tissue mass.
2. **Aneurysmal bone cyst (ABC):** An ABC is usually expansile with multiloculated blood-fluid levels. It does not show corticomedullary continuity (*Fig. 55-5*).
3. **Osteoblastoma:** An osteoblastoma is an expansile lesion of the neural arch. It does not show corticomedullary continuity (*Fig. 55-6*).

TREATMENT

1. **Scheduled observation:** If an osteochondroma is found incidentally and is asymptomatic, the lesion can be followed with occasional imaging.
2. **Surgery:** Surgery is the treatment of choice if an osteochondroma becomes symptomatic, rapidly increases in size, has recurred, or is needed for cosmetic reasons.[1,8] Osteochondromas are radioresistant.[1] Surgical excision of the entire cartilaginous cap is essential to prevent a recurrence.[6,16] Some clinicians purport aggressive surgical treatment, even if it compromises the stability of the vertebral column,[13] whereas others purport surgical treatment to remove as much of the tumor as possible without creating functional deficits.[17] The risk of recurrence is stated to be 2% to 4%, with subtotal resection with a disease-free interval of from 1 to 26 years.[2,13] Any recurrence should raise the suspicion for malignant degeneration and should be surgically removed and submitted to pathology for signs of malignancy.

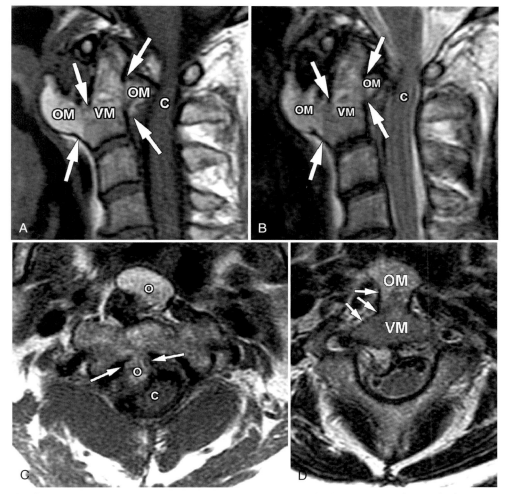

Figure 55-4 ► **Osteochondroma, MRI.** Same patient as in Figures 55-1 to 55-3. Sagittal T1-weighted image **A**, sagittal T2-weighted image **B**, axial T1-weighted image **C**, and axial T2-weighted image **D**. Continuity of the parent vertebral body cortex with that of the osteochondroma (*arrows*) and the continuity of the medullary cavities of the osteochondromas (*OM*) and vertebral body (*VM*) are readily identified by MR imaging. One is also able to better appreciate the affect of the posterior osteochondroma (*O*) on the spinal cord (*C*). The medullary cavity of the ventral osteochondroma is of increased T1 and T2 signal intensity.

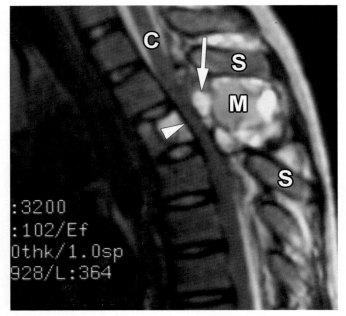

Figure 55-5 ▶ Aneurysmal Bone Cyst. Sagittal T1-weighted image. Multiloculated isointense to hyperintense expansile mass of the spinous process (*M*) with extension into the posterior epidural space (*arrow*) and compressing the spinal cord (*arrowhead*). C = Spinal cord; S = spinous process.

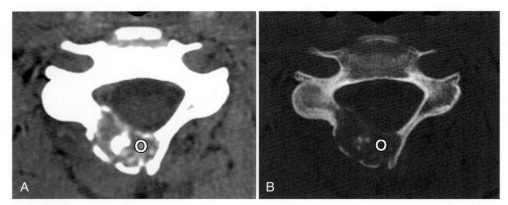

Figure 55-6 ▶ Osteoblastoma. Axial CT of the cervical spine using soft tissue window (image **A**) and bone window (image **B**). Expansile mass (*O*) of the right posterior neural arch with a calcific inner matrix.

References

1. Khosla A, Martin DS, Awwad EE. The solitary intraspinal vertebral osteochondromas: An unusual cause of compressive myelopathy: features and literature review. *Spine.* 1999;24:77-81.
2. Dahlin DC, Unni KK. *Bone Tumors.* 4th ed. Springfield, IL: Charles C. Thomas; 1986:19-22,228-229.
3. Soloman L. Hereditary multiple exostosis. *J Bone Joint Surg Br.* 1963;45:292-304.
4. Jayakumar PN, Indira Devi B, Shenoy SN, et al. Thoracic spinal osteochondromas causing cord compression: A report of five cases. *Indian J Radiol Imag.* 1998;8:117-120.
5. Cree AK, Hadlow AT, Taylor TK, Chapman GK. Radiation-induced osteochondroma in the lumbar spine. *Spine.* 1994;19:376-379.
6. Sharma MC, Arora C, Deol PS, et al. Osteochondroma of the spine: An enigmatic tumor of the spinal cord. A series of 10 cases. *J Neurol Sci.* 2002;46:66-70.
7. d'Ambrosia R, Rergusson AB. The formation of osteochondroma by epiphyseal cartilage transplantation. *Clin Orthop.* 1968;61:103-115.
8. Albrecht S, Crutchfield JS, SeGall GK. On spinal osteochondromas. *J Neurosurg.* 1992;77:247-252.
9. Rose EG, Fekete A. Odontoid osteochondroma causing sudden death. *Am J Clin Pathol.* 1964;42:606-609.
10. Quirini GE, Meyer JR, Herman M, Russel EJ. Osteochondroma of the thoracic spine: An unusual cause of spinal cord compression. *AJNR Am J Neuroradiol.* 1996;17:961-964.
11. Prasad A, Renjen PN, Prasad ML, et al. Solitary spinal osteochondroma causing neural syndromes. *Paraplegia.* 1992;30:678-680.

12. Srikantha U, Devi Bhagavatula I, Satyanarayana S, et al. Spinal osteo-chondromas: Spectrum of a rare disease. *J Neurosurg Spine*. 2008;8: 561-566.
13. Gille O, Pointillart V, Vital JM. Course of spinal solitary osteochondromas. *Spine*. 2004;30:13-19.
14. Hudson TM, Springfield DS, Spanier SS, et al. Benign exostoses and exos-totic chondrosarcomas: Evaluation of cartilage cap thickness by CT. *Radiology*. 1984;152:595-599.
15. Calhoun JM, Chadduck WM, Smith JL. Single cervical exostosis: Report of a case and review of the literature. *Surg Neurol*. 1992;37:26-29.
16. Yukawa Y, Kato F, Sugiura H. Solitary osteochondroma of the lower cervical spine. *Orthopedics*. 2001;24:292-293.
17. Maheshwari AV, Jain AK, Dhammi IK. Osteochondroma of C7 vertebra presenting as compressive myelopathy in a patient with nonhereditary (nonfamilial/sporadic) multiple exostoses. *Arch Orthop Trauma Surg*. 2006;126:654-659.

OSTEOMYELITIS AND DISCITIS (SPONDYLODISCITIS)

Leo F. Czervionke, M.D.

CLINICAL PRESENTATION

The patient is a 39-year-old otherwise healthy woman who developed a papulopustular skin eruption/infection attributed to MRSA (methicillin-resistant *Staphylococcus aureus*). One month later, she developed pleuritic chest pain and a cough and was diagnosed with pneumonia. The symptoms resolved, but pleuritic chest pain recurred along with back pain. The patient was afebrile. Magnetic resonance (MR) imaging of the thoracic spine was ordered.

IMAGING PRESENTATION

MR imaging of the thoracic spine revealed signal abnormalities consistent with T5-6 discitis and vertebral osteomyelitis (*Figs. 56-1 to 56-4*). A paraspinal phlegmon was also demonstrated (*Fig. 56-5*). A percutaneous paraspinal computed tomography (CT)–guided biopsy was performed at the T5-6 level, which yielded no viable organisms (*Fig. 56-6*). This was followed with a percutaneous transpedicular biopsy (*Fig. 56-7*). A diagnosis of MRSA osteomyelitis and discitis was made based on the culture of biopsy tissue.

DISCUSSION

Spondylodiscitis is an infectious process involving the vertebra (*osteomyelitis*) and adjacent intervertebral disc (*discitis*). Rarely, tuberculosis and other granulomatous infections can cause vertebral infection without invading the intervertebral disc, but the vast majority of cases of osteomyelitis penetrate the vertebral endplate to involve the intervertebral disc.[1] The vertebral-disc infection frequently extends into the paraspinal and epidural space forming a phlegmon, which may cavitate to form an abscess. Rarely, the infection infiltrates the thecal sac where it can cause arachnoiditis, meningitis, or an intramedullary spinal cord abscess.

Pyogenic and granulomatous spondylodiscitis occurs more frequently in patients with a chronic illness, including patients with diabetes mellitus, chronic renal failure, or chronic liver disease; immunocompromised patients; and IV drug abusers. Spondylodiscitis also occurs in patients with chronic nutritional deficiencies such as those in chronic alcoholics.[2]

Most vertebral infections occur from blood-borne pathogens that preferentially settle in the hypervascular marrow adjacent to the vertebral endplates. In adults, the disc is an avascular structure and becomes secondarily involved after the infectious process destroys the vertebral endplates.[3] The vertebral cortical and cartilaginous endplates represent the nutritional conduit for the intervertebral disc. When the cortical and cartilaginous endplate becomes disrupted, the infection can enter directly into the disc. In children, the intervertebral disc may still be vascularized, so the infectious process can begin primarily within the disc.[3] Infections can also invade the vertebra by direct extension from infections in adjacent organs such as infections originating in the genitourinary or gastrointestinal tract. Infections may also occur in the vertebra after trauma, surgery, or percutaneous spine interventional procedures.

Vertebral infections are most commonly caused by pyogenic bacteria. The most common pathogen is *Staphylococcus aureus* (see Figs. 56-1 to 56-5). However, other organisms may cause pyogenic spine infections, including coagulase negative *Staphylococcus* (*Figs. 56-8 and 56-9*), *Streptococcus, Pneumococcus, Hemophilus, Enterococcus, Escherchia coli, Salmonella,* and rarely anaerobic organisms.[2,4] Granulomatous spinal infections are seen with increasing frequency, especially in immunocompromised patients. Granulomatous spondylodiscitis is most commonly produced by *Mycobacterium tuberculosis* (*Fig. 56-10*). However, atypical mycobacteria (*Figs. 56-11 to 56-13*), *Brucella, Streptomyces,* parasites, and fungal organisms can also cause granulomatous spine infections.[1] Fungal spondylodiscitis is a rare spinal infection, usually occurring in immunocompromised patients.[5] Infections produced by both common and uncommon pathogens more frequently occur in immunocompromised patients.

The diagnosis of spondylodiscitis should be made based on clinical information and the imaging appearance. Patients with spine infections typically present with acute or progressively worsening back pain. The pain tends to have an acute onset with pyogenic infections and a more insidious onset in granulomatous infections, but in both cases, the pain becomes progressively worse.[6] Constitutional symptoms may be present including fever, chills, malaise, and night sweats. These patients may present with myelopathic symptoms if the cord is compressed by epidural phlegmon or abscess. If the phlegmon extends into the neural foramen or paraspinal soft tissues, they may have radicular symptoms.

Leukocytosis with a high neutrophil count, markedly elevated ESR (erythrocyte sedimentation rate), and C-reactive protein levels are strongly suggestive of a pyogenic infection.[2] In granulomatous infections (e.g., tuberculosis, *Brucella*), the ESR is usually elevated out of proportion to the degree of leukocytosis.

Text continued on page 431

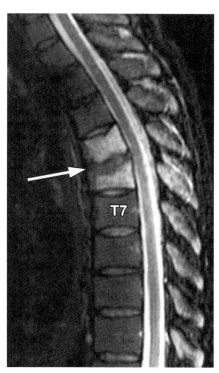

Figure 56-1 ▶ Spondylodiscitis at T5-6 Level. Sagittal T2-weighted MR image reveals partial collapse of the T5 and T6 vertebral bodies. Abnormal T2 hyperintensity visible throughout the T5 and T6 vertebral body marrow. The T5-6 vertebral endplates are indistinct and ill-defined tissue is located within the T5-6 intervertebral disc (*arrow*). T7 = T7 vertebral body.

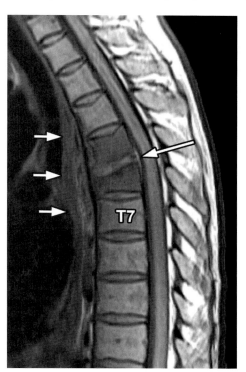

Figure 56-2 ▶ Spondylodiscitis at T5-6 Level. A prevertebral soft tissue mass (*short arrows*) is evident on this sagittal T1-weighted MR image in same slice location as in Figure 56-1. The T5 and T6 vertebral marrow is relatively T1 hypointense compared to the marrow signal intensity in normal adjacent vertebrae. The T5-6 vertebral endplates are poorly defined and the intervertebral disc (*long arrow*) contains tissue that is slightly T1 hyperintense relative to adjacent vertebral bodies. T7 = T7 vertebral body.

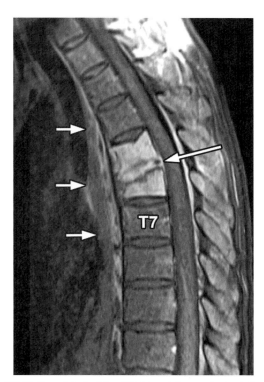

Figure 56-3 ▶ Spondylodiscitis at T5-6 Level. Same patient as in Figures 56-1 and 56-2. Sagittal contrast-enhanced fat-saturated T1-weighted MR image. The prevertebral phlegmonous soft tissue mass (*short arrows*) enhances following IV contrast. Intense enhancement is seen throughout the T5 and T6 vertebral bodies. There is diffuse enhancement of inflammatory tissue in the T5-6 intervertebral disc and minimal enhancement of inflammatory tissue in the ventral epidural space (*long arrow*). T7 = T7 vertebral body.

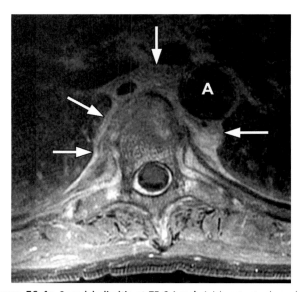

Figure 56-4 ▶ Spondylodiscitis at T5-6 Level. Axial contrast-enhanced fat-saturated T1-weighted MR image at the T6 level in same patient as in Figures 52-1 to 52-3, shows contrast enhancement of the T6 vertebral body and paraspinal phlegm (*arrows*). A = aorta.

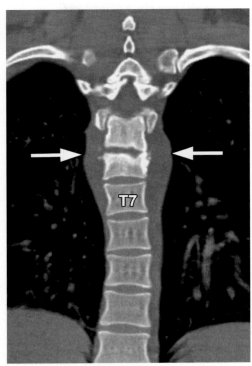

Figure 56-5 ▶ Spondylodiscitis at T5-6 Level. Corona CT image obtained through thoracic vertebral bodies in same patient as in Figures 56-1 to 56-4. Paraspinal soft tissue mass (*arrows*) represents paravertebral phlegmon, which extends from C5 to C7 level. Note partial collapse of vertebral body superiorly and increased bone density in C5 and C6 vertebral bodies. T5-6 vertebral endplates are slightly indistinct, irregular and sclerotic.

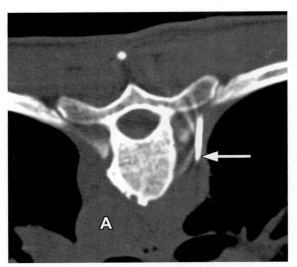

Figure 56-6 ▶ Spondylodiscitis at T5-6 Level, CT-Guided Biopsy. Axial CT image obtained through C6 level with patient prone during CT guided percutaneous biopsy in same patient as in Figures 56-1 to 56-5. The biopsy needle (*arrow*) is positioned in the right paraspinal soft tissue mass. A = aorta.

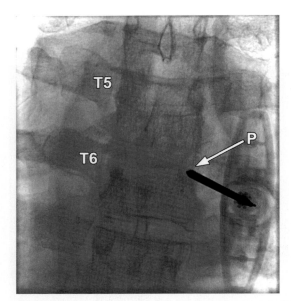

Figure 56-7 ▶ Spondylodiscitis at T5-6 Level, X-Ray Fluoroscopic-Guided Biopsy. PA radiograph of the mid-thoracic spine with patient prone during percutaneous fluoroscopic-guided needle biopsy performed using right T6 transpedicular approach. The needle tip projects over the right T6 pedicle (*P*). T5 and T6 lettering overly the right T5 and T6 transverse processes, respectively.

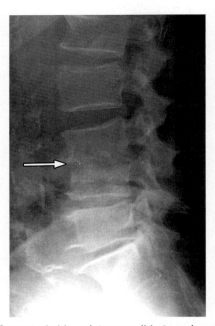

Figure 56-8 ▶ L3-4 Discitis and Osteomyelitis Secondary to Coagulase Negative *Staphylococcus*. Lateral radiograph of lumbar spine reveals obscure intervertebral disc space (*arrow*) and indistinct vertebral endplates, secondary to vertebral bone destruction on either side of L3-4 intervertebral disc. Reduction in vertebral body height of L3 and L4 is also demonstrated. Note narrowed L4-5 and L5-S1 intervertebral disc spaces associated with well-defined, sclerotic endplates, secondary to intervertebral disc degeneration.

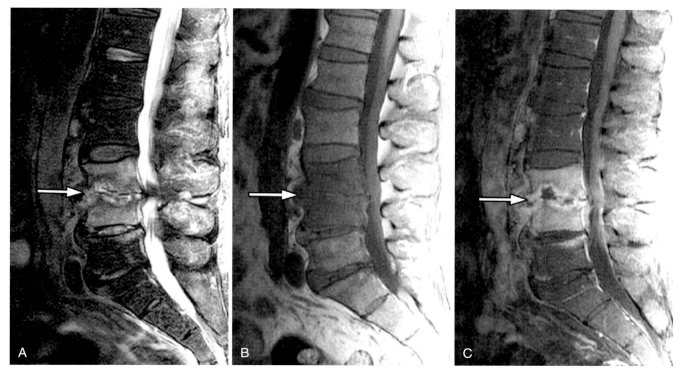

Figure 56-9 ▶ **L3-4 Discitis and Osteomyelitis.** Same patient as in Figure 56-8. Sagittal fat-saturated T2-weighted MR image **A**. T1-weighted image **B**, and contrast-enhanced fat-saturated T1-weighted MR image **C**. The L3-4 intervertebral disc (*arrow in images* **A**, **B**, and **C**) is narrowed and adjacent vertebral endplates are irregular and enhance intensely. The L3-4 intervertebral disc contains T1 hypointense and heterogeneous T2 hyperintense tissue. On image **C**, intradiscal inflammatory tissue enhances but intradiscal fluid does not enhance. The L3 and L4 vertebra are T1 hypointense and T2 hyperintense relative to other vertebral bodies, due to presence of marrow edema. The L3 and L4 vertebral bodies enhance diffusely indicating presence of vertebral inflammation secondary to osteomyelitis.

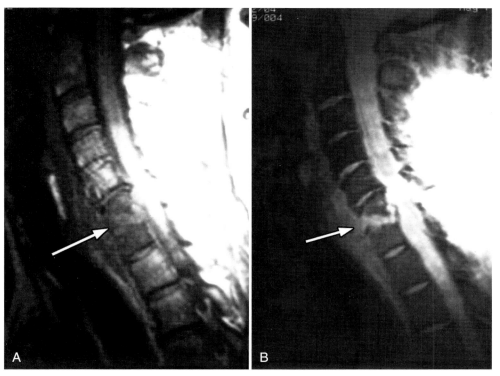

Figure 56-10 ▶ **C6-7 Spondylodiscitis Secondary to *Mycobacterium Tuberculosis* Infection.** On sagittal T1-weighted MR image **A**, the C6-7 intervertebral disc space has been replaced by heterogeneous tissue and adjacent endplates are indistinct. On sagittal gradient echo images, the C6-7 intervertebral disc space contains hyperintense tissue and adjacent vertebral endplates and vertebral bodies are destroyed. The MR appearance in this case of tuberculous spondylodiscitis is nonspecific and could be produced by almost any organism capable of producing discitis.

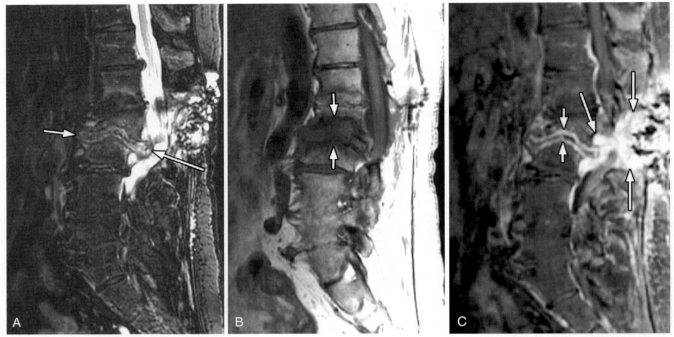

Figure 56-11 ▶ L2-3 Spondylodiscitis, Epidural and Paraspinal Abscesses Caused by Atypical Mycobacterium (*M. Abscessus*). On sagittal T2-weighted MR image **A**, the L2-3 intervertebral disc is narrowed, undulating and contains ill-defined T2 hyperintense tissue (*arrows*). The posterior disc margin (*long arrow*) protrudes into the spinal canal. The anterior disc margin (*short arrow*) protrudes into the prevertebral tissues. Heterogeneous T2 hyperintense tissue is seen in the posterior paraspinal region from L1-3. On sagittal T1-weighted image **B**, the disc space appears widened, but in reality is not widened, due to presence of T1 hypointense tissue between T1 hypointense curvilinear areas of bony reactive response (*arrows*) in the L2 and L3 vertebral bodies. On sagittal contrast-enhanced fat-saturated T1 weighted MR image **C**, the upper and lower margins of the tissue within the L2-3 intervertebral disc display intense, uniform, curvilinear enhancement (*short arrows*). Enhancing epidural and posterior paraspinal tissues enhance intensely (*long arrows*), representing epidural and paraspinal inflammatory tissue (phlegmon).

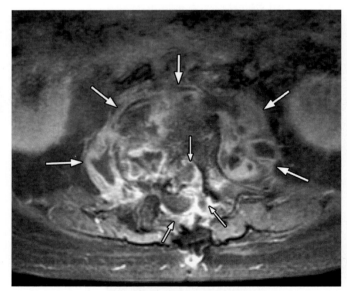

Figure 56-12 ▶ L2-3 Spondylodiscitis, Epidural and Paraspinal Abscesses Caused by Atypical Mycobacterium. Same patient as in Figure 56-11. On this axial contrast-enhanced fat-saturated T1-weighted MRI, a large paravertebral phlegmon (*large arrows*) contains multiple small fluid collections representing multiple abscesses. The thecal sac is displaced to the right by epidural phlegmon (*small arrows*) which contains several small abscesses.

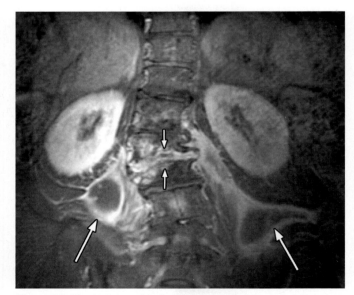

Figure 56-13 ▶ L2-3 Spondylodiscitis, Epidural and Paraspinal Abscesses Caused by Atypical Mycobacterium. Same patient as in Figures 56-11 and 56-12. Coronal contrast-enhanced fat-saturated T1-weighted MRI. Lumbar dextroscoliosis. The tissue at the superior and inferior margin of the L2-3 intervertebral disc (*small arrows*) enhances intensely due to discitis. Both psoas muscles enhance diffusely and contain non-enhancing fluid filled cavities (*long arrows*), which represent abscesses in the psoas muscles.

If a disc infection is suspected, it is important to perform percutaneous needle aspiration biopsy of the disc, adjacent vertebra, and/or phlegmonous tissue to culture the offending organism and determine the most effective antibiotic for treatment (see Figs. 56-6 and 56-7). However, one should not rely on a positive culture after aspiration biopsy to initiate therapy because the results are commonly negative for a variety of reasons.[6] The disc aspiration may yield negative results if the patient has already received antibiotic therapy or if samples are taken only from the disc center, which may contain only noninfectious liquid and necrotic debris. It is important that aspiration samples be obtained from inflamed, contrast-enhancing tissue in the involved vertebral body, adjacent to a bony sequestrum or in a paravertebral phlegmon. Disc aspiration biopsy often yields negative results in patients with mycobacterial infections, so it is important to always consider tuberculosis as a possible cause of the infection.[6]

It requires about 4 weeks to culture *M. tuberculosis,* so it is not practical to withhold therapy while waiting for culture results. However, the diagnosis of tuberculosis can also be made if acid-fast bacilli are detected in the tissue samples (using an enzyme-linked immunosorbent assay for tuberculous bacilli) or if characteristic Langhans giant cells are seen in the tissue. If tuberculosis is suspected, a positive Mantoux (purified protein derivative [PPD]) skin test supports the diagnosis of tuberculosis. A PCR (polymerase chain reaction) test should be performed on the biopsy tissue samples. PCR is a quick, reliable DNA test that is used to confirm the diagnosis of tuberculosis.[6] However, the PCR may be, in a minority of cases, falsely negative, so a negative PCR does not exclude the diagnosis of tuberculous spondylitis. If caseating granulomas are observed histologically in the tissues, this indicates either tuberculosis or brucellosis.

IMAGING FEATURES

Radiographs, CT, and MR imaging are important in the initial diagnosis of spondylodiscitis, and MRI is valuable for determining the extent of the paraspinal or epidural infection if present.[7] Serial follow-up MRI studies in these patients are routinely obtained to monitor their progress and guide the clinical management if complications arise. On these follow-up examinations, special attention should be given to the paraspinal or epidural extent of the infection. However, it is important to bear in mind that the imaging appearance of the infection on radiographs, CT, and MRI does not correlate well with the degree of clinical improvement, because clinical improvement often precedes signs of improvement as demonstrated by imaging.[7,8]

The hallmark of early stage pyogenic osteomyelitis/discitis is erosion or destruction of the vertebral endplate. Although endplate erosion or destruction is highly specific for discitis, the endplates rarely may be completely normal in appearance in pyogenic infection and in a minority of patients with granulomatous spondylodiscitis.[1] Vertebral endplate erosion or destruction is best demonstrated on plain radiographs and with CT (see Figs. 56-5, 56-8, and ***56-14***). With MR imaging, endplate destruction can also be readily detected and is best demonstrated on T1-weighted

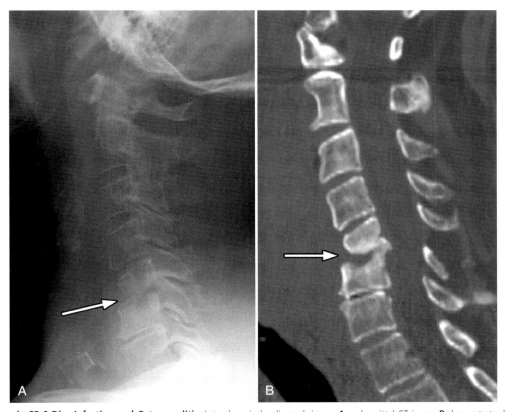

Figure 56-14 ► **Chronic C5-6 Disc Infection and Osteomyelitis.** Lateral cervical radiograph image **A** and sagittal CT image **B** demonstrate destruction of the C5-6 vertebral endplates and vertebral bone adjacent to the endplates (*arrow in images* **A** *and* **B**). The bone adjacent to the widened C5-6 intervertebral disc space is slightly sclerotic.

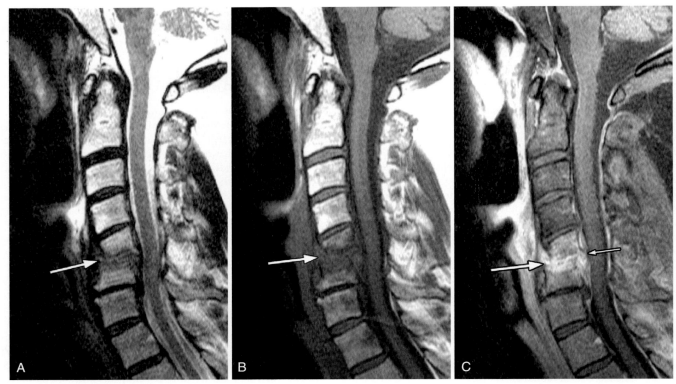

Figure 56-15 ▶ **Chronic C5-6 Disc Infection and Osteomyelitis.** Same patient as in Figure 56-14. On sagittal T2-weighted MR image **A** and T1-weighted image **B**, there is heterogeneous T1 hypointense and slightiy T2 hyperintense tissue (relative to normal disc T2 intensity) replacing the intervertebral disc (*arrow in* **A** *and* **B**) associated with destruction of the adjacent C5-6 vertebral endplates and vertebral bodies. On sagittal contrast-enhanced fat-saturated T1-weighted MR image **C**, the intervertebral disc tissue enhances (*large arrow*), the adjacent vertebral bodies enhance, and an enhancing phlegmon (*small arrow*) occupies the epidural space posterior to the C5 and C6 vertebral bodies.

images (see *Figs.* 56-9, 56-11, and *56-15*). MRI has the additional advantage of defining the extent of the inflammatory process into the disc, paraspinal tissues, and epidural space (see Figs. 56-11, 56-12, 56-13, and 56-15). Therefore, MRI is an valuable imaging tool for following these patients over time. In the early stages of discitis, the disc space is usually narrowed or collapsed, but the disc stature may be expanded if the disc is filled with an inflammatory effusion or intradiscal abscess.

On MR imaging, the most sensitive signs of vertebral osteomyelitis/discitis in general are with decreasing frequency: (1) presence of an epidural or paraspinal inflammatory mass, (2) intradiscal contrast enhancement, (3) intradiscal T2 signal hyperintensity, (4) erosion or destruction of at least one endplate, and (5) obscuration of the intranuclear cleft.[9]

With MR imaging, initially the intervertebral disc and vertebral bone adjacent to involved endplates are classically T1 hypointense and T2 hyperintense, compared with intensity of normal disc, degenerated disc, or normal marrow, because of fluid and inflammation in the disc and marrow edema in the adjacent vertebra (see Figs. 56-1, 56-2, 56-9, 56-11, and 56-15).[1,10,11] T2-weighted images obtained with fat-saturation technique are more sensitive for detecting osteomyelitis/discitis.[12] The same regions that are abnormal on the fat-saturated, T2-weighted images are also hyperintense on short tau inversion recovery (STIR) images. The intranuclear cleft normally visible on MR images is usually obliterated by the inflammatory process in the disc, but this is not always the case in disc infections, so the presence of an intranuclear cleft does not exclude discitis.[9]

Following IV contrast administration, the disc will enhance intensely if filled with inflammatory tissue, which is the most common imaging pattern (see Figs. 56-3, 56-9, 56-11, and 56-15).[10] However, the infected disc will enhance only at its periphery if filled with fluid and/or debris.[9] Sometimes the infected disc space contains enhancing inflammatory tissue intermixed with nonenhancing fluid-filled cavities (see Fig. 56-9).

In some patients with *Mycobacterium tuberculosis* infection or early, acute staphylococcal infection, the intervertebral disc may enhance minimally or not at all. The adjacent endplates may be intact and slightly irregular. In this situation, the imaging appearance may simulate that seen with Modic type 1 degenerative discogenic vertebral endplate disease (*Fig. 56-16*).

Unless the bone is sclerotic, the infected vertebral bone enhances intensely after IV contrast administration. Vertebral and disc enhancement is most conspicuous when fat-saturated MRI techniques are used (see Figs. 56-3, 56-9, 56-11, and 56-15).[1,9] Paraspinal phlegmons and abscesses frequently accompany both pyogenic and granulomatous infections of the spine. Phlegmonous tissue enhances homogeneously, whereas abscesses enhance peripherally (see Figs. 56-3, 56-4, 56-9, 56-11, 56-12, 56-13, and 56-15).[10] In chronic osteomyelitis, the involved bone often becomes sclerotic and is T1 and T2 hypointense on MR imaging.

In the healing or chronic phases of osteomyelitis, the vertebral destruction is replaced by hyperdense, sclerotic bone that is shown best on radiographs or CT. Eventually fusion may occur across the disc space in chronic, late stage osteomyelitis-discitis.

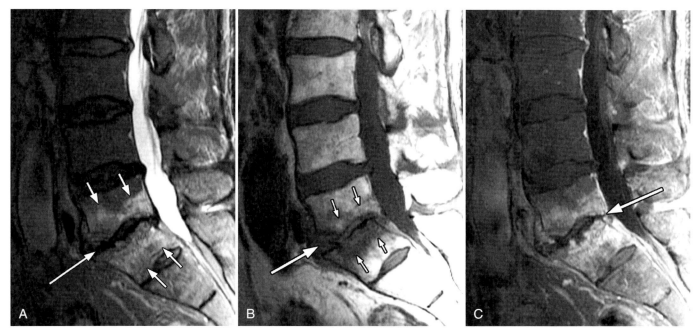

Figure 56-16 ▶ **Atypical Acute *Staphylococcus Aureas* Discitis and Osteomyelitis at L5-S1 Level Simulating Modic Type 1 Degenerative Discogenic Endplate Disease.** (Note: some cases of tuberculous discitis/osteomyelitis may present with a similar imaging appearance). On sagittal T1-weighted MR image **A** and sagittal fat-saturated T2-weighted image **B**, the intervertebral disc is narrowed and T2 hypointense (*long arrow in* **A** *and* **B**), vertebral endplates appear intact but slightly irregular. T1 hypointense and T2 hyperintense marrow signal is demonstrated adjacent to the endplates. On contrast-enhanced fat-saturated T1-weighted MR image **C**, the intervertebral disc (*arrow*) does not enhance, but the adjacent vertebral bodies do enhance.

Several unique imaging features of granulomatous infections of the spine deserve special mention. Tuberculous infections are usually slowly developing infections that more commonly arise in the thoracic spine or thoracolumbar junction, whereas pyogenic osteomyelitis has a more rapid onset and more frequently occurs in the lumbar region.[1,2] The majority of patients with granulomatous osteomyelitis/discitis have similar imaging features as in pyogenic spondylodiscitis, including endplate destruction, intradiscal T2 hyperintensity, and contrast enhancement of the intervertebral disc and adjacent vertebrae (see Figs. 56-10 to 56-13). In most cases of tuberculous spondylitis, the infection begins in the anterior portion of the spine and progresses posteriorly.[1] In some cases of mycobacterial or other granulomatous infections, the vertebral endplates are spared completely, which is believed to be the result of a lack of proteolytic enzymes in the case of mycobacterial infections.[1,13,14] In tuberculous spine infections, the disc is involved in 50% to 70% of patients.[13] If the disc is involved in mycobacterial spondylodiscitis, the intradiscal contents are usually T2 hyperintense (similar to pyogenic infections), but in some cases, the intradiscal T2 signal intensity may be relatively low, simulating degenerative discogenic endplate disease (vertebral osteochondrosis).

Both pyogenic and tuberculous infections commonly extend into the subligamentous space, and this involvement may extend over several vertebral levels.[13,15] Multilevel involvement can occur with pyogenic and tuberculous infections but is more common in tuberculous spondylitis. Tuberculous osteomyelitis may involve a solitary vertebral body or two adjacent vertebral bodies without involving the adjacent disc.[1,13] Osteomyelitis involving an entire vertebral body or three or more vertebral bodies is more commonly observed in tuberculosis.[16]

Focal areas of tuberculous osteomyelitis may occur in the posterior vertebral arch or vertebral bodies without any disc involvement.[13,16] Posterior vertebral arch involvement (pedicle, lamina, or transverse or spinous process) by tuberculosis is not uncommon, more commonly occurring in the thoracic region.[12]

Paraspinal abscesses commonly occur with pyogenic, tuberculous, and atypical mycobacterial infections of the spine (see Fig. 56-13). When pyogenic paraspinal abscesses occur, they may extend into the psoas muscles, but tend to be fairly localized. Only 10% of patients with *Brucella* spondylodiscitis develop a paraspinal abscess.[4] Mycobacterial abscesses often involve the psoas muscles over several levels and characteristically have thin enhancing walls (see Fig. 56-13), whereas pyogenic paraspinal abscesses tend to have shaggy, irregularly enhancing margins and tend to stay confined to the level of the disc infection.[1,6,16] The presence of multifocal paraspinal abscesses (skip lesions) or a cold abscess (an abscess that lacks surrounding inflammation) are characteristic of mycobacterial paraspinal abscesses **(Figs.** 56-13 and **56-17)**.[16] The presence of calcification in or adjacent to the paraspinal abscess is highly suggestive of a mycobacterial infection **(Fig. 56-18)**.[1] Severe deformities of the spine commonly result from chronic tuberculous spondylodiscitis (Pott's disease). The affected vertebrae may become fused together into a globular vertebral mass, with associated severe kyphotic spinal deformity **(Figs.** 56-18 and **56-19)**.

Brucellosis is also a granulomatous infection caused by a gram negative bacillus (*Brucella melitensis*), which has worldwide distribution, although is rarely seen in North America.[4] Brucellosis is more common in Middle Eastern and Mediterranean countries and in portions of Central and South America. *Brucella* spondylodiscitis has a predilection for the lower lumbar spine, but can occur in the thoracic and cervical spine. The intervertebral disc is involved in 80% of cases.[4] When the disc is involved, it usually causes vertebral endplate erosion or destruction, and the disc space is usually T2 hyperintense. Although the adjacent vertebral body may be extensively involved by osteomyelitis, brucellosis does not usually result in vertebral collapse or kyphotic deformity, as is so common with chronic tuberculous spondylitis.[1] Small paraspinal abscesses may occur with *Brucella* spondylodiscitis. Coexistent infection involving the facet joints may also occur with this organism.

Fungal spondylodiscitis may occur in immunocompromised patients as a result of fungi such as *Candida albicans* and *Aspergillus fumigatus*. The MRI appearance is similar to that seen in granulomatous osteomyelitis/discitis.[5] Although the MRI appearance may resemble that seen in pyogenic infections, typically the intradiscal T2 signal is not as hyperintense or is T2 hypointense, so the appearance may be more similar to that seen with degenerative discogenic vertebral osteochondrosis described by deRoos and Modic.[17,18] The intervertebral disc may be spared, which may also be the case in some cases of tuberculous osteomyelitis and in early *Staphylococcus aureus* discitis (see Fig. 56-19).

Radionuclide bone scanning may be useful for determining other sites of skeletal infection, but radionuclide uptake is nonspecific and false-negative bone scans may occur in elderly patients.[19] A three-phase bone scan that includes a flow study is more specific because there will be increased blood flow to regions of active infection.

Single photon emission computed tomography (SPECT) gallium-67 scanning is specific and reliable for demonstrating active sites of inflammation and infection in the axial skeleton.[20] The sensitivity of gallium scanning and MR imaging are comparable in detecting spondylodiscitis, both modalities having a 91% sensitivity in one study.[20] Gallium scanning is helpful in differentiating noninfectious, noninflammatory conditions that resemble spondylodiscitis on MR imaging. MRI is slightly more sensitive than gallium scanning for detecting paraspinal soft tissue infection.[20]

White blood cell radionuclide scanning may also be useful for detecting areas of pyogenic infection, particularly if there is abscess formation, but can be negative if the infection is nonpyogenic or in cases of chronic spondylodiscitis.

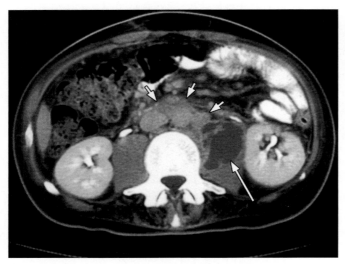

Figure 56-17 ▶ *Mycobacterium Tuberculosis* **Psoas Abscess.** Axial contrast-enhanced CT image through abdomen at level of kidneys. A thin rim of subtle contrast enhancement is located along the margin of the centrally hypodense left psoas abscess (*long arrow*). Note phlegmonous tissue (*short arrows*) in retroperitoneum adjacent to abdominal aorta and inferior vena cava.

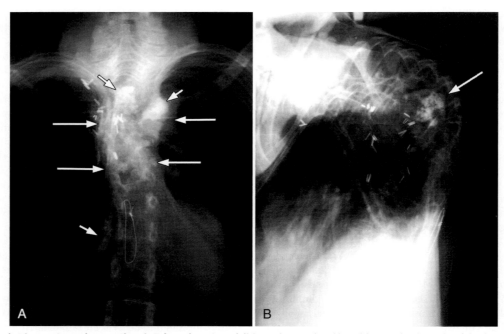

Figure 56-18 ▶ Pott's Disease Secondary to Chronic Tuberculous Spondylitis. AP (image **A**) and lateral (image **B**) radiographs of the thoracic spine. Several upper thoracic vertebrae are fused together into a dense bony "mass" (*long arrows in image* **A**). Three calcified paraspinal abscesses are indicated by short arrows in image **A**. Severe kyphotic deformity (*arrow in image* **B**) of the thoracic spine is demonstrated at this level.

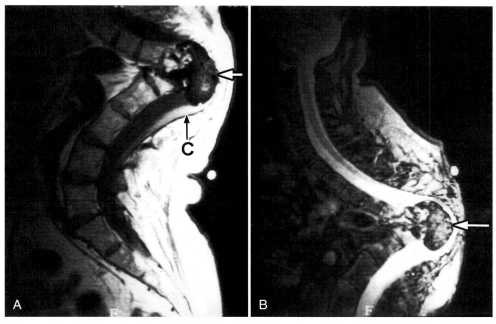

Figure 56-19 ► Pott's Disease, Chronic Tuberculous Spondylitis. (A different patient than shown in Figure 56-18). Sagittal T2-weighted MR image **A** and T1-weighted image **B**. Several low thoracic vertebral bodies are fused together into a bony "mass" (*arrow in images* **A** *and* **B**) with resulting extreme kyphosis. The spinal cord (**C**) in image **B** is draped posteriorly and compressed by the fused bone mass (*arrow*).

DIFFERENTIAL DIAGNOSIS

1. **Degenerative discogenic vertebral endplate disease (vertebral osteochondrosis, Modic type 1):** The endplates in this very common condition may be irregular but are not destroyed.[17,18] Intradiscal T2 signal intensity is usually low due to intervertebral disc degeneration, unless multiple annular fissures are present within the disc. The vertebral body marrow on either side of the disc is T1 hypointense and T2 hyperintense relative to normal marrow signal, and this same region may enhance intensely with contrast (*Fig. 56-20*). It may be difficult to differentiate this condition from some cases of granulomatous spondylodiscitis or early *Staphylococcus aureus* spondylodiscitis (see Fig. 56-9).

2. **Ankylosing spondylitis:** Vertebral pseudoarthrosis may occur in ankylosing spondylitis with endplate irregularities resembling spondylodiscitis (*Fig. 56-21*).[21] On T2-weighted MR images, the intradiscal T2 signal is usually hypointense.

3. **Neuropathic spondyloarthropathy:** This condition most commonly occurs at the thoracolumbar junction in diabetics or in patients with post-traumatic paralysis or syringohydromyelia. Previous spinal cord infarction may have occurred. Vertebral manifestations include vertebral body destruction and/or collapse and disc space collapse. The involved vertebral endplates become very irregular, resembling the endplate destruction in discitis. The neuropathic disc does not enhance centrally, but some enhancement may be seen at its periphery. The involved disc is most often T2 hypointense but can be T2 hyperintense.[22,23] Vacuum disc phenomena (intradiscal gas) and vertebral bone disorganization are commonly present in the neuropathic joint.[1,23] (The authors of this book have never seen intradiscal gas formation in disc infections, not even in rare cases of clostridial disc infection.) Vertebral pseudoarthrosis, spondylolisthesis, and severe kyphosis represent end-stage manifestations of neuropathic spondyloarthropathy.[22] The articular facets often show severe degeneration with facet subluxation.[23]

4. **Hemodialysis-related spondyloarthropathy:** This occurs more commonly in the cervical region, but can occur in the lumbar spine. The imaging appearance simulates spondylodiscitis or a neuropathic joint.[24,25] The disc is usually T2 hypointense in this condition and filled with amyloid material, mainly composed of B-2 microglobulin.[26] There may be a paraspinal soft tissue mass present, which is predominantly composed of amyloid.

5. **SAPHO (synovitis-acne-pustulosis hyperostosis-osteomyelitis) syndrome:** The majority of patients with this condition have chest wall involvement, but one-third of patients have spinal involvement with focal vertebral body abnormalities and endplate irregularities resembling spondylodiscitis.[27] No epidural or paravertebral abscess formation occurs.

PROGNOSIS AND TREATMENT

1. **Prognosis:** The prognosis in patients with vertebral osteomyelitis/discitis depends on early diagnosis and treatment with the appropriate antibiotic agent or surgical drainage of a paraspinal or epidural abscess if present. Up to 45% of patients require some type of surgical treatment eventually.[2]

2. **Initial broad-spectrum antibiotic therapy:** A broad-spectrum antibiotic, effective against a variety of aerobic and anaerobic bacteria, should be given initially when osteomyelitis/discitis is suspected. Optimally, percutaneous needle aspiration biopsy of the offending disc and adjacent

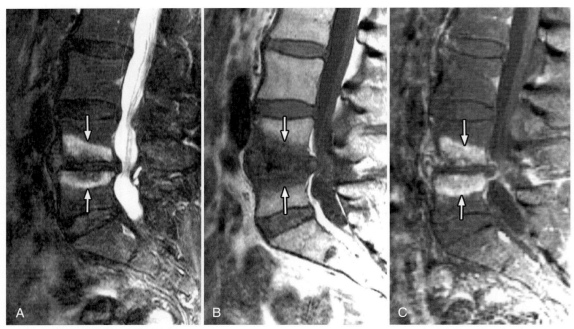

Figure 56-20 ▶ Degenerative Discogenic Vertebral Endplate Disease (Modic Type 1) Simulating Spondylodiscitis at L4-5 Level. The L4-5 intervertebral disc is narrowed and hypointense relative to normal intervertebral disc signal on sagittal fat-saturated. T2-weighted MR image **A** and T1-weighted image **B**. Note T2 hyperintense and T1 hypointense marrow signal intensity (*arrows in* **A** *and* **B**) in vertebral body marrow on either side of the L4-5 disc, consistent with marrow edema. On contrast-enhanced fat-saturated T1-weighted MR image **C**, intense enhancement is located in the vertebral body marrow (*arrows*) adjacent to the L4-5 intervertebral disc indicating presence of nonspecific inflammation.

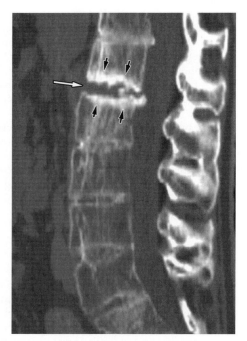

Figure 56-21 ▶ Chronic Noninfectious Spondylodiscitis in Patient with Longstanding Ankylosing Spondylitis. The L1-2 intervertebral disc space is widened (*white arrow*). The adjacent cortical vertebral endplates are irregular and sclerotic (*black arrows*). Note classic squared off configuration of the lumbar vertebral bodies, intradiscal calcifications at multiple levels, and generalized osteopenia, all of which commonly occur in patients with ankylosing spondylitis.

vertebra or phlegmon should be performed before initiating the antibiotic therapy to identify the causative pathogen.

3. **Intravenous antibiotic therapy:** A 6- to 8-week course of intravenous antibiotic therapy directed at the causative pathogen is the standard treatment. A rapid decline in the ESR after the first month of medical therapy is a positive prognostic indicator.[28]

4. **Surgery:** Surgery may be required urgently to evacuate an epidural or paraspinal abscess and to alleviate cord compression. In later stages of the disease, surgery may be necessary to restore spine stability if vertebral collapse has occurred or to correct chronic spinal deformities resulting from the infection.

References

1. Hong SH, Choi JY, Lee JW, et al. MR imaging assessment of the spine: infection or an imitation? *Radiographics.* 2009;29:599-612.
2. Colmenero JD, Jimenez-Mejias ME, Sanchez-Lora FJ, et al. Pyogenic, tuberculous, and brucellar vertebral osteomyelitis: A descriptive and comparative study of 219 cases. *Ann Rheum Dis.* 1997;56:709-715.
3. Ratcliffe JF. Anatomic basis for the pathogenesis and radiologic features of vertebral osteomyelitis and its differentiation from childhood discitis: A microarteriographic investigation. *Acta Radiol Diagn (Stockh).* 1985;26:137-143.
4. Colmenero JD, Ruiz-Mesa JD, Plata A, et al. Clinical findings, therapeutic approach, and outcome of brucellar vertebral osteomyelitis. *Clin Infect Dis.* 2008;46:426-433.
5. Lang EW, Pitts LH. Intervertebral disc space infection caused by Aspergillus fumigatus. *Eur Spine J.* 1996;5:207-209.
6. Wang D. Diagnosis of tuberculous vertebral osteomyelitis (TVO) in a developed country and literature review. *Spinal Cord.* 2005;43:531-542.

7. Carragee EJ. The clinical use of magnetic resonance imaging in pyogenic vertebral osteomyelitis. *Spine.* 1997;22:780-785.
8. Kowalski TJ, Layton KF, Berbari EF, et al. Follow-up MR imaging in patients with pyogenic spine infections: Lack of correlation with clinical features. *AJNR Am J Neuroradiol.* 2007;28:693-699.
9. Ledermann HP, Schweitzer ME, Morrison WB, Carrino JA. MR imaging findings in spinal infections: Rules or myths? *Radiology.* 2003;228:506-514.
10. Dagirmanjian A, Schils J, McHenry M, Modic MT. MR imaging of vertebral osteomyelitis revisited. *AJR Am J Roentgenol.* 1996;167:1539-1543.
11. Modic MT, Feiglin DH, Piraino DW, et al. Vertebral osteomyelitis: Assessment using MR. *Radiology.* 1985;157:157-166.
12. Narlawar RS, Shah JR, Pimple MK, et al. Isolated tuberculosis of posterior elements of spine: Magnetic resonance imaging findings in 33 patients. *Spine.* 2002;27:275-281.
13. Arizono T, Oga M, Shiota E, et al. Differentiation of vertebral osteomyelitis and tuberculous spondylitis by magnetic resonance imaging. *Int Orthop.* 1995;19:319-322.
14. Chapman M, Murray RO, Stoker DJ. Tuberculosis of the bones and joints. *Semin Roentgenol.* 1979;14:266-282.
15. Smith AS, Weinstein MA, Mizushima A, et al. MR imaging characteristics of tuberculous spondylitis vs vertebral osteomyelitis. *AJR Am J Roentgenol.* 1989;153:399-405.
16. Jung NY, Jee WH, Ha KY, et al. Discrimination of tuberculous spondylitis from pyogenic spondylitis on MRI. *AJR Am J Roentgenol.* 2004;182:1405-1410.
17. de Roos A, Kressel H, Spritzer C, Dalinka M. MR imaging of marrow changes adjacent to end plates in degenerative lumbar disk disease. *AJR Am J Roentgenol.* 1987;149:531-534.
18. Modic MT, Steinberg PM, Ross JS, et al. Degenerative disk disease: Assessment of changes in vertebral body marrow with MR imaging. *Radiology.* 1988;166:193-199.
19. Schlaeffer F, Mikolich DJ, Mates SM. Technetium Tc 99m diphosphonate bone scan: False-normal findings in elderly patients with hematogenous vertebral osteomyelitis. *Arch Intern Med.* 1987;147:2024-2026.
20. Love C, Patel M, Lonner BS, et al. Diagnosing spinal osteomyelitis: A comparison of bone and Ga-67 scintigraphy and magnetic resonance imaging. *Clin Nucl Med.* 2000;25:963-977.
21. Resnick D. *Ankylosing spondylitis.* In: Diagnosis of Bone and Joint Disorders. 4th ed. Philadelphia: Saunders; 2002:1023-1081.
22. Park YH, Taylor JA, Szollar SM, Resnick D. Imaging findings in spinal neuroarthropathy. *Spine.* 1994;19:1499-1504.
23. Wagner SC, Schweitzer ME, Morrison WB, et al. Can imaging findings help differentiate spinal neuropathic arthropathy from disk space infection? Initial experience. *Radiology.* 2000;214:693-699.
24. Kaplan P, Resnick D, Murphey M, et al. Destructive noninfectious spondyloarthropathy in hemodialysis patients: A report of four cases. *Radiology.* 1987;162:241-244.
25. Chin M, Hase H, Miyamoto T, et al. Radiological grading of cervical destructive spondyloarthropathy in long-term hemodialysis patients. *J Spinal Disord Tech.* 2006;19:430-435.
26. Niu CC, Chen WJ, Chen LH, Shih CH. Destructive spondyloarthropathy mimicking spondylitis in long-term hemodialysis patients. *Arch Orthop Trauma Surg.* 2000;120:594-597.
27. Toussirot E, Dupond JL, Wendling D. Spondylodiscitis in SAPHO syndrome: A series of eight cases. *Ann Rheum Dis.* 1997;56:52-58.
28. Carragee EJ, Kim D, van der Vlugt T, Vittum D. The clinical use of erythrocyte sedimentation rate in pyogenic vertebral osteomyelitis. *Spine.* 1997;22:2089-2093.

OSTEOSARCOMA—VERTEBRAL

Leo F. Czervionke, M.D.

CLINICAL PRESENTATION

The patient is a 23-year-old man who presented with severe progressive neck pain, left arm pain, and symptoms of cord compression. The patient had received a course of radiotherapy 8 years previously for a malignant neck soft tissue tumor.

IMAGING PRESENTATION

Computed tomography (CT) images reveal bone destruction of the C3 and C4 vertebral bodies and near complete collapse of the C4 vertebral body. There is a large area of tumoral bone formation along the left anterolateral aspect of the C4 vertebral body (*Fig. 57-1*). Magnetic resonance (MR) imaging revealed heterogeneous enhancement of a large paraspinal mass at C3-4 on the left with encasement of the left vertebral artery (*Figs. 57-2 to 57-4*). There was enhancing tumor extending into the left C3-4 neural foramen and into the epidural space anteriorly and on the left (see Fig. 57-4). The spinal cord was compressed from the left and displaced posteriorly and to the right by the epidural tumor (see Figs. 57-3 and 52-4). Surgery was performed to decompress the spinal cord and remove the tumor, which proved to be osteosarcoma. Because of the history of radiation therapy, this was presumed to be a radiation-induced vertebral osteosarcoma.

DISCUSSION

Osteosarcoma, also known as *osteogenic sarcoma*, is a highly malignant primary tumor of bone that produces immature osteoid matrix.[1] No more than 3% of osteosarcomas originate in the spine, so these are very uncommon vertebral tumors.[2] Osteosarcomas represent up to 5% of primary malignant spine tumors, vertebral myeloma/plasmacytoma, and lymphoma being far more common.[2] Most vertebral osteosarcomas manifest in the second through fifth decades of life. The much more common appendicular skeleton osteosarcomas usually occur in children or adolescents. Most primary vertebral osteosarcomas arise in the vertebral body but often infiltrate the pedicles and can involve the posterior arch.[2] Only 10% to 17% of osteosarcomas are reported to occur primarily in the posterior vertebral arch.[2-4] Primary vertebral osteosarcomas most commonly occur in the lumbar spine, followed by the thoracic spine, sacrum, and least commonly in the cervical spine.[1]

Most primary vertebral osteosarcomas have a bulky, lobulated soft tissue component that breaks through the cortex and commonly extends into the spinal canal or paraspinal soft tissues (see Figs. 57-1 to 57-4).

The majority of vertebral osteosarcomas are metastatic tumors that originate from primary osteosarcomas in the appendicular skeleton or adjacent soft tissues of the extremities in children, adolescents, or young adults (*Figs. 57-5 to 57-7*). These patients often have hepatic and pulmonary metastases in addition to vertebral metastases.

Osteosarcoma usually manifests clinically with slow onset of back pain, which is reported by some to be worse at night. Radicular pain, myelopathy, paraplegia, and bladder and bowel dysfunction may be present, depending on the location of the tumor; 80% of patients have sensory deficits.[3] Patients may present with cauda equina syndrome if the tumor invades the epidural space.[5] A chest radiograph should be obtained in all patients with known or suspected osteosarcoma.

Patients with osteosarcomas may present with ossified pulmonary metastases that can be associated with a pneumothorax. The pleural surfaces may contain ossifications as well. Rarely, vertebral osteosarcomas can invade the paravertebral venous system, extend into the inferior vena cava, and extend into the right atrium.[5] The serum alkaline phosphatase is often elevated in patients with osteosarcoma.[3,6]

Regulatory genes are involved in the pathogenesis of osteosarcomas in some patients.[7] Overexpression of the oncogene *erbB-2* is believed to be responsible for some cases of osteosarcoma.[8] There is a well known association of osteosarcoma and retinoblastoma, because both can arise secondary to an alteration or mutation at the RB gene locus (chromosome *13q 14*).

Osteosarcomas are classified into one of seven histologic subtypes: osteoblastic (most common), fibroblastic, chondroblastic, epithelioid, telangiectatic, small cell, and giant cell. Osteosarcomas of all types have a poor prognosis. All telangiectatic osteosarcomas manifest as osteolytic lesions, but the other histologic types of osteosarcomas may also manifest as predominantly osteolytic vertebral lesions.[1] Parosteal osteosarcomas are not known to occur in the spine.[1]

Metachronous spinal and/or skeletal osteosarcomas occur in up to 3% of patients.[9] Osteosarcomas may arise in vertebra with Paget disease, which accounts for some osteosarcomas in the elderly population. Sarcomatous degeneration of pagetoid bone may be multicentric.[10] Osteosarcomas can also occur in bone previously treated with radiotherapy for other disorders,

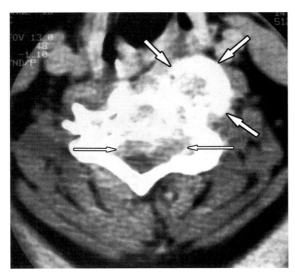

Figure 57-1 ► Radiation Induced Cervical Vertebral Osteosarcoma. Axial CT image, C4 level. Heterogeneous bone destruction resulting in vertebral collapse and tumoral bone formation (*short thick arrows*) projects anterolateral to the vertebral body on the left. Heterogeneous epidural tumor (*long thin arrows*) displaces the cord posteriorly to the right.

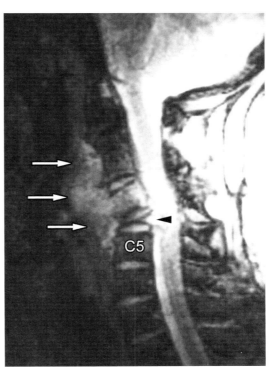

Figure 57-2 ► Radiation Induced Cervical Vertebral Osteosarcoma. Same patient as in Figure 57-1. Sagittal fat-saturated T2-weighted image. Tumor has destroyed the C4 and C5 vertebral bodies. The C4 vertebral body has collapsed resulting in C4 vertebral planum (*black arrowhead*). C4-5 ventral epidural tumor displaces the cord posteriorly. Prevertebral soft tissue mass (*arrows*) extends from C2 to C5 level. C5 = C5 vertebral body.

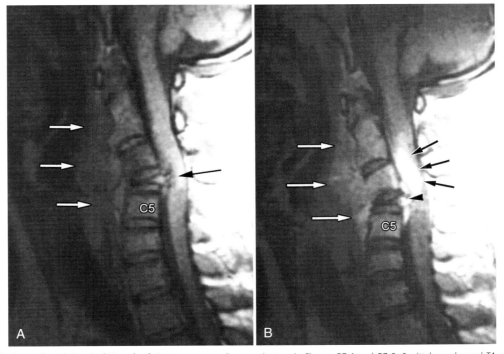

Figure 57-3 ► Radiation Induced Cervical Vertebral Osteosarcoma. Same patient as in Figures 57-1 and 57-2. Sagittal unenhanced T1-weighted image **A** and contrast-enhanced T1-weighted image **B**. The prevertebral mass (*white arrows*), adjacent infiltrated vertebrae and anterior epidural mass (*black arrows*) enhance following IV contrast. Collapsed, posteriorly displaced C4 vertebral body (*black arrow* in **A**, *arrowhead* in **B**) and epidural tumor (*black arrows in image* **B**) displace the spinal cord posteriorly. C5 = C5 vertebra body.

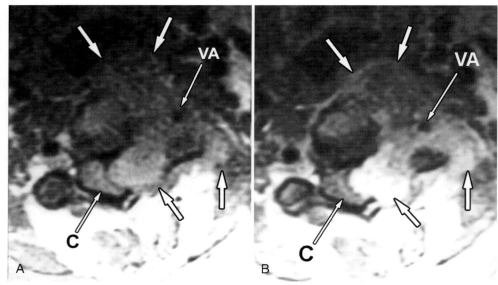

Figure 57-4 ▶ Radiation Induced Cervical Vertebral Osteosarcoma. Same patient as in Figures 57-1 to 57-3. Axial unenhanced MR image **A** and contrast-enhanced image **B**, at C3-4 level. The patient's neck is turned toward the right. Heterogeneously enhancing mass encases the left vertebral artery (*VA*) and extends into the C3-4 foraminal and paraspinal soft tissues on the left (*arrows*). The epidural tumor on the left displaces the spinal cord (*C*) to the right of midline.

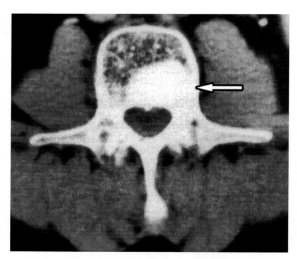

Figure 57-5 ▶ Metastatic Osteosarcoma to T12 Vertebral Body from Lower Extremity Primary Osteosarcoma. Axial CT image shows sclerotic metastasis (*arrow*) in T12 vertebral body. This may be mistaken for a bone island or osteoblastic metastasis from another type of primary tumor.

occurring 5 to 20 years after radiation therapy.[3,11] Malignant fibrous histiocytoma may also occur in tissues several years after radiotherapy.[12]

Primary spinal or sacral osteosarcomas are difficult to resect and carry a much poorer prognosis than osteosarcomas of the appendicular skeleton, especially when the vertebral tumor is large, when the sacrum is involved, and when distant metastases are present;[3,13] 10% to 20% of patients with appendicular primary osteosarcomas metastasize to other portions of the skeleton including the spine.[9] Patients with appendicular primary osteosarcomas with spine metastases have a higher incidence of local

recurrence of tumor and a worse prognosis than patients with lung metastases.[14]

IMAGING FINDINGS

Imaging is important in diagnosing and assessing the extent of primary vertebral tumors, for tumor staging, and for detecting recurrent local or metastatic tumor. In the majority of osteosarcomas, the osteoid matrix calcifies, and the tumor is densely sclerotic or contains sclerotic regions; 80% of vertebral osteosarcomas have a dense, sclerotic bone matrix or a mixed osteolytic and sclerotic appearance.[15] In the remainder of cases of vertebral osteosarcoma, the matrix does not calcify, resulting in a perceptive or moth-eaten osteolytic region of expansion and bone destruction in the vertebra. Osteosarcomas may manifest with an "ivory vertebra" appearance on spine radiographs.[1] However, bone sclerosis and osteolysis are best demonstrated on CT (see Fig. 57-1), although the extent of the soft tissue in the spinal canal, neural foramen, or paraspinal soft tissues is best visualized with MRI (see Figs. 57-2 to 57-4). Associated pathologic fractures of the vertebrae are also best shown on CT but well demonstrated on MRI as well.

On MRI, sclerotic osteosarcomas are classically markedly T1 hypointense and T2 hypointense relative to normal vertebrae (see Figs. 57-5 and 57-6).[3] Predominantly osteolytic osteosarcomas are T1 hypointense to isointense and T2 hyperintense tumors. If fluid/fluid levels are visible in the tumor, this is characteristic of the telangiectatic type of osteosarcomas; these tumors are permeative, osteolytic tumors on CT and can resemble aneurysmal bone cysts, except that osteosarcomas usually have poorly defined margins. Primary osteosarcomas often extend into the paravertebral soft tissues, neural foramina, and epidural space, where they may compress the spinal cord (see Figs. 57-1 to 57-4). Metastatic osteosarcomas may appear as discrete ovoid T1 and T2

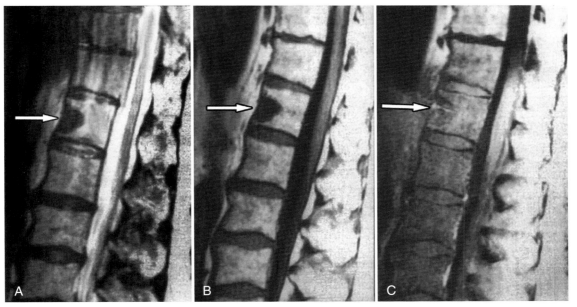

Figure 57-6 ▶ Metastatic Osteosarcoma to T12 Vertebral Body. Sagittal MR images in same patient as in Figure 57-5. A well-defined sclerotic osteosarcoma metastasis (*arrow*) is T2 hypointense in image **A** and T1 hypointense in image **B** and enhances slightly so that it is nearly isointense relative to adjacent marrow on contrast enhanced image **C**. Bone islands may have a similar CT, T1, and T2 MR appearance, but bone islands do not enhance following IV contrast.

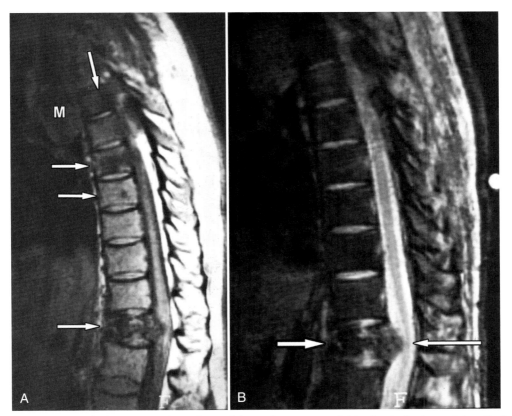

Figure 56-7 ▶ Multiple Thoracic Vertebral Metastases Secondary to Primary Osteosarcoma Originating in the Lower Extremity. On sagittal T1-weighted image **A**, T1 hypointense metastases in the T5, T6, T7, T8, and T12 vertebral bodies (*arrows*) are seen. A pleural based lung mass (*M*) is located anterior to the spine in at the T5-6 level. The T12 vertebral metastasis (*short thick arrow in image* **B**) is T2 hypointense. Tumor has resulted in a pathologic fracture of the T12 vertebral body. Tumor has broken through the posterior T12 vertebral cortex into the ventral epidural space where it compresses and posteriorly displaces the spinal cord (*long thin arrow in image* **B**).

hypointense lesions in the vertebrae (see Figs. 57-5 and 57-6) or can cause vertebral bone destruction or pathologic fracture and may extend into the epidural space or paraspinal soft tissues (see Fig. 57-7).

Osteosarcomas usually display increased uptake on radionuclide bone scans and have avid fluorodeoxyglucose (FDG) uptake on positron emission tomography (PET) scans. Bone and PET scanning are especially useful in restaging to detect local recurrence of tumor and dissemination of tumor.[9,16]

DIFFERENTIAL DIAGNOSIS

1. **Osteoblastic metastases:** These commonly arise secondary to prostate carcinoma, treated breast cancer, or gastrointestinal (GI) tract malignancies. Osteoblastic metastases have an "ivory vertebral body" appearance that is nonspecific, also seen in patients with osteoblastic metastases, lymphoma, Paget disease, and vertebral osteosarcoma.[1] The soft tissue components of osteoblastic metastases usually lack matrix bone formation.

2. **Large vertebral enostosis (bone island):** These manifest as ovoid, sclerotic, well-circumscribed areas in the vertebra and are composed of mature bone.[3] They are hypointense on all pulse sequences but do not enhance after IV contrast administration as osteosarcomas typically do (see Figs. 57-5 and 57-6).

3. **Chronic vertebral osteomyelitis:** This commonly manifests with sclerosis involving adjacent vertebral bodies, but usually the adjacent disc space has previously been destroyed, distorted, or fused. Osteosarcoma may involve contiguous vertebral bodies.

4. **Osteoblastoma:** This is an expansile tumor that typically arises in the posterior vertebral elements but may extend anteriorly to involve the vertebral body.[15] Osteosarcomas may secondarily involve the posterior arch but rarely are confined only to the posterior vertebral arch. Osteoblastomas may contain areas of new bone formation, so aggressive osteoblastoma can have the appearance of vertebral osteosarcoma.[3]

5. **Aneurysmal bone cyst:** This may resemble the telangiectatic type of osteosarcoma, which contains blood-filled cystic areas displaying fluid/fluid levels on CT or MR imaging. Both aneurysmal bone cysts and osteosarcomas can have an expansile appearance with cortical disruption, but osteosarcomas have a more aggressive appearance.[3,15] The margins of aneurysmal bone cysts tend to be well defined, whereas osteosarcoma usually has an ill-defined bony margin. Aneurysmal bone cysts can be primary or can occur secondarily in other tumors such as osteoblastoma, chondroblastoma, and osteosarcoma (especially telangiectatic type).[3,15]

6. **Malignant giant cell tumors:** Most giant cells arise in the sacrum as expansile lesions that may contain areas of calcification or bone formation. Giant cell tumors may rarely undergo malignant sarcomatous degeneration.[15] Malignant giant cell tumors may look identical to giant cell type osteosarcoma histologically and radiographically.

7. **Chondrosarcoma:** These are expansile lesions that may involve the vertebral bodies. The matrix of these tumors is cartilaginous and classically calcifies in arcuate or ringlike configuration.[15]

8. **Ewing sarcoma:** This is typically a permeative, osteolytic tumor that infiltrates the vertebra without gross bone destruction as in osteosarcoma. They rarely contain areas of sclerosis.[15]

9. **Lymphoma:** Vertebral lymphoma is usually an infiltrative bone tumor but can be sclerotic in some cases, manifesting with an "ivory vertebral body" appearance.[15]

TREATMENT

1. **Surgery:** Surgical en bloc resection of the vertebral tumor is the treatment of choice with removal of a wide margin of bone and soft tissue.[13] Osteosarcomas in the vertebrae and sacrum are difficult to resect completely and therefore recurrence is common.

2. **Neoadjuvant and adjuvant chemotherapy:** Neoadjuvant chemotherapy is given prior to surgery with the goal of reducing tumor size prior to surgery.[11,14] The use of aggressive neoadjuvant and postsurgical adjuvant chemotherapy has been shown to be effective in reducing the rate of recurrence and metastases.[7,9] A potential long-term complication of neoadjuvant chemotherapy is the development of a second tumor of a different nature, such as leukemia or Ewing sarcoma.[17]

3. **Immunotherapy:** Immunomodulation with agents such as cytokines (such as interleukin 2), ifosfamide, and interferon has been used with limited success in some cases.[18,19] Gene therapy is also under investigation.[19]

4. **Radiotherapy:** Osteosarcoma is generally very resistant to radiation therapy. However, in patients who have unresectable osteosarcomas, such as in the spine, radiotherapy is sometimes used with adjuvant chemotherapy.[13,18]

References

1. Ilaslan H, Sundaram M, Unni KK, Shives TC. Primary vertebral osteosarcoma: imaging findings. *Radiology.* 2004;230:697-702.
2. Knoeller SM, Uhl M, Gahr N, et al. Differential diagnosis of primary malignant bone tumors in the spine and sacrum: The radiological and clinical spectrum: mini review. *Neoplasma.* 2008;55:16-22.
3. Murphey MD, Andrews CL, Flemming DJ, et al. From the archives of the AFIP: Primary tumors of the spine: radiologic pathologic correlation. *Radiographics.* 1996;16:1131-1158.
4. Wright NB, Skinner R, Lee RE, Craft AW. Osteogenic sarcoma of the neural arch. *Pediatr Radiol.* 1995;25:62-63.
5. Hines N, Lantos G, Hochzstein J, et al. Osteosarcoma of the lumbosacral spine invading the central venous pathways, right-sided cardiac chambers, and pulmonary artery. *Skeletal Radiol.* 2007;36:1091-1096.
6. Bacci G, Longhi A, Versari M, et al. Prognostic factors for osteosarcoma of the extremity treated with neoadjuvant chemotherapy: 15-year experience in 789 patients treated at a single institution. *Cancer.* 2006;106:1154-1161.
7. Bramwell VH. Osteosarcomas and other cancers of bone. *Curr Opin Oncol.* 2000;12:330-336.
8. Peabody TD, Gibbs CP Jr, Simon MA. Evaluation and staging of musculoskeletal neoplasms. *J Bone Joint Surg Am.* 1998;80:1204-1218.
9. Bearcroft PW, Davies AM. Follow-up of musculoskeletal tumours. 2. Metastatic disease. *Eur Radiol.* 1999;9:192-200.
10. Vuillemin-Bodaghi V, Parlier-Cuau C, Cywiner-Golenzer C, et al. Multifocal osteogenic sarcoma in Paget's disease. *Skeletal Radiol.* 2000;29:349-353.
11. Bacci G, Longhi A, Forni C, et al. Neoadjuvant chemotherapy for radioinduced osteosarcoma of the extremity: The Rizzoli experience in 20 cases. *Int J Radiat Oncol Biol Phys.* 2007;67:505-511.
12. Patel SR. Radiation-induced sarcoma. *Curr Treat Options Oncol.* 2000;1:258-261.
13. Ozaki T, Flege S, Liljenqvist U, et al. Osteosarcoma of the spine: Experience of the Cooperative Osteosarcoma Study Group. *Cancer.* 2002;94:1069-1077.
14. Bacci G, Longhi A, Bertoni F, et al. Bone metastases in osteosarcoma patients treated with neoadjuvant or adjuvant chemotherapy: The Rizzoli experience in 52 patients. *Acta Orthop.* 2006;77:938-943.

15. Rodallec MH, Feydy A, Larousserie F, et al. Diagnostic imaging of solitary tumors of the spine: What to do and say. *Radiographics*. 2008;28:1019-1041.

16. Bredella MA, Caputo GR, Steinbach LS. Value of FDG positron emission tomography in conjunction with MR imaging for evaluating therapy response in patients with musculoskeletal sarcomas. *AJR Am J Roentgenol*. 2002;179: 1145-1150.

17. Ferrari C, Bohling T, Benassi MS, et al. Secondary tumors in bone sarcomas after treatment with chemotherapy. *Cancer Detect Prev*. 1999;23:368-374.

18. Longhi A, Errani C, De Paolis M, et al. Primary bone osteosarcoma in the pediatric age: State of the art. *Cancer Treat Rev*. 2006;32:423-436.

19. Mori K, Redini F, Gouin F, et al. Osteosarcoma: Current status of immunotherapy and future trends (Review). *Oncol Rep*. 2006;15:693-700.

PAGET DISEASE

Douglas S. Fenton, M.D.

CLINICAL PRESENTATION

The patient is a 67-year-old man who presented with a chief complaint of low back pain that had been worsening over the last 2 years. The pain radiates down both legs and is worse with walking. He must sit down in order to gain relief. The patient also complains of midline upper thoracic spinal pain that has been occurring for the last month. The patient has a history of bladder cancer. Laboratory evaluation demonstrates elevated alkaline phosphatase.

IMAGING PRESENTATION

Sagittal and axial T1-weighted images demonstrate enlargement of the L5 vertebral body in its anterior-posterior dimension but not in height. On the sagittal image, the L5 vertebral body has a characteristic picture-frame appearance and loss of its typical trabecular pattern. These findings are characteristic of Paget disease of bone (*Fig. 58-1*).

DISCUSSION

Paget disease (PD) is a chronic metabolically active bone disease, characterized by a disturbance in both bone modeling and remodeling secondary to increased osteoblastic and osteoclastic activity.[1] PD of bone can be a monostotic (single bone) or polyostotic (multiple bones) nonhormonal disorder. PD was originally described by Sir John Paget in 1877.[2]

PD, also known as *osteitis deformans*, is a common metabolically active bone disease, second only to osteoporosis. It is more common in people of Anglo-Saxon origin. Radiographic studies have revealed a prevalence of 3.5%.[3,4] A recent study of radiographic examinations of the pelvis demonstrated an overall prevalence of 1% to 2% in the United States,[5] with near equal distribution in whites and African Americans and between men and women. By the age of 90 years, the prevalence jumps to approximately 10%.[6] Recent studies have demonstrated several interesting findings. First the incidence and prevalence of PD are declining.[7] Second, the severity of the disease is decreasing as measured by serum alkaline phosphatase levels.[8] Third, there has been a rise of the age at presentation by approximately 4 years per decade,[7] and lastly, the proportion of patients with monostotic disease is increasing.[7]

The etiology of PD remains debatable. Because Paget disease can undergo sarcomatous transformation (0.7% of cases,[9] some believe that PD is a benign neoplasm of the mesenchymal osteoprogenitor cell.[10] Others have postulated that PD is caused by a viral disease[11] or a zoonosis associated with ownership of birds, dogs, cats, or cattle.[12]

Paget disease most commonly involves the pelvis, with the spine being the second most common site.[13] Hartman and Dohn[14] demonstrated that approximately 15% of patients with PD, either monostotic or polyostotic, have vertebral involvement. Polyostotic PD is seen in 66% of cases[15] with between 35% and 50% of the total having spine involvement.[16] The L4 and L5 levels are the most frequently involved sites of spine involvement, closely followed by thoracic involvement.[17] Cervical involvement is much less common.

Spine involvement predisposes patients to low back pain and spinal stenosis. Back pain is the most common clinical symptom associated with PD of the spine. The back pain of PD can be due to the disease itself or its complications, including periosteal stretching, vascular engorgement, microfractures, facet arthritis, intervertebral disc disease, overt fractures, spondylolysis, spondylolisthesis, and sarcomatous transformation.[1] The spine pain of PD is often a deep, dull ache that is unrelated to activity and not relieved by rest or anti-inflammatory medications.[1] The most common complication in PD of the spine is a vertebral compression fracture, which manifests with an acute onset of back pain.[1] Approximately one third of patients with spine involvement exhibit symptoms of clinical spinal stenosis.[18] Spinal stenosis can be caused by three different methods: (1) posterior expansion of the vertebral body (*Fig. 58-2*), (2) expansion of the neural arch with overgrowth of the facet joints (*Fig. 58-3*), or (3) a combination of the two.[18] The bone enlargement can cause classic symptoms of neurogenic claudication or if there is neural foraminal encroachment, radicular pain. Not all patients with spinal stenosis secondary to PD have clinical symptoms. Some patients with severe spinal stenosis may be asymptomatic, whereas some patients with mild spinal stenosis may have significant back pain.[15]

IMAGING FEATURES

With spinal PD, the vertebral body is nearly always involved in conjunction with a portion of the neural arch. The radiologic appearance of PD is enlargement of vertebra characterized by

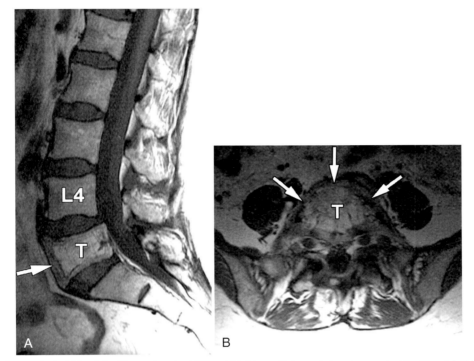

Figure 58-1 ▶ Paget Disease. Sagittal T1-weighted image **A** and axial T1-weighted image **B** demonstrate enlargement of the L5 vertebral body in the anteroposterior dimension but not in height. On the sagittal image, the L5 vertebral body has a picture-frame appearance with loss of the anterior concave margin. Both images reveal thickened cortical bone (*arrows*) and hypertrophy of the trabecular bone (*T*).

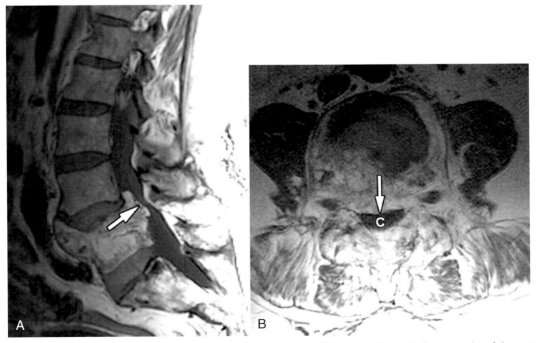

Figure 58-2 ▶ Paget Disease with Spinal Stenosis. Sagittal T1-weighted image **A** and axial T1-weighted image **B**. Note expansion of the posterior margin of the pagetoid L5 vertebral body (*arrow*) causing severe narrowing of the central spinal canal (*C*).

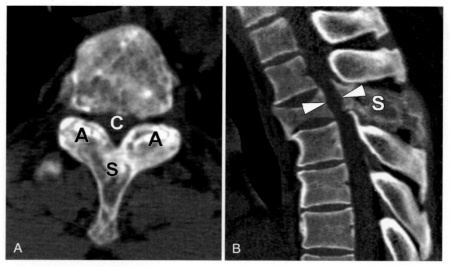

Figure 58-3 ▶ Paget Disease with Spinal Stenosis. Axial CT image **A** and sagittal image **B**. Note hypertrophy of the neural arch (*A*) including the facet joints, lamina, and spinous process (*S*) with severe narrowing of the central spinal canal (*C*, image **A**; *between arrowheads*, image **B**).

enlargement in the anteroposterior and lateral dimensions but not in the overall height of the vertebral body (see Fig. 58-1).[1] There are three phases of PD; an active/osteolytic phase, a mixed osteoblastic/osteolytic phase, and an inactive phase. PD is usually not discovered until the mixed phase in which there is a combination of trabecular bone hypertrophy and thickening at the end-plates with apposition/absorption on the periosteal/endosteal surfaces at the anterior and posterior vertebral borders leading to the "picture-frame" appearance.[19] At this stage, the vertebra has a squared appearance with a thickened cortex and loss of the anterior concave margin (see Fig. 58-1). As the process moves into a more sclerotic phase, one may see an "ivory vertebra" resulting from an increase in overall vertebral density. At this stage, one could mistake PD for a metastasis or primary neoplasm; however, the increased size of the vertebra is an important clue to the actual diagnosis. Occasionally, one may see PD in its early osteolytic phase with the appearance of a "ghost vertebra".[20]

Imaging with computed tomography (CT) or magnetic resonance imaging (MRI) depends upon the phase in which one discovers PD. In the lytic phase, there is loss of much of the trabecular pattern. On MRI, the marrow is hypointense on T1-weighted imaging and hyperintense on T2-weighted sequences secondary to the fibrovascular marrow. On CT, there is absence of the trabecular pattern *(Fig. 58-4)*. In the mixed (blastic-lytic) phase, there is thickening of the cortex, enlargement of the vertebral body, and a coarsened, disorganized trabecular pattern with focal areas of fat density/intensity.[1] This phase is often seen as combinations of hyperintensity and hypointensity on T1- and T2-weighted acquisitions *(Fig. 58-5)*. The late phase is characterized by gradual decrease in both osteoclastic and osteoblastic activity, with residual smoldering osteoblastic activity. MR imaging in the late phase may demonstrate enlarged, thickened vertebra with decreased T1 and T2 signal intensity and sclerosis on CT *(Fig. 58-6)*. Nuclear medicine bone scan will demonstrate increased radiotracer uptake in the pathologic vertebra in the active phase *(Fig. 58-7)*, but may not demonstrate any abnormality in the inactive phase. Plain films are the most cost effective imaging tool to diagnose and follow PD.

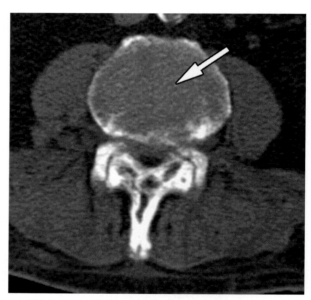

Figure 58-4 ▶ Paget Disease, Absent Trabecular Pattern. Axial CT demonstrates the featureless appearance of the vertebral body (*arrow*) due to loss and hypertrophy of trabecular bone. Note severe central canal spinal stenosis.

CT can be obtained if there is concern related to possible bone destruction. CT or MRI can be reserved to evaluate claudication and/or radicular symptoms. Nuclear medicine bone scan can be used to evaluate the overall extent of the disease process.

DIFFERENTIAL DIAGNOSIS

1. **Vertebral hemangioma**: There is no vertebral enlargement or cortical thickening as seen with Paget disease. A vertebral

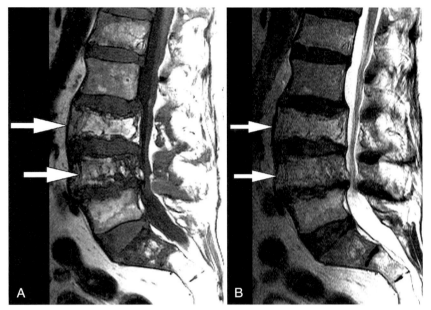

Figure 58-5 ▶ Paget Disease, Mixed Phase. Sagittal T1-weighted image **A** and T2-weighted image **B**. Enlargement of the L3 and L4 vertebral bodies (*arrows*) in the anteroposterior dimension causing moderate to severe central canal narrowing. Both vertebral bodies demonstrate varying amounts of increased and decreased signal intensity compatible with the mixed (blastic/lytic) phase of Paget disease.

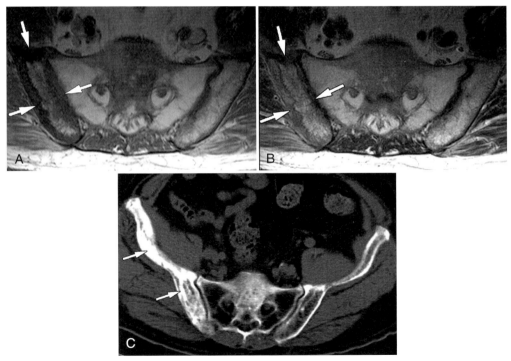

Figure 58-6 ▶ Paget Disease, Late Phase. Axial T1-weighted MR image **A**, axial T2-weighted image **B**, and axial CT image **C**. Cortical thickening and decreased T1 and T2 signal intensity on images **A** and **B** (*arrows*) is seen. This same region shows sclerosis on CT image **C** (*arrows*).

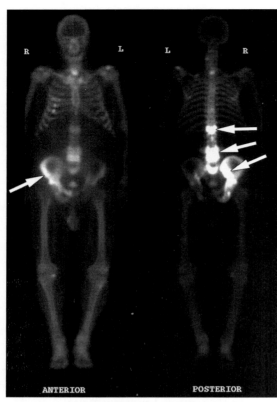

Figure 58-7 ▶ Paget Disease, Active Phase. Nuclear medicine bone scan, anterior and posterior projections. Increased radiotracer activity is seen in the lumbar spine, sacrum, and left iliac bone (*arrows*).

hemangioma has a stippled appearance on axial CT due to thickened trabecula and is usually hyperintense on both T1- and T2-weighted MR imaging (*Fig. 58-8*).

2. **Osteoblastic metastases**: These can look similar to the late phase of Paget disease with decreased T1 and T2 signal intensity. The picture-frame appearance is uncommon (*Fig. 58-9*) and enlargement of the vertebral body is uncommon. Metastases are often multilevel.

3. **Primary neoplasm: Neoplasms** such as osteosarcoma, carcinoid, and Hodgkin's lymphoma can have a similar appearance; however, one does not usually see the typical squaring of vertebral bodies or picture-frame appearance.

TREATMENT

1. **Antipagetic medical therapy:** PD can be treated with antipagetic medical therapy such as the bisphosphates, calcitonin, and mithramycin to reduce osteoclastic bone resorption and pain.

2. **Nonsteroidal anti-inflammatory medications:** If antipagetic medical therapy does not ameliorate the symptoms within 3 months, then nonsteroidal anti-inflammatory medications can be prescribed.

3. **Additional drug therapy:** The spinal stenosis of PD can also be treated with nonsteroidal anti-inflammatory medications in addition to sodium etidronate, pamidronate disodium, and clondronate.[1,21]

4. **Surgical management:** If spinal stenosis is severe enough and antipagetic therapy fails, then surgical decompression should be considered.

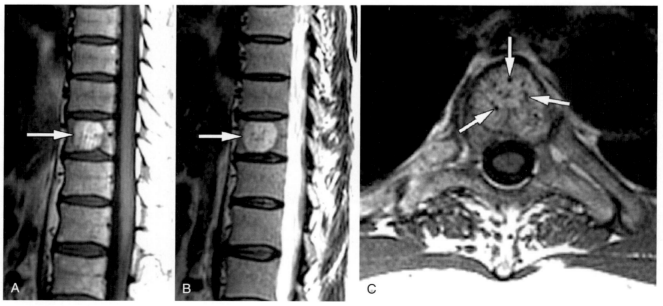

Figure 58-8 ▶ Hemangioma of Bone. Rounded region of increased signal intensity on both sagittal T1-weighted image **A** (*arrow*) and sagittal T2-weighted image **B** (*arrow*). Note the thickened trabecula of a typical hemangioma (*arrows*) on axial T1-weighted image **C**.

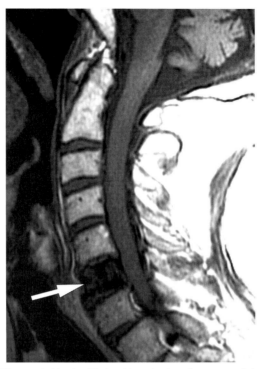

Figure 58-9 ▶ Sclerotic Metastasis. Very low T1 signal intensity throughout a normal-sized C6 vertebral body (*arrow*).

References

1. Dell'Atti C, Cassar-Pullicino VN, Lalam RK, et al. The spine in Paget's disease. *Skeletal Radiol.* 2007;36:609-626.
2. Paget J. On a form of chronic inflammation of bone (osteitis deformans). *Trans R Med Chir Soc Lond.* 1877;60:36-43.
3. Maldaque B, Malghem J. Dynamic radiologic patterns of Paget's disease of bone. *Clin Orthop.* 1987;217:126-151.
4. Pygott F. Paget's disease of bone: The radiological incidence. *Lancet.* 1957;1:1170-1179.
5. Altman RD, Bloch DA, Hochberg MC, Murphy WA. Prevalence of pelvic Paget's disease of bone in the United States. *J Bone Miner Res.* 2000;15:461-465.
6. Schmorl G. Uber osteitis deformans Paget. *Virchows Arch Pathol Anat Physiol.* 1932;238:694-751.
7. Cundy T. Is Paget's disease of bone disappearing? *Skeletal Radiol.* 2006;6:350-351.
8. Cundy T, McAnulty K, Wattie D, et al. Evidence for secular change in Paget's disease. *Bone.* 1997;1:69-71.
9. Hadjipavlou A, Lander P, Srulovitz H, Enker P. Malignant transformation in Paget's disease of bone. *Cancer.* 1992;70:2802-2808.
10. Ramussen H, Bordeier P. The physiological cellular basis of metabolic bone disease. *N Engl Med J.* 1973;184:25-29.
11. Baslé MF, Rebel A, Fournier JG, Russell WC, Malkani K. On the trail of paramyxoviruses in Paget's disease of bone. *Clin Orthop.* 1987;217:9-15.
12. López-Abente G, Morales-Piga A, Elena-Ibáñez A, et al. Cattle, pets, and Paget's disease of bone. *Epidemiology.* 1997;8:247-251.
13. Altman RD. Musculoskeletal manifestation of Paget's disease of bone. *Arthritis Rheum.* 1980;23:1121-1127.
14. Hartman JT, Dohn DF. Paget's disease of the spine with cord or nerve root compression. *J Bone Joint Surg Am.* 1966;48:1079-1084.
15. Hadjipavlou A, Lander P, Srolovitz H. Pagetic arthritis: Pathophysiology and management. *Clin Orthop Relat Res.* 1986;208:15-19.
16. Mirra JM, Brien EW, Tehranzadeh J. Paget's disease of bone: Review with emphasis on radiologic features. *Skeletal Radiol.* 1995;3:163-171.
17. Guyer PB, Shepherd DF. Paget's disease of the lumbar spine. *Br J Radiol.* 1980;628:286-288.
18. Hadjipavlou A, Lander P. Paget's disease of the spine. *J Bone Joint Surg Am.* 1991;73:1376-1381.
19. Graham TS. The ivory vertebra sign. *Radiology.* 2005;2:614-615.
20. Sprecher S, Steinberg R, Lichtenstein D, et al. Magnetic resonance imaging presentation of lytic Paget's disease of the cervical spine. *J Bone Miner Res.* 2002;11:1929-1930.
21. Chen JR, Rhee RS, Wallach S, et al. Neurologic disturbances in Paget's disease of bone: Response to calcitonin. *Neurology.* 1979;29:448-457.

POST RADIATION EFFECTS

Douglas S. Fenton, M.D.

CLINICAL PRESENTATION

The patient is a 70-year-old woman with metastatic breast cancer who presented with paresthesias with a cold sensation and burning dysesthesias in both feet. Decreased sensation in both legs extends from her feet to her groin. Paresthesias also involve the left forearm. She has difficulty buttoning clothing. The patient has had two recurrences of metastatic adenopathy in the supraclavicular, mediastinal, and perihilar regions bilaterally for which she received two courses of chemotherapy and radiation therapy. These treatments were completed approximately 1 year ago.

IMAGING PRESENTATION

Sagittal T1-weighted image reveals homogeneous increased signal intensity throughout the vertebral marrow and a mildly enlarged cervical spinal cord. Sagittal T2-weighted image shows a long segment of abnormal increased T2 signal intensity within the cervical spinal cord from C3-C7. These findings are consistent with radiation-induced spinal cord edema causing myelopathy (*Fig. 59-1*).

DISCUSSION

Radiation therapy is a mainstay in the treatment of neoplasms of the spine. However, the use of radiation must be balanced with its potential side effects. Radiation can cause disturbance in bone growth in the immature skeleton. Complications in the mature skeleton include osteoradionecrosis, radiation-induced fractures, and radiation-induced neoplasms. Radiation can also have an effect on the intraspinal and paraspinal soft tissues. Radiation myelopathy/myelitis is a very serious complication.

Histologically, there are two phases of bone marrow changes from radiation. In the acute phase, radiation causes edema, vascular congestion, and capillary injury.[1] These changes can be seen within 1 to 3 days of the initiation of radiation therapy. In the chronic phase, hematopoietic cells and blood vessels are depleted and replaced by yellow fat cells.[1-3] These changes can be seen within 2 to 6 weeks of the initiation of radiation therapy.[1,2] Radiation changes in bone depend on the patient's age, absorbed dose, size of the radiation field, beam energy, and fractionation.[4]

Radiation to the immature skeleton can cause asymmetric vertebral growth and fibrosis of the overlying soft tissues.[5,6] This asymmetry can lead to scoliosis. Radiation-induced scoliosis is convex to the side opposite the radiation port and occurs in up to 80% of skeletally immature patients.[7] The degree of scoliosis is related to the dose of radiation and is more severe in patients who have received radiation under 2 years of age.[8]

In skeletally mature patients, radiation impairs osteoblast function resulting in decreased matrix production. Radiographically, this is seen as osteopenia, which is typically seen 1 year after radiation and can lead to bone atrophy.[9] Attempts at repair of the damaged bone result in deposition of new bone on ischemic trabecula.[10] Fractures may occur through this weakened bone. The constellation of radiographic findings of osteopenia, areas of increased density from attempts at repair, and coarsened trabecula has been called *radiation osteitis, radiation necrosis,* or *osteoradionecrosis*).[10] These findings can appear similar to radiation-induced sarcoma; however, osteoradionecrosis can be differentiated from sarcoma by the absence of soft tissue mass seen with osteoradionecrosis, changes confined to the radiation field, and its stability over time.[10]

Radiation can give rise to benign and malignant neoplasms. Osteochondromas are the most common benign radiation-induced tumor and are histologically and radiographically identical to spontaneously occurring osteochondromas.[11] Radiation-induced osteochondromas are most commonly found in children who were irradiated at less than 2 years of age, with a latent period from 17 months to 9 years.[11-13] Radiation can rarely give rise to malignant sarcomas, the majority of which are osteosarcomas followed by fibrosarcomas.[14] They can arise in both preexisting bone lesions and in bones that were normal prior to radiation therapy. The latency period is from 11 to 14 years.[15] The diagnosis of radiation-induced sarcoma is established by four criteria: (1) a long latency period, (2) malignancy with the radiation field, (3) pathologic evaluation demonstrating sarcomatous change, and (4) the radiation-induced sarcoma must differ histologically from the original lesion that was treated with radiation.[16] Patients with sarcomas are often symptomatic, presenting with pain and swelling, often with a palpable soft-tissue mass.[13]

Radiation myelopathy causes injury to the white matter of the spinal cord. Patients usually present 9 to 15 months after the end of radiation.[17] Clinically, the patient can present early on with paresthesia (particularly with an inability to perceive pain and temperature). As it progresses, the patient can experience various symptoms including gait abnormalities and hemiplegia.[18] Several factors influence the development of radiation myelopathy including the total delivered dose of radiation, fractionation of the

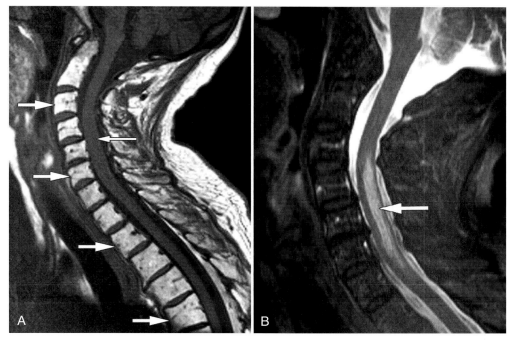

Figure 59-1 ▶ Radiation-Induced Spinal Cord Edema. Diffuse increased T1 signal intensity throughout all cervical and visualized thoracic vertebral bodies (*large arrows*, image **A**) and mild, nonspecific enlargement of the spinal cord (*small arrow*). Long segment region of abnormal increased T2 signal intensity within the spinal cord (*arrow*, image **B**).

radiation dose (fractionation increases the latent period), the volume of the irradiated tissue (larger volumes decrease the latent period), the linear energy transfer (the greater the transfer the more likely myelopathy is going to occur), and the level of the spinal cord irradiated (posterior and lateral spinal cord involvement in the cervical/upper thoracic region, anterior and lateral spinal cord involvement in the lower thoracic/lumbar region).[18-20] Three criteria must be satisfied to diagnose radiation myelopathy: (1) the affected spinal cord must have been within the radiation field, (2) the neurologic deficit must correspond to the affected spinal cord segment, and (3) metastases or other primary spinal cord lesions must have been excluded.[21]

IMAGING FEATURES

Marrow-related changes from radiation therapy are best seen with magnetic resonance imaging (MRI). Within the first 6 weeks after radiation, the marrow signal reflects changes of bone edema and vascular congestion. Therefore, the marrow may demonstrate slightly decreased to no change on T1-weighted images and hyperintensity on short tau inversion recovery (STIR) or T2-weighted images, particularly if a fat-suppression technique is used. There is also enhancement of the marrow in the early stages. After 6 weeks, the more typical appearance of increased T1 signal secondary to fatty marrow and intermediate signal intensity on T2-weighted images is found (Fig. 59-1). There is no contrast enhancement in the late phase. One also finds that there is a sharply demarcated bandlike appearance on T1-weighted images of the portions of the spine that are within the radiation field *(Fig. 59-2)*. This same radiation portal can be "seen" as a sharp region of photopenia on bone scan.

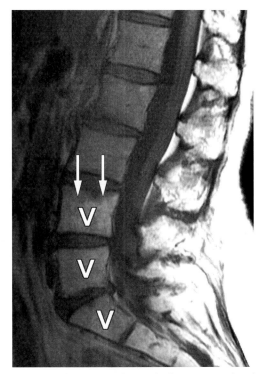

Figure 59-2 ▶ Radiation-Induced Vertebral Marrow Related Change. Sagittal T1-weighted MR image. Increased T1 signal intensity within the L4 and L5 vertebral bodies and the visualized sacrum (*V*). There is a sharply marginated line in the superior portion of the L4 vertebral body (*arrows*), which demarcates the upper aspect of the radiation port.

Radiation myelopathy is also best seen with MRI. In the acute phase of radiation myelopathy, the spinal cord is expanded and demonstrates decreased to intermediate T1 signal and increased T2 signal (see Fig. 59-1). Contrast enhancement is variable and may be patchy or ringlike *(Fig. 59-3)*. In the chronic phase of radiation myelopathy, the affected portions of the spinal cord (often the regions that enhanced) can become atrophic.

Radiation-induced osteochondromas are identical to spontaneous osteochondromas. Corticomedullary continuity of the osteochondroma with the parent bone is pathognomonic *(Fig. 59-4)*. An osteochondroma appears as a pedunculated or sessile bony projection. At the point of attachment, the cortex of the bone of origin flares into the cortex of the osteochondroma. This is further elaborated in Chapter 50, "Osteochondroma."

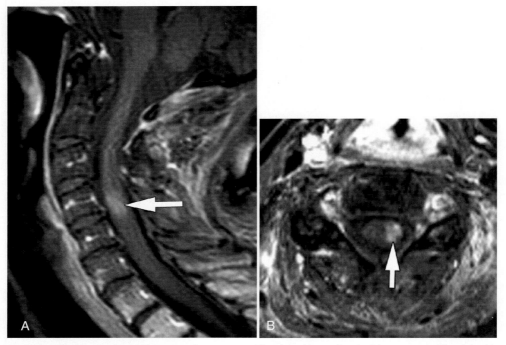

Figure 59-3 ▶ **Acute Radiation Myelopathy.** Sagittal fat-saturated, post-contrast, T1-weighted image **A** and axial post-contrast, T1-weighted image **B**. Patchy enhancement within the left side of the cervical spinal cord at the C4-5 level (*arrow*) in a patient who received radiation to the neck.

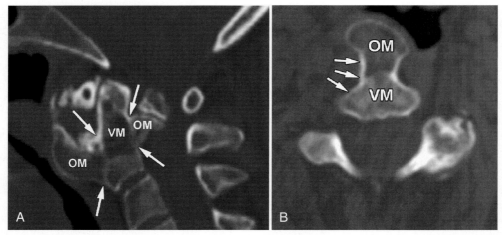

Figure 59-4 ▶ **Osteochondroma.** Sagittal CT image **A** and axial CT image **B** reveal pedunculated bone lesions from the anterior and posterior C2 vertebra. The medullary cavities of the vertebral body (*VM*) and bone lesions (*OM*) are in continuity as are their cortices (*arrows*), which are the pathognomonic findings of an osteochondroma.

Osteosarcomas are rare. They are of decreased T1 signal and can have variable T2 signal intensity and enhancement. They are aggressive tumors that demonstrate a soft tissue mass and cortical breakthrough that can cause spinal canal or neural foraminal compromise. Noncontrast computed tomography (CT) can narrow the differential of this neoplasm because most osteosarcomas have an internal bone matrix.

DIFFERENTIAL DIAGNOSIS

Radiation Change

1. **Normal fatty marrow** can have an appearance similar to radiation-induced change. One should look for the sharp demarcation of the radiation field.
2. **Hemangiomas of bone** are typically round, well-circumscribed lesions without the sharp demarcation of radiation-induced marrow changes *(Fig. 59-5)*. Hemangiomas also demonstrate avid contrast enhancement.

Radiation Myelopathy

1. **Transverse myelitis** can have an identical appearance to radiation change; however, it often has a rapid onset and is associated with infection and recent vaccination *(Fig. 59-6)*.

2. **Multiple sclerosis** may be multifocal with waxing and waning symptoms. Lesions are typically discrete and in the posterolateral aspect of the spinal cord *(Fig. 59-7)*.
3. **Primary neoplasm** such as astrocytoma can be difficult to distinguish from radiation myelopathy. A history of radiation to the affected spinal cord segment tends to steer the diagnosis away from primary neoplasm.
4. **Spinal cord infarction** has an acute onset of paralysis. It is often limited to the gray matter *(Fig. 59-8)*.

TREATMENT

1. **No treatment:** There is no need to treat the changes of fatty marrow replacement.
2. **Bracing:** Scoliosis, if mild, can be treated with bracing. More severe cases of scoliosis may require surgery.
3. **Stabilization:** Radiation-induced fractures can be treated with rest, bracing, vertebroplasty/kyphoplasty, or surgical stabilization.
4. **Surgery:** Osteochondromas or fractures that are causing spinal canal compromise should be surgically treated.
5. **Radiation therapy:** Sarcomatous change can be treated with additional radiation therapy and/or surgery. However, one must consider that additional radiation therapy increases the risk of radiation myelopathy.
6. **Hyperbaric oxygen:** Radiation myelopathy, unfortunately, tends to be progressive, without much improvement. There has been some success with hyperbaric oxygen in early cases.[22]

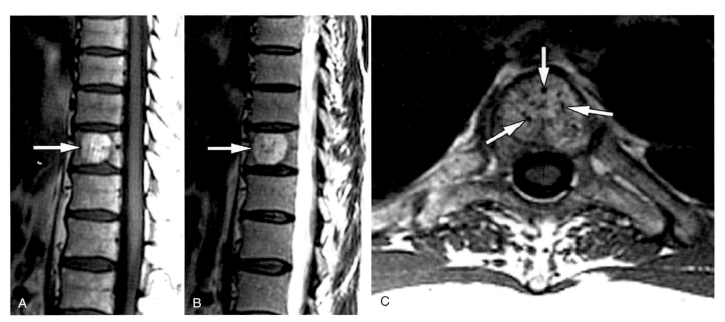

Figure 59-5 ▶ Hemangioma of Bone. Rounded region of increased signal intensity on both sagittal T1-weighted image **A** *(arrow)* and sagittal T2-weighted image **B** *(arrow)*. Note the thickened trabecula of a typical hemangioma *(arrows)* on axial T1-weighted image **C**.

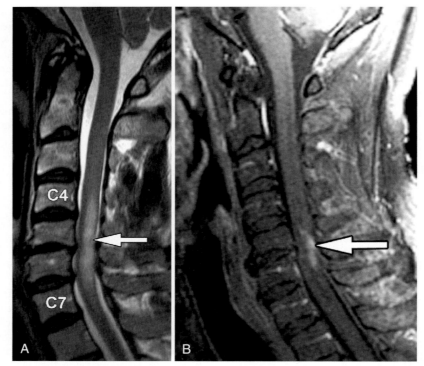

Figure 59-6 ▸ Transverse Myelitis. Sagittal T2-weighted image **A** demonstrates a long segment region of abnormal increased cord signal intensity (*arrow*) with a normal-sized spinal cord. There is patchy enhancement in the dorsal inferior aspect of this lesion on sagittal post-contrast, T1-weighted image **B** (*arrow*).

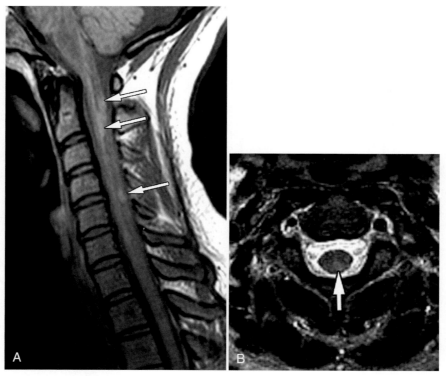

Figure 59-7 ▸ Multiple Sclerosis. Sagittal proton density image **A** reveals multiple short-segment hyperintensities primarily in the dorsal spinal cord (*arrows*). Axial T2-weighted image **B** shows a solitary demyelinating lesion of multiple sclerosis (*arrow*).

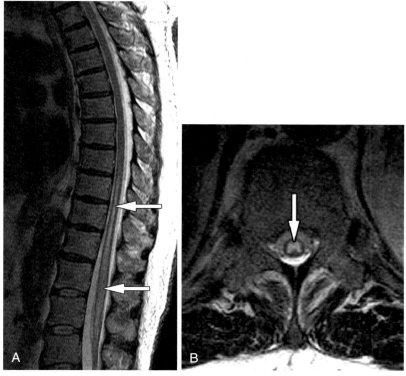

Figure 59-8 ▶ Spinal Cord Infarction. Early spinal cord infarction demonstrates increased T2 signal intensity in the central spinal cord gray matter on sagittal T2 image **A** and axial T2 image **B** (*arrows*).

References

1. Stevens SK, Moore SG, Kaplan ID. Early and late bone-marrow changes after irradiation: MR evaluation. *AJR Am J Roentgenol.* 1990;154:745-750.
2. Yankelevitz DF, Henschke CI, Knapp PH, et al. Effect of radiation therapy on thoracic and lumbar bone marrow: evaluation with MR imaging. *AJR Am J Roentgenol.* 1991;157:87-92.
3. Otake S, Mayr NA, Ueda T, et al. Radiation-induced changes in MR signal intensity and contrast enhancement of lumbosacral vertebrae: Do changes occur only inside the radiation therapy field? *Radiology.* 2002;222: 179-183.
4. Dalinka MK, Haygood TM. Radiation changes. In: Resnick D, ed. *Diagnosis of bone and joint disorders.* Philadelphia, PA: Saunders; 1995:3276-3308.
5. Parker RG, Berry HC. Late effects of therapeutic irradiation on the skeleton and bone marrow. *Cancer.* 1976;37:1162-1171.
6. Arken AM, Simon N. Radiation scoliosis: An experimental study. *J Bone Joint Surg Am.* 1950;32:396-401.
7. Heaston DK, Libshitz HI, Chan RC. Skeletal effects of megavoltage irradiation in survivors of Wilms' tumor. *AJR Am J Radiol.* 1979;133:389-395.
8. Neuhauser EBD, Wittenborg MH, Berman CZ, Cohen J. Irradiation effects of roentgen therapy on the growing spine. *Radiology.* 1952;59: 637-650.
9. Rutherford H, Dodd GD. Complications of radiation therapy: Growing bone. *Semin Roentgenol.* 1974;9:15-27.
10. Mitchell MJ, Logan PM. Radiation-induced changes in bone. *Radiographics.* 1998;18:1125-1136.
11. Murphy FD, Blount WP. Cartilaginous exostoses following irradiation. *J Bone Joint Surg Am.* 1962;44:662-668.
12. El Mahdi AM, Marks R Jr, Thorton WN, Constable WC. Sequelae of pelvic irradiation in infancy. *Radiology.* 1974;110:665-666.
13. Bluemke DA, Fishman EK, Scott WW. Skeletal complications of radiation therapy. *Radiographics.* 1994;14:111-121.
14. Smith J. Radiation-induced sarcoma of bone: clinical and radiographic findings in 43 patients irradiated for soft tissue neoplasms. *Clin Radiol.* 1982; 33:205-221.
15. Seatherby RP, Dahlin DC, Ivins JC. Postradiation sarcoma of bone: Review of 78 Mayo Clinic cases. *Mayo Clin Proc.* 1981;56:294-306.
16. Cahan WG, Woodard HQ, Higinbotham NL, et al. Sarcoma arising in irradiated bone: Report of eleven cases. *Cancer.* 1948;1:3-29.
17. Schultheiss TE, Higgins EM, el-Mahdi AM. The latent period in clinical radiation myelopathy. *Int J Radiat Oncol Biol Phys.* 1984;10:1109-1115.
18. Okada S, Okeda R. Pathology of radiation myelopathy. *Neuropathology.* 2001;21:247-265.
19. van der Kogel AJ. Radiation tolerance of the rat spinal cord: Time-dose relationships. *Radiology.* 1977;122:505-509.
20. Mastaglia FL, McDonald WI, Watson JV, Yogendran K. Effect of X-radiation on the spinal cord: An experimental study of the morphological changes in central nerve fibers. *Brain.* 1976;99:101-122.
21. Pallis CA, Louis S, Morgan RL. Radiation myelopathy. *Brain.* 1961;84: 460-479.
22. Calabró F, Jinkins JR. MRI of radiation myelitis: A report of a case treated with hyperbaric oxygen. *Eur Radiol.* 2000;10:1079-1084.

RETROPHARYNGEAL ABSCESS

Douglas S. Fenton, M.D.

CLINICAL PRESENTATION

The patient is a 5-year-old boy who presented to the emergency department in respiratory distress. The patient has a 2-day history of sore throat and fever and a several hour history of stiff neck, difficulty breathing, and drooling.

IMAGING PRESENTATION

Lateral radiograph of the neck shows abnormal widening of the soft tissues between the posterior airway and the ventral vertebral bodies. Given the patient's clinical history, one should suspect a retropharyngeal inflammatory process and obtain more specific imaging if the patient is stable (*Fig. 60-1*).

DISCUSSION

Retropharyngeal abscess (RPA) is a deep neck space infection that has the potential for very serious complications including airway compromise and sepsis. RPA used to be exclusively a disease of young children; however, it has been increasing in frequency in adults.

An RPA is a collection of pus within lymph nodes in the back of the throat. RPAs are believed to occur as a consequence of infections of the nasopharynx, paranasal sinuses, tonsils, adenoids, or middle ear. The infection then spreads to retropharyngeal lymph nodes that lie between the posterior pharyngeal wall and the prevertebral fascia. It is believed that these lymph nodes atrophy by the third or fourth year of life, which is why the typical nontraumatic RPA is seen in young children.[1] The incidence of RPA decreases in children over 3 years of age.[2] Although rare, the majority of adult cases arise from localized trauma, foreign body ingestion, complications from procedures such as intubation or endoscopy, or in immunocompromised patients.[3-5] The incidence of RPAs has decreased since the advent of antibiotics.[3] A new subset of patients at risk for RPAs is intravenous drug abusers who inject the vessels in their neck.[6]

Whether in children or adults, RPAs can manifest with a sore throat, difficulty swallowing, nuchal pain, fever, and an elevated white blood cell count.[5] Less common symptoms include stridor and respiratory difficulty. Because stridor and respiratory difficulty are rare, limited neck mobility is an important clinical clue in diagnosing RPA. Torticollis can result if the inflammatory process irritates the cervical muscles or nerves.[7]

IMAGING FEATURES

The lateral radiograph was the single most important imaging tool to aid in the diagnosis of retropharyngeal abscess prior to the advent of advanced imaging. If one uses the lateral radiograph as a diagnostic tool, it is important to ensure that it is a true lateral radiograph with the neck in extension and with full inspiration so as to not falsely thicken the retropharyngeal soft tissues.[8,9] Computed tomography (CT) and magnetic resonance imaging (MRI) are now the preferred imaging techniques.[10] Although these advanced imaging modalities are used to confirm the diagnosis, they more importantly localize the infectious process and search for and define an abscess cavity.[11] However, CT scanning has been shown to have significant false-negative (13%) and false-positive (10%) rates in predicting pus at surgery.[12] The distinction between retropharyngeal abscess (RPA) and retropharyngeal cellulitis (RPC) or phlegmon is important. One study used this difference in its treatment decision.[13] Patients with RPA underwent surgical intervention and antibiotics, whereas those with RPC were treated with antibiotics alone. There were no treatment failures in either arm of this study.

The lateral radiograph is often used as a screening examination and will demonstrate thickening of the prevertebral soft tissues (Fig. 60-1). CT will demonstrate a region of fluid density in the retropharyngeal space (*Fig. 60-2*). There is variable peripheral enhancement of the fluid collection. A mature retropharyngeal abscess is suggested by thick enhancement of the wall. MRI is more sensitive in differentiating the fluid signal intensity abscess (decreased T1, increased T2 signal and peripheral enhancement) from cellulitis. Depending on operator experience, ultrasound is more accurate than either CT or MRI in differentiating RPA from cellulitis.

DIFFERENTIAL DIAGNOSIS

1. **Longus colli tendonitis** demonstrates a typical calcific density immediately anterior to the dens (*Fig. 60-3*). Longus colli tendonitis does not enhance and the associated effusion is more diffuse and tracks craniocaudally.
2. **Nonabscess fluid** due to pharyngitis, internal jugular vein thrombosis, or chemotherapy can be present.
3. **Cervical discitis** is centered on the intervertebral disc with enhancement of the disc (*Fig. 60-4*).

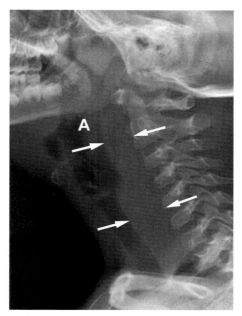

Figure 60-1 ► **Retropharyngeal Edema Secondary to Abscess.** Lateral radiograph shows significant widening of the prevertebral soft tissues (*between arrows*) compatible with edema causing ventral bowing of the posterior wall of the airway (*A*).

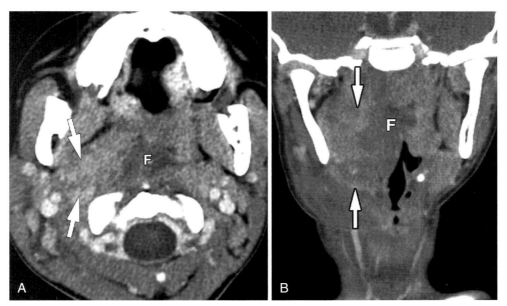

Figure 60-2 ► **Retropharyngeal Abscess.** Axial CT image **A** and coronal CT image **B**. Midline retropharyngeal fluid collection (*F*) with obliteration of the soft tissue/fat planes on the right (*between arrows*) compatible with edema and enlarged lymph nodes.

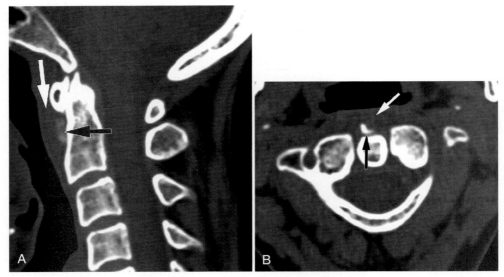

Figure 60-3 ► **Longus Colli Tendonitis.** Sagittal CT image **A** and axial CT image **B** demonstrate a small amorphic region of calcification in the midline just anterior to the dens (*black arrow*) with mild edematous changes in the prevertebral soft tissues (*white arrow*) with very slight mass effect on the posterior oral airway.

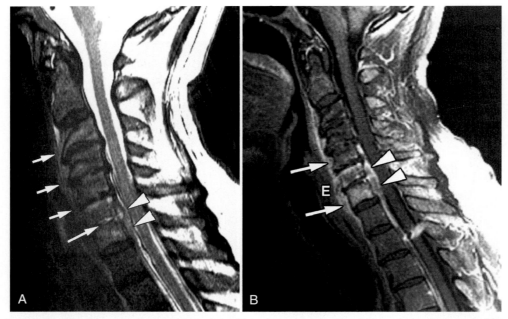

Figure 60-4 ► **Cervical Discitis with Phlegmon.** Abnormal increased signal intensity involving the C6 and C7 vertebral bodies on sagittal fat-saturated, T2-weighted image **A**. There is also increased signal intensity within the C6-7 disc (*large arrow*) and ventral epidural soft tissue (*arrowheads*). Prevertebral increased T2 signal intensity (*small arrows*). Post-contrast, fat-saturated, T1-weighted image **B** shows diffuse enhancement of the C6 and C7 vertebral bodies consistent with discitis/osteomyelitis. There is enhancement of the ventral epidural soft tissue (*arrowheads*) and the prevertebral soft tissue (*arrows*) compatible with phlegmon. Nonenhancing soft tissue is seen posterior to the airway (*E*) compatible with retropharyngeal edema.

TREATMENT

1. **Surgical drainage of pus and antibiotics:** The traditional treatment of RPA has been surgical drainage of the pus collection with intraoral incision and drainage,[14] along with antibiotic therapy to prevent abscess rupture, which could lead to meningitis or osteomyelitis of the cervical spine.

2. **Antibiotics alone:** There have been some cases that have been successfully managed with antibiotic therapy alone.

References

1. Asmar BI. Bacteriology of retropharyngeal abscess in children. *Pediatr Infect Dis J.* 1990;9:595-597.
2. Nario K, Miyahara H, Sasai H, Matsushiro N. A case of retropharyngeal abscess with trismus. *Pract Otol (Kyoto).* 2005;98:483-492.
3. Goldenberg D, Golz A, Joachims HZ. Retropharyngeal abscess: A clinical review. *J Laryngol Otol.* 1997;111:546-550.
4. Sethi DS, Stanley RE. Deep neck abscesses-changing trends. *J Laryngol Otol.* 1994;108:138-143.
5. Tannebaum RD. Adult retropharyngeal abscess: A case report and review of the literature. *J Emerg Med.* 1995;14:147-158.
6. Beasley DJ, Amedee RG. Deep neck space infections. *J La State Med Soc.* 1995;147:181-184.
7. Harries PG. Retropharyngeal abscess and acute torticollis. *J Laryngol Otol.* 1997;111:1183-1185.
8. Haug RH, Wible RT, Lieberman J. Measurement standards for the prevertebral region in the lateral soft-tissue radiograph of the neck. *J Oral Maxillofac Surg.* 1991;49:1149-1151.
9. Brechtelsbauer PB, Garetz SL, Gebarski SS, Bradford CR. Retropharyngeal abscess: Pitfalls of plain films and computed tomography. *Am J Otolaryngol.* 1997;18:258-262.
10. Craig F, Schunk J. Retropharyngeal abscess in children: Clinical presentation, utility of imaging, and current management. *Pediatrics.* 2003;111:1394-1398.
11. Weber AL, Siciliano A. CT and MR imaging evaluation of neck infections with clinical correlations. *Radiol Clin North Am.* 2000;38:941-968.
12. Lazor JB, Cunningham MJ, Eavey RD, Weber AL. Comparison of computed tomography and surgical findings in deep neck infections. *Otolaryngol Head Neck Surg.* 1994;111:746-750.
13. Broughton RA. Nonsurgical management of deep neck infections in children. *Pediatr Infect Dis J.* 1992;11:14-18.
14. Haug RH, Picard U, Indresano AT. Diagnosis and treatment of the retropharyngeal abscess in adults. *Br J Oral Maxillofac Surg.* 1990;28:34-38.

RHEUMATOID ARTHRITIS

Douglas S. Fenton, M.D.

CLINICAL PRESENTATION

The patient is a 76-year-old woman who presented with high cervical neck pain and headache. These symptoms have been ongoing for 6 months. There are no radicular features or myelopathic symptoms. There was no antecedent trauma. On physical examination, there is moderate limitation of neck movement in all directions. The patient is also noted to have moderate degenerative changes in both hands.

IMAGING PRESENTATION

Sagittal fat-saturated, T2- and T1-weighted images demonstrate soft tissue proliferation around the dens, more prominent posteriorly, with some mild mass effect upon the upper cervical spinal cord. There is some increased T2 signal intensity along the margin of the soft tissue. The findings are compatible with pannus formation with some surrounding bone marrow edema and/or inflammation (*Fig. 61-1*).

DISCUSSION

Rheumatoid arthritis (RA) is a common systemic autoimmune process that causes chronic inflammation of the joint. It was first described by Garrod in 1890.[1] A distinguishing feature of RA is symmetric and erosive synovitis of peripheral joints.[2] RA has a predilection for cervical spine involvement and is the most common inflammatory disorder to affect the spine.[3] RA never involves the spine without concomitant involvement of the hands and/or feet. It is estimated that RA affects approximately 1.3 million adults in the United States, with a worldwide prevalence of approximately 0.5% to 1% in developed countries.[4,5] RA is more common in women by a ratio of 2 to 3:1, and although men are the minority of cases, they have a greater risk of more advanced cervical disease.[5-7] Other risk factors that are associated with progressive disease include rheumatoid factor seropositivity, severe peripheral disease, and the prolonged use of steroids.[3] RA demonstrates an increasing prevalence with older age, but interestingly, has been showing a progressive decrease in incidence in the younger age groups since the 1960s, making RA more and more a disease of older adults.[5] Despite how common RA is, the etiology of this process remains unclear. Currently, it is thought that RA is an immune response to an antigenic expression by synovial cells.[2]

Neck pain is a common symptom in patients with RA. The neck pain is often found at the craniocervical junction and may be associated with occipital headaches. The incidence of neck pain ranges from 40% to 88%. Other symptoms include mastoid pain, ear pain, migraine, and facial pain from compression of local nerves. There may also be myelopathic symptoms including weakness, gait disturbance, and paresthesia of the hands. If there is basilar invagination, the patient can present with vertigo, loss of equilibrium, or tinnitus.[3]

The most serious complication of RA in the cervical spine is compression of the spinal cord or brainstem. This can occur from either subluxation of the spine or from direct pressure from pannus formation. Pannus formation around the dens may loosen or destroy the ligamentous structures, particularly the transverse ligament of the atlas and to a lesser extent the alar ligaments and apical dental ligament.[8] This can lead to atlantoaxial subluxation, or horizontal instability, which is defined as a greater than 3 mm distance between the midpoint of the posterior aspect of the anterior arch of the atlas and the anterior aspect of the dens (*Fig. 61-2*).[8] There can also be vertical instability, leading to basilar impression in which the dens extends through the foramen magnum (*Fig. 61-3*).[8]

The upper cervical spine is most commonly affected in RA for two reasons: (1) the C0-C1 and C1-2 articulations are purely synovial and are therefore primary targets for RA, and (2) the C1-2 facet joint is oriented in the axial plane, and therefore, there is no bony interlocking to prevent subluxation.[2] Cervical subluxations have been reported in 40% to 80% of patients on radiographs; however, neurologic deficits are seen in only 10% to 30% of patients.[9,10]

The diagnosis of rheumatoid arthritis is made by a combination of clinical, physical, and/or radiologic findings as delineated in the revised 1987 *Criteria for the Classification of Acute Arthritis of Rheumatoid Arthritis* by the American Rheumatism Association.[11] A patient must satisfy four of the seven criteria, and criteria 1 to 4 must have been present for at least 6 weeks.

1. **Morning stiffness**—Morning stiffness in and around the joints, lasting at least 1 hour before maximal improvement
2. **Arthritis of three or more joint areas**—At least three joint areas simultaneously have had soft tissue swelling or fluid (not bony overgrowth alone) observed by a physician. The 14 possible areas are the right or left proximal interphalangeal joint, metacarpal phalangeal joint, wrist, elbow, knee, ankle, and metatarsal phalangeal joints
3. **Arthritis of hand joints**—At least one hand joint area swollen (as defined in #2)

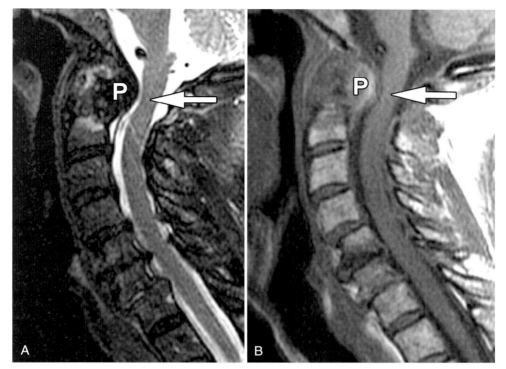

Figure 61-1 ▶ Rheumatoid Arthritis with Pannus Formation. Sagittal fat-saturated, T2-weighted image **A** and T1-weighted image **B**. Large intermediate T1 signal intensity, decreased T2 signal intensity soft tissue mass (*P*) involving the posterior dens compatible with pannus. There is mass effect on the ventral upper cervical spinal cord (*arrow*) with mild central canal narrowing.

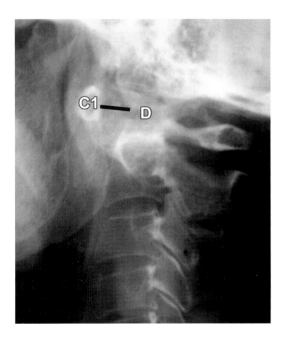

Figure 61-2 ▶ Atlantoaxial Subluxation. Lateral radiograph. The distance (*black line*) between the midpoint of the posterior aspect of the anterior arch of C1 (*C1*) and the ventral dens (*D*) exceeds 3 mm compatible with atlantoaxial subluxation or horizontal instability.

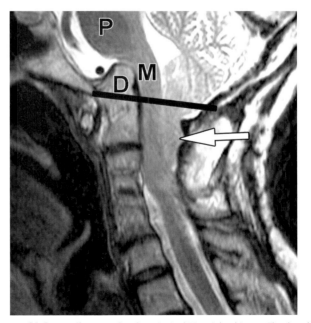

Figure 61-3 ▶ Basilar Invagination. Sagittal T2-weighted image. The dens (*D*) is subluxed superiorly through the floor of the skull base/foramen magnum (*black line* extending from the basion anteriorly to the opisthion posteriorly) compatible with basilar invagination or vertical instability. The dens is compressing the medulla (*M*) but remains inferior to the pons (*P*). Note the inferior cerebellar tonsillar herniation (*arrow*) compatible with Chiari 1 malformation.

4. **Symmetric arthritis**—Symmetric to nearly symmetric simultaneous involvement of the same joint areas (as defined in #2) on both sides of the body
5. **Rheumatoid nodules**—Subcutaneous nodules over bony prominences, extensor surfaces, or in juxtaarticular regions
6. **Serum rheumatoid factor**—Demonstration of abnormal amounts of serum rheumatoid factor by any method
7. **Radiographic changes**—Erosions or unequivocal bony decalcification of the hands or wrists

IMAGING FEATURES

Plain radiographs of the cervical spine should be obtained in neutral, flexion, and extension to assess for motion and instability. The odontoid should be evaluated for evidence of erosions. One may see multilevel ("stepladder") subluxations (*Fig. 61-4*).[8] The distance between the midpoint of the posterior margin on the anterior C1 ring and the dens should be measured. A distance of 3 mm or less is normal. Greater than 3 mm may suggest instability (see Fig. 61-2).[8] If rheumatoid arthritis is suspected from imaging of the spine, additional radiographs of the patient's hands and feet should be performed to evaluate for typical rheumatoid changes because rheumatoid arthritis never involves the spine without involving the hands and feet (*Fig. 61-5*). Computerized tomography (CT) can demonstrate pannus around the dens and the degree of spinal stenosis or narrowing of the foramen magnum caused by the pannus (*Fig. 61-6*). Erosive changes of the dens and facet joints

are well visualized (*Fig. 61-7*). Magnetic resonance imaging (MRI) demonstrates the pannus as low T1 signal intensity and heterogeneous signal intensity on T2-weighted images.[12] Pannus demonstrates avid enhancement (*Fig. 61-8*). Erosions are well seen on MRI in both the dens and facet joints.[12] Bone marrow edema and facet joint effusions can be seen.[12] MRI demonstrates not only the degree of spinal stenosis or narrowing of the foramen magnum caused by pannus but also the direct relationship of the pannus to the spinal cord and whether or not there are compressive changes within the spinal cord or brainstem.

DIFFERENTIAL DIAGNOSIS

1. **Seronegative spondyloarthropathy** (psoriatic arthritis, ankylosing spondylitis, and Reiter disease): An evaluation of the sacroiliac joints should be made because the sacroiliac joints are always involved with seronegative spondyloarthropathy if there is cervical spine involvement. Rheumatoid arthritis rarely has sacroiliac joint involvement.
2. **Infection:** Patients with discitis/osteomyelitis are usually sick with elevated white blood cell counts and sedimentation rates. Infection is often centered on the disc and is more typically found in the lumbar and thoracic regions.
3. **Degenerative disc disease:** One may see endplate sclerosis, Schmorl's nodes, osteophyte formation, and disc space narrowing with degenerative disc disease. Erosions of the dens

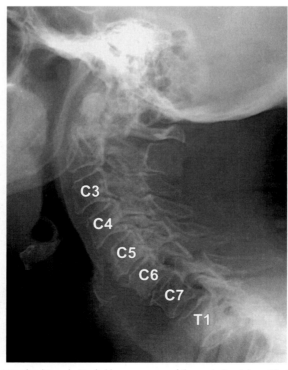

Figure 61-4 ▶ "Stepladder" Subluxations. Lateral radiograph. Stepladder appearance of the cervical vertebra with slight anterior subluxations of each cervical vertebra with the one inferior from C3 to C7.

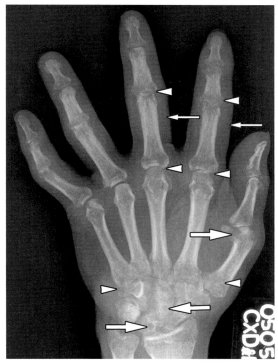

Figure 61-5 ► Rheumatoid Arthritis of the Hand and Wrist. Anteroposterior radiograph of the hand and wrist. Several of the typical findings of rheumatoid arthritis of the hand and wrist are seen including periarticular osteoporosis (*arrowheads*), erosions (*large arrows*), and soft tissue thickening (*small arrows*).

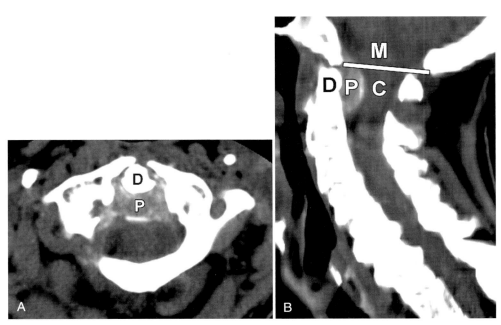

Figure 61-6 ► Rheumatoid-Arthritis and Pannus Formation. Axial CT image **A** and sagittal image **B**. Thick soft tissue along the posterior aspect of the dens (*D*) compatible with pannus (*P*). The pannus impresses the ventral surface of the upper cervical spinal cord (*C*). In this patient, the pannus does not extend through the foramen magnum (*bounded by white line*), and there is no evidence of compression of the medulla (*M*).

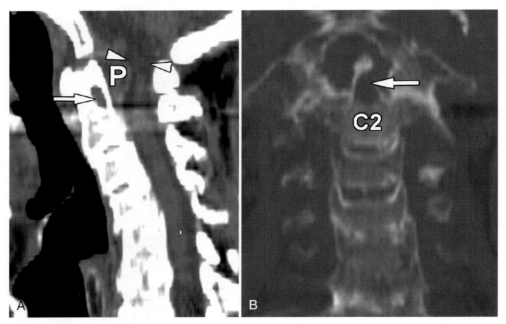

Figure 61-7 ► **Rheumatoid Arthritis Erosions.** Sagittal CT image **A** and coronal image **B**. Erosion in the dorsal dens (*arrow*) with prominent pannus (*P*) along the dorsal dens causing spinal canal narrowing (*arrowheads*).

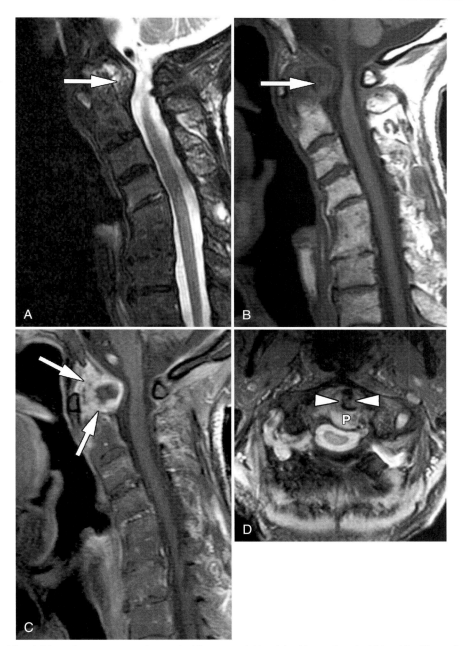

Figure 61-8 ▶ Rheumatoid Arthritis and Pannus Formation. Sagittal fat-saturated, T2-weighted image **A**, sagittal T1-weighted image **B**, sagittal fat-saturated, post-contrast, T1-weighted image **C**, and axial T2-weighted image **D**. Pannus demonstrates decreased T1 signal, increased T2 signal, and avid enhancement (*arrow*). Axial image at the atlantoaxial level shows pannus (*P*) surrounding and causing erosive changes of the dens (*arrowheads*).

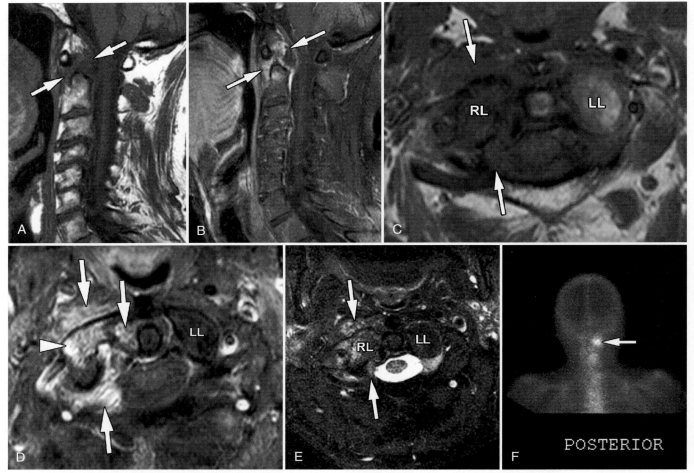

Figure 61-9 ▶ C1-2 Inflammatory Facet Synovitis. Sagittal (**A**) and axial (**C**) T1-weighted images; sagittal (**B**) and axial (**D**) fat-saturated, post-contrast, T1-weighted images; axial fat-saturated, T2-weighted image (**E**). Decreased T1 signal, increased T2 signal, and enhancement centered on the right C1-2 facet articulation involving both the bones on either side of the joint space including the right C1 lateral mass (*RL*) and periarticular soft tissues (*arrows*). Note the normal marrow signal intensity of the left C1 lateral mass (*LM*). There are no erosive changes of the dens. A nuclear medicine bone scan (image **F**) of the same patient demonstrates an intense focus of radiotracer uptake in the upper posterior right neck (*arrow*) corresponding to the MR signal abnormality.

and facet joints are not typical of degenerative disc disease. With advancing age, it is common to see degenerative disc disease changes in patients with rheumatoid arthritis.

4. **Cervical facet synovitis**: MR imaging demonstrates decreased T1, increased T2 signal intensity, and enhancement of and around the joint. Nuclear medicine bone scan demonstrates increased radiotracer activity (***Fig. 61-9***). Pannus formation is not found.

TREATMENT

Treatment of RA in the cervical spine lies in the prevention of irreversible deficits and to avoid sudden death secondary to spinal cord compression.[3] Approximately 10% of patients with RA die of unrecognized spinal cord or brainstem compression.[13]

1. **Surgical management**: It has been demonstrated that earlier surgical intervention when a patient has less severe neurologic deficits has a better outcome. However, 50% of patients with radiographic instability are asymptomatic.[10] A patient with radiographic instability and a neurologic deficit should have surgical intervention. Surgery should also be performed if the patient has cord compression. The controversy lies with the patient who has radiographic instability but no neurologic deficit.

2. **Disease-modifying antirheumatic drugs (DMARDs)**: Treatment of mild to moderate systemic RA is not curative; however, the symptoms can be ameliorated with DMARDs, such as methotrexate and gold therapy. More severe systemic disease is treated by biologic response modifiers that target the parts of the immune system that lead to inflammation.[14]

References

1. Zeidman SM, Ducker TB. Rheumatoid arthritis. *Spine*. 1994;19: 2259-2266.
2. Nguyen HV, Ludwig SC, Silber J, et al. Rheumatoid arthritis of the cervical spine. *Spine J*. 2004;4:329-334.
3. Reiter MF, Boden SD. Inflammatory disorders of the cervical spine. *Spine*. 1998;23:2755-2766.

4. MacGregor AJ, Silman AJ. A reappraisal of the measurement of disease occurrence in rheumatoid arthritis. *J Rheumatol.* 1992;19:1163-1165.
5. Gabriel SE, Crowson CS, O'Fallon WM. The epidemiology of rheumatoid arthritis in Rochester, Minnesota, 1955-1985: *Arthritis Rheum.* 1998;27:325-334.
6. Dreyer SJ, Boden SD. Natural history of rheumatoid arthritis of the cervical spine. *Clin Orthop.* 1999;366:98-106.
7. Weissman BN, Aliabadi P, Weinfield MS, et al. Prognostic features of atlantoaxial subluxation in rheumatoid arthritis patients. *Radiology.* 1982;144:745-751.
8. Castro S, Verstraete K, Mielants H, et al. Cervical spine involvement in rheumatoid arthritis: A clinical, neurological and radiological evaluation. *Clin Exp Rheumatol.* 1994;12:369-374.
9. Boden SD, Dodge LD, Bohlman HH, Rechtine GR. Rheumatoid arthritis of the cervical spine. *J Bone Joint Surg Am.* 1993;75:1282-1297.
10. Pellicci PM, Ranawat CS, Tsairis P, Bryan WJ. A prospective study of the progression of rheumatoid arthritis of the cervical spine. *J Bone Joint Surg Am.* 1981;63:342-350.
11. Arnett FC, Edworthy SM, Bloch DA, et al. The American Rheumatism Association 1987 revised criteria for the classification of rheumatoid arthritis. *Arthritis Rheum.* 1988;31:315-324.
12. Hermann KA. Magnetic resonance imaging of the axial skeleton in rheumatoid disease. *Baillieres Best Pract Res Clin Rheumatol.* 2004;18:881-907.
13. Mikulowski P, Wollheim FA, Rotmil P, Olsen I. Sudden death in rheumatoid arthritis with atlanto-axial dislocation. *Acta Med Scand.* 1975;198:445-451.
14. Ruderman E, Tambar S. Rheumatoid Arthritis. June 2008. http://www.rheumatology.org/practice/clinical/patients/diseases_and_coditionsra.asp. Accessed April 29, 2009.

SACRAL INSUFFICIENCY FRACTURE

Leo F. Czervionke, M.D.

CLINICAL PRESENTATION

The patient is a 79-year-old woman who presented with progressive gait disturbance, low back pain, right groin pain, bilateral lower extremity pain, and left shoulder pain. Patient has remote history of breast cancer with prior radiation therapy to the pelvis for previous metastasis, but no objective evidence of tumor recurrence.

IMAGING PRESENTATION

Magnetic resonance (MR) imaging of the lumbosacral spine reveals abnormal signal intensity in both iliac wings consistent with bilateral sacral insufficiency fractures (*Figs. 62-1 and 62-2*). Radionuclide bone scan reveals intense bilaterally symmetric uptake in the sacral wings consistent with sacral insufficiency fractures (*Fig. 62-3*). Computed tomography (CT) scan of the pelvis reveals fractures of both sacral wings and comminuted fracture to the right of the symphysis pubis (*Fig. 62-4*).

DISCUSSION

Sacral stress fractures are estimated to occur in up to 1% of women over 55 years of age.[1] Sacral stress fractures often go undiagnosed clinically because back pain associated with this condition is attributed to other more common conditions of the spine in the elderly. These fractures are also overlooked during image interpretation, especially when the imaging study obtained does not focus specifically on the sacrum. Sacral stress fractures are of two types: (1) *Insufficiency fractures* are stress fractures of the sacrum resulting from normal stress on abnormal or demineralized bone and (2) *fatigue fractures* are stress fractures that occur when abnormal or demineralized bone is subjected to abnormal stress.[2] Both types of stress fractures have the same imaging appearance and clinical presentation.

The underlying process responsible for the development of sacral stress fractures is an abnormality of bone mineralization. Many conditions can be associated with abnormal bone density resulting in weakening of the sacrum and other bones. This abnormal "insufficient" bone can be subjected to normal axial loading stress; minor or major trauma or repeated trauma can eventually cause fracture. The most common predisposing condition is osteoporosis, which usually develops in post-menopausal females, so sacral stress fractures are far more common in elderly females. The second most common predisposing condition is post-radiotherapy osteoporosis.[3-6] Other conditions that predispose to insufficiency fractures include osteomalacia, long-term steroid therapy, renal osteodystrophy, rheumatoid arthritis, Paget's disease, chronic bed rest, chronic nutritional disorders, and hyperaldosteronism.[2]

Post-menopausal women are most commonly afflicted by sacral stress fractures, but these may also occur in elderly men. Some cases have been reported in pregnant or postpartum women and in long-distance runners.[7] Rarely sacral stress fractures have been reported in the pediatric population, even in nonathletes.[8]

Sacral insufficiency fractures are commonly overlooked initially in the elderly population, the low back pain often being attributed to SI joint arthritis, lumbar spine disc disease, facet arthropathy, or spinal stenosis.[2] Some stress fractures of the sacrum are asymptomatic.[5] However, patients with sacral insufficiency fractures most commonly present with severe low back pain, but also complain of pain in the buttocks, hips, or groin region.[9] The sacrum is often tender to palpation. Radicular symptoms may or may not be present. The back pain is typically worse during activity and usually improves with rest. Rarely, patients with sacral stress fractures present with or develop cauda equina syndrome, which could occur secondary to nerve root traction, nerve root compression, epidural hematoma formation, or perineural inflammation.[9-11]

IMAGING FEATURES

Sacral stress fractures are usually bilateral but can be unilateral. The fractures usually are oriented vertically within the sacral wings but may involve the sacral vertebral bodies, especially in the midsacral region. Occasionally the stress fracture involves only the lower portion of the sacrum. When a sacral stress fracture is discovered, the thoracolumbar spine and other portions of the pelvis should be imaged to rule out other insufficiency fractures. In the pelvis, stress fractures also occur in the pubic rami and in the supra-acetabular region.[5,12,13]

Sacral stress fractures may or may not be visible on radiographs of the pelvis as vague vertical regions of increased bone density (sclerosis) in the sacral wings (ala). Normal radiographs of the sacrum do not exclude the presence of sacral insufficiency fractures.[2] Bowel gas frequently obscures the sacrum rendering subtle fractures difficult to visualize.[14] Vertically oriented fracture lines through the sacral ala may be visible on radiographs, but this is not common. Rarely, cortical disruption of the sacral foraminal roofs is visible, but this finding is more commonly observed with

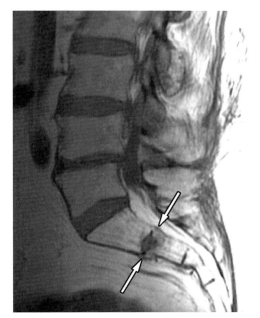

Figure 62-1 ► **Sacral Insufficiency Fractures.** Minimal anterior and posterior cortical disruption (*arrows*) at the S1-2 level is visible on sagittal T1-weighted MRI.

traumatic sacral fractures. Radiographs of the spine and pelvis may show other insufficiency fractures.[4]

With CT, vertically oriented fracture lines, if present, are more readily seen (*Figs. 62-5 and 62-6*). The sacrum is optimally scanned with thin section helical imaging so reformatted oblique coronal images can be generated, which often display the fracture lines optimally. The fracture lines usually extend through the anterior and posterior cortex, although occasionally the anterior or posterior sacral cortex is spared. As the fracture heals, broad regions of heterogeneous sclerosis form in the sacral wings adjacent to the fracture lines (see Fig. 62-5), and the sclerosis may partially obscure the fractures (see Fig. 62-6).

Sacral stress fractures are often diagnosed in patients with low back pain undergoing lumbar MR imaging. However, occasionally the sacral insufficiency goes undetected on routine MR imaging of the lumbar spine if careful attention is not given to examining the sacrum or if one relies on sagittal MR images of the sacrum to make the diagnosis (*Fig. 62-7*). Sacral fractures are best demonstrated with dedicated axial or oblique coronal MRI or CT images of the sacrum (*Figs.* 62-2 and *62-8*). The earliest imaging signs of sacral insufficiency fracture are visible with MR imaging as broad regions of heterogeneous T1 hypointensity and T2 hyperintensity in the sacral wings, which often extend to the sacral cortical margin of the sacroiliac (SI) joints (see Fig. 62-8). The signal disturbance is most conspicuous on fat-saturated or short tau inversion recovery

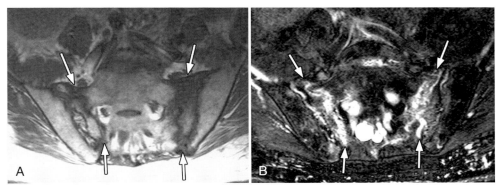

Figure 62-2 ► **Sacral Insufficiency Fractures.** Oblique coronal T1-weighted MR image **A** and axial T2-weighted image **B** in same patient as in Figure 62-1. A large region of irregular T1 hypointensity and T2 hyperintensity (*arrows in image **A** and **B***) is demonstrated in both sacral wings.

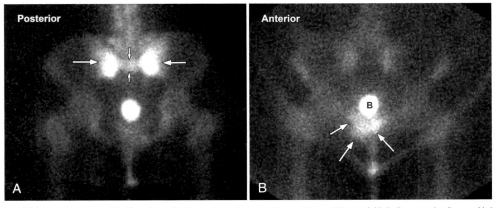

Figure 62-3 ► **Sacra Insufficiency Fractures.** 99mTc-radionuclidebone scan in same patient as Figures 62-1 and 62-2. On posterior (image **A**), intense uptake is present in both sacral ala (*long arrows*) with faint uptake (*short arrows*) in the adjacent vertebral bodies, resulting in a classic H-shaped pattern of increased uptake. On anterior view (image **B**), there is increased activity in the symphysis pubis region, right more than left (*arrows*). B = bladder activity in image **B**.

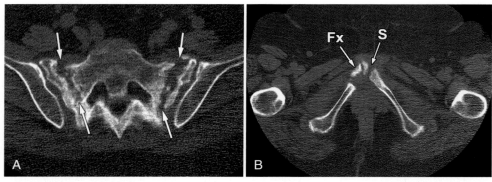

Figure 62-4 ► Sacral Insufficiency Fractures. Axial CT images **A** and **B** in same patient as Figures 62-1 to 62-3. Fracture defects (*arrow*) are well demonstrated in both sacral wings on image **A**. Adjacent sclerosis suggests chronic attempt at bone repair. Findings consistent with chronic sacral fractures with non-osseous union. On axial image **B**, there is a comminuted fracture (*Fx*) to the right of the symphysis pubis (*S*) which is rotated and displaced to the left of midline.

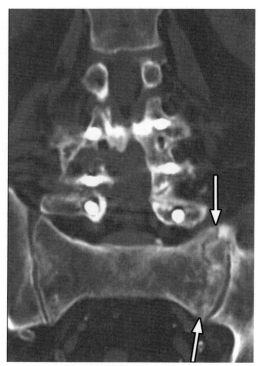

Figure 62-5 ► Sacral Insufficiency Fractures. 76-year-old male patient with severe bilateral low back pain. Coronal CT image reveals distinct fracture line (*between arrows*) extending through left sacral wing. Right sacral wing appears slightly heterogeneous in density, but no distinct fracture line is seen on the right.

(STIR) MR images attributed to presence of bone marrow edema (see Figs. 62-2 and 62-8).[14] Sacral insufficiency fractures usually involve the upper portion of the sacral wings, but uncommonly the lower portion of the sacrum may be involved (*Fig. 62-9*). Sacral insufficiency fractures are usually bilateral but may be unilateral (*Figs. 62-10 to 62-12*). Vertebral insufficiency fractures commonly coexist with sacral insufficiency fractures (see Fig. 62-10).

Following administration of paramagnetic contrast agent, the sacral stress fractures may enhance heterogeneously or homogeneously (see Fig. 62-11). Contrast enhancement may render fracture lines more conspicuous within the larger adjacent zones of abnormal signal intensity.[14] Occasionally, a peripheral zone of contrast enhancement may surround the region of abnormal signal in the sacral wings (*Fig. 62-13*).

The cortex on either side of the SI joints nearly always remains intact, and typically there is no edema on the iliac side of the SI joint. Usually there is no expansion of the involved portions of the sacrum as is often present with sacral neoplasms. A sacral stress or insufficiency fracture rarely results in epidural hematoma formation, which can result in severe neurologic compromise including cauda equina syndrome. The epidural hematoma, if present, is readily visible on sagittal MR images.[10]

Tc-99m radionuclide bone scanning is often positive in patients with sacral stress fractures. However, bone scanning in general may be nonspecific, occurring in any condition where bone repair is taking place including fractures, inflammation, SI joint disease, and neoplasia.[4] A classic H-shaped pattern of increased uptake is present in approximately 40% of patients with bilateral sacral alar fractures (see Fig. 62-3).[15] Increased uptake may be visible only in the sacral wings (*Fig. 62-14*). However, many sacral stress fractures are in various stages of healing at the time of bone scanning and therefore the classic H pattern may not be present or it may assume a uniform *bar shape* if the sacrum is extensively involved.[16] A similar H pattern may be visible in the sacrum on fluorodeoxyglucose positron emission tomography (FDG-PET) scans in patients with sacral stress fractures.[15] However, it may be difficult to differentiate neoplastic involvement of the sacrum and stress fractures because both conditions would result in increased FDG uptake.[17] Therefore, one should always obtain MR imaging for comparison when bone scan uptake or PET scan activity is positive in the sacrum.

Patients with sacral insufficiency fractures nearly always have abnormal bone densitometry related to osteoporosis, which is the most common predisposing factor for development of insufficiency fractures.

DIFFERENTIAL DIAGNOSIS

1. **Traumatic sacral fractures:** Usually traumatic sacral fractures present immediately after pelvic trauma with acute low back pain. Sacral insufficiency fractures develop slowly and present with slow onset of low back pain. Traumatic sacral fractures often extend through the sacral neural foramina, and distinct

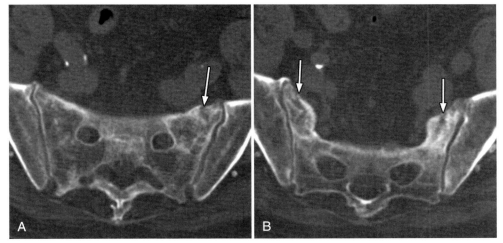

Figure 62-6 ▶ Sacral Insufficiency Fractures. Axial CT images **A** and **B** in same patient as in Figure 62-5. In image **A**, the anterior cortex of the left sacral ala (*arrow*) is disrupted and both sacral wings contain bone of heterogeneous density. On image **B**, the anterior cortex of both sacral wings is disrupted (*arrows*) indicating presence of bilateral sacral insufficiency fractures. Note sclerosis adjacent to fractures.

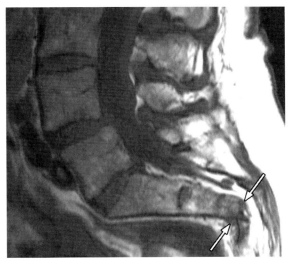

Figure 62-7 ▶ Bilateral Sacral Insufficiency Fractures. In 77-year-old female with severe low back pain. Sagittal T1-weighted MRI reveals acute angular deformity (*arrows*) at the S3 level.

fracture lines are usually visible with acute fractures. The sacral fractures may extend through the cortical margins of the SI joint and other pelvic fractures, or symphysis pubis diastasis may be present with acute sacral fractures.[18]

2. **Sacral neoplasm:** The most common sacral neoplasm is a sacral metastasis.[19] Other sacral tumors metastasis, lymphoma, plasmacytoma, teratoma, giant cell tumor, osteoblastoma, and other tumors also arise in the sacrum. Aneurysmal bone cyst can also occur in the sacrum. These conditions usually cause bone osteolysis, destruction, or expansion. There may be an extraosseous soft tissue mass component in the adjacent soft tissues with neoplasm.

3. **Sacral osteomyelitis:** Sacral osteomyelitis is a rare condition that can cause bone marrow edema, but sacral involvement tends to be asymmetric and there is associated cortical bone destruction. Usually there is infection involving the soft tissues

adjacent to the sacrum such as an abscess, cellulitis, or disc infection.[19]

4. **Sacroiliitis:** Sacroiliitis may be unilateral or bilateral.[19] Unilateral sacroiliitis may be secondary to infectious disease. Bilateral SI joint disease occurs in patients with noninfectious spondyloarthropathies such as ankylosing spondylitis or inflammatory bowel disease. Osteoarthritis of the SI joints may be unilateral or bilateral. Inflammation of the SI joints is often associated with cortical erosions on one or both cortical surfaces of the SI joint. Marrow edema is usually present in the acute stage on both the sacral and iliac sides of the SI joint. In later stages, the adjacent bone margins become sclerotic. With SI joint osteoarthritis, there is usually little if any adjacent bone marrow edema, the SI joint cortex is sclerotic, and osteophytes bridge across the SI joint, especially anteriorly.

TREATMENT

Most patients improve considerably with resolution of the low back pain within a few to several months after conservative therapy.

1. **Conservative therapy:** Conservative therapy includes bed rest, external bracing during weight-bearing activities, gradual mobilization with crutches, analgesic medications, and graduated physical therapy.[14,20] Prolonged bed rest should be avoided if possible to minimize complications of long-term immobilization such as respiratory and urinary tract infections, deep venons thrombosis, and bed sores.

2. **Osteoporosis treatment:** The underlying bone condition, most often osteoporosis, should be treated.

3. **Sacroplasty:** The goal of percutaneous sacroplasty is performed to alleviate the back pain and restore the patient to a functional state of activity more quickly than with conservative therapy.[1,20-23] Similar to vertebroplasty, polymethylmethacrylate cement is injected into the involved portion of the sacrum, usually the sacral ala. This can result in more rapid pain relief. Both short axis (localized cement deposition) and long axis (more diffuse cement deposition) sacroplasty techniques have been shown to be effective in reducing pain associated with sacral stress fractures.[3] Sacroplasty is believed to

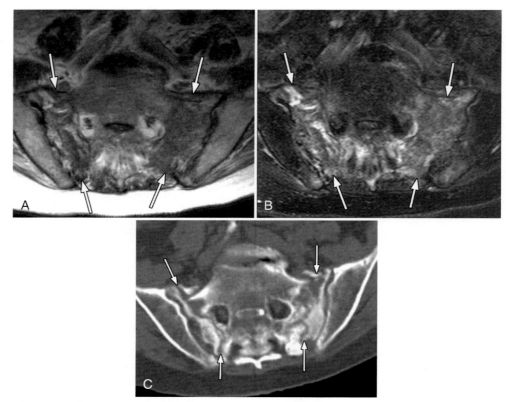

Figure 62-8 ▶ **Bilateral Sacral Insufficiency Fractures.** Axial MR and CT images in same patient as in Figure 62-7. Diffuse heterogeneous signal intensity is present in both sacral wings (*between arrows*) on T1-weighted MR image **A** and T2-weighted image **B**. Corresponding axial CT image C reveals irregular, well-defined fracture lines in both sacral ala with cortical disruption anteriorly and posteriorly (*arrows*).

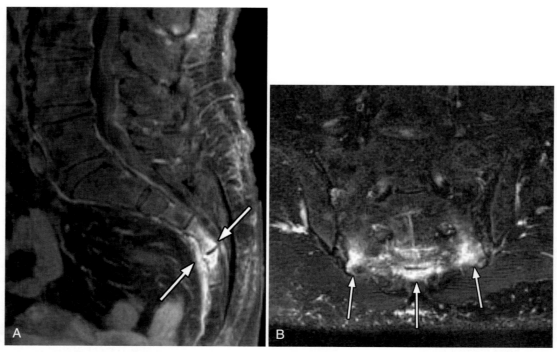

Figure 62-9 ▶ **Lower Sacral Insufficiency Fracture.** 64-year-old female with severe low back pain. Abnormal contrast enhancement is demonstrated in the lower sacrum (*arrows*) at the S3-4 level in sagittal fat saturated contrast enhanced MR image **A** and in axial image **B**.

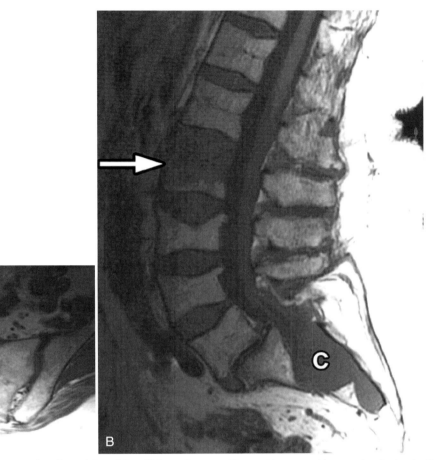

Figure 62-10 ▶ L2 Vertebral Insufficiency Fracture and Unilateral Sacral Insufficiency Fracture. 73-year-old woman with severe low back pain. On axial T1-weighted MR image **A**, there is abnormal T1 hypointense signal intensity in the right sacral wing (*arrows*) consistent with bone marrow edema secondary to unilateral right sacral insufficiency fracture. On sagittal T1-weighted MR image, the L2 vertebra is T1 hypointense (*arrow*) secondary to acute insufficiency fracture. There are old compression deformities of the L3 and L4 vertebral bodies. C = large Tarlov cyst or intrasacral meningocele in sacral spinal canal on image **A** and image **B**.

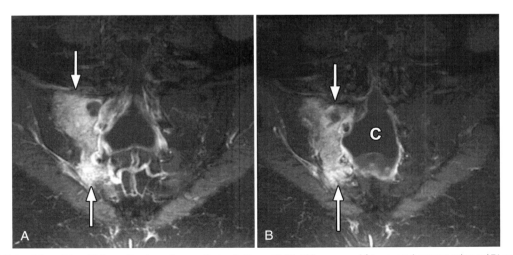

Figure 62-11 ▶ Unilateral Sacral Insufficiency Fracture. Same patient as in Figure 62-10. Oblique coronal fat saturated contrast-enhanced T1-weighted MR images **A** and **B** reveal diffuse enhancement of the right sacral wing (*arrows*) secondary to insufficiency fracture. No abnormal contrast enhancement in left sacral wing. C = Cyst in sacral spinal canal.

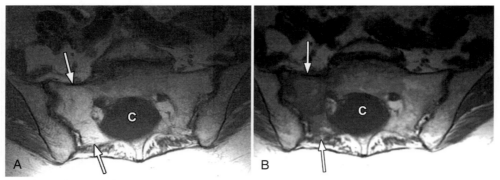

Figure 62-12 ► **Unilateral Sacral Insufficiency Fracture.** Same patient as in Figures 62-10 and 62-11. Axial T1-weighted MR image **A**, obtained 2 years later, shows complete healing of right sacral insufficiency fracture with marrow signal entirely normal. Compare with abnormal signal intensity in right sacral wing on corresponding axial T1-weighted MR image **B** obtained 2 years prior the time when images shown in Figures 62-10 and 62-11 were obtained.

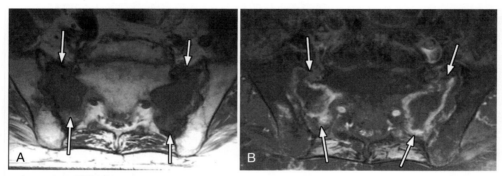

Figure 62-13 ► **Bilateral Sacral Insufficiency Fractures.** Ring-like contrast enhancement of bilateral sacral insufficiency fractures in 75-year-old male patient with severe low back pain. On axial T1-weighted MR image **A**, large homogenous areas of T1 hypointensity (*arrows*) are demonstrated in both sacral ala. On axial fat-saturated T1-weighted MR image **B**, peripheral contrast-enhancement (*arrows*) is demonstrated at the margins of the sacral insufficiency fractures.

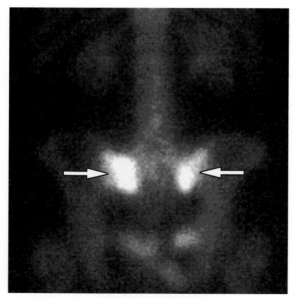

Figure 62-14 ► **Unilateral Sacral Insufficiency Fracture.** Technetium-99m radionuclide bone scan image, posterior view, in same patient as in Figure 62-13. Increased bilateral activity (*arrows*) is visible in the sacral wings in this patient with bilateral sacral insufficiency fractures.

reduce painful micromotion in the affected sacral bone, but there is evidence that it does not increase the overall bone strength by increasing bone stiffness.[24,25]

4. **Surgical instrumentation augmentation:** Surgical instrumentation augmentation, for example by insertion of a transiliosacral rod or screws, represents a last resort therapeutic procedure in cases where the above methods fail or when a highly unstable sacrum requires stabilization.[26] Polymethylmethacrylate cement can be inserted adjacent to the rods or screws to help fixate the hardware within the insufficient bone.[26]

5. **Bone allograft:** Surgical stabilization of the sacrum can also be achieved by insertion of a bone allograft such as a fibular strut.[27]

References

1. Grasland A, Pouchot J, Mathieu A, et al. Sacral insufficiency fractures: An easily overlooked cause of back pain in elderly women. *Arch Intern Med.* 1996;156(6):668-674.
2. Lee YJ, Bong HJ, Kim JT, Chung DS. Sacral insufficiency fracture, usually overlooked cause of lumbosacral pain. *J Korean Neurosurg Soc.* 2008;44(3):166-169.
3. Kamel EM, Binaghi S, Guntern D, et al. Outcome of long-axis percutaneous sacroplasty for the treatment of sacral insufficiency fractures. *Eur Radiol.* 2009; June 16. [E-pub ahead of print.]

4. Kwon JW, Huh SJ, Yoon YC, et al. Pelvic bone complications after radiation therapy of uterine cervical cancer: Evaluation with MRI. *AJR Am J Roentgenol.* 2008;191(4):987-994.
5. Otte MT, Helms CA, Fritz RC. MR imaging of supra-acetabular insufficiency fractures. *Skeletal Radiol.* 1997;26(5):279-283.
6. Blomlie V, Lien HH, Iversen T, et al. Radiation-induced insufficiency fractures of the sacrum: Evaluation with MR imaging. *Radiology.* 1993; 188(1):241-244.
7. Major NM, Helms CA. Sacral stress fractures in long-distance runners. *AJR Am J Roentgenol.* 2000;174(3):727-729.
8. Patterson SP, Daffner RH, Sciulli RL, Schneck-Jacob SL. Fatigue fracture of the sacrum in an adolescent. *Pediatr Radiol.* 2004;34(8):633-635.
9. Muthukumar T, Butt SH, Cassar-Pullicino VN, McCall IW. Cauda equina syndrome presentation of sacral insufficiency fractures. *Skeletal Radiol.* 2007;36(4):309-313.
10. Cronin CG, Lohan DG, Swords R, et al. Sacral insufficiency fracture complicated by epidural haematoma and cauda equina syndrome in a patient with multiple myeloma. *Emerg Radiol.* 2007;14(6):425-430.
11. Martineau PA, Ouellet J, Reindl R, Arlet V. Surgical images: Musculoskeletal. Delayed cauda equina syndrome due to a sacral insufficiency fracture missed after a minor trauma. *Can J Surg.* 2004;47(2):117-118.
12. Grangier C, Garcia J, Howarth NR, et al. Role of MRI in the diagnosis of insufficiency fractures of the sacrum and acetabular roof. *Skeletal Radiol.* 1997;26(9):517-524.
13. Peh WC, Khong PL, Yin Y, et al. Imaging of pelvic insufficiency fractures. *Radiographics.* 1996;16(2):335-348.
14. Blake SP, Connors AM. Sacral insufficiency fracture. *Br J Radiol.* 2004;77(922):891-896.
15. Finiels H, Finiels PJ, Jacquot JM, Strubel D. [Fractures of the sacrum caused by bone insufficiency. Meta-analysis of 508 cases]. *Presse Med.* 1997; 26(33):1568-1573.
16. Fujii M, Abe K, Hayashi K, et al. Honda sign and variants in patients suspected of having a sacral insufficiency fracture. *Clin Nucl Med.* 2005; 30(3):165-169.
17. Halac M, Mut SS, Sonmezoglu K, et al. Avoidance of misinterpretation of an FDG positive sacral insufficiency fracture using PET/CT scans in a patient with endometrial cancer: A case report. *Clin Nucl Med.* 2007;32(10): 779-781.
18. White JH, Hague C, Nicolaou S, et al. Imaging of sacral fractures. *Clin Radiol.* 2003;58(12):914-921.
19. Diel J, Ortiz O, Losada RA, et al. The sacrum: pathologic spectrum, multimodality imaging, and subspecialty approach. *Radiographics.* 2001; 21(1):83-104.
20. Beall DP, Datir A, D'Souza SL, et al. Percutaneous treatment of insufficiency fractures: Principles, technique and review of literature. *Skeletal Radiol.* 2009.
21. Whitlow CT, Mussat-Whitlow BJ, Mattern CW, et al. Sacroplasty versus vertebroplasty: Comparable clinical outcomes for the treatment of fracture-related pain. *AJNR Am J Neuroradiol.* 2007;28(7):1266-1270.
22. Pommersheim W, Huang-Hellinger F, Baker M, Morris P. Sacroplasty: A treatment for sacral insufficiency fractures. *AJNR Am J Neuroradiol.* 2003;24(5):1003-1007.
23. Garant M. Sacroplasty: a new treatment for sacral insufficiency fracture. *J Vasc Interv Radiol.* 2002;13(12):1265-1267.
24. Anderson DE, Cotton JR. Mechanical analysis of percutaneous sacroplasty using CT image based finite element models. *Med Eng Phys.* 2007;29(3): 316-325.
25. Richards AM, Mears SC, Knight TA, et al. Biomechanical analysis of sacroplasty: Does volume or location of cement matter? *AJNR Am J Neuroradiol.* 2009;30(2):315-317.
26. Sciubba DM, Wolinsky JP, Than KD, et al. CT fluoroscopically guided percutaneous placement of transiliosacral rod for sacral insufficiency fracture: case report and technique. *AJNR Am J Neuroradiol.* 2007;28(8):1451-1454.
27. Khanna AJ, Kebaish KM, Ozdemir HM, et al. Sacral insufficiency fracture surgically treated by fibular allograft. *J Spinal Disord Tech.* 2004;17(3): 167-173.

SACROILIITIS

Douglas S. Fenton, M.D.

CLINICAL PRESENTATION

The patient is a 49-year-old woman who presented with intermittent low back pain, right more than left, with radiation to the lateral hips but no radiation below the knee. This started without precipitating event as best as she is able to recall. It has gotten worse over the past 10 months. She describes intermittent dull discomfort that can sometimes be burning. The severity fluctuates from mild to quite severe. Prolonged standing, walking, and transitional movements make her symptoms worse. She has tried several over-the-counter and narcotic medications without benefit. She denies any paresthesias, weakness, or radicular features. She denies any bowel or bladder dysfunction and no saddle anesthesia. No recent fevers or infection. She has had a 40-pound weight gain since her pain complaints started.

IMAGING PRESENTATION

Frontal radiograph of the pelvis reveals sclerosis about both sacroiliac joints. There are also small irregularities along the margin of both sacroiliac joints consistent with erosions (*Fig. 63-1*).

DISCUSSION

The sacroiliac joint (SIJ) is the largest joint in the axial skeleton. The inferior two thirds of the SIJ are lined by articular cartilage and the upper third is a syndesmosis. The lower portion is often called a *diarthrodial joint*, however, only a portion of the SIJ has a true synovial-lined joint capsule. The majority of the lower SIJ is like a symphysis, lined with hyaline cartilage and held together by fibrous tissues. The cartilage is thinner on the iliac side of the joint, which is why degenerative change is seen much earlier on the iliac side of the joint. Only the inferior few centimeters is a true chondral joint from front to back. The sacrum and ilium are held together in the syndesmotic portion by the interosseous ligament. The entire joint is also supported by strong anterior and posterior sacroiliac ligaments and the sacrospinous and sacrotuberous ligaments. The SIJ ligamentous structure is more extensive dorsally because a posterior capsule is either absent or rudimentary. The main function of the SIJ ligamentous structure is to limit motion in all directions. This ligamentous structure is weaker in women to allow mobility for birthing. Several muscles, including the gluteus maximus, piriformis, and biceps femoris muscles, help stabilize the SIJ and are

connected to SIJ ligaments.[1,2] The innervation of the SIJ is often debated. Most agree that the lateral branches of the L4-S3 dorsal rami supply innervation to the posterior joint; however, some believe L3 and S4 also give posterior joint supply.[3,4] Multiple studies debate anterior innervation ranging from L2-S2, L4-S2, and L5-S2, and some who believe there is no innervation anteriorly.[3,5-7]

Pain related to the SIJ is not uncommon. Studies based solely on physical examination,[8] fluoroscopically guided SIJ injections of local anesthetics in joints that were abnormal on post-arthrography computed tomography (CT) and with concordant pain during joint distension,[9] and unilateral SIJ blocks using International Spine Intervention Society guidelines[10] place the prevalence of SIJ dysfunction from 15% to 30% of patients presenting with chronic low back pain.

Studies have shown that examination the patient history and physical are unable to consistently identify patients with SIJ pain. SIJ pain crosses over with many other causes of low back pain. The most common pain pattern for SIJ dysfunction is radiation into the buttocks (94%), lower lumbar region (72%), lower extremity (50%), pain radiating below the knee (28%), groin (14%), foot pain (12%), upper lumbar region (6%), and abdomen (2%).[1,9] The most common finding in SIJ dysfunction is unilateral pain below the level of L5.[9] "Risk factors associated with SIJ pain include leg length discrepancy,[1,11] gait abnormalities,[1,12] prolonged vigorous exercise,[1,13] scoliosis,[1,14] spinal fusion to the sacrum,[15] and pregnancy because of increased weight gain, exaggerated lordosis, hormonal ligamentous laxity, and trauma from birth."[1,16]

Osteoarthritis is one of the most common disorders to affect the SIJ. Osteoarthritis is usually seen in patients older than 40 years of age.[17] The main findings of osteoarthritis of the SIJ are joint space narrowing, subchondral sclerosis, and anterior osteophytes. When the osteophytes get larger, they can fuse anteriorly. Osteoarthritis is distinguished from the inflammatory arthritides in that intra-articular ankylosis is not a feature of osteoarthritis. Gas can be seen in the SIJ space in osteoarthritis.

The SIJ is often involved with the HLA-B27 inflammatory arthritides, most commonly ankylosing spondylitis (AS). The sacroiliitis related to AS is usually bilateral and symmetric. Patients with inflammatory bowel disease and approximately 5% to 15% of patients with Crohn's disease and ulcerative colitis can develop a sacroiliitis indistinguishable from AS.[17] Interestingly, 50% of patients with Crohn's disease and ulcerative colitis carry the HLA-B27 antigen.[17] Sacroiliitis is also seen in patients with psoriatic arthritis and Reiter's syndrome, but is distinguished from AS by being bilateral and asymmetric. Sacroiliitis is unusual with rheumatoid arthritis. People with Behçet's syndrome, relapsing polychondritis, and systemic lupus erythematosus can also demonstrate sacroiliitis.[17] Infection can cause a septic arthritis that is usually unilateral.[17]

IMAGING FEATURES

The imaging findings of sacroiliitis are erosions along the joint margin. The erosions are identified earlier on the iliac side of the joint because the cartilage is thinner on the iliac side. The joint can have a fuzzy appearance on plain radiographs (see Fig. 63-1). There may be pseudo joint space widening due to the erosions. In the late stages, ankylosis of the joint can be seen. Plain radiographs are widely used and most cost-effective in the screening for sacroiliac joint disease. However, there are significant interobserver and intraobserver variations in interpretation. In one study, 20% of radiographs incorrectly underdiagnosed sacroiliitis when compared with computed tomography (CT) results.[18] Plain radiographs also have very poor sensitivity in the early stages of sacroiliitis, which is why, in the past, there was between a 2- to 7-year lag between the diagnosis and presentation. SIJ radiographs are used to categorize sacroiliitis into five grades: grade 0 (normal), grade 1 (suspicious, unclear), grade 2 (small erosions, hypersclerosis), grade 3 (definite erosions, pseudodilitation of the joint space), and grade 4 (ankylosis).[19,20]

Nuclear medicine bone scan has been used in the past in the diagnosis of SIJ inflammatory disease; however, it has been shown to be too nonspecific of an examination and has many factors that can influence the imaging interpretation. "For example, hopping on one leg before an examination will increase the uptake of the radionuclide."[19]

CT is more sensitive and specific in evaluating the early erosions and sclerosis seen with sacroiliitis *(Fig. 63-2)*. However, two disadvantages of CT are the radiation dose and the inability to detect changes of synovitis and marrow edema that can be detected with magnetic resonance imaging (MRI). Both CT and MRI can demonstrate the anterior osteophytes commonly associated with SIJ osteoarthritis.

MR imaging is the imaging modality of choice in the evaluation of sacroiliitis. T1-weighted images demonstrate the synovial compartment cartilage as a thin zone of intermediate signal intensity with an adjacent low signal intensity cortex.[21] MR imaging nicely distinguishes the ligamentous from the synovial portions of the SIJ by its signal intensities. The ligamentous portion contains fatty tissue, and the synovial compartment has cartilage signal intensity *(Fig. 63-3)*. The addition of a fat-saturated, T1-weighted contrast acquisition and a fat-saturation, T2-weighted or short tau inversion recovery (STIR) technique can assist in demonstrating the marrow edema within and inflammation within and surrounding the SIJ *(Fig. 63-4)*.[2,19,22] MRI can be used not only to identify active disease but also to follow response to treatment.[23,24] In the case of an infectious SIJ process, MRI can demonstrate infiltration of the adjacent musculature. A nuclear medicine bone scan can be used in patients who are unable to undergo MR imaging. With active SIJ disease, increased radiotracer uptake is seen along the joint(s) *(Fig. 63-5)*.

DIFFERENTIAL DIAGNOSIS

1. **Calcium pyrophosphate disease (CPPD):** People with CPPD can have changes that appear like sacroiliitis with

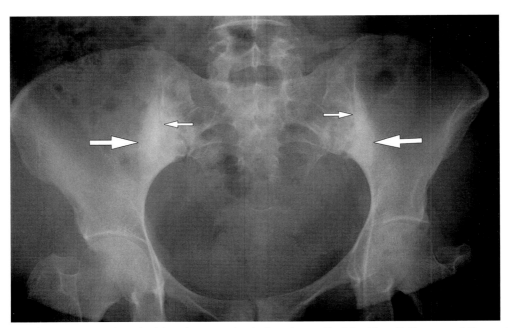

Figure 63-1 ▶ Sacroiliitis. Anteroposterior radiograph of the pelvis. Note sclerosis about the sacroiliac joints bilaterally (*large arrows*). The sacroiliac joint is ill-defined bilaterally (*small arrows*)

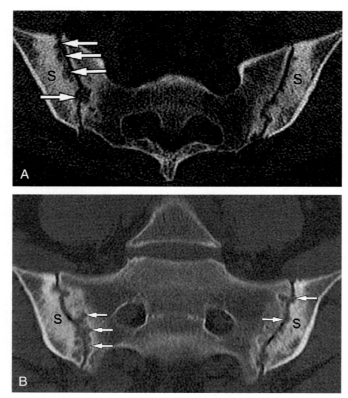

Figure 63-2 ▶ **Sacroiliitis, CT.** Same patient as in Figure 63-1. Oblique axial CT (image **A**) and oblique coronal CT (image **B**). Sclerosis (*S*) on both the sacral and iliac sides of the sacroiliac joint as well as multiple erosions (*arrows*).

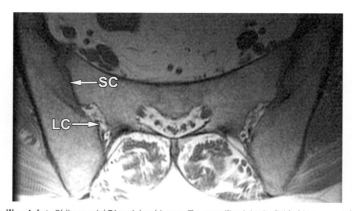

Figure 63-3 ▶ **Anatomy of the Sacroiliac Joint.** Oblique axial T1-weighted image. The sacroiliac joint is divided into synovial (*SC*) and ligamentous (*LC*) compartments. The ligamentous compartment contains fat. The synovial compartment has cartilage signal intensity.

bilateral SIJ erosion, sclerosis, and joint space narrowing, but they also often have anterior osteophytes.[17]

2. **Hyperparathyroidism:** People with hyperparathyroidism can have SIJ bone resorption leading to joint space widening or an ill-defined joint.[17] This can be bilateral and symmetric; however, joint space narrowing or ankylosis does not develop.

3. **Radiation therapy:** Radiation therapy to the pelvis can cause widening and irregularity of the SIJ *(Fig. 63-6).*[17] A

history of radiation therapy is necessary to entertain this diagnosis.

4. **Sports-related sacral abnormalities:** Erosions and sclerosis of the SIJ can occur in athletes, particularly long-distance runners and soccer players.[25]

5. **Pregnancy-related SIJ changes:** After pregnancy, some women develop a pattern of SIJ sclerosis called *osteitis condensans ilii.* This appears as a bilateral triangle of sclerosis in the

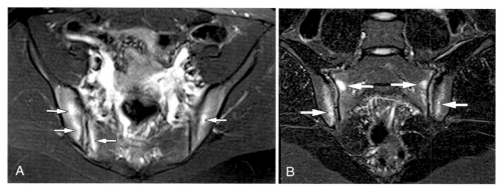

Figure 63-4 ▶ Marrow Edema from Sacroiliitis. Oblique axial fat-saturated, T2-weighted image **A** and oblique coronal fat-saturated, T2-weighted image **B**. Increased signal intensity seen along both sides of the sacroiliac joint compatible with marrow edema (*arrows*).

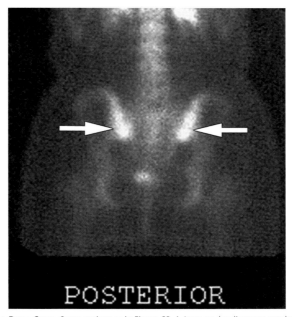

Figure 63-5 ▶ Sacroiliitis, Nuclear Medicine Bone Scan. Same patient as in Figure 63-4. Increased radiotracer uptake along both sides of both sacroiliac joints (*arrows*) compatible with active inflammation.

ilium adjacent to the inferior SIJ. There are no erosions and the joint space is not narrowed.[2]

TREATMENT

1. **Rest:** Resting the joint can decrease pain symptoms.
2. **Nonsteroidal anti-inflammatory drugs (NSAIDs):** Pain relief may be obtained with NSAIDs and if necessary a mild-narcotic medication.
3. **Shoe inserts:** If the patient has a leg length discrepancy, then a shoe insert may stabilize the SIJ joint leading to pain relief.
4. **Physical therapy or chiropractic manipulation:** In patients with abnormal gait or spine malalignment, physical therapy or chiropractic manipulation may reduce symptoms.[26]

5. **Anesthetic and steroid:** Intra-articular injection of anesthetic and steroid serves both a diagnostic and therapeutic function. If this procedure is carefully performed under fluoroscopic or CT guidance, demonstrating intraarticular placement of the needle in the synovial portion of the joint through the injection of contrast media, then a diagnosis of SIJ abnormality is evident if the patient has a positive response to the anesthetic portion of the injection. Several clinicians have found that therapeutic SIJ injections can give sustained relief in patients with painful inflammatory sacroiliitis.[27,28]
6. **Radiofrequency denervation:** Radiofrequency denervation has been used by many physicians; however, there is access to only posterior innervation and therefore relief should not be expected to occur in pain related to the ventral SIJ.
7. **Proliferative therapy:** Some authors advocate proliferative therapy ("prolotherapy") for SIJ pain.[29] The rationale of this

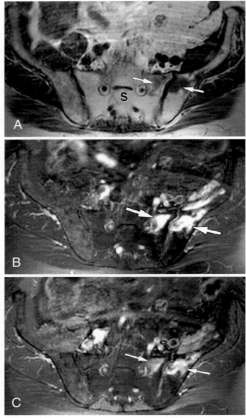

Figure 63-6 ▶ Sacral Marrow Changes from Radiation Therapy. Oblique coronal T1 image **A**, fat-saturated T2 image **B**, and fat-saturated, post-contrast T1 image **C**. Similar changes of decreased T1 signal intensity, increased T2 signal intensity, and enhancement on both sides of the left sacroiliac joint (*arrows*); however, one notes the generalized increased T1 signal intensity throughout the sacrum (*S*) and left iliac bone in this patient that has received pelvic irradiation.

procedure is that the ligaments around the SIJ are important in the development of low back pain; therefore, an injection of a substance that strengthens and reduces sensitization of the ligaments should alleviate SIJ pain.

8. **Surgical fixation:** There are several clinicians who advocate surgical fixation of the SIJ in patients with SIJ pain that have not responded to conservative therapy; however, most studies are small case series.

References

1. Cohen SP. Sacroiliac joint pain: a comprehensive review of anatomy, diagnosis and treatment. *Anesth Analg.* 2005;101:1440-1453.
2. Tuite MJ. Sacroiliac joint imaging. *Semin Musculoskelet Radiol.* 2008;12: 72-82.
3. Bernard TN, Cassidy JD. The sacroiliac syndrome: Pathophysiology, diagnosis and management. In: Frymoyer JW, ed. *The adult spine: Principles and practice.* New York: Raven; 1991;2107-2130.
4. Murata Y, Takahashi K, Yamagata M, et al. Sensory innervation of the sacroiliac joint in rats. *Spine.* 2000;25:2015-2019.
5. Solonen KA. The sacroiliac joint in the light of anatomical, roentgenological and clinical studies. *Acta Orthop Scand.* 1957;27:1-27.
6. Ikeda R. Innervation of the sacroiliac joint: Macroscopic and histological studies. *J Nippon Med Sch.* 1991;58:587-596.
7. Fortin JD, Kissling RO, O'Connor BL, Vilensky JA. Sacroiliac joint innervation and pain. *Am J Orthop.* 1999;28:68-90.
8. Bernard TN, Kirkaldy-Willis WH. Recognizing specific characteristics of nonspecific low back pain. *Clin Orthop.* 1987;217:266-280.
9. Schwarzer AC, Aprill CN, Bogduk N. The sacroiliac joint in chronic low back pain. *Spine.* 1995;20:31-37.
10. Maigne JY, Aivaliklis, Pfefer F. Results of sacroiliac joint double block and value of sacroiliac pain provocation tests in 54 patients with low back pain. *Spine.* 1996;21:1889-1892.
11. Schuit D, McPoil TG, Mulesa P. Incidence of sacroiliac joint malalignment in leg length discrepancies. *J Am Podiatr Med Assoc.* 1989;79: 380-383.
12. Herzog W, Conway PJ. Gait analysis of sacroiliac joint patients. *J Manipulative Physiol Ther.* 1994;17:124-127.
13. Marymont JV, Lynch MA, Henning CE. Exercise-related stress reaction of the sacroiliac joint: An unusual cause of low back pain in athletes. *Am J Sports Med.* 1986;14:320-323.
14. Schoenberger M, Hellmich K. Sacroiliac dislocation and scoliosis. *Hippokrates.* 1964;35:476-479.
15. Katz V, Schofferman J, Reynolds J. The sacroiliac joint: A potential cause of pain after lumbar fusion to the sacrum. *J Spinal Disord Tech.* 2003;16: 96-99.
16. Berg G, Hammar M, Möller-Nielsen J, et al. Low back pain during pregnancy. *Obstet Gynecol.* 1988;71:71-75.
17. Resnick D. *Diagnosis of Bone and Joint Disorders.* 4th ed. Philadelphia: Saunders; 2002.
18. Ryan L, Carrera G, Lightfoot RW, et al. The radiographic diagnosis of sacriliitis: A comparison of different views with computed tomograms of the sacroiliac joint. *Arthritis Rheum.* 1983;26:760-763.
19. Braun J, Sieper J, Bollow M. Imaging of sacroiliitis. *Clin Rheumatol.* 2000;19:51-57.
20. van der Linden S, Valkenburg HA, Cats A. Evaluation of diagnostic criteria for ankylosing spondylitis: A proposal for modification of the New York criteria. *Arthritis Rheum.* 1984;27:361-368.

21. Murphey MD, Wetzel LH, Bramble JM, et al. Sacroiliitis: MR imaging findings. *Radiology.* 1991;180:239-244.
22. Wittram C, Whitehouse GH, Bucknall RC. Fat suppressed contrast enhanced MR imaging in the assessment of sacroiliitis. *Clin Radiol.* 1996;51:554-558.
23. Bredella MA, Steinbach LS, Morgan S, et al. MRI of the sacroiliac joints in patients with moderate to severe ankylosing spondylitis. *AJR Am J Roentgenol.* 2006;187:1420-1426.
24. Jee WH, McCauley TR, Lee SH, et al. Sacroiliitis in patients with ankylosing spondylitis: Association of MR findings with disease activity. *Magn Reson Imaging.* 2004;22:245-250.
25. Brolinson PG, Kozar AJ, Cibor G. Sacroiliac joint dysfunction in athletes. *Curr Sports Med Rep.* 2003;2:47-56.
26. Osterbauer PJ, De Boer KF, Widmaier R, et al. Treatment and biomechanical assessment of patients with chronic sacroiliac joint syndrome. *J Manipulative Physiol Ther.* 1993;16:82-90.
27. Maugars Y, Mathis C, Vilon P, Prost A. Corticosteroid injection of the sacroiliac joint in patients with seronegative spondyloarthropathy. *Arthritis Rheum.* 1992;35:564-568.
28. Bollow M, Braun J, Taupitz M, et al. CT-guided intraarticular corticosteroid injection into the sacroiliac joints in patients with spondyloarthropathy: indication and follow-up with contrast-enhanced MRI. *J Comput Assist Tomogr.* 1996;20:512-521.
29. Ongley MJ, Klein RG, Dorman TA, et al. A new approach to the treatment of chronic low back pain. *Lancet.* 1987;2:143-146.

SCHMORL'S NODE

Leo F. Czervionke, M.D.

CLINICAL PRESENTATION

The patient is a 21-year-old man who has had intermittent severe low back pain for 2 years. Pain began immediately after lifting a heavy object. Patient has not been completely pain free for 2 years. Presented with low back pain; the reported visual analog scale (VAS) was 6/10 with pain medication (hydrocodone 4 times daily), and VAS was reported to be 9/10 with no pain medication. Physical therapy, vertebral axial decompression (VAX-D) therapy, and three epidural steroid injections did not relieve the pain. The patient had been told he had an incidental cyst in the L3 vertebral body that required no therapy.

IMAGING PRESENTATION

Computed tomography (CT) reveals a small Schmorl's node at the superior endplate of L2 and a large cystlike Schmorl's node in the superior portion of the L3 vertebral body (Fig. 64-1). A rim of sclerosis is seen adjacent to both Schmorl's nodes. On T1-weighted images (Fig. 64-2), zones of variable signal intensity surround the nodes. T2-weighted magnetic resonance (MR) images (Fig. 64-3) show a fluid-level within the large cystic Schmorl's node, with surrounding marrow edema. A peripheral rim of contrast enhancement surrounds the larger Schmorl's node, whereas the smaller Schmorl's node enhances centrally (Fig. 64-4).

CLINICAL COURSE

Both the small L2 and larger L3 Schmorl's nodes were proved to be major low back pain generators by discography. During discographic injection, the patient reported intense back pain precisely when the intradiscal contrast agent entered the Schmorl's node (Fig. 64-5). The cystic L3 Schmorl's node was treated by a transpedicular injection of 2 mL of methylmethacrylate cement directly into and around the cystic cavity. The L2 Schmorl's node was treated 3 months later using a transpedicular approach to inject cement into the marrow substance adjacent to the node. The patient's pain level 3 weeks after treatment was VAS = 2/10 with no pain medication.

DISCUSSION

Schmorl's nodes represent focal protrusions or herniations of the intervertebral disc through the vertebral endplate. This localized vertebral endplate deformity was first described by the German pathologist Christian G. Schmorl in 1927. Schmorl's nodes may occur in either the inferior or superior endplate, although the inferior endplate is said to be a more common site. They reportedly occur more frequently in males and more commonly near the thoracolumbar junction. The "classic" Schmorl's occurs in the middle one third of the vertebral endplate and is most commonly located slightly posterior to the central axis of the vertebral endplate (Fig. 64-6).[1] The typical Schmorl's node occurs near the midline, but paramidline locations are also common.[2] Over time, the usage of the term Schmorl's node has expanded in scope and now is used to describe nearly any endplate depression, focal or diffuse, regardless of location.

The pathogenesis of the Schmorl's node remains controversial. Schmorl's nodes may be idiopathic, developmental, or acquired.[3] The etiology of so-called idiopathic and developmental Schmorl's nodes are likely the same, probably arising from some preexisting endplate deformity, anomaly, or subchondral osteonecrosis (ischemic necrosis) that weakens the endplate, predisposing it to herniation of the nucleus pulposus through the endplate.[3-6] These endplate anomalies can be small ossifications, pits, or defects that arise where endplate vascular or nutrient channels exist or once existed. The nucleus pulposus is a remnant of the notochord.

Incomplete notochordal regression may also leave behind endplate defects, which are typically midline and slightly posterior to the central axis of the vertebral body. Such congenital Schmorl's nodes can be seen on images early in life as isolated or multiple vertebral endplate defects adjacent to the nucleus and may be associated with abnormally shaped vertebral bodies (Fig. 64-7). Scheuermann-type vertebrae (juvenile kyphosis) may have Schmorl's nodes along their vertebral endplates, usually located anteriorly. The limbus vertebra, rarely seen in children but not uncommonly seen in adults, is thought to result from herniation of the nucleus pulposus through the ring apophysis prior to fusion, resulting in an isolated anterior ring apophyseal fragment.

Vertebral trauma, not disc degeneration, is the likely etiology of Schmorl's node development in the younger age groups and in some older adults with the nucleus pulposus herniating through an endplate fracture or preexisting developmental endplate defect[7,8] that have been opened by trauma. There is a high incidence of Schmorl's node development in vertebrae adjacent to vertebral fractures in childhood.[6,7] Schmorl's nodes associated with vertebral trauma have been shown to go through distinct phases of evolution, typically regressing in size over time. It has been suggested that Schmorl's nodes developing later in life could also be secondary to trauma, but other factors such as disc degeneration,

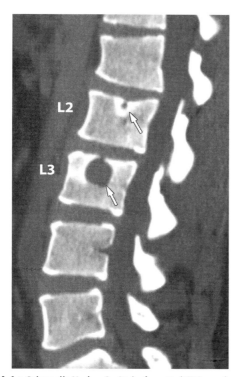

Figure 64-1 ▶ Schmorl's Nodes. Sagittal reformatted CT image lumbar spine. A large cystic Schmorl's node (*arrow*) in the superior portion of L3 vertebral body is connected to the L2-L3 intervertebral disc narrow by a narrow isthmus. Small Schmorl's node (*arrow*) in superior portion of L2 vertebral body. Hyperdense (sclerotic) bone density is seen adjacent to both Schmorl's nodes.

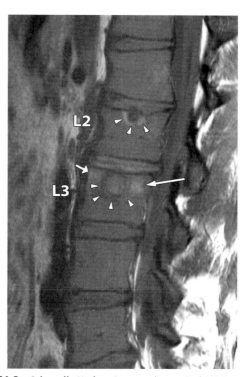

Figure 64-2 ▶ Schmorl's Nodes. Corresponding sagittal MR images in same patient as in Figure 64-1. Sagittal T1-weighted MR image reveals a T1 hyperintense rim (*arrowheads*) surround the small T2 hypointense Schmorl's node in superior endplate of L2. The larger Schmorl's node in the L3 vertebral body is T1 hyperintense centrally and is surrounded by a small rim of T1 hypointensity (*arrowheads*). A large region of T1 hyperintensity (*long arrow*) is located in the cancellous bone posterior to the Schmorl's node, and a smaller region of T1 hyperintensity (*short arrow*) is located in the cancellous bone anterior to the Schmorl's node.

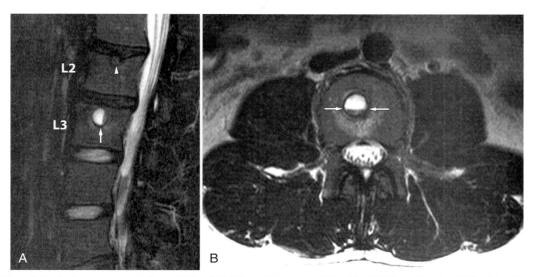

Figure 64-3 ▶ Schmorl's Node. Same patient as in Figures 64-1 and 64-2. Sagittal fat-saturated T2-weighted MR image **A** and axial T2-weighted image **B** shows a fluid/fluid level in the cystic Schmorl's node, the T2 hyperintense fluid anteriorly and the hypointense fluid posteriorly. A T2 hypointense rim (*arrow*) surrounds the Schmorl's node and is surrounded by a larger region of relative T2 hyperintensity. Note small smaller Schmorl's node (*arrowhead*) in superior portion of L2 vertebral body in image **A**.

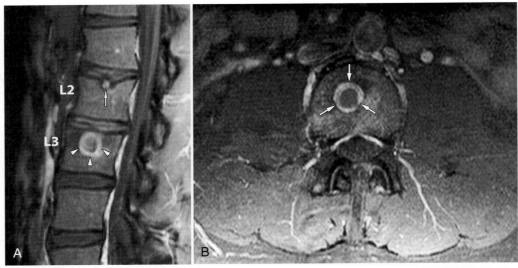

Figure 64-4 ▶ Schmorl's node. Fat-saturated contrast-enhanced sagittal MR image **A** and axial image **B**. The small Schmorl's node in L2 (*arrow*) enhances with contrast. The large Schmorl's node in L3 is hypointense centrally and surrounded by a rim of contrast enhancement (*arrowheads in image **A***). In image **B**, the Schmorl's node is positioned to the right of midline and has an intense enhancing rim (*arrows*).

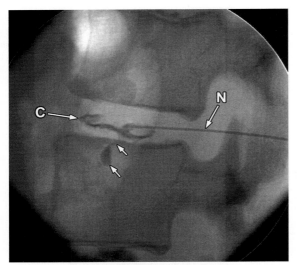

Figure 64-5 ▶ Percutaneous Treatment of Symptomatic Schmorl's Node. Same patient as in Figures 64-1 to 64-4. Lateral spot radiograph obtained at fluoroscopy during discogram. Discographic needle (*N*) has been inserted into L2-L3 intervertebral disc. Injected contrast (*C*) is located within intervertebral disc space. Patient experienced intense pain while the contrast agent (*small arrows*) was entering the Schmorl's node.

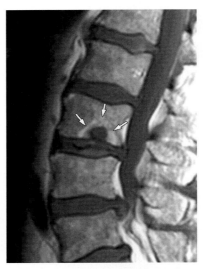

Figure 64-6 ▶ Classic Schmorl's Node Location. Sagittal T1-weighted MRI. Schmorl's node positioned slightly posterior to central axis of inferior L3 vertebral endplate. A region of T1 hyperintensity (*arrows*) surrounds the Schmorl's node.

metabolic disease, infection, or neoplasm may play a causative role in older persons. Schmorl's nodes are commonly seen in the elderly population, the incidence reported as being approximately 30% to 75% of the population.[4] The vast majority of Schmorl's nodes in older adults remains stable or changes very little with time[3,6] and are usually asymptomatic. Although Schmorl's nodes and disc degeneration frequently coexist in older persons, there is a paucity of evidence supporting disc degeneration as a cause of Schmorl's node formation.[3] Acquired metabolic conditions, such as osteoporosis, osteomalacia, and hyperparathyroidism can also weaken the

vertebral endplate, resulting in smooth, broad endplate concavities at multiple levels.

The incidence of symptomatic Schmorl's nodes in adults is unknown, but likely small. Most Schmorl's nodes seen in adults are asymptomatic. However, it is likely that symptomatic Schmorl's nodes are more common than one would expect, but because the symptomatic phase is short-lived or self-limited, go unrecognized as a cause of back pain. Symptomatic Schmorl's nodes that produce back pain are more likely to occur in younger individuals, often developing after an episode of acute vertebral trauma. Symptomatic

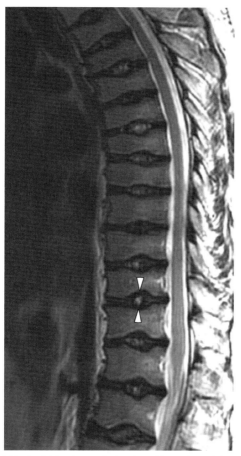

Figure 64-7 ▸ Multiple Congenital Schmorl's Nodes. Likely secondary to incomplete notochord regression. Sagittal T2-weighted MRI. Schmorl's node with associated vertebral endplate concavities (*arrowheads at one level*) are present at all visualized vertebral levels. The nucleus pulposus is T2 hyperintense at nearly every disc level. Multiple flat vertebral bodies (platyspondyly).

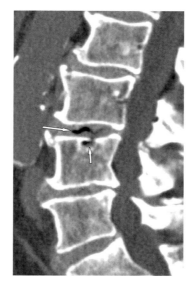

Figure 64-8 ▸ Gas-Filled Schmorl's Node, Vacuum Disk Phenomenon. Sagittal reformatted CT image lumbar spine. L2-3 intervertebral disc degeneration with intradiscal gas formation (i.e., vacuum disc phenomenon—*long arrow*) with extension of gas into a Schmorl's node (*short arrow*) through a defect in the superior L3 vertebral endplate.

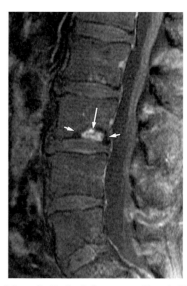

Figure 64-9 ▸ Schmorl's Node, Subacute to Chronic Phase. Sagittal fat-saturated T1-weighted contrast-enhanced lumbar MRI. Subacute to chronic phase of Schmorl's node evolution. The intranodal tissue (*long arrow*) enhances fairly homogeneously with contrast. There is a nonenhancing hypointense rim (*short arrows*) surrounding a Schmorl's node. The adjacent intervertebral disc does not enhance.

Schmorl's nodes occurring in older adults are likely related to endplate disruption by trauma, disc degeneration, infection, or neoplasm. Larger Schmorl's nodes and those with surrounding bone marrow edema are more likely to be symptomatic.[6,9-11] Large Schmorl's nodes are more frequently symptomatic.[12]

IMAGING FEATURES

On CT, the Schmorl's node is a well-defined focal endplate defect often with adjacent dense, sclerotic bone (see Fig. 64-1). Gas may be present in the node if there is an adjacent vacuum disc phenomenon *(Fig. 64-8)*. Schmorl's nodes have been shown to go through evolutional stages of development,[10] displaying variable MRI signal intensity characteristics (see Fig. 64-2) similar to the reactive signal disturbance occurring adjacent to degenerated intervertebral discs in vertebral osteochondrosis, which has been classified by Modic.[13] On T2-weighted images, the intranodal tissue is often T2 hypointense but may be T2 hyperintense (see Fig. 64-3). There is usually a zone of variable T1 and T2 signal disturbance adjacent to the Schmorl's node (see Figs. 64-2, 64-3, and 64-6). In the early phase of Schmorl's node development, there is typically a surrounding concentric ring of reactive hyperemia, marrow edema,

and inflammation that is T1 hypointense and T2 hyperintense.[3,5] The zone surrounding the nodal tissue often enhances after IV contrast in the early development of the Schmorl's node, indicating the presence of active perinodal inflammation (see Fig. 64-4). In this early phase, Schmorl's nodes are frequently symptomatic.[14] Months after the acute phase, the Schmorl's node usually regresses and becomes asymptomatic. In this stage of evolution, enhancement is no longer present in the bone surrounding the node. However, the tissue within the Schmorl's node at this time may enhance uniformly *(Fig. 64-9)*, in a ringlike fashion or not at all, depending on the stage of evolution. In the later stages, the peripheral zone of T2 signal intensity diminishes and the node decreases in size. There is no intranodal or peripheral contrast enhancement in the late stage of Schmorl's node evolution, usually only a small T1 and T2 hypointense endplate defect remains.

Giant Schmorl's nodes, as in this case, are rare but more commonly occur in the lumbar spine and are said to be more common in men. These may contain disc material, fluid, blood, or granulation tissue. Symptomatic giant Schmorl's nodes have a concentric rim of T2 hyperintensity (marrow edema) that enhances with contrast, likely representing perinodal inflammation.[15] Giant Schmorl's nodes may be replaced entirely by fat.[16] These are usually asymptomatic and may represent an end stage in the evolution of giant Schmorl's nodes.

Discography is the procedure of choice to determine whether a Schmorl's node is symptomatic. In these cases, injection of the contrast agent into the adjacent disc elicits a strong pain response when the contrast material enters the Schmorl's node during fluoroscopy (see Fig. 64-5).

DIFFERENTIAL DIAGNOSIS

1. **Balloon disc**: A developmental deformity of the inferior vertebral endplate. This is most commonly located in the lower lumbar inferior endplates (Incidence L5 > L4 > L3 > L2). Approximately 15% of the general population has this endplate deformity. Balloon discs are smooth, broad, bilateral, paramidline concavities centered in the posterior one-third of the inferior endplate. The inferior endplate of the balloon disc typically has a *cupid's bow deformity* when viewed on anteroposterior (AP) radiographs of the lumbar spine.[1,17]

2. **Metabolic disorders**: Metabolic disorders such as osteoporosis, osteomalacia, or hyperparathyroidism can result in diffuse weakening of the vertebral endplates resulting in smooth, uniform depression or concavity of the superior and inferior vertebral endplates at multiple vertebral levels. The resulting radiographic appearance of the vertebral endplate concavities have been referred to as resembling *fish vertebrae* or *fish mouth intervertebral discs*.[18-20]

3. **Spondylodiscitis**: Spondylodiscitis can certainly weaken the endplate resulting in disc protrusion through the endplate. Discitis usually has typical imaging features, including endplate destruction, intradiscal edema, and a characteristic contrast enhancement within the disc and vertebra, allowing differentiation from Schmorl's node.

4. **Metastasis**: A well-defined vertebral metastasis adjacent to the endplate can be confused with the imaging appearance of a Schmorl's node *(Fig. 64-10)*. One should look for other signs of metastatic disease elsewhere in the spine or paraspinal soft tissues. Metastases typically enhance after IV contrast administration and their margins are poorly defined.

5. **Other tumors**: Cystic hemangiomas, chondromas, giant cell tumor, aneurysmal bone cyst, osteoblastoma, and plasmacytoma could be confused with giant, cystic Schmorl's nodes.[15]

TREATMENT

1. **Conservative therapy**: Painful Schmorl's nodes are often self-limited, the symptoms controlled by pain medications, or

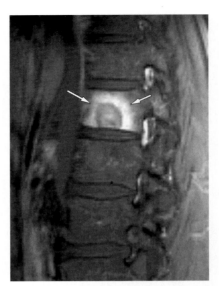

Figure 64-10 ► Vertebral Body Metastasis Simulating Schmorl's Node. Sagittal fat-saturated T1-weighted contrast-enhanced image. A large well-defined lung carcinoma vertebral metastasis abuts the inferior vertebral endplate of L1 and is surrounded by an intense ring of contrast enhancement (*arrows*). A Schmorl's node may mimic a vertebral body metastasis, especially in the early phase of Schmorl's node development.

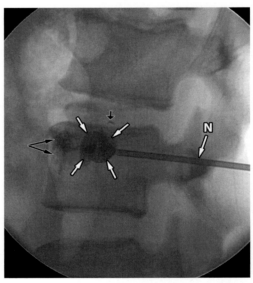

Figure 64-11 ► Percutaneous Treatment of Symptomatic Schmorl's Node. Lateral radiograph lumbar spine. A 13-gauge needle cannula (*N*) has been inserted percutaneously directly into the L3 cystic Schmorl's node using a transpedicular approach. Methylmethacrylate cement was injected to fill the cystic nodal cavity (*white arrows*) until a tiny amount of cement (*small black arrow*) was seen in the disc space to seal the communication between the cystic cavity and the disc. Additional cement (*long black arrows*) was injected into the cancellous bone anterior to the Schmorl's node to provide additional support to the bone adjacent to the cystic Schmorl's node.

anti-inflammatory agents. The symptoms often resolve spontaneously within weeks to months.

2. **Cement injection**: Direct percutaneous injection of cement into and around symptomatic Schmorl's nodes can be effective in extremely painful Schmorl's nodes as in the cystic L3 node in this case. The Schmorl's node must be large enough to facilitate needle placement *(Fig. 64-11)*.

3. **Vertebroplasty:** Injecting cement adjacent to the Schmorl's node can be effective when the symptomatic node is small in size and difficult to precisely target percutaneously, as was done in the symptomatic L2 node in this case.
4. **Lumbar fusion:** A last resort therapy for refractory severely painful Schmorl's nodes that do not respond to above therapies.

References

1. Dietz GW, Christensen EE. Normal "Cupid's bow" contour of the lower lumbar vertebrae. *Radiology.* 1976;121:577-579.
2. Saluja G, Fitzpatrick K, Bruce M, Cross J. Schmorl's nodes (intravertebral herniations of intervertebral disc tissue) in two historic British populations. *J Anat.* 1986;145:87-96.
3. Wu HT, Morrison WB, Schweitzer ME. Edematous Schmorl's nodes on thoracolumbar MR imaging: Characteristic patterns and changes over time. *Skeletal Radiol.* 2006;35:212-219.
4. Hamanishi C, Kawabata T, Yosii T, Tanaka S. Schmorl's nodes on magnetic resonance imaging: Their incidence and clinical relevance. *Spine.* 1994;19:450-453.
5. Peng B, Wu W, Hou S, et al. The pathogenesis of Schmorl's nodes. *J Bone Joint Surg Br.* 2003;85:879-882.
6. Wagner AL, Murtagh FR, Arrington JA, Stallworth D. Relationship of Schmorl's nodes to vertebral body endplate fractures and acute endplate disk extrusions. *AJNR Am J Neuroradiol.* 2000;21:276-281.
7. Moller A, Maly P, Besjakov J, et al. A vertebral fracture in childhood is not a risk factor for disc degeneration but for Schmorl's nodes: A mean 40-year observational study. *Spine.* 2007;32:2487-2492.
8. Oner FC, van der Rijt RR, Ramos LM, et al. Changes in the disc space after fractures of the thoracolumbar spine. *J Bone Joint Surg Br.* 1998;80:833-839.
9. Hasegawa K, Ogose A, Morita T, Hirata Y. Painful Schmorl's node treated by lumbar interbody fusion. *Spinal Cord.* 2004;42:124-128.
10. Park P, Tran NK, Gala VC, et al. The radiographic evolution of a Schmorl's node. *Br J Neurosurg.* 2007;21:224-227.
11. Lipson SJ, Fox DA, Sosman JL. Symptomatic intravertebral disc herniation (Schmorl's node) in the cervical spine. *Ann Rheum Dis.* 1985;44:857-859.
12. Martel W, Seeger JF, Wicks JD, Washburn RL. Traumatic lesions of the discovertebral junction in the lumbar spine. *AJR Am J Roentgenol.* 1976;127:457-464.
13. Modic MT, Ross JS. Lumbar degenerative disk disease. *Radiology.* 2007;245:43-61.
14. Takahashi K, Miyazaki T, Ohnari H, et al. Schmorl's nodes and low-back pain: Analysis of magnetic resonance imaging findings in symptomatic and asymptomatic individuals. *Eur Spine J.* 1995;4:56-59.
15. Hauger O, Cotten A, Chateil JF, et al. Giant cystic Schmorl's nodes: Imaging findings in six patients. *AJR Am J Roentgenol.* 2001;176:969-972.
16. Coulier B. Giant fatty Schmorl's nodes: CT findings in four patients. *Skeletal Radiol.* 2005;34:29-34.
17. Tsuji H, Yoshioka T, Sainoh H. Developmental balloon disc of the lumbar spine in healthy subjects. *Spine.* 1985;10:907-911.
18. Mulligan ME. Regarding "fish" or "fish mouth" vertebrae. *AJR Am J Roentgenol.* 2004;182:1600.
19. Resnick DL. Fish vertebrae. *Arthritis Rheum.* 1982;25:1073-1077.
20. Rexroad JT, Moser IR, Georgia JD. "Fish" or "fish mouth" vertebrae? *AJR Am J Roentgenol.* 2003;181:886-887.

INTRADURAL SCHWANNOMA

Leo F. Czervionke, M.D.

CLINICAL PRESENTATION

The patient is a 32-year-old man with a history of low back and left hip pain that developed 9 months prior and diffuse back pain and back throbbing over the past 3 months. The patient has recently developed lower extremity numbness and burning in the feet and occasionally experiences a sharp radiating pain down the spine (L'Hermitte's sign). He has been unable to walk any distance and experiences occasional urinary and fecal urgency. He reports one episode of urinary incontinence. Physical examination reveals diminished sensation to pinprick in the lower trunk and below. He has moderately reduced strength in the hip flexors and mildly reduced strength in the feet dorsiflexors. The clinical findings are those of myelopathy with a sensory level in the mid to lower thoracic region.

IMAGING PRESENTATION

Magnetic resonance (MR) imaging was obtained and revealed a lobulated, dumbbell-shaped, 4 cm in maximal dimension mass located at the T11 level. The mass has a large intradural component and smaller extradural component extending into and enlarging the right T11-12 neural foramen, consistent with nerve sheath tumor (schwannoma or neurofibroma) (*Figs. 65-1 to 65-4*).

DISCUSSION

A schwannoma is a nerve sheath tumor arising from Schwann cells in the nerve sheath.[1] Sometimes referred to as *neurilemmoma* or *neurinoma*, a schwannoma is the most common intradural-extramedullary tumor originating within the thecal sac (meningioma is the second most common intradural-extramedullary tumor) (*Fig. 65-5*). Approximately 75% of spinal schwannomas arise intradurally; 15% of spinal schwannomas are located in both the intradural and extradural compartments.[2] The majority of other spinal schwannomas are entirely extradural, located in the paraspinal region (*Fig. 65-6*). Rarely, intradural schwannomas occur that have an intramedullary component.[3]

Those schwannomas with intradural and extradural components characteristically have a *dumbbell* configuration. Small to medium-sized schwannomas are commonly discovered as incidental findings within the thecal sac arising from the cauda equina on routine MR imaging (Figs. 65-5, *65-7, and 65-8*). Intradural nerve sheath tumors can be lobulated (see Figs. 65-7 and 65-8) or spherical in configuration (*Fig. 65-9*). So called *giant schwannomas* may also occur, which are large tumors that can extend for a variable distance into the paraspinal soft tissues (*Fig. 65-10*).

Schwannoma is the second most common nerve sheath tumor, the neurofibroma being the most common nerve sheath tumor.[4] Far less common nerve sheath tumors include ganglioneuromas and malignant nerve sheath tumors.[5] Schwannomas arise in the nerve sheath eccentric to the adjacent nerve and are slowly growing tumors. These tumors manifest as isolated masses or as multiple masses anywhere along the spinal axis. Schwannomas are usually isolated lesions except when associated with neurofibromatosis type-2 (NF-2).[6] Most patients with a schwannoma have the sporadic form of the disease; 50% or more of the patients with the more common (sporadic) form have gene mutations that inactivate a portion of chromosome 22. However, the patients with the sporadic form do not have the other manifestations of neurofibromatosis type 2 (NF-2).

Most schwannomas, solitary or multiple, occur sporadically. The presence of multiple schwannomas does not necessarily mean the patient has NF-2, although multiple schwannomas almost always occur in patients with NF-2. Neurofibromatosis type 2 is an autosomal dominant condition associated with mutations in chromosome 22q (long arm) that occurs in approximately 1 in 30,000 people. Patients with NF-2 usually have multiple schwannomas either intracranially, in the spinal canal, or neural foramina, along with other tumors, including meningiomas and ependymomas, which may occur in the spine or intracranially in NF-2 patients (*Figs. 65-11 to 65-14*). The presence of bilateral cranial nerve VIII schwannomas is pathognomonic of NF-2 (see Fig. 65-11), but cranial nerve VIII schwannomas may be absent in patients with NF-2.[7,8] The intradural and paraspinal nerve sheath tumors in NF-2 are usually schwannomas, but some patients with this condition have both nerve sheath schwannomas and neurofibromas.[7] However, the majority of nerve sheath tumors in patients with neurofibromatosis type 1 (NF-1, von Recklinghausen disease) are neurofibromas or plexiform neurofibromas.[1] However, schwannomas can also occur in patients with NF-1.[4]

Most patients with schwannomas present between the ages of 30 and 50 with radicular pain or paresthesias, but can present with myelopathy, including progressive paraparesis, if they occur in the cervical or thoracic region. Depressed motor function resulting in weakness can occur later in the course of the disease. Most

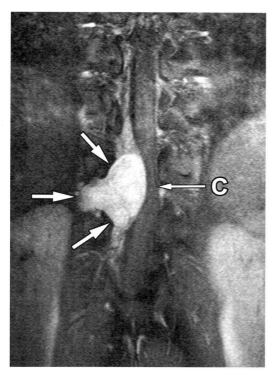

Figure 65-1 ▸ **"Dumbbell" Schwannoma, T11 Level.** A large lobulated mass (*arrows*) enhances homogeneously following IV contrast on coronal T1-weighted MRI. The intradural component of the mass is larger, compressing and displacing the spinal cord (*C*) to the left. The extradural component of the mass has enlarged the right T11-12 neural foramen.

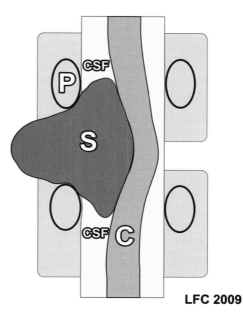

Figure 65-2 ▸ **Illustration of Thoracic Dumbbell Schwannoma.** Similar to that depicted in Figure 65-1. The schwannoma (*S*) has intradural and extradural components. A large intradural component compresses the spinal cord (*C*) on the right and displaces the cord to the left of midline. The extradural component of the tumor extends out the right T11 neural foramen. P = vertebral pedicle.

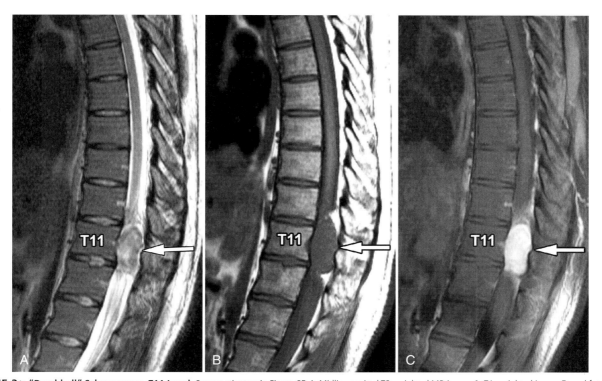

Figure 65-3 ▸ **"Dumbbell" Schwannoma, T11 Level.** Same patient as in Figure 65-1. Midline sagittal T2 weighted MR image **A**, T1-weighted image **B**, and fat-saturated contrast enhanced T1-weighted image **C**. The mass (*arrow*) is slightly heterogeneous but predominantly isointense relative to the spinal cord on T1- and T2-weighted images. In image **C** the mass (*arrow*) enhances intensely and homogeneously. T11 = T11 vertebral body.

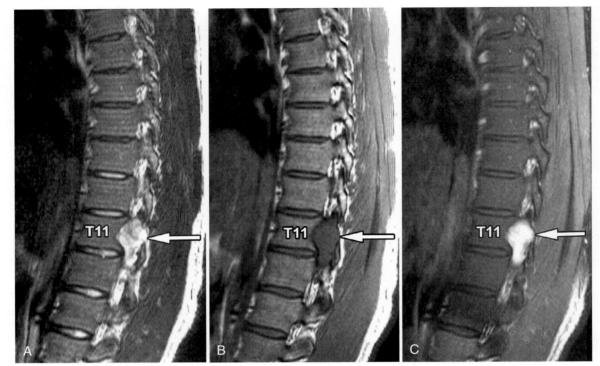

Figure 65-4 ▶ "Dumbbell" Schwannoma, T11 Level. Same patient as in Figures 65-1 and 65-3. Parasagittal T2-weighted image **A**, T1-weighted image **B**, and fat-saturated contrast enhanced T1-weighted image **C**. The mass (*arrow*) is slightly heterogeneous on T2-weighted image **A**. On image T1-weighted image **B**, the mass (*arrow*) appears more homogeneous and enlarges the right T11-12 neural foramen. On image **C**, the mass (*arrow*) enhances intensely and homogeneously following IV contrast administration.

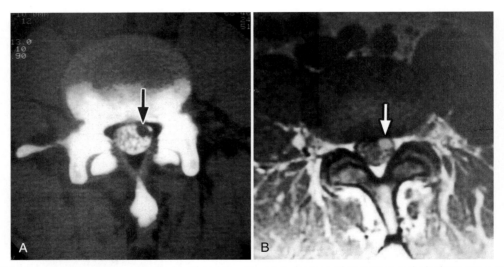

Figure 65-5 ▶ Small Intradural Schwannoma within Lumbar Thecal Sac. On post-myelogram axial CT image **A** in the lumbar region, a small, round, dark filling defect (*arrow*), representing an intradural mass, is located within the contrast filled thecal sac. On corresponding contrast enhanced axial T1-weighted MR image **B**, the mass (*arrow*) within the thecal sac enhances with contrast and is larger than adjacent normal cauda equina nerve roots. Small intradural schwannomas such as this are often discovered as incidental findings on routine MR imaging studies of the lumbar spine.

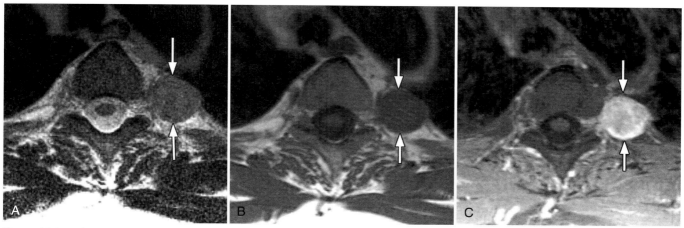

Figure 65-6 ▶ Left Paraspinal Schwannoma, Upper Thoracic Level. Axial T2-weighted image **A**. T1-weighted image **B**, and fat saturated contrast enhanced T1-weighted image **C**. The schwannoma (*arrows in image* **A** *and* **B**) is hypointense relative to paraspinal fat on T2-weighted and T1-weighted images. On contrast-enhanced fat-saturated T1-weighted MR image **C**, the schwannoma enhances intensely and is slightly heterogeneous.

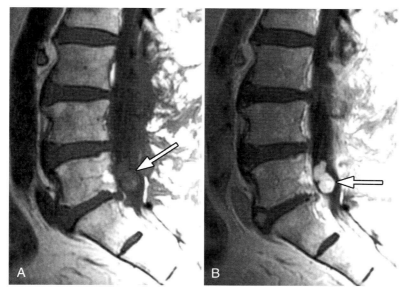

Figure 65-7 ▶ Lobulated Intradural Schwannoma. Patient with left S1 radiculopathy. Sagittal unenhanced T1-weighted image **A** and contrast enhanced T1-weighted image **B**. The mass (*arrow in image* **A** *and* **B**) enhances homogeneously following IV contrast.

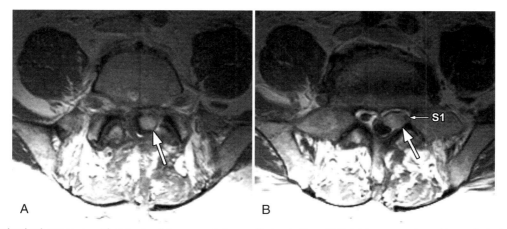

Figure 65-8 ▶ Intradural Schwannoma with Extradural Component. Same patient as in Figure 65-7. Axial contrast enhanced image **A** obtained at L5-S1 level, and contrast-enhanced image **B** obtained at level of S1 lateral recess. A homogeneously enhancing intradural mass (*arrow in image* **A**) is demonstrated within the thecal sac on the left. The tumor has an extradural component (*large arrow in* **B**) which compresses and displaces the left S1 nerve root (*S1*).

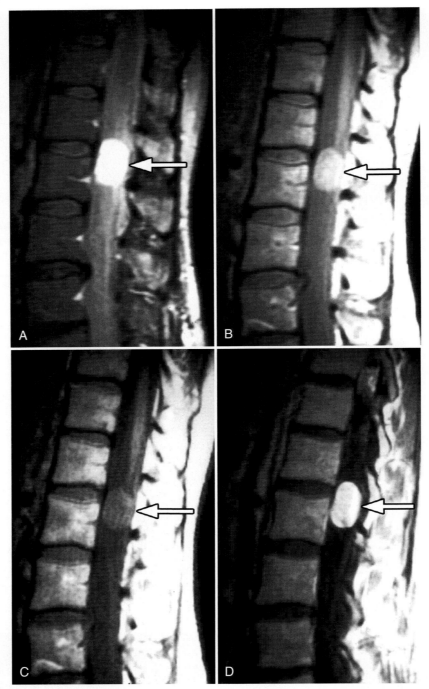

Figure 65-9 ▸ Intradural Schwannoma Adjacent to Conus Medullaris. Ovoid intradural mass at L1-2 level simulates a myxopapillary ependymoma. The intradural mass (*arrow*) is hyperintense relative to CSF on sagittal conventional T2-weighted MR image **A** and on proton density-weighted image **B**. The mass (*arrow*) is isointense relative to the spinal cord on unenhanced sagittal T1-weighted image **C**. On sagittal contrast-enhanced image **D**, the schwannoma (*arrow*) enhances intensely and nearly homogeneously.

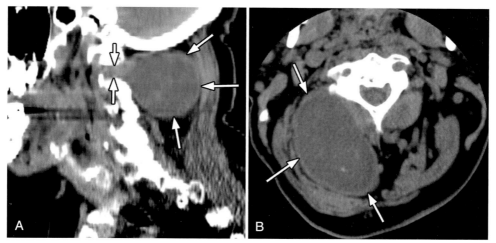

Figure 65-10 ▶ Giant Paraspinal Schwannoma at C2-3 Level. Achondroplastic dwarf. Large paraspinal mass demonstrated on unenhanced parasagittal CT image **A** and axial CT image **B**. The schwannoma has a slightly hyperdense rim (*long arrows in* **A** *and* **B**) and is relatively hypodense centrally. A component of the mass enlarges the right C1-2 neural foramen (*short arrows in image* **A**).

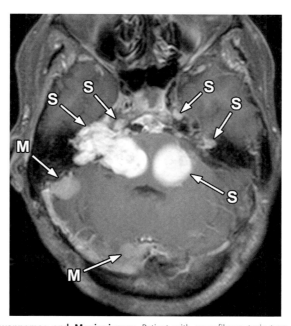

Figure 65-11 ▶ Multiple Intracranial Schwannomas and Meningiomas. Patient with neurofibromatosis type 2 (NF-2). Axial fat-saturated contrast enhanced T1-weighted MRI obtained through posterior fossa reveals multiple enhancing intracranial schwannomas (*S*) involving cranial nerves V and VIII bilaterally. A meningioma (*M*) is located along the posterior slope of the right petrous bone and another meningioma (*M*) is located to the right of the torcula.

schwannomas arise in the lumbar spinal canal between the ages of 30 and 50.[2] Schwannoma has a slightly higher male predilection.[2]

The vast majority of schwannomas are classified by the WHO (World Health Organization) as WHO grade 1 tumors. Histologically, schwannomas usually contain cells of two types. Antoni A cells are compact, elongated cells that are often found in the solid portion of the schwannoma. Antoni B cells are less cellular, loosely arranged cells in the tumoral tissue that may contain lipids. The myxoid tissue containing Antoni B cells also has a high water content.[1] Schwannomas are usually solid cellular tumors

containing mainly Antoni type A cells.[2] Intradural-extramedullary plexiform schwannomas rarely occur and are far less common than the common plexiform neurofibroma that is pathognomonic of NF-1.[9]

Immunohistochemical staining of the cells in the nerve sheath tumor is often performed in an attempt to differentiate schwannoma from neurofibroma, although there is overlap in the immunostaining characteristics of these tumors. Schwannomas and neurofibromas are S-100 protein positive.[1,9] Glut 1, a glucose transporter protein, and EMA (epithelial membrane antigen) are specific to

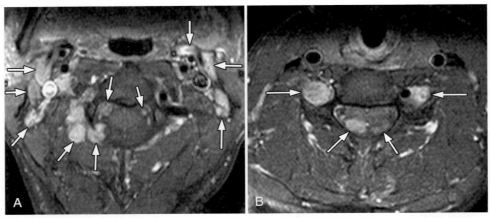

Figure 65-12 ▶ Neurofibromatosis Type 2 (NF-2). Same patient as in Figure 65-11. Axial contrast enhanced fat-saturated T1-weighted MR images **A** and **B**, obtained through the upper and mid-cervical region, respectively. Multiple enhancing nerve sheath tumors (*arrows*), most likely schwannomas, are located within the spinal canal paraspinal tissues and adjacent to the carotid sheath bilaterally.

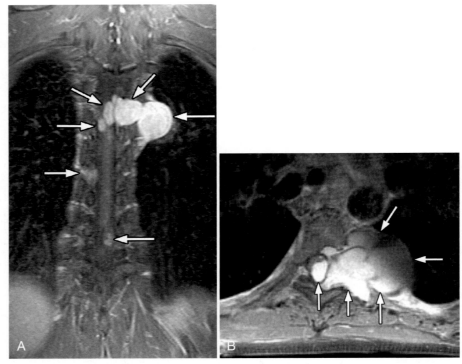

Figure 65-13 ▶ Neurofibromatosis Type 2 (NF-2). Same patient as in Figures 65-11 and 65-12. Coronal contrast-enhanced fat-saturated T1-weighted MR image **A**, obtained through the thoracic spine, demonstrates multiple intraspinal and paraspinal nerve sheath tumors (*arrows*). Axial fat saturated T1-weighted image **B**, obtained through upper thoracic spine, shows lobulated intraspinal and left paraspinal masses (*arrows*). The intradural mass is displacing the spinal cord anteriorly and to the right.

perineural cells and therefore schwannomas usually stain positive for these substances.[10] Calretinin, a calcium-binding protein, is more commonly found in schwannomas.[11] Neurofibromas usually stain positive for CD34, which is found in endoneural fibroblasts.[10]

The morphologic features of schwannomas and neurofibromas are usually different. Schwannomas are surrounded by a true capsule composed of epineurium.[12] Neurofibromas do not usually

have a true capsule and cannot be separated from the nerve.[12] Neurofibromas tend to extend beyond the epineurium.[1] Rarely, schwannomas contain areas of hemorrhage, and this instance can be a cause of subarachnoid hemorrhage.[13] Schwannomas rarely undergo infarction and central necrosis.[14]

Melanotic schwannoma is a rare subtype of schwannoma. Most melanotic schwannomas are benign,[15,16] but even histologically benign melanotic melanomas have a tendency to recur.[17]

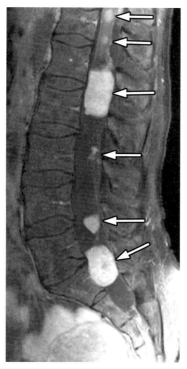

Figure 65-14 ▶ **Neurofibromatosis Type 2 (NF-2).** Same patient as in Figures 65-11 to 65-13. Multiple schwannomas (*arrows*) of varying sizes are demonstrated in the lumbar spinal canal on sagittal fat-saturated contrast enhanced T1-weighted image.

Melanotic schwannoma can become malignant and should be followed closely with imaging.[17,18] Melanotic schwannomas usually contain areas of hemorrhage and cystic degeneration and may occur as isolated tumors or as part of the *Carney complex.*[19] Patients with this autosomal dominant condition may also have cardiac myxomas, cutaneous myxomas, pituitary tumors, and pigmented adrenal gland tumors.[20,21] Genetic abnormalities have been discovered in chromosomes *2* and *17* in patients with Carney complex.[22,23]

IMAGING FEATURES

A schwannoma, if sufficiently large, usually expands the spinal canal or neural foramen, causing bone remodeling of the spinal canal or involved neural foramen, which may be visible on spine radiographs, CT, or MRI. On CT images, schwannomas are usually slightly hypodense relative to the paraspinal musculature (see Fig. 65-10). Calcification rarely occurs in schwannomas, but if present, is visible on CT. Giant schwannomas can occur within the lumbar spinal canal that cause marked bone remodeling of the spinal canal and neural foramina (see Figs. 65-10 and 65-12).[24] Intradural schwannomas at myelography have a characteristic *cap sign*, where the contrast-filled intrathecal cerebrospinal fluid (CSF) forms a meniscal cap above and/or below the intradural tumor *(Fig. 65-15)*. This sign is nonspecific, seen at myelography with any intradural tumor including schwannoma, meningioma, and arachnoid cyst *(Fig. 65-16)*.

MRI is the modality of choice for diagnosing and assessing the extent of schwannomas. These tumors are typically T1 hypointense or isointense relative to the spinal cord. Schwannomas can be T2 hypointense, isointense, or hyperintense relative to the spinal cord, but most schwannomas are T2 hyperintense relative to the cord (see Figs. 65-3, 65-6, 65-9, and 65-17)[4]. T2 hypointense regions are usually centrally located in the schwannoma and are attributed to the presence of densely cellular tissue composed of Antoni A cells *(Fig. 65-17)*. T2 hyperintense regions in the tumor are usually located in the periphery of the schwannoma and are associated with loosely arranged myxoid cellular tissue composed of Antoni B cells (see Fig. 65-17).[4] This classic arrangement of cells imparts a *target appearance* to the schwannoma on T2-weighted images.[4] However, in most cases, it is usually not possible to differentiate regions of Antoni A and Antoni B cellularity based on the imaging appearance.

Foraminal schwannomas often have an intradural component giving them a dumbbell-shaped configuration (see Figs. 65-1, 65-13, and 65-17). Neurofibromas may have an identical dumbbell configuration and therefore usually cannot be differentiated from schwannoma based on imaging alone.[1] Plexiform neurofibromas are pathognomonic of NF-1 and have a fusiform beaded appearance that often extends over a considerable distance along the peripheral nerve. Plexiform neurofibromas are characteristically more conspicuous on T2-weighted images and usually have a T2 hypointense focus centrally *(Fig. 65-18)*. They may not enhance appreciably on contrast-enhanced MR images, but enhancing plexiform neurofibromas characteristically enhance more at their periphery (Fig. 65-18).[1] Plexiform schwannomas are rare but have an identical appearance. Neurofibromas and rarely schwannomas can degenerate into malignant nerve sheath tumors. When this occurs, these tumors have avid fluorodeoxyglucose (FDG) uptake

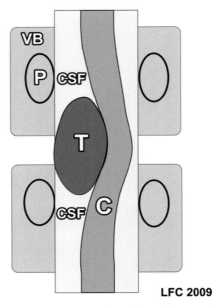

LFC 2009

Figure 65-15 ▶ Illustration of Intradural-Extramedullary Tumor. The spinal canal, depicted in coronal plane, contains an intradural-extramedullary tumor (*T*). The intrathecal CSF (*yellow region*) surrounds the spinal cord (*C*) and forms a meniscal "cap" above and below the tumor. VB = vertebral body. P = pedicle.

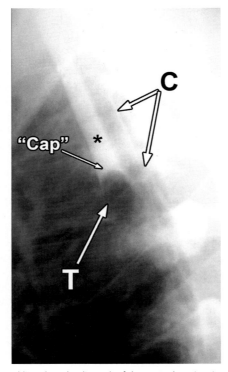

Figure 65-16 ▶ Myelographic Intradural *Cap Sign*. Oblique lateral radiograph of the upper thoracic spine obtained during myelography in patient with an intradural arachnoid cyst. Opaque intrathecal contrast (*asterisk*) surrounds the spinal cord (*C*) and forms a meniscal "Cap" above the intradural lesion. The same myelographic appearance can be seen with any intradural mass including schwannoma and meningioma.

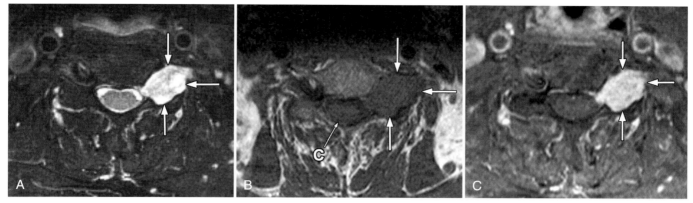

Figure 65-17 ▶ Schwannoma Producing Enlargement of Left C5-6 Neural Foramen, Secondary to Chronic Bone Remodeling. On axial T2-weighted MR image **A**, the schwannoma (*arrows*) is heterogeneous. The mass is hyperintense peripherally and contains hypointense areas centrally, likely due to mixture of Antoni types A and B cells. Overall, the schwannoma is T2 hyperintense relative to the spinal cord. On axial T1-weighted MR image **B**, the schwannoma (*arrows*) is more homogeneous in intensity. The mass is isointense relative to the spinal cord (*C*) and is slightly hyperintense relative to the vertebra on T1-weighted image **B**. On axial fat saturated contrast enhanced T1 weighted image **C**, the schwannoma (*arrows*) enhances diffusely and is slightly heterogeneous.

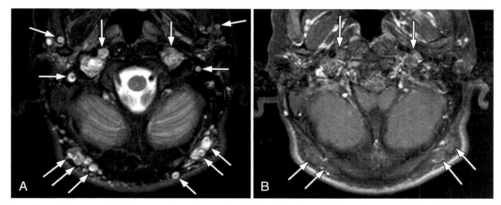

Figure 65-18 ▶ Plexiform Neurofibromas. Multiple tumors located near the skull base in patient with Neurofibromatosis Type 1 (NF-1). Axial T2-weighted MR image **A** and contrast-enhanced fat-saturated T1-weighted MR image **B**. Multiple bead-like plexiform neurofibromas (*arrows*) are located in the subcutaneous soft tissues, in the parotid regions, and in the jugular foramina bilaterally. The plexiform neurofibromas (*arrows*) are far more conspicuous on T2-weighted image **A**. These lesions characteristically contain a T2 hypointense focus centrally. On contrast-enhanced fat-saturated T1-weighted MR image **B**. The plexiform neurofibromas (*arrows*) enhance either minimally at their periphery or not at all.

on positron emission tomography (PET) scanning. Approximately 2% of nerve sheath tumors are malignant. Bone destruction (not merely bone remodeling) should always raise suspicion that one is dealing with a malignant nerve sheath tumor or neurofibrosarcoma (*Fig. 65-19*).

The solid portions the of intradural or intraforaminal schwannomas usually enhance homogeneously after IV contrast administration.[25] Some schwannomas enhance slightly more at their periphery. A cystic area commonly occurs within an intradural schwannoma and does not enhance (*Fig. 65-20*). About one half of schwannomas contain cysts and one half are completely solid. Intratumoral hemorrhage occurs in approximately 5% of cases. Rarely, subarachnoid hemorrhage can occur secondary to hemorrhage of an intradural schwannoma.[13]

In patients with multiple intradural nerve sheath tumors or if neurofibromatosis NF-1 or NF-2 is suspected, the entire neuroaxis should be imaged to exclude the presence of other nerve sheath tumors or other tumors such as coexistent ependymomas.

DIFFERENTIAL DIAGNOSIS

1. **Meningioma:** A meningioma tumor is usually benign, but can be malignant. Meningiomas arise from arachnoid cap cells and are the second most common intradural tumor. These tumors are more common in females, most commonly arising as intradural masses in the thoracic spinal canal or at the foramen magnum level (*Fig. 65-21*). They rarely have an intradural-extradural location, but if so, do have a dumbbell configuration. They rarely occur in the lumbar spinal canal, 80% of spinal lesions occurring in the thoracic intradural-extramedullary compartment.[4] They are usually T2 isointense or hypointense relative to the spinal cord and slightly heterogeneous in signal intensity. Calcification is much more common in meningiomas.[4]

2. **Neurofibroma:** The majority of neurofibromas occur as isolated, sporadic tumors in patients without neurofibromatosis type 1 (NF-1).[1] The presence of solitary or multiple

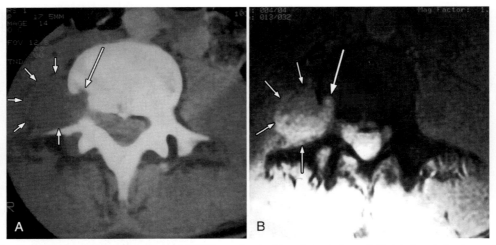

Figure 65-19 ▶ Lumbar Intraforaminal Neurofibrosarcoma. Axial CT image **A** and axial gradient echo image **B**. The intraforaminal and paraspinal tumor (*small arrows in image* **A** *and* **B**) enlarges the right L3-4 neural foramen and extends into the right paraspinal soft tissues. The tumor causes localized vertebral bone erosion (*long arrow*) on images **A** and **B**.

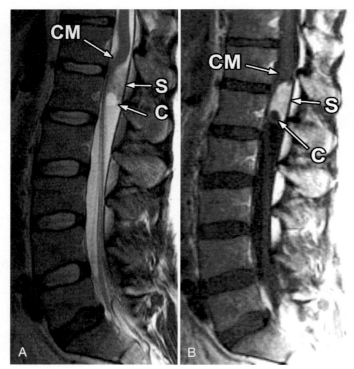

Figure 65-20 ▶ Schwannoma in Conus Medullaris Region. Sagittal T2-weighted image **A** and contrast enhanced T1-weighted image **B**. The predominantly solid schwannoma (*S*) displaces the conus medullaris (*CM*) anteriorly and contains a small T2 hyperintense, nonenhancing cyst (*C*) at its caudal pole.

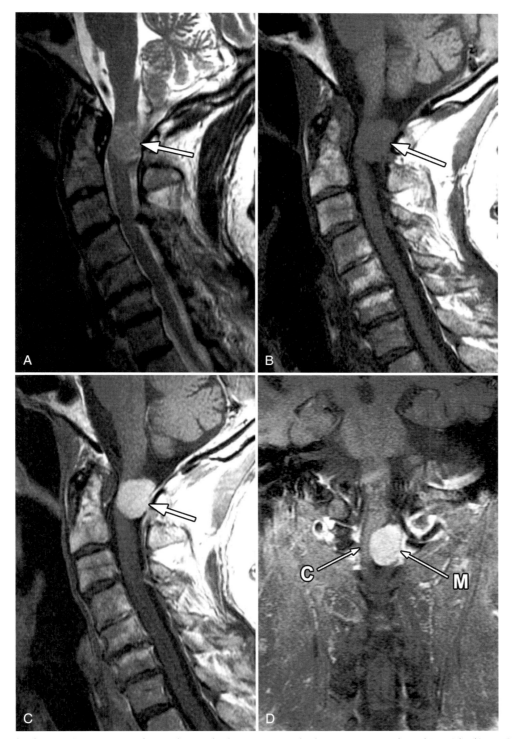

Figure 65-21 ▶ Intradural Meningioma at C1 Level. Sagittal T2-weighted image **A**, T1-weighted image **B**, contrast enhanced T1-weighted image **C**, and coronal contrast-enhanced image **D**. The meningioma (*arrow in image* **A** *and* **B**) is slightly T2 hyperintense and T1 isointense relative to the spinal cord. On image **C**, the meningioma (*arrow*) enhances homogeneously following IV contrast administration. On image **D**, the spinal cord (*C*) is compressed and displaced to the right by the meningioma (M).

neurofibromas, however, should initiate a search for stigmata of NF-1 (von Recklinghausen disease) including café-au-lait spots, subcutaneous neurofibromas, plexiform neurofibromas, and Lisch nodules, which is a hamartomatous pigmented nevus in the iris.[1] Neurofibromas typically have a fusiform configuration. However, isolated neurofibromas may be difficult or impossible to differentiate from schwannomas by imaging. Dumbbell-shaped spinal nerve sheath tumors may appear identical to schwannomas and may occur in the same location as schwannomas in the spinal canal, neural foramen, or paraspinal tissues. Plexiform neurofibromas have a lobulated, beaded appearance and tend to be more T2 hypointense centrally and T2 hyperintense at their periphery giving them a *target appearance* (see Fig. 65-18).

3. **Malignant nerve sheath tumor or neurofibrosarcoma:** It may not be possible to differentiate a schwannoma from a malignant nerve sheath tumor or neurofibrosarcoma. Approximately 2% of nerve sheath tumors are malignant. Indeed, malignant nerve sheath tumors are believed to develop within previously benign nerve sheath tumors, usually from neurofibromas.[12] Malignant nerve sheath tumors rarely develop from schwannomas. Imaging features that should raise concern of a possible malignant nerve sheath tumor include (1) loss of the classic T2 target appearance in the nerve sheath tumor, (2) increasing tumor size over time, (3) tumor diameter greater than 5 cm, and (4) development of central necrosis in the tumor,[4] associated vertebral bone destruction (see Fig. 65-19). Malignant tumors usually grow rapidly and have avid FDG uptake on PET images.

4. **Foraminal disc herniation:** This is the most common differential diagnostic consideration when an intraforaminal *mass* is present. A dumbbell-shaped configuration is usually not seen with foraminal herniated discs because intradural disc herniation is rare. Herniated discs that extend into the neural foramen are usually T2 hypointense. Herniated disc fragments do not enhance centrally but nearly all display a thin rim of peripheral contrast enhancement, because of inflammation surrounding the disc fragment. Unless a cyst is present in the schwannoma, foraminal schwannomas usually enhance homogeneously. Chronic intraforaminal disc herniations may cause slight enlargement of the neural foramen by slow remodeling bone.

5. **Myxopapillary ependymoma:** This tumor usually arises at the level of the conus medullaris or within the upper portion of the cauda equina and can have an imaging appearance very similar to intradural schwannomas. The tumor does not extend out the neural foramen and usually arises from the conus medullaris or in the upper portion of the cauda equina. Myxopapillary ependymomas tend to have more heterogeneous signal intensity on T1- and T2-weighted images and also enhance heterogeneously. The incidence of intratumoral hemorrhage is much higher in ependymomas but can occur in schwannomas.[13]

6. **Meningocele:** Cerebrospinal fluid–filled outpouchings of the dura may occur in patients with or without NF-1. They can enlarge the neural foramen by bone remodeling. They have the same intensity as fluid on all MR imaging sequences and do not enhance with IV contrast.

7. **Hemangiopericytoma and hemangioblastoma:** Rarely, these tumors can arise within the neural foramen and can have a similar configuration and imaging appearance on MR imaging as schwannoma, although usually they have a more heterogeneous signal intensity on T1- and T2-weighted images, tend to be larger at time of presentation, and typically grow at a faster rate than schwannoma. They usually display heterogeneous contrast enhancement because of a variable degree of vascularity in these tumors. Associated bone erosion or bone destruction may be present.

8. **Other intradural tumors:** Epidermoid, dermoid, paraganglioma, lipoma, plasmacytoma, melanocytoma, and chloroma may also manifest as intradural masses that should be considered in the differential diagnosis of schwannoma.[4]

9. **Extraosseous cavernous hemangioma:** These hemangiomas may rarely arise in the neural foramen simulating an intraforaminal nerve sheath tumor.[26]

TREATMENT

1. **Conservative approach:** Tiny or small intradural schwannomas found incidentally in the cauda equina are usually not treated unless they become symptomatic.

2. **Surgical excision:** Surgical removal of schwannomas is reserved for patients with significant neurologic dysfunction or uncontrollable pain or in the rare case of malignant degeneration. Postoperative kyphosis is a potential complication of removal of nerve sheath tumors related to facetectomy.[2,27] Small schwannomas can sometimes be removed from the nerve sheath in their entirety with preservation of neural function. However, larger schwannomas may be difficult to remove completely without causing some damage to the adjacent nerve root or spinal cord. Intradural schwannomas in particular are difficult to remove because they are often adherent to the pial surface of the spinal cord because of adhesions, which presumably developed because of prior inflammation or hemorrhage.[2] Neurofibromas are intimately intertwined with the nerve and nerve sheath and therefore cannot be separated from the involved nerve root surgically. When a nerve sheath neurofibroma is removed, the nerve is removed along with the tumor.[4]

3. **Radiotherapy:** Giant intradural schwannomas are treated by subtotal resection and/or radiotherapy.[24]

References

1. Murphey MD, Smith WS, Smith SE, et al. From the archives of the AFIP. Imaging of musculoskeletal neurogenic tumors: Radiologic-pathologic correlation. *Radiographics.* 1999;19(5):1253-1280.
2. Jeon JH, Hwang HS, Jeong JH, et al. Spinal schwannoma: Analysis of 40 cases. *J Korean Neurosurg Soc.* 2008;43(3):135-138.
3. Kono K, Inoue Y, Nakamura H, et al. MR imaging of a case of a dumbbell-shaped spinal schwannoma with intramedullary and intradural-extramedullary components. *Neuroradiology.* 2001;43(10):864-867.
4. Beall DP, Googe DJ, Emery RL, et al. Extramedullary intradural spinal tumors: A pictorial review. *Curr Probl Diagn Radiol.* 2007;36(5):185-198.
5. Halliday AL, Sobel RA, Martuza RL. Benign spinal nerve sheath tumors: their occurrence sporadically and in neurofibromatosis types 1 and 2. *J Neurosurg.* 1991;74(2):248-253.
6. Rodallec MH, Feydy A, Larousserie F, et al. Diagnostic imaging of solitary tumors of the spine: What to do and say. *Radiographics.* 2008;28(4):1019-1041.
7. Mautner VF, Tatagiba M, Lindenau M, et al. Spinal tumors in patients with neurofibromatosis type 2: MR imaging study of frequency, multiplicity, and variety. *AJR Am J Roentgenol.* 1995;165(4):951-955.
8. Evans DG, Huson SM, Donnai D, et al. A clinical study of type 2 neurofibromatosis. *Q J Med.* 1992;84(304):603-618.
9. Sakaura H, Ohshima K, Iwasaki M, Yoshikawa H. Intra-extradural plexiform schwannoma of the cervical spine. *Spine.* 2007;32(21):E611-614.

10. Hirose T, Tani T, Shimada T, et al. Immunohistochemical demonstration of EMA/Glut1-positive perineurial cells and CD34-positive fibroblastic cells in peripheral nerve sheath tumors. *Mod Pathol.* 2003;16(4):293-298.

11. Fine SW, McClain SA, Li M. Immunohistochemical staining for calretinin is useful for differentiating schwannomas from neurofibromas. *Am J Clin Pathol.* 2004;122(4):552-559.

12. Beaman FD, Kransdorf MJ, Menke DM. Schwannoma: Radiologic-pathologic correlation. *Radiographics.* 2004;24(5):1477-1481.

13. Parmar H, Pang BC, Lim CC, et al. Spinal schwannoma with acute subarachnoid hemorrhage: A diagnostic challenge. *AJNR Am J Neuroradiol.* 2004; 25(5):846-850.

14. Shrier DA, Rubio A, Numaguchi Y, Powers JM. Infarcted spinal schwannoma: An unusual MR finding. *AJNR Am J Neuroradiol.* 1996;17(8):1566-1568.

15. Zhang HY, Yang GH, Chen HJ, et al. Clinicopathological, immunohistochemical, and ultrastructural study of 13 cases of melanotic schwannoma. *Chin Med J (Engl).* 2005;118(17):1451-1461.

16. Er U, Kazanci A, Eyriparmak T, et al. Melanotic schwannoma. *J Clin Neurosci.* 2007;14(7):676-678.

17. Vallat-Decouvelaere AV, Wassef M, Lot G, et al. Spinal melanotic schwannoma: A tumour with poor prognosis. *Histopathology.* 1999;35(6):558-566.

18. Noubari BA, Chiaramonte I, Magro G, et al. Spinal malignant melanotic schwannoma: Case report. *J Neurosurg Sci.* 1998;42(4):245-249.

19. Carney JA, Swee RG. Carney complex. *Am J Surg Pathol.* 2002;26(3):393.

20. Mees ST, Spieker T, Eltze E, et al. Intrathoracic psammomatous melanotic schwannoma associated with the Carney complex. *Ann Thorac Surg.* 2008; 86(2):657-660.

21. Watson JC, Stratakis CA, Bryant-Greenwood PK, et al. Neurosurgical implications of Carney complex. *J Neurosurg.* 2000;92(3):413-418.

22. Sandrini F, Stratakis C. Clinical and molecular genetics of Carney complex. *Mol Genet Metab.* 2003;78(2):83-92.

23. Malchoff CD. Editorial: Carney complex–clarity and complexity. *J Clin Endocrinol Metab.* 2000;85(11):4010-4012.

24. Kagaya H, Abe E, Sato K, et al. Giant cauda equina schwannoma: A case report. *Spine.* 2000;25(2):268-272.

25. Demachi H, Takashima T, Kadoya M, et al. MR imaging of spinal neurinomas with pathological correlation. *J Comput Assist Tomogr.* 1990;14(2):250-254.

26. Carlier R, Engerand S, Lamer S, et al. Foraminal epidural extra osseous cavernous hemangioma of the cervical spine: A case report. *Spine.* 2000; 25(5):629-631.

27. Lonstein JE. Post-laminectomy kyphosis. *Clin Orthop Relat Res.* 1977(128): 93-100.

LUMBAR SCOLIOSIS

Douglas S. Fenton, M.D.

CLINICAL PRESENTATION

The patient is a 70-year-old woman with a 1-year history of left hip and groin pain. There was no antecedent trauma. She underwent injection therapy, particularly epidurals, for which she stated she would have anywhere from 6 weeks to up to 4 months relief. She states that her pain is most significant when walking. The pain becomes intense after walking approximately 50 feet or standing longer than 15 minutes. The pain is present but decreases when sitting, particularly in the reclined position with the left leg elevated. She is rarely pain free, only when lying supine and remaining motionless. Her pain is described as both aching and sharp with activities.

IMAGING PRESENTATION

Sagittal T1-weighted midline image does not demonstrate the L2 and L3 vertebral bodies because they are not in the midsagittal plane secondary to scoliosis. The axial T2-weighted image reveals moderate narrowing of the left neural foramen *(Fig. 66-1)*.

DISCUSSION

Scoliosis, historically, has been defined as an abnormal coronal curvature of the spine of 10 degrees or more.[1] However, through a better understanding of biomechanics, spinal anatomy, and imaging techniques, it has been discovered that scoliosis is not merely coronal imbalance. Scoliosis is a three-dimensional rotational deformity that affects the coronal balance, sagittal balance, and axial rotation of the spine.[2]

There are many different types of scoliosis. They can be classified by curve location, age at onset, and curve type. Typically, they are classified by their etiology—congenital, idiopathic—and their part in other diseases and syndromes—traumatic or degenerative.[3] Each type has its own natural history, methods of treatment, and prognosis.

Curve location is defined by its apex. The apex of a curve is the most lateral vertebral body on frontal radiographs. A scoliosis is considered cervical if its apex is between C2-C6, cervicothoracic if between C7-T1, thoracic if between T2-T11, thoracolumbar if between T12-L1, lumbar if between L2-L4, or lumbosacral if at L5 or below.[3]

Scoliosis can be defined by age at presentation. Type 1 (infantile) is from 0 to 3 years of age, type 2 (juvenile) is from 4 to 10 years of age, type 3 (adolescent) is from 11 to 17 years of age, and type 4 (adult) is 18 years of age or older.[3]

Curve types are defined as either primary, those that first develop, or secondary, those that develop as a "means to balance the head and trunk over the pelvis, not only in the frontal but also in the sagittal plane."[3]

Congenital scoliosis is the most frequent congenital spinal deformity. The curvature is not present at birth. The vertebral anomalies are present at birth, but the spinal deformity does not reveal itself until later childhood after the spine grows.[4] Congenital scoliosis is commonly associated with cardiac and/or urologic abnormalities.[3] Congenital scoliosis progresses in 75% of cases.

Idiopathic scoliosis is the most common type of scoliosis in skeletally immature patients. Idiopathic scoliosis can be classified as infantile, juvenile, or adolescent forms. The infantile and juvenile forms of idiopathic scoliosis are less prevalent than the adolescent form. The prevalence of adolescent scoliosis is 2% to 3%. Males are more affected than females in the infantile form.[5] This reverses in the juvenile form, where there is a female preponderance, although this depends on curve magnitude. For curves closer to 10 degrees, there is no significant gender difference with juvenile scoliosis. With curves greater than 30 degrees, the ratio of female : male is 10:1.[6] There appears to be a genetic predisposition to the development of scoliosis. Monozygotic twin studies show an increased prevalence of scoliosis as opposed to dizygotic twins, and is also greater in family members with scoliosis as compared with the general population.[7,8] Idiopathic scoliosis appears to be due to a failure of adequate control of spinal growth with differential growth between left and right sides of the spine and/or differential growth between the anterior and posterior aspects of the spine. The infantile form of idiopathic scoliosis rarely progresses. The juvenile form progresses in 70% of cases with the potential for cardiac and pulmonary compromise secondary to trunk deformity.[9] Only 2% of adolescents have scoliosis (curve of 10 degrees), but only 5% of these have a progression of their curve beyond 30 degrees.[10]

Scoliosis is associated with other diseases and syndromes. **Cerebral palsy** and **muscular dystrophy** are associated with scoliosis. Scoliosis is seen in nearly 10% of patients with **trisomy 21**.[11] Scoliosis is also associated with **Chiari malformations, syrinx, spinal tumors,** and generalized diseases and syndromes such as **Marfan syndrome, neurofibromatosis**, and **rheumatoid disease**.[12,13]

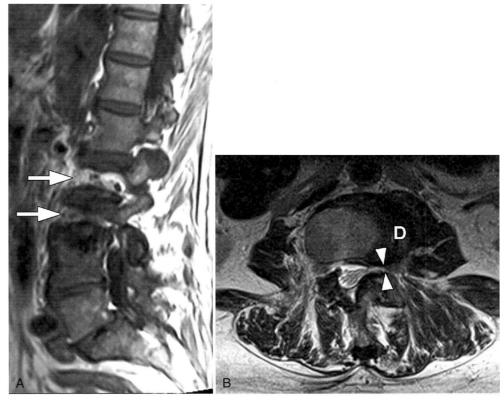

Figure 66-1 ▶ Lumbar Scoliosis. Sagittal T1-weighted image **A** is obtained near the midline; however, the L2 and L3 vertebral bodies (*arrows*) are not visualized because they are out of the midsagittal plane secondary to scoliosis. Axial T2-weighted image **B** is obtained at the L3-4 disc level. There is a large amount of uncovering of the disc (*D*) as a result of the scoliosis and right lateral listhesis of L3 relative to L4. There is also moderate narrowing of the left L3-4 neural foramen, which could potentially affect the exiting left L3 nerve root and cause the patient's symptoms.

Traumatic scoliosis is a compensatory mechanism to fractures and/or dislocations or to soft tissue injuries such as burns.[3]

Adult scoliosis can be divided into type 1 adult scoliosis, which is degenerative; type 2 idiopathic adolescent scoliosis, which progresses into adulthood; and type 3 secondary adult scoliosis, which may be due to a leg length discrepancy, hip pathology, or may be secondary to a metabolic bone disease such as osteoporosis combined with asymmetric arthritic disease.[14] Adult idiopathic scoliosis generally does not progress if curves are less than 30 degrees. Curves that are between 30 and 50 degrees at skeletal maturity tend to progress an average of 10 to 15 degrees over their lifetime. Curves between 50 and 75 degrees progress at an average of 1 degree per year.[14,15] **Degenerative scoliosis** usually develops after the age of 50 and is typically associated with disc degeneration, facet arthritis, thickening/hypertrophy of the ligamentum flava, loss of lumbar lordosis, and lateral listhesis.[3] Degenerative scoliosis can lead to neurogenic claudication, radicular pain, and back pain.

IMAGING FEATURES

Computed tomography (CT) and magnetic resonance imaging (MRI) can be used to demonstrate the effects of scoliosis in relation to the spinal canal, spinal cord, and neural foramen. CT can be used to evaluate more subtle bone abnormalities such as hemivertebrae and butterfly vertebrae and is particularly useful in computer-assisted placement of pedicle screws because there is a much greater difficulty and thus a greater morbidity with "blind" screw placement secondary to the three-dimensional abnormalities of scoliosis. By far, the most useful imaging technique in the evaluation of scoliosis is plain film radiographs. Many advocate upright and supine frontal and lateral long-cassette (36-inch) radiographs that include the occiput to the femoral heads (*Fig. 66-2*). The greatest magnitude of a patient's spinal deformity is best seen on the weight-bearing upright images. By convention, scoliosis radiographs are evaluated as if the physician were looking at the patient from the back (the left side of the radiograph is the left side of the patient), and the lateral view is with the physician looking at the patient's right side (patient looking to the right). Four measurements are typically calculated from the plain radiographs; the Cobb angle, the apical vertebral translation, the coronal balance, and the sagittal balance.

1. **The Cobb angle** measures the angular magnitude of a spinal deformity and is calculated by using the end vertebrae (the vertebrae that are maximally tilted at each end of the curve). Lines are drawn parallel to the superior endplate of the cranial end vertebrae and parallel to the inferior endplate of the

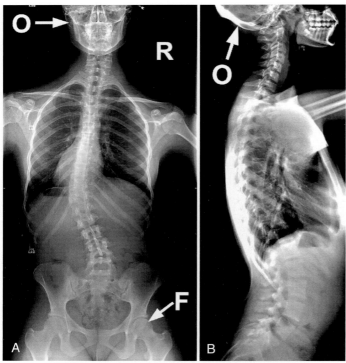

Figure 66-2 ▶ Routine Scoliosis Images. Frontal radiograph image **A** and lateral radiograph image **B** are obtained from the occiput (*O*) to the femoral heads (*F*). The convention for scoliosis imaging is that the radiographs are obtained and viewed as if one was looking at the patient's back and that the patient is looking to the right.

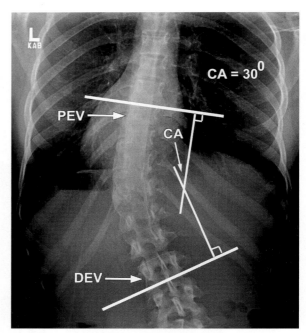

Figure 66-3 ▶ Cobb Angle. The Cobb angle (*CA*) is obtained on the frontal radiograph. The Cobb angle is calculated by finding the proximal (*PEV*) and distal (*DEV*) end vertebrae; the vertebrae that are maximally tilted at the cranial and caudal portions of the curve being evaluated. Lines are drawn parallel to the superior endplate of the proximal end vertebrae and parallel to the inferior endplate of the of the distal end vertebrae; 90-degree perpendicular lines are then drawn for each of these lines so that they intersect. The angle created by these two intersecting lines is the Cobb angle. A Cobb angle should be obtained for each spinal curve.

caudal end vertebrae; 90-degree perpendicular lines are then drawn for each of these lines so that they intersect. The angle created by these two intersecting lines is the Cobb angle *(Fig. 66-3)*.[16] A Cobb angle measurement is obtained for each curve present. It is very important to make sure that positioning of the patient is consistent, because measurements have been shown to differ by more than 20% secondary to positioning variances.[17]

2. **The apical vertebral translation (AVT)** is the lateral displacement of the apex of a coronal curve relative to the center sacral vertical line (CSVL) on the frontal radiograph.[16] The CSVL is a line, on the frontal radiograph, perpendicular to the floor, drawn through the midline of the sacrum *(Fig. 66-4)*. The AVT is calculated as the horizontal distance between the CSVL and the centroid of the apex of the curve.

3. **Coronal balance** is measured on the frontal radiograph. A line, perpendicular to the floor, is drawn through the middle of the C7 vertebral body (C7 plumb line). Distance from the left edge of the radiograph to the C7 line (A) is measured as well as from the left edge of the radiograph to the CSVL (B). By convention, the coronal balance is measured using the formula coronal balance = A − B *(Fig. 66-5)*. A positive result is obtained for a coronal balance to the right and a negative balance for a displacement to the left.[16]

4. **Sagittal balance** is obtained from the lateral radiograph. Sagittal balance is the alignment of the C7 vertebral body to the posterior superior corner of the S1 segment. A line, perpendicular to the floor, is drawn from the center of the C7 vertebral body. The horizontal distance from the left edge of the radiograph to the C7 line is measured (A). A second line, perpendicular to the floor, is drawn through the posterior superior corner of the S1 segment. The horizontal distance between the left edge of the radiograph and this sacral line is measured (B). Sagittal balance is measured as A−B *(Fig. 66-6)*. A positive result (positive sagittal balance) is seen if the C7 line falls anterior to the sacral promontory. The C7 line should normally pass within ±2 cm of the posterior superior aspect of the sacrum (sacral promontory). Positive sagittal balance greater than 2 cm is more significantly associated with pain and disability than curve magnitude, curve location, or coronal imbalance.[18]

DIFFERENTIAL DIAGNOSIS

Scoliosis is not an imaging finding that has a wide differential. Scoliosis is simply a finding. The type of scoliosis can be discovered

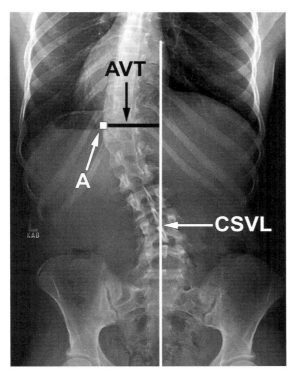

Figure 66-4 ▶ Apical Vertebral Translation. The apical vertebral translation (*AVT*) is obtained on the frontal radiograph. The AVT is the lateral displacement of the apex of a coronal curve relative to the center sacral vertical line (*CSVL*) on the frontal radiograph. The CSVL is obtained by drawing a line, perpendicular to the floor, through the midline of the sacrum. The AVT is calculated as the horizontal distance (*black line*) between the CSVL and the centroid of the apex of the curve (*A*).

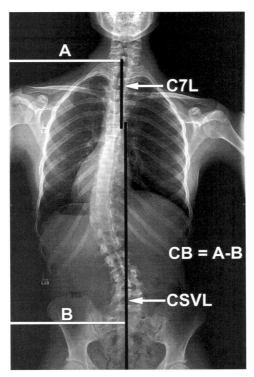

Figure 66-5 ▶ Coronal Balance. Coronal balance (*CB*) is obtained on the frontal radiograph. A line, perpendicular to the floor, is drawn through the middle of the C7 vertebral body (*C7L*). The center sacral vertical line (*CSVL*) is obtained by drawing a line, perpendicular to the floor, through the midline of the sacrum. Distance from the left edge of the radiograph to the C7L (*A*) is measured as well as from the left edge of the radiograph to the CSVL (*B*). By convention, the coronal balance is measured using the formula coronal balance = A − B. A positive result is obtained for a coronal balance to the right and a negative balance for a displacement to the left.

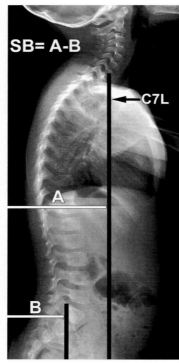

Figure 66-6 ▸ Sagittal Balance. Sagittal balance (*SB*) is obtained on the lateral radiograph. Sagittal balance is the alignment of the C7 vertebral body to the posterior superior corner of the S1 segment. A line, perpendicular to the floor, is drawn from the center of the C7 vertebral body (*C7L*). The horizontal distance from the left edge of the radiograph to the C7 line is measured (*A*). A second line, perpendicular to the floor is drawn through the posterior superior corner of the S1 segment. The horizontal distance between the left edge of the radiograph and this sacral line is measured (*B*). Sagittal balance is measured as A − B. A positive result (positive sagittal balance) is seen if the C7 line falls anterior to the sacral promontory. The C7 line should normally pass within ±2 cm of the posterior superior aspect of the sacrum.

based on the etiology, age at onset, and patient history or other disease processes or trauma.

1. **Congenital scoliosis**
2. **Idiopathic scoliosis**
3. **Scoliosis associated with other diseases and syndromes**
4. **Traumatic scoliosis**
5. **Degenerative scoliosis**

TREATMENT

1. **Bracing:** Bracing is performed to avoid spinal surgery. Bracing will not reduce the curve present, but can maintain the degree of curvature that is present. Bracing does not impact curves greater than 45 degrees. Bracing is used only in patients that have significant spinal growth remaining. Braces are worn nearly all day long and should be used for several years until the curve is stabilized. With strict bracing, curves can be limited to 5 degrees of progression in 75% of patients.[3]
2. **Surgery:** Curves greater than 45 degrees in patients with spinal growth remaining should be surgically corrected.[3] Patients with greater than 30 degrees of curvature at puberty should also be considered for surgery.[3] Adult degenerative scoliosis is surgically challenging given a complication rate of 56% to 75%.[19]

References

1. Cowell HR, Hall JN, MacEwen GD. Genetic aspects of idiopathic scoliosis: A Nicholas Andry award essay, 1970. *Clin Orthop Relat Res.* 1972;86: 121-131.
2. Birknes JK, White AP, Albert TJ, et al. Adult degenerative scoliosis: A review. *Neurosurgery.* 2008;63:94-103.
3. Van Goethem J, Van Campenhout A, van den Hauvve L, Parizel PM. Scoliosis. In: Van Goethem J, ed. *Neuroimaging Clinics of North America.* Elsevier; 2007;17:105-115.
4. McMaster M. Spinal growth and congenital deformity of the spine. *Spine.* 2006;31:2284-2287.
5. Fernandes P, Weinstein SL. Natural history of early onset scoliosis. *J Bone Joint Surg Am.* 2007;89:21-33.
6. Weinstein SL. Adolescent idiopathic scoliosis: Natural history. In: Weinstein SL, eds. *The Pediatric Spine: Principles and Practice.* ed 2. Philadelphia: Lippincott Williams & Wilkins; 2001:355-369.
7. Carr AJ. Adolescent idiopathic scoliosis in identical twins. *J Bone Joint Surg Br.* 1990;72:1077.
8. Kesling KL, Reinker KA. Scoliosis in twins: A meta-analysis of the literature and report of six cases. *Spine.* 1997;22:2009-2015.
9. Charles YP, Daures JP, de Rosa V, Diméglio A. Progression risk of idiopathic juvenile scoliosis during pubertal growth. *Spine.* 2006;31:1933-1942.
10. Lonstein JE, Carlosn JM. The prediction of curve progression in untreated idiopathic scoliosis during growth. *J Bone Joint Surg.* 1984;667:1061-1071.
11. Milbrandt TA, Johnston CE II. Down syndrome and scoliosis: A review of 50-year experience at one institution. *Spine.* 2005;30:2051-2055.
12. Spiegel DA, Flynn JM, Stasikelis PJ, et al. Scoliotic curve patterns in patients with Chiari I malformation and/or syringomyelia. *Spine.* 2003;28: 2139-2146.

13. Morcuende JA, Dolan LA, Vazquez JD, et al. A prognostic model for the presence of neurogenic lesions in atypical idiopathic scoliosis. *Spine.* 2004;29:51-58.
14. Aebi M. The adult scoliosis. *Eur Spine J.* 2005;14:925-948.
15. Tribus CB. Degenerative lumbar scoliosis: evaluation and management. *J Am Acad Orthop Surg.* 2003;11:174-183.
16. Angevine PD, Kaiser MG. Radiographic measurement techniques. *Neurosurgery.* 2008;63:40-45.
17. Gocen S, Havitcioglu H. Effect on rotation on frontal plane deformity in idiopathic scoliosis. *Orthopedics.* 2001;24:265-268.
18. Glassman SD, Bridwell K, Dimar JR. The impact of positive sagittal balance in adult spinal deformity. *Spine.* 2005;30:2024-2029.
19. Akbarnia BA, Ogilvie JW, Hammerberg KW. Debate: Degenerative scoliosis: to operate or not to operate. *Spine.* 2006;31:S195-S201.

SPINAL CORD CAVERNOUS ANGIOMA

Leo F. Czervionke, M.D.

CLINICAL PRESENTATION

The patient is a 70-year-old woman with a long history of progressive neck pain and bilateral shoulder pain, right more than left, and right arm numbness. She has a mild gait disturbance requiring use of a cane. She underwent right rotator cuff surgery 7 months prior, with no improvement in symptoms. In fact, the neck and right shoulder pain has progressively worsened since the surgery. She has moderate right deltoid and biceps weakness on physical examination.

IMAGING PRESENTATION

Magnetic resonance (MR) imaging reveals an ovoid lesion in the posterior portion of the spinal cord at the C4-5 level associated with mild cord enlargement *(Fig. 67-1)*. The lesion is T2 hyperintense centrally and surrounded by a well-defined region of T2 hypointensity *(Figs. 67-1 and 67-2)*. The lesion is slightly hyperintense at its periphery on T1-weighted images *(Fig. 67-3)* and displays subtle enhancement after administration of IV paramagnetic contrast agent *(Fig. 67-4)*. The imaging appearance is classic for a spinal cord cavernous angioma (cavernoma).

DISCUSSION

Cavernous malformations are also called *cavernous malformations, cavernous hemangiomas, cavernomas, "cryptic" malformations,* or *angiographically occult vascular malformations*.[1] Cavernous angiomas are uncommon spinal cord lesions, comprising 5% of intramedullary cord lesions.[2] These lesions commonly occur in the brain and much less commonly in the spinal cord.[3] Half of the cases arise in the cervical cord and the other half in the thoracic cord *(Figs. 67-5 to 67-7)*, or in the conus medullaris. They are more common in females and usually manifest in young to middle-aged adults. Cavernous angiomas can be isolated lesions or can be one of multiple lesions occurring in the brain and spinal cord. Up to 40% of patients with spinal cord cavernous angiomas have at least one brain cavernous angioma.[4] Multiple brain and cord cavernous angiomas may occur sporadically or can be associated with a familial syndrome that is autosomal dominant with variable penetrance in a minority of cases.[4,5] In familial cases, spinal cord cavernomas may coexist with cavernomas in the brain, retina, and skin as well as cavernous hemangiomas in the vertebral bodies.[5] Cavernous angiomas manifesting in the pediatric patient are more likely to manifest with acute symptoms, more likely to hemorrhage, and

more likely to be familial.[1] Up to 50% of pediatric patients with spinal cord cavernomas have associated hemorrhage.[1] Rarely, spinal cord angiomas can occur in patients with Klippel-Trénaunay-Weber syndrome.[6]

Cavernous angiomas in adults usually manifest clinically with slowly evolving sensory or motor deficits or slowly progressive myelopathy that may progress to paraparesis. Up to 40% of patients with intramedullary cavernous angiomas report episodes of neck, back, or extremity pain.[7] Acute onset of symptoms is most commonly associated with hemorrhage.[8] If the lesion hemorrhages, all symptoms tend to be accentuated, including acute onset of neck, back, or extremity pain, and paraplegia or quadriplegia may develop.[7,9] Rarely, patients with cervical cord cavernomas present with shoulder or upper arm pain and a coexistent neurologic "itch."[2] Uncommonly, patients with spinal cord cavernomas present with sudden onset of symptoms with rapid progression of neurologic deficits, especially if acute hemorrhage occurs. However, the majority of cord cavernomas do not have a frank hemorrhagic episode, even when followed over many years.[10] If hemorrhage does occur and the blood leaks into the subarachnoid space, they may present with symptoms of subarachnoid hemorrhage, and these patients can eventually develop superficial siderosis. Rarely, hemorrhage from a cervical cord cavernous hemangioma can cause a Brown-Séquard syndrome.[11]

Cavernous angiomas grossly are well-circumscribed, ovoid or lobulated lesions, composed of vascular sinusoids interspersed with connective tissue, but no neural tissue is located between the vascular channels,[12] as is the case with capillary telangiectasias. The vascular channels are lined by a single layer of endothelial cells. The walls of these sinusoidal channels resemble neither veins nor arteries, lacking smooth muscle and elastin. The nidus of the angioma contains blood metabolites in different stages of evolution and thrombosis.[3] Calcification may occur in spinal cavernomas but is more common in brain cavernous malformations. There is no true capsule surrounding a cavernous angioma. The tissue at the margins of the cavernoma is gliotic and contains hemosiderin-laden macrophages and calcification in varying amounts.[3]

IMAGING FEATURES

MR imaging is the modality of choice for detecting and following spinal cord cavernous angiomas. The entire spinal cord and brain should be imaged with MRI if a cavernous angioma is detected because multiple cavernomas are common.[1] The MRI appearance is classic and the same as those cavernomas that occur in the brain.[9] The typical cavernoma is ovoid, fairly well defined, containing a

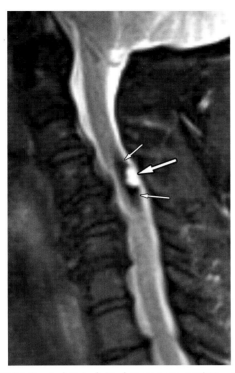

Figure 67-1 ► **Cervical Spinal Cord Cavernous Angioma C4-5 Level.** Sagittal fat-saturated T2-weighted image. T2 hyperintense focus (*long arrow*) positioned along dorsal surface of cord, which appears slightly enlarged. Peripheral T2 hypointense hemosiderin (*short arrows*) in cord adjacent to focal hyperintensity.

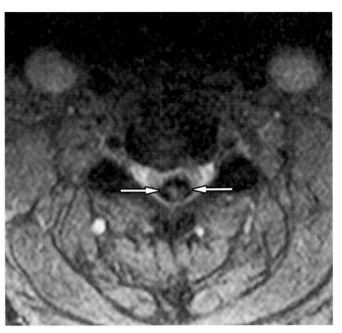

Figure 67-2 ► **Cervical Spinal Cord Cavernous Angioma C4-5 Level.** Axial Gradient echo image C4-5 level in same patient as in Figure 67-1. Small central hyperintense focus surrounded by hemosiderin ring (*arrows*) in posterior portion of cord.

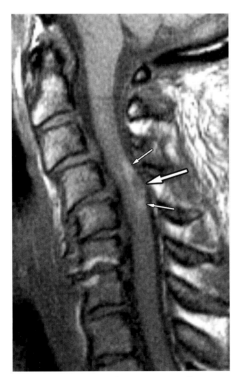

Figure 67-3 ► **Cervical Spinal Cord Cavernous Angioma C4-5 level.** Same patient as in Figures 67-1 to 67-2. T1-weighted sagittal image. T1 hypointense focus (*long arrow*) with T1 hyperintense region (*short arrows*) likely represent subacute blood metabolites.

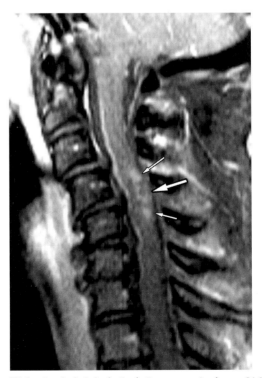

Figure 67-4 ► **Cervical Spinal Cord Cavernous Angioma C4-5 level.** Corresponding T1-weighted sagittal image following IV contrast, in same patient as in Figures 67-1 to 67-3. The cord lesion centrally (*long arrow*) and peripherally (*short arrows*) enhances slightly with contrast.

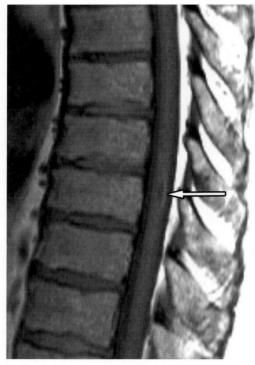

Figure 67-5 ▶ Thoracic Spinal Cord Cavernous Angioma. T1-weighted sagittal image. Small ovoid T1 hypointense intramedullary lesion (*arrow*). contains a tiny T1 hyperintense focus.

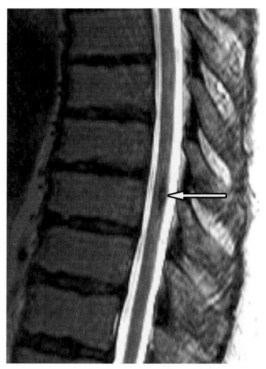

Figure 67-6 ▶ Thoracic Spinal Cord Cavernous Angioma. Corresponding sagittal T2-weighted sagittal image to Figure 67-5. Tiny T2 hyperintense central focus (*arrow*) surrounded by T2 hypointense zone. No associated cord enlargement.

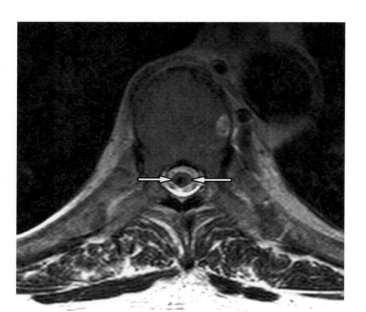

Figure 67-7 ▶ Thoracic Spinal Cord Cavernous Angioma. T2-weighted axial image through lesion shown in Figure 67-1. The cavernoma (*arrows*) is seen as a T2 hypointense "bull's eye" in the center of the thoracic spinal cord.

focal or speckled T1 and T2 hyperintense central region surrounded by a rim of T2 hypointensity representing hemosiderin deposition in macrophages on the surface of the lesion (see Figs. 67-1 to 67-4).[3] Some spinal cord cavernous angiomas contain a T1 hypointense focus (see Fig. 67-5) that is hyperintense on

T2-weighted MR images (see Fig. 67-6). A hypointense rim that is usually apparent on T2-weighted images (see Figs. 67-1, 67-6 and 67-7). This hypointense rim is characteristically more conspicuous on gradient echo MR images (see Fig. 67-2).[9,13] The hemosiderin ring is most often secondary to blood pigments chronically leeching out of the vascular sinusoids into the surrounding tissues where it is consumed by macrophages.[3] Edema surrounding the cord cavernoma is rarely seen unless a recent hemorrhage has occurred. Cavernous angiomas may or may not enhance after IV contrast. When enhancement does occur, the intensity of enhancement tends to be minimal (see Fig. 67-4). Vascular flow voids are typically not observed in cavernous angiomas.

DIFFERENTIAL DIAGNOSIS

The imaging appearance of cavernous malformations is quite characteristic.[12] However, the following disorders should be considered when the classic MRI appearance of a cord cavernoma is observed:

1. **Intramedullary Arterial-Venous Malformation (AVM):** Look for a cluster of flow voids within the cord representing the vascular nidus of the AVM (*Figs.* 67-7 and *67-8*).
2. **Ependymoma:** Commonly contains an area of hemorrhage or hemosiderin deposition at the inferior or superior pole of the intramedullary tumor. Astrocytomas are less likely to contain hemorrhage.
3. **Hemangioblastoma:** Can be associated with hypervascularity and hemorrhage. Look for intensely enhancing intramedullary nodule-associated syrinx cavity that frequently accompanies these tumors. Cord edema, adjacent to the enhancing lesion, is a common finding.

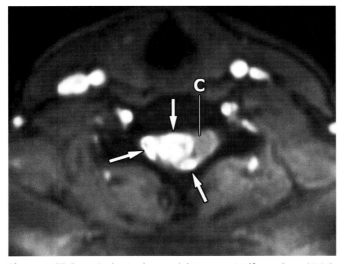

Figure 67-8 ▶ Spinal Cord Arterial-Venous Malformation (AVM). Sagittal T1-weighted image through cervical cord. No IV contrast. Serpentine T1 hypointense vessels (*arrows*) display signal "flow void" represent intramedullary AVM nidus in the lower cervical cord.

Figure 67-9 ▶ Spinal Cord Arterial-Venous Malformation (AVM). Corresponding to Figure 65-8, axial gradient echo image obtained through cord AVM at C5-6 level. No IV contrast. The AVM nidus within the cord has a hyperintense vascular nidus (*arrows*), similar to the intensity of other vessels elsewhere in the neck soft tissues. The normal portion of the spinal cord (C) is displaced to the left of midline.

4. **Intramedullary metastasis**: Extensive edema often is out of proportion to the size of the enhancing mass. Associated hemorrhage is rare.

5. **Multiple sclerosis (MS)**: Patients with MS and spinal cord cavernous angiomas may present with similar clinical features,[8,9] but these disorders can be differentiated with MR imaging, because MS plaques lack significant T1 hyperintensity and have no T2 hypointense rim because hemosiderin is not present in MS plaques.

TREATMENT

1. **No treatment:** If asymptomatic, a conservative approach is taken. The cord lesion is followed with sequential MR imaging.[10]

2. **Carefully considered treatment:** Complete resection of the cord cavernoma can be achieved in most patients using microsurgical techniques, especially when the lesion abuts the posterior surface of the spinal cord (see Figs. 67-1 and 67-6), damage to the cord at surgery then being less likely.[8,12] The chance of cord hemorrhage is nearly eliminated by complete excision of the cord lesion.[14] However, clinical improvement postoperatively varies.[1,14] In a study of pediatric patients with spinal cord cavernomas, 83% of patients with neurologic deficits either improved or stabilized after surgery.[1] There is often a transient worsening of motor symptoms in the immediate postoperative period, which usually resolves. Surgery may or may not alleviate the pain that may accompany spinal cord cavernous angiomas.[7]

References

1. Deutsch H, Shrivistava R, Epstein F, Jallo GI. Pediatric intramedullary spinal cavernous malformations. *Spine.* 2001;26:E427-431.
2. Dey DD, Landrum O, Oaklander AL. Central neuropathic itch from spinal-cord cavernous hemangioma: A human case, a possible animal model, and hypotheses about pathogenesis. *Pain.* 2005;113:233-237.
3. Fontaine S, Melanson D, Cosgrove R, Bertrand G. Cavernous hemangiomas of the spinal cord: MR imaging. *Radiology.* 1988;166:839-841.
4. Cohen-Gadol AA, Jacob JT, Edwards DA, Krauss WE. Coexistence of intracranial and spinal cavernous malformations: A study of prevalence and natural history. *J Neurosurg.* 2006;104:376-381.
5. Toldo I, Drigo P, Mammi I, et al. Vertebral and spinal cavernous angiomas associated with familial cerebral cavernous malformation. *Surg Neurol.* 2009;71:167-171.
6. Pichierri A, Piccirilli M, Passacantilli E, et al. Klippel-Trénaunay-Weber syndrome and intramedullary cervical cavernoma: A very rare association. Case report. *Surg Neurol.* 2006;66:203-206; discussion 206.
7. Kim LJ, Klopfenstein JD, Zabramski JM, et al. Analysis of pain resolution after surgical resection of intramedullary spinal cord cavernous malformations. *Neurosurgery.* 2006;58:106-111; discussion 106-111.
8. Labauge P, Bouly S, Parker F, et al. Outcome in 53 patients with spinal cord cavernomas. *Surg Neurol.* 2008;70:176-181; discussion 181.
9. Chabert E, Morandi X, Carney MP, et al. Intramedullary cavernous malformations. *J Neuroradiol.* 1999;26:262-268.
10. Kharkar S, Shuck J, Conway J, Rigamonti D. The natural history of conservatively managed symptomatic intramedullary spinal cord cavernomas. *Neurosurgery.* 2007;60:865-872; discussion 865-872.
11. Mathews MS, Peck WW, Brant-Zawadzki M. Brown-Sequard syndrome secondary to spontaneous bleed from postradiation cavernous angiomas. *AJNR Am J Neuroradiol.* 2008;29:1989-1990.
12. Weinzierl MR, Krings T, Korinth MC, et al. MRI and intraoperative findings in cavernous haemangiomas of the spinal cord. *Neuroradiology.* 2004;46:65-71.
13. Maeda K, Kawai H, Sanada M. Thoracic cavernous malformations on T2*-weighted MR images. *Intern Med.* 2008;47:1073-1074.
14. Santoro A, Piccirilli M, Frati A, et al. Intramedullary spinal cord cavernous malformations: Report of ten new cases. *Neurosurg Rev.* 2004;27:93-98.

SPINAL CORD GLIOMA

Leo F. Czervionke, M.D.

CLINICAL PRESENTATION

The patient is a 62-year-old man with 3-year history of progressive neck pain, low back pain, bilateral shoulder pain, proximal muscle pain and weakness, and paresthesias. The patient had difficulty elevating his upper extremities on physical examination. The initial clinical diagnosis was cervical and lumbar osteoarthritis, shoulder capsulitis and bursitis, and possible fibromyalgia.

IMAGING PRESENTATION

Magnetic resonance (MR) imaging revealed a diffuse expansile process involving the medulla and cervical spinal cord extending inferiorly to approximately the C5 level. The intramedullary process is T1 isointense and T2 hyperintense, with no distinct margins between the abnormal process and the normal spinal cord (*Figs. 68-1 and 68-2*). There were no areas of contrast enhancement visible within the lesion (*Fig. 68-3*).

DISCUSSION

Only 5% of spine tumors are intramedullary in location.[1] However, 90% of all intramedullary cord tumors are gliomas, either astrocytomas or ependymomas.[2] In adults, 60% of these are ependymomas and approximately 30% are astrocytomas.[3] Hemangioblastoma is the third most common intramedullary tumor,[4] accounting for approximately 5%. Intramedullary metastases comprise 4% of intramedullary tumors. Ganglioglioma, oligodendroglioma, xanthoastrocytoma, paraganglioma, primitive neuroectodermal tumor (PNET), and lymphoma can also arise within the spinal cord but are rare.[4]

Intramedullary spinal cord astrocytoma is the most common intramedullary tumor in a child and the second most common intramedullary tumor in an adult. In children, 60% of intramedullary tumors are astrocytomas.[1] These tumors range from WHO (World Health Organization) grade 1 to grade 4; 90 % of intramedullary astrocytomas are low-grade tumors (grade 1 or 2). WHO grade 1 astrocytomas are usually pilocytic astrocytomas and typically involve the spinal cord over multiple vertebral segments and may involve the entire spinal cord.[5] The majority of intramedullary astrocytomas are WHO grade 2 fibrillary astrocytomas. WHO grade 3 and grade 4 tumors are uncommon, representing less than 10% of intramedullary gliomas. Most high-grade astrocytomas are

WHO grade 3 anaplastic astrocytomas. WHO grade 4 cord astrocytoma, glioblastoma multiforme, is rare. The 5-year survival rate for cord astrocytoma is 75% to 80% for low-grade tumors, and the prognosis for high-grade tumors is extremely poor.[4,6-8] Pilocytic astrocytomas have the best prognosis.[9]

Cellular ependymomas are the most common subtype; these are malignant tumors, usually classified as WHO grade 2, but sometimes as grade 3. Anaplastic (WHO grade III) ependymomas have a tendency to disseminate throughout the central nervous system (CNS), often depositing tumors in multiple locations within the spinal canal, resulting in so called *drop metastases*. Intracranial seeding from spinal cord gliomas rarely occurs.[10,11]

Intramedullary gliomas most commonly arise in the cervical cord, and less frequently in the thoracic spinal cord; 50% of cord astrocytomas occur in the upper thoracic cord.[2] Ependymomas can occur throughout the cord. The myxopapillary ependymoma is the most common tumor occurring in the conus/cauda equina region. Cord astrocytomas and ependymomas usually have a slow, insidious clinical onset with myelopathy, neck pain, and stiffness, and may cause scoliosis in a child, adolescent, or young adult. These patients may present with progressive paraparesis and paresthesias. In children, back or neck pain and lower extremity paresis are the most common manifesting symptoms. Gait disturbance, occipital headache,[12] kyphoscoliosis, torticollis,[13] and bladder/bowel dysfunction may also occur.

There are six histologic subtypes of ependymomas: cellular (most common type), papillary, clear cell, tanycytic, myxopapillary, and melanotic (the least common).[4] Ependymomas histologically display characteristic perivascular pseudorosettes or less commonly perivascular rosettes.[4,14] Cord gliomas may have positive immunohistochemical markers including GFAP (glial fibrillary acid protein), S-100 protein, and synaptophysin.[15] Mitoses are usually lacking in ependymomas. Astrocytomas have variable mitoses and usually high cellularity. Rosenthal fibers and hyalinized vessels are characteristically present in pilocytic astrocytomas.

IMAGING FEATURES

It may not be possible to differentiate an intramedullary astrocytoma from an ependymoma based on imaging features alone. Both can cause enlargement of the spinal canal, visible on radiographs. Tumoral cysts may be associated with spinal cord astrocytoma or ependymoma, but are more commonly associated with

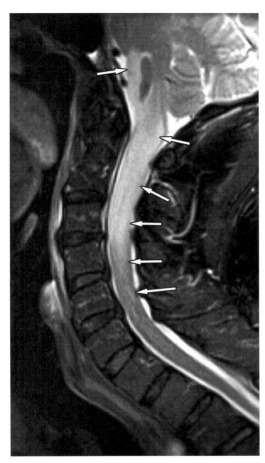

Figure 68-1 ▸ Spinal Cord and Brainstem Astrocytoma. T2-weighted sagittal image. The tumor is represented as an ill-defined region of T2 hyperintensity (*arrows*) that involves the medulla and majority of the cervical spinal cord to approximately the C6 level. The lower extent of the tumor is not well defined.

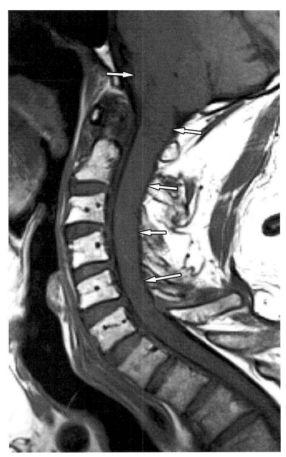

Figure 68-2 ▸ Diffuse Cervical-medullary Astrocytoma. (Same patient as in Fig. 68-1.) Sagittal T1-weighted image. The medulla and upper cervical cord are enlarged and slightly T1 hypointense by diffusely infiltrating tumor (*arrows*), but no localized mass lesion is demonstrated.

ependymoma, typically occurring rostral or caudal to the solid, enhancing portion of the tumor (*Figs. 68-4 to 68-6*).

Syringohydromyelia is often associated with intramedullary gliomas, more common with ependymomas. The extent of the hydromyelic cavity is often much greater than the extent of the actual tumor. The margins of the syrinx do not enhance (*Fig. 68-7*).[6] The syrinx usually involutes after removal of the tumor.[1]

Hemorrhage may occur in astrocytomas or ependymomas but is much more common in spinal cord ependymoma, the hemorrhage typically occurring rostral or caudal to the enhancing portion of the tumor (see Figs. 68-4 and 68-6).[14,16] Astrocytomas and ependymomas both cause fusiform cord expansion and are usually isointense to hypointense on T1-weighted images and usually hyperintense on proton density or T2-weighted images (see Figs. 68-1 to 68-6).[4,6] These tumors usually extend cephalocaudally two to four vertebral segments, but can involve the cord over many vertebral segments, especially pilocytic astrocytomas, which can involve the entire spinal cord.[17] A portion of the intramedullary glioma usually enhances after IV contrast administration (*Figs. 68-6 and 68-8*).

Astrocytomas tend to be more eccentrically located in the cord, display patchy enhancement, and the margins of the enhancing region tends to be ill-defined.[4] A minority of low-grade

astrocytomas do not enhance with contrast (see Fig. 68-3).[18] Ependymomas are typically centrally located in the cord and almost always contain an ovoid, well-defined region of intense contrast enhancement within the T2 hyperintense tumor (see Fig. 68-8).[14,16,19] Ependymomas can be a cause of subarachnoid hemorrhage and subsequently superficial siderosis.[4] Intramedullary spinal cord ependymomas may occur in patients with type 2 neurofibromatosis,[4] along with intracranial schwannomas and meningiomas.

DIFFERENTIAL DIAGNOSIS

1. **Spinal cord metastasis:** Intramedullary metastases most commonly arise from primary lung or breast tumors.[20] Intramedullary metastases may occur anywhere in the cervical cord, but more commonly arise in the lower thoracic cord or conus medullaris. Associated spinal cord edema is usually out of proportion to the size of the enhancing intramedullary metastasis (*Fig. 68-9*).[20] Look for other metastases in the vertebrae.

2. **Transverse myelitis:** Can simulate an intramedullary tumor (*Fig. 68-10*). The cord is enlarged by T2 hyperintense edema

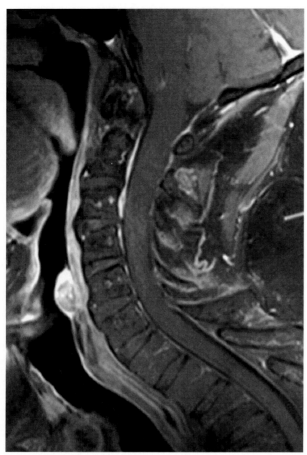

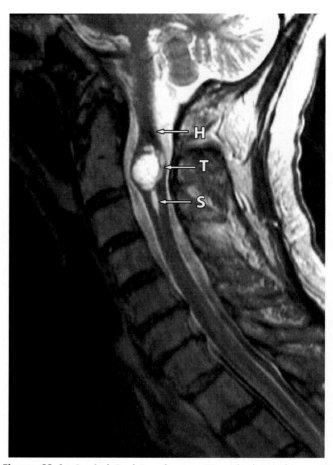

Figure 68-3 ► Diffuse Cervical-medullary Astrocytoma. (Same patient as in Fig. 68-1.) Sagittal contrast-enhanced, T1-weighted image acquired with fat saturation. The tumor causes diffuse enlargement of the cervical spinal cord but does not enhance after IV contrast.

Figure 68-4 ► Cervical Cord Ependymoma. T2-weighted sagittal image. T2 hyperintense cystlike tumor (*T*) expands the cervical cord. A linear cyst or syrinx cavity (*S*) extends below the tumor. T2 hypointense old blood metabolites, likely hemosiderin (*H*), located superior to intramedullary tumor.

and may or may not contain an ovoid area of enhancement.[20] Several viral agents can produce this appearance, including HIV, which causes a so called *vacuolar myelopathy/myelitis*. Myelitis may involve the cervical or thoracic cord.

3. **Neuromyelitis optica (Devic's disease):** This condition has an imaging appearance that may simulate an intramedullary tumor or transverse myelitis. A more rapid clinical onset with visual disturbance secondary to optic neuritis is characteristic of neuromyelitis optica. Multiple sclerosis or acute disseminated encephalomyelitis (ADEM) can manifest with multiple focal lesions in the cord, but these usually are more widely scattered and less *tumor-like* in appearance.[20] Look for other demyelinating periventricular lesions in the brain, but brain lesions are not always present along with demyelinating cord lesions. Multiple sclerosis is a multi-episodic, remitting illness. ADEM is a monophasic disorder clinically.

4. **Hemangioblastoma:** May manifest as a small intramedullary mass within the cord but more commonly is an intensely enhancing pial-based mass on the surface of the spinal cord. Tumor recurrence is common and often manifests as multiple pial-based nodules.

5. **Granulomatous disease:** Sarcoidosis and syphilis can involve the spinal cord, simulating the imaging appearance of an intramedullary glioma.

6. **Cord infarction:** Sudden onset of acute myelopathy, often in a patient with diabetes, endocarditis, or prior aortic graft or stent placement. Cord infarctions most commonly occur in the lower thoracic cord.

7. **Atrioventricular (AV) malformation:** Intramedullary cord AV malformations are rare. Look for a tangle of vessels within the cord displaying flow voids on MRI. Cavernous hemangioma (cavernous angioma) can occur in the cervical or thoracic spinal cord and have MRI signal characteristics identical to those cavernomas that occur commonly in the brain with a central T1 hyperintense nidus (extracellular methemoglobin) surrounded by a T2 hypointense rim (hemosiderin).

TREATMENT

1. **Watchful waiting:** Often, no treatment is given initially. Patients should be followed with clinical examination and MR imaging to assess for tumor progression.

2. **Surgical biopsy:** May be performed for tissue diagnosis.

3. **Microsurgical resection:** May be considered for low-grade tumors, with intraoperative ultrasound and evoked potentials.[6] Diffusion tensor imaging of the spinal cord with fiber
Text continued on page 518

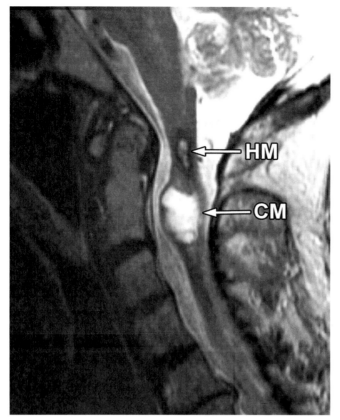

Figure 68-5 ► **Cervical Cord Ependymoma.** (Same patient as in Fig. 68-4.) T2-weighted parasagittal image. T2 hyperintense cystic expansile intramedullary mass (*CM*). Mixed intensity (centrally hyperintense and peripherally hypointense) old hemorrhagic metabolites (*HM*), located superior to the intramedullary tumor.

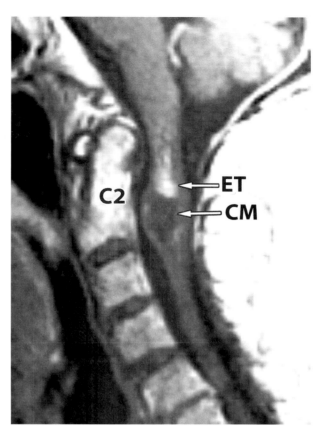

Figure 68-6 ► **Cervical Cord Ependymoma.** Parasagittal T1-weighted image corresponding to Figure 68-5 reveals small enhancing solid tumor (*ET*) superior to nonenhancing T1 hypointense predominantly cystlike mass (*CM*) at the C2 vertebral level.

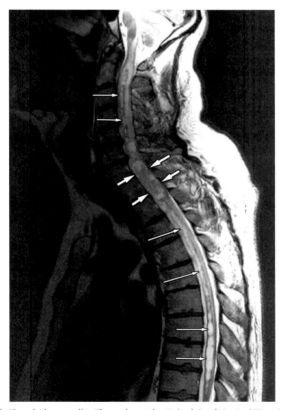

Figure 68-7 ► **Ependymoma Associated with Signal Abnormality Throughout the Spinal Cord.** Sagittal T2-weighted image. The tumor is an ovoid mass (*thick short arrows*) within the cord extending from the C7 to T2 level. A lobulated hydromyelic cavity of variable size (*long thin arrows*) extends above and below the tumor in the upper cervical cord and throughout much of the thoracic spinal cord. The T2 hyperintensity adjacent to the hydromyelic cavity represents cord edema that extends the length of the spinal cord.

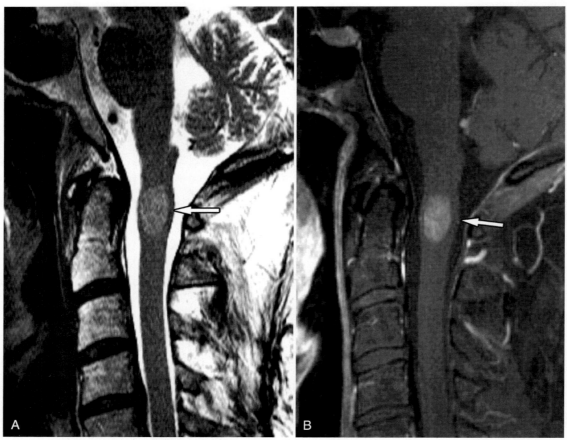

Figure 68-8 ▶ Small Well-Circumscribed Ependymoma in Upper Cervical Cord. Well-defined homogeneous T2 hyperintense slightly expansile mass (*arrow*) in spinal cord on sagittal T1-weighted image **A** and on contrast-enhanced image **B**. No associated cyst or hemorrhage.

Figure 68-9 ▶ Spinal Cord Metastasis in Patient with Lung Carcinoma. On sagittal T2-weighted MR image **A**, the spinal cord is diffusely enlarged and contains a T2 hypointense intramedullary mass (*long arrow*) at the C6-7 level. A large amount of edema (*short arrows*) involves the spinal cord for many levels above and below the intramedullary tumor. On sagittal contrast-enhanced, fat-saturated, T1-weighted MR image **B**, the intramedullary cord metastasis enhances in a concentric ringlike or *target* pattern (*arrow*). Edematous portions of the spinal cord do not enhance.

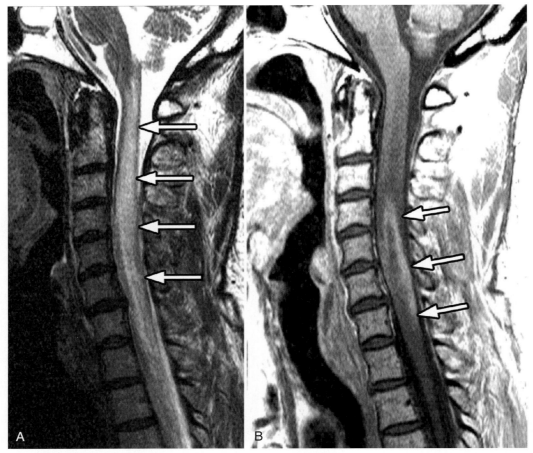

Figure 68-10 ▶ **Probable Transverse Myelitis.** On axial T2-weighted MR image **A**, the cervical spinal cord is enlarged and is T2 hyperintense (*arrows*) because of edema throughout the cervical spinal cord. On contrast-enhanced, T1-weighted MR image **B**, a fusiform contrast-enhancing lesion (*arrows*) is located in the spinal cord from C4 to C7 level. A similar imaging appearance may be seen in neuromyelitis optica. The patient had no evidence of optic neuritis on clinical examination or by imaging. The cord lesion resolved almost completely within 10 days.

tracking may have some value for presurgical planning, but its role is not clearly established.[21,22]

4. **Radiotherapy and chemotherapy:** The role of radiotherapy and chemotherapy is controversial.[7] Adjuvant radiotherapy and chemotherapy is often used for higher grade astrocytomas, but their role in treatment of ependymoma is not clear.[23] Radiotherapy after surgery does not improve outcome in pilocytic astrocytoma, but may improve survival in patients with higher grade astrocytomas.[9] Postradiation necrosis is a potential complication of spinal cord radiotherapy and can simulate recurrent tumor.[24] Several chemotherapeutic agents have been used in treatment of high-grade astrocytomas.[23] Temozolomide has been used in the management of progressive recurrent low-grade spinal cord astrocytomas with favorable results in some cases.[25]

References

1. Baleriaux DL. Spinal cord tumors. *Eur Radiol*. 1999;9:1252-1258.
2. Brinar M, Rados M, Habek M, Poser CM. Enlargement of the spinal cord: Inflammation or neoplasm? [see comment]. *Clin Neurol Neurosurg*. 2006;108:284-289.
3. Afshani E, Kuhn JP. Common causes of low back pain in children. *Radiographics*. 1991;11:269-291.
4. Koeller KK, Rosenblum RS, Morrison AL. Neoplasms of the spinal cord and filum terminale: Radiologic-pathologic correlation. *Radiographics*. 2000;20:1721-1749.
5. Schittenhelm J, Ebner FH, Tatagiba M, et al. Holocord pilocytic astrocytoma: Case report and review of the literature. *Clin Neurol Neurosurg*. 2009;111:203-207.
6. Houten JK, Cooper PR. Spinal cord astrocytomas: Presentation, management and outcome. *J Neurooncol*. 2000;47:219-224.
7. Innocenzi G, Salvati M, Cervoni L, et al. Prognostic factors in intramedullary astrocytomas. *Clinical Neurology & Neurosurgery*. 1997;99:1-5.
8. Kopelson G, Linggood RM. Intramedullary spinal cord astrocytoma versus glioblastoma: The prognostic importance of histologic grade. *Cancer*. 1982;50:732-735.
9. Minehan KJ, Brown PD, Scheithauer BW, et al. Prognosis and treatment of spinal cord astrocytoma. *Int J Radiat Oncol, Biol, Phys*. 2009;73:727-733.
10. Hely M, Fryer J, Selby G. Intramedullary spinal cord glioma with intracranial seeding. *J Neurol Neurosurg Psych*. 1985;48:302-309.
11. Peraud A, Herms J, Schlegel J, et al. Recurrent spinal cord astrocytoma with intraventricular seeding. *Childs Nerv Syst*. 2004;20:114-118.
12. Tsutsumi S, Higo T, Kondo A, et al. Atypical cervical astrocytoma manifesting as occipitalgia. *Neurologia Medico-Chirurgica*. 2007;47:371-374.
13. Kumandas S, Per H, Gumus H, et al. Torticollis secondary to posterior fossa and cervical spinal cord tumors: report of five cases and literature review. *Neurosurg Rev*. 2006;29:333-338; discussion 338.
14. Kahan H, Sklar EM, Post MJ, Bruce JH. MR characteristics of histopathologic subtypes of spinal ependymoma. *AJNR Am J Neuroradiol*. 1996;17:143-150.
15. Santi M, Mena H, Wong K, et al. Spinal cord malignant astrocytomas: Clinicopathologic features in 36 cases. *Cancer*. 2003;98:554-561.

16. Nemoto Y, Inoue Y, Tashiro T, et al. Intramedullary spinal cord tumors: Significance of associated hemorrhage at MR imaging. *Radiology.* 1992;182: 793-796.

17. Mauser HW, Dokkum TA. Astrocytomas involving the whole spinal cord: Two case reports. *Clinical Neurology & Neurosurgery.* 1981;83: 239-245.

18. Larson DB, Hedlund GL. Non-enhancing pilocytic astrocytoma of the spinal cord. *Pediatric Radiology.* 2006;36:1312-1315.

19. Fine MJ, Kricheff II, Freed D, Epstein FJ. Spinal cord ependymomas: MR imaging features. *Radiology.* 1995;197:655-658.

20. Bourgouin PM, Lesage J, Fontaine S, et al. A pattern approach to the differential diagnosis of intramedullary spinal cord lesions on MR imaging. *AJR Am J Roentgenol.* 1998;170:1645-1649.

21. Ducreux D, Lepeintre JF, Fillard P, et al. MR diffusion tensor imaging and fiber tracking in 5 spinal cord astrocytomas. *AJNR: Am J Neuroradiol.* 2006;27:214-216.

22. Vargas MI, Delavelle J, Jlassi H, et al. Clinical applications of diffusion tensor tractography of the spinal cord. *Neuroradiology.* 2008;50:25-29.

23. Nishio S, Morioka T, Fujii K, et al. Spinal cord gliomas: Management and outcome with reference to adjuvant therapy. *J Clin Neurosci.* 2000;7:20-23.

24. Phuphanich S, Jacobs M, Murtagh FR, Gonzalvo A. MRI of spinal cord radiation necrosis simulating recurrent cervical cord astrocytoma and syringomyelia. *Surg Neurol.* 1996;45:362-365.

25. Chamoun RB, Alaraj AM, Al Kutoubi AO, et al. Role of temozolomide in spinal cord low grade astrocytomas: Results in two paediatric patients. *Acta Neurochirurgica.* 2006;148:175-179; discussion 180.

SPINAL CORD INFARCTION

Leo F. Czervionke, M.D.

CLINICAL PRESENTATION

The patient is a 70-year-old man who had open surgical repair of an abdominal aortic aneurysm with bilateral aortoiliac bypass graft, bypass of the right renal, and surgical exploration of the superior mesenteric artery. The patient had a hypotensive episode during the surgical procedure. He awoke from anesthesia with flaccid paralysis of both lower extremities and diminished sensation to pinprick at the T11 level. He reported abdominal pain but no back pain or lower extremity pain. A magnetic resonance (MR) image was obtained to rule out either epidural hematoma or spinal cord infarction.

IMAGING PRESENTATION

MR imaging revealed a region of abnormal T2 signal hyperintensity involving gray matter in the central portion of the lower spinal cord extending from the T9 level to the L1 level consistent with acute anterior spinal artery territory infarction *(Figs. 69-1 and 69-2)*.

DISCUSSION

Spinal cord transient ischemic attacks or infarction occur when the blood supply to the spinal cord is compromised.[1] Infarction most often occurs in the lower thoracic spinal cord. The precise etiology is not always known, but a variety of conditions can predispose to spinal cord infarction including aortic or vertebral atherosclerotic disease, aortic dissection, after aortic surgery, aortic stenting, cardioembolic disease, arteritis, cocaine usage, coagulopathy, lupus erythematosus, sickle cell disease, hypotensive episode, spinal infection, sepsis, after spinal cord trauma, and decompression sickness.[1-7] Smoking, diabetes, atherosclerotic disease, and hypertension are believed to be predisposing factors in many patients who develop spinal cord infarction. Cervical osteophytosis and spinal cord ischemia can also result from spinal atrioventricular (AV) fistula or AV malformation, which shunt blood from the spinal cord parenchyma. Spinal cord infarction can occur rarely after spinal surgery[2] or during embolization of spinal AV fistulas.[8] Spinal cord infarction rarely occurs as a complication of epidural anesthesia or epidural catheter placement.[9] Rare cases of cord infarction may be associated with disc herniation.[10] A case of spinal cord infarction secondary to fibrocartilaginous embolization of the

nucleus pulposus has been reported.[11] Despite the many possible causes of spinal cord infarctions, some patients with spinal cord infarction have no known cause or apparent risk factors.

Percutaneous spinal interventional procedures, including epidural injections, celiac plexus blocks, transforaminal epidural injection, or nerve blocks may predispose to AV fistula formation in some cases. Possible etiologies for iatrogenic AV fistula formation include inadvertent injection of the anesthetic and/or steroidal agent into a radiculomedullary artery, injection-related arterial dissection, or injection-induced arterial spasm.[1,12-14] Cord infarction should be considered a possibility when cervical, thoracic, or upper lumbar injections are performed. Vertebrobasilar infarction is also a possibility after cervical injections.[14,15] Even though the reported complication rate is very small with transforaminal epidural injections, to minimize the chance of complication, it is recommended that the injection be performed after digital subtraction angiography (DSA), that a nonparticulate or small particulate diameter steroidal agent be used, and that the patient receive minimal or no sedation for the procedure.[12,13,15]

Most spinal cord infarcts involve the anterior spinal artery territory, the gray matter of the anterior horns being most susceptible to ischemia *(Figs. 69-1 to 69-7)*.[6] This can be understood if one considers the spinal cord arterial supply in cross section. The relatively large but solitary anterior spinal artery generally supplies the anterior two thirds of the spinal cord, whereas the paired smaller posterior spinal arteries supply the posterior one third of the spinal cord.[6] The central portion anterior spinal artery territory is usually supplied by central sulcal arteries originating from the anterior spinal artery that extends into the anterior midline fissure of the cord.[16] There is a rich network of tiny arteries along the surface of the spinal cord, the vasa corona, which anastomose with branches of the anterior and posterior spinal arteries. This peripheral arterial network is more prominent posterolaterally. Penetrating arteries from this network supply the periphery of the spinal cord.[6] There are watershed zones between the peripheral and central cord arterial supply in the anterolateral aspect of the anterior horn gray matter and central portion of the dorsal horn gray matter.[6,17] A rich venous network also surrounds the spinal cord that drains into the paravertebral venous plexus.[1]

The cervical and upper most portion of the thoracic spinal cord is supplied predominantly by the anterior spinal artery from the vertebral arteries and branches of the thyrocervical trunks bilaterally. The rich vascular supply to the cervical cord accounts for the fact that cord infarction is least common in the cervical region.[5] For this reason, unilateral vertebral artery dissection rarely results

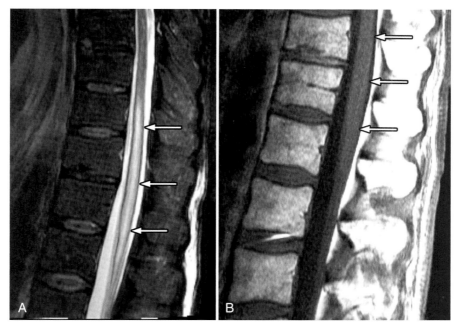

Figure 69-1 ▶ Acute Lower Thoracic Spinal Cord Infarction Post Abdominal Aortic Aneurysm (AAA) Repair. Diffuse enlargement of the lower thoracic spinal cord (*arrow*) is evident on sagittal T2-weighted image **A** and T1-weighted image **B**. Note diffuse T2 signal hyperintensity in the lower thoracic cord (*arrows*) on image **A** due to cord edema and/or infarction.

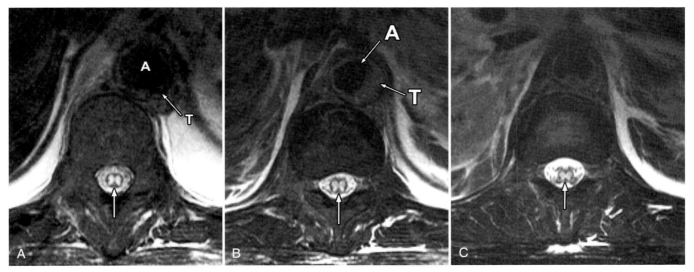

Figure 69-2 ▶ Acute Lower Thoracic Spinal Cord Infarction Post AAA Repair. Same patient as in Figure 69-1. Shown here are a series of 3 axial T2-weighted images obtained through lower thoracic spinal cord. Note "owl eye" appearance within the spinal cord (*arrows in images* **A**, **B**, *and* **C**) due to abnormal T2 signal hyperintensity in the central gray matter of the spinal cord secondary to anterior spinal artery infarction. There is crescentic thrombus (*T*) along the wall of the lower thoracic aortic lumen (*A*).

in cord infarction.[5] If an infarct is to occur in the cervical cord, it is more likely to occur at the C2-3 level, especially after bilateral vertebral artery dissection.[6] The upper and midthoracic spinal cord is fed by relatively small radiculomedullary arteries and is considered to be a watershed zone, and therefore may be more susceptible to cord infarction after hypotensive episodes.[1,5] Sometimes a prominent radiculomedullary feeder is present at approximately the T7 level. The lower thoracic spinal cord is supplied by radiculomedullary arteries from the lower intercostals arteries or upper lumbar arteries. The largest radiculomedullary artery and predominant arterial supply to the lower thoracic cord is the artery of Adamkiewicz, which arises 90% of the time from intercostal or lumbar arteries from the T5 to the L2 level on the left (most commonly from the T9 to T12 intercostal on the left), but can arise from intercostal or lumbar arteries on the right, more superior intercostal arteries, or from upper lumbar arteries.[1] Arterial occlusion from thrombosis, embolism, arteritis, or trauma to the artery of Adamkiewicz is probably responsible for the high incidence of cord infarction in the lower thoracic spinal cord.[5] Spinal cord infarction can also result from compression of the spinal cord (see Figs. 69-6 and 69-7). The most common level to be involved clinically with cord infarction is the T9 level.[1]

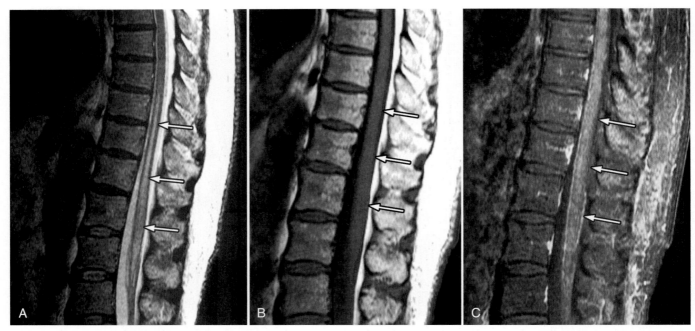

Figure 69-3 ▶ Acute Spinal Cord Infarction. 67-year-old diabetic patient with severe atherosclerotic disease who developed acute paraplegia secondary to acute spinal cord infarction which occurred following an episode of superior mesenteric artery thrombosis and gastrointestinal bleeding. On sagittal T2-weighted image **A**, diffuse hyperintensity is demonstrated in the spinal cord (*arrows*). On T1 weighted image **B**, the lower thoracic spinal cord (*arrows*) is slightly enlarged. On contrast enhanced fat saturated sagittal T1-weighted image **C**, slight heterogeneous enhancement is demonstrated in the lower spinal cord (*arrows*).

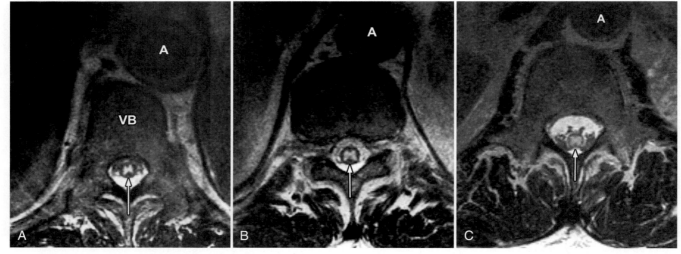

Figure 69-4 ▶ Acute Spinal Cord Infarction. Shown are a series of axial T2-weighted images obtained through the lower thoracic spinal cord in same patient as in Figure 69-3. Classic "owl eye" appearance (*arrow in images* **A**, **B**, *and* **C**) is demonstrated in the spinal cord, representing T2 hyperintensity of accentuated central cord gray matter, secondary to anterior spinal artery infarction. Note circumferential atheromatous plaque along the margins of the lower thoracic aorta (*A*).

The typical patient presenting with spinal cord infarction is older than 50, usually with significant atherosclerotic risk factors including smoking, diabetes, and chronic hypertension. Patients usually present with acute onset of weakness and loss of sensation, depending on the vascular territory involved. With anterior spinal artery infarction, patients present with paraparesis or flaccid paralysis, loss of pain and temperature sensation, and bladder and bowel dysfunction.[18] Posterior spinal artery infarction causes loss of proprioception, inability to detect vibration, weakness, and sphincter dysfunction. Patients may present with Brown-Séquard syndrome

if an anterior median sulcal artery (sulcocommissural artery) is involved.[1] Rapid neurologic deterioration occurs as the cord swells. In fact the majority of patients with cord infarction characteristically report no back pain at time of presentation, although some patients with anterior spinal artery territory cord infarction may complain of *girdle-like* back pain or painful dysesthesias.[6,18-20] Patients with posterior spinal artery territory infarctions usually do not report associated pain.[8] Spinal cord transient ischemic attacks are said to occur when the neurologic deficit resolves within 1 day.[1]

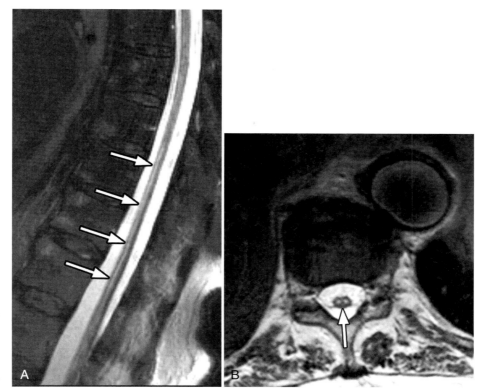

Figure 69-5 ► **Chronic Lower Thoracic Spinal Cord Infarction.** On sagittal T2-weighted image **A**, the lower thoracic spinal cord (*arrows*) is diffusely atrophic and contains a linear band of T2 hyperintensity. On axial T2-weighted image **B**, two bilaterally symmetric hyperintense foci (*arrows*) are demonstrated within the atrophic spinal cord, which imparts an "owl eye" appearance to the cord. Findings are secondary to old spinal cord infarction affecting predominantly the central gray matter.

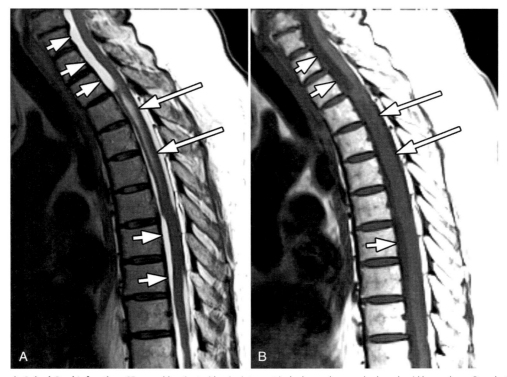

Figure 69-6 ► **Thoracic Spinal Cord Infarction.** 65-year-old patient with prior intraventricular hemorrhage and subarachnoid hemorrhage. Paraplegia developed 6 months following intracranial subarachnoid hemorrhage. Multiple intracranial and spinal intradural adhesions developed, resulting in loculated CSF cavities (*short arrows*) that cause posterior spinal cord displacement as shown on sagittal T2-weighted image **A** and T1-weighted image **B**. In images **A** and **B**, The spinal cord infarction is seen as a region of T2 hyperintensity and vague T1 hypointensity within the spinal cord (*long arrows in images **A** and **B***).

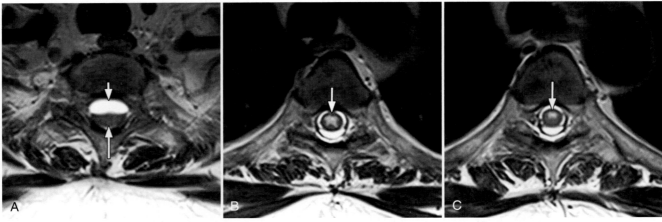

Figure 69-7 ▶ Thoracic Spinal Cord Infarction. Series of three axial T2-weighted MR images through the upper thoracic spine in same patient as in Figure 69-6. In image **A**, loculated CSF (*short arrow*) compresses and displaces the spinal cord (*long arrow*) posteriorly. In axial images **B** and **C**, obtained through the region of cord infarction, there is abnormal T2 signal hyperintensity in the central gray matter of the cord (*arrow on image* **A** *and* **B**), more pronounced anteriorly. Presumably the spinal cord infarction occurred secondary to compression of the anterior spinal artery.

IMAGING FEATURES

MRI is the modality of choice for imaging detection and evaluation of spinal cord infarction. Diffusion-weighted images may show restricted diffusion in the infarcted portion of the spinal cord.[21] T1-weighted images may reveal slight cord swelling but usually the acute infarct is T1 isointense (see Figs. 69-1 and 69-3). The infarcted region is hyperintense on T2-weighted images and short tau inversion recovery (STIR) images (*see* Figs. 69-1, 69-3, and 69-5). The cephalocaudal extent of cord infarction, as seen on T2-weighted images, is usually one to three vertebrae in length but can be smaller or larger. Anterior spinal artery territory infarction involves the anterior two-thirds of the spinal cord, often affecting the central cord gray matter. In anterior spinal artery territory infarction on MR imaging, bilaterally symmetric foci of T2 hyperintense foci are frequently seen in the spinal cord, which has an *owl eye* appearance.[7] In other cases, the T2 signal abnormality associated with cord infarction involves the cord center.[7,18] In some patients, nearly the entire cord cross-sectional diameter is T2 hyperintense due to associated cord edema.[7] The greater the extent of the cord T2 signal hyperintensity due to infarction and/or edema, the worse is the prognosis in these patients.[5] Spinal cord transient ischemic attacks are said to occur when the neurologic deficits resolve within 1 day and there is no discernable MR imaging T2 signal abnormality in the spinal cord.

Special attention should be given to the MR imaging appearance of adjacent vertebral bodies, because these may also undergo infarction at the same time as the spinal cord, because they share a common radicular arterial supply.[16,19] The signal disturbance is usually located in the posterior portion of the adjacent vertebral bodies and is manifested as a region of T2 signal hyperintensity that may enhance with IV contrast.[10,19,22] In a minority of cases, the T2 signal disturbance is adjacent to the vertebral endplate or in the anterior portion of the vertebral body.[10] The vertebral marrow signal disturbance is nonspecific, indicating presence of bone marrow edema and/or inflammation. The absence of signal abnormality in the adjacent vertebral body of course does not exclude cord infarction.[16] Vertebral infarction may be a source of back pain in patients with spinal cord infarction.[19]

If the infarct becomes hemorrhagic, this will be evident on the T1- and T2-weighted MR images depending on the stage of hemorrhage. The presence of hemorrhage carries a worse prognosis.[5] Acute cord hemorrhage is hypointense to isointense on T1-weighted images and usually hypointense on T2-weighted images. Subacute hemorrhage is typically T1 and T2 hyperintense. Old hemorrhage is T2 hypointense and dark on gradient echo images if hemosiderin deposition is present. The region of infarction does not enhance after IV contrast initially, but in the subacute phase may enhance heterogeneously as a result of disruption of the blood/neuron barrier in the cord (see Fig. 69-3).[6] Enhancement may also be seen in the cauda equina in the subacute phase after lower thoracic spinal cord infarction.[9] In the chronic stage of cord infarction, the cord becomes atrophic with a varying degree of myelomalacia observed in the infarcted region of the spinal cord (see Fig. 69-5).

MR angiography (MRA) and computed tomography (CT) angiography (CTA) are usually not helpful in the workup of thoracic spinal cord infarction, because it is difficult to define the small radicular arteries that supply the spinal cord. It is possible to visualize the anterior spinal artery with MRA or CTA. These techniques are helpful to evaluate the aorta for severe atherosclerotic disease or to rule out a thoracic aortic dissection or vertebral artery dissection as a possible cause of either a thoracic or cervical cord infarction.

Conventional angiography is usually not used in the routine workup of possible spinal cord infarction, although it is possible to detect small vessel occlusion or occlusion of the anterior spinal artery with spinal angiography. Angiography, CTA, or MRA, can also be helpful for identifying the location of the artery of Adamkiewicz preoperatively, so this vessel can be avoided when lower thoracic spinal surgery is performed.

DIFFERENTIAL DIAGNOSIS

1. **Dural AV fistula:** On T2-weighted images, spinal cord dural AV fistula may have the same appearance as spinal cord infarction (**Figs. 69-8 and 69-9**). Indeed, cord ischemia may result

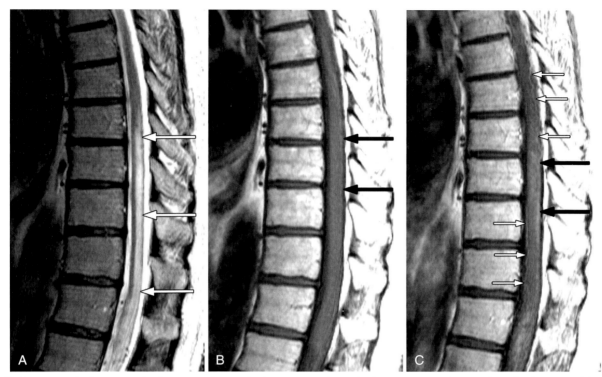

Figure 69-8 ▶ Type I Spinal Dural AV Fistula. On sagittal T2-weighted MR image **A**, abnormal T2 hyperintense signal intensity (*arrows*) is demonstrated throughout the lower thoracic spinal cord. Corresponding sagittal T1-weighted image **B** reveals mild diffuse cord enlargement (*black arrows*) in this region. On sagittal contrast enhanced T1-weighted image **C**, subtle heterogeneous enhancement (*black arrows*) is demonstrated in the cord in this region. Note enhancement of tortuous intradural vessels (*white arrows*) adjacent to the anterior and posterior margins of the spinal cord.

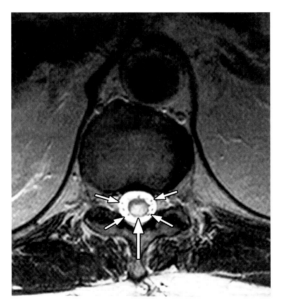

Figure 69-9 ▶ Type I Spinal Dural AV Fistula. Same patient as in Figure 69-8. Axial T2-weighted MR image reveals an ill-defined region of T2 hyperintensity (*long arrow*) in the posterior portion of the lower thoracic spinal cord, likely representing myelomalacia and/or edema secondary to chronic ischemia. Small T2 hypointense intradural vessels (*short arrows*) represent tortuous arterialized veins within the subarachnoid space.

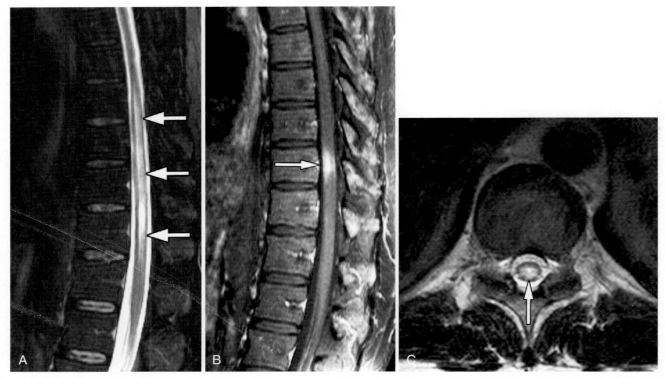

Figure 69-10 ▶ Transverse Myelitis. On sagittal T2-weighted image **A**, a region of T2 hyperintensity (*arrows*) is located within the spinal cord from the T8 through T11 level. On fat saturated contrast enhanced sagittal T1 weighted image **B**, a focal area of contrast enhancement (*arrow*) is located predominantly in the anterior portion of the spinal cord at the T9 level. On axial T2-weighted image **C**, a region of abnormal T2 hyperintensity occupies the majority of the cord cross section (*arrow*).

from spinal AV fistula secondary to a *steal* phenomenon. Look for prominent vessels adjacent·to the cord, representing arterialized veins that typically enhance after IV contrast administration.

2. **"Transverse" myelitis:** Inflammatory conditions of the spinal cord in the acute phase often cause cord swelling and edema that is T2 hyperintense. The cord may or may not enhance *(Fig. 69-10)*. In the later phases, the spinal cord becomes atrophic. Acute demyelinating encephalomyelitis (ADEM), a postviral condition may also involve the spinal cord.

3. **Devic's disease (neuromyelitis optica):** Usually involves the cervical spinal cord. The cord is heterogeneous on T2-weighted images and usually contains a flame-shaped region of heterogeneous contrast enhancement *(Fig. 69-11)*.

4. **Multiple sclerosis:** The plaques in multiple sclerosis most commonly occur in the dorsal or lateral white matter columns.[6] Cord ischemia more commonly results in T2 signal abnormality in the anterior portion of the cord or in the central zone of the spinal cord.

5. **Spinal cord neoplasm:** Intramedullary cord neoplasms may be primary tumors, most commonly astrocytomas or ependymomas, which most commonly involve the cervical spinal cord. An intramedullary spinal cord metastasis may also simulate cord infarction, although a spinal cord metastasis usually enhances intensely and is associated with localized cord enlargement.

TREATMENT

1. **Supportive treatment:** The treatment of spinal cord infarction is mainly supportive.[22] The systemic blood pressure should be maintained at a constant normal level.

2. **Corticosteroid therapy:** Corticosteroids are useful for reducing cord swelling, protecting cell membranes, and inhibiting free radical formation after cord infarction or spinal cord injury.[20,23,24]

3. **Anticoagulation or use of intra-arterial thrombolytic agents:** This may be considered in the acute phase, but their efficacy in improving clinical outcome in the setting of cord infarction is unknown.[22]

4. **Long-term rehabilitation**

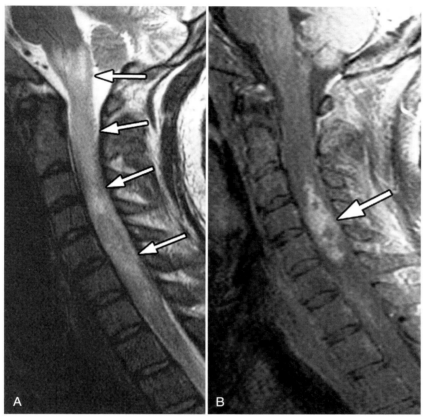

Figure 69-11 ► **Devic's Disease (Neuromyelitis Optica).** On sagittal T2-weighted image **A**, a heterogeneous region of hyperintense signal (*arrows*) involves the medulla and entire cervical spinal cord. On sagittal contrast-enhanced image **B**, a flame-shaped heterogeneous region of contrast enhancement (*arrow*) is located within the cervical cord, centered at the C4-5 level.

References

1. Cheshire WP, Santos CC, Massey EW, Howard Jr JF. Spinal cord infarction: Etiology and outcome. *Neurology.* 1996;47(2):321-330.
2. Weber P, Vogel T, Bitterling H, et al. Spinal cord infarction after operative stabilisation of the thoracic spine in a patient with tuberculous spondylodiscitis and sickle cell trait. *Spine.* 2009;34(8):E294-E297.
3. Morales JP, Taylor PR, Bell RE, et al. Neurological complications following endoluminal repair of thoracic aortic disease. *Cardiovasc Intervent Radiol.* 2007;30(5):833-839.
4. Etz CD, Halstead JC, Spielvogel D, et al. Thoracic and thoracoabdominal aneurysm repair: Is reimplantation of spinal cord arteries a waste of time? *Ann Thorac Surg.* 2006;82(5):1670-1677.
5. White ML, El-Khoury GY. Neurovascular injuries of the spinal cord. *Eur J Radiol.* 2002;42(2):117-126.
6. Weidauer S, Nichtweiss M, Lanfermann H, Zanella FE. Spinal cord infarction: MR imaging and clinical features in 16 cases. *Neuroradiology.* 2002;44(10):851-857.
7. Mawad ME, Rivera V, Crawford S, et al. Spinal cord ischemia after resection of thoracoabdominal aortic aneurysms: MR findings in 24 patients. *AJR Am J Roentgenol.* 1990;155(6):1303-1307.
8. Mascalchi M, Cosottini M, Ferrito G, et al. Posterior spinal artery infarct. *AJNR Am J Neuroradiol.* 1998;19(2):361-363.
9. Chan LL, Kumar AJ, Leeds NE, Forman AD. Post-epidural analgesia spinal cord infarction: MRI correlation. *Acta Neurol Scand.* 2002;105(4):344-348.
10. Yuh WT, Marsh EE 3rd, Wang AK, et al. MR imaging of spinal cord and vertebral body infarction. *AJNR Am J Neuroradiol.* 1992;13(1):145-154.
11. Toro G, Roman GC, Navarro-Roman L, et al. Natural history of spinal cord infarction caused by nucleus pulposus embolism. *Spine.* 1994;19(3):360-366.
12. Malhotra G, Abbasi A, Rhee M. Complications of transforaminal cervical epidural steroid injections. *Spine.* 2009;34(7):731-739.
13. Lyders EM, Morris PP. A case of spinal cord infarction following lumbar transforaminal epidural steroid injection: MR imaging and angiographic findings. *AJNR Am J Neuroradiol.* 2009.
14. Scanlon GC, Moeller-Bertram T, Romanowsky SM, Wallace MS. Cervical transforaminal epidural steroid injections: More dangerous than we think? *Spine.* 2007;32(11):1249-1256.
15. Ludwig MA, Burns SP. Spinal cord infarction following cervical transforaminal epidural injection: A case report. *Spine.* 2005;30(10):E266-E268.
16. Faig J, Busse O, Salbeck R. Vertebral body infarction as a confirmatory sign of spinal cord ischemic stroke: Report of three cases and review of the literature. *Stroke.* 1998;29(1):239-243.
17. Turnbull IM, Brieg A, Hassler O. Blood supply of cervical spinal cord in man: A microangiographic cadaver study. *J Neurosurg.* 1966;24(6):951-965.
18. Suzuki K, Meguro K, Wada M, et al. Anterior spinal artery syndrome associated with severe stenosis of the vertebral artery. *AJNR Am J Neuroradiol.* 1998;19(7):1353-1355.
19. Bornke C, Schmid G, Szymanski S, Schols L. Vertebral body infarction indicating midthoracic spinal stroke. *Spinal Cord.* 2002;40(5):244-247.
20. Gaeta TJ, LaPolla GA, Balentine JR. Anterior spinal artery infarction. *Ann Emerg Med.* 1995;26(1):90-93.
21. Bammer R, Fazekas F, Augustin M, et al. Diffusion-weighted MR imaging of the spinal cord. *AJNR Am J Neuroradiol.* 2000;21(3):587-591.
22. Suzuki T, Kawaguchi S, Takebayashi T, et al. Vertebral body ischemia in the posterior spinal artery syndrome: Case report and review of the literature. *Spine.* 2003;28(13):E260-E264.
23. Satran R. Spinal cord infarction. *Stroke.* 1988;19(4):529-532.
24. Bracken MB, Shepard MJ, Collins WF, et al. A randomized, controlled trial of methylprednisolone or naloxone in the treatment of acute spinal-cord injury. Results of the Second National Acute Spinal Cord Injury Study. *N Engl J Med.* 1990;322(20):1405-1411.

SPINAL CORD METASTASIS

Leo F. Czervionke, M.D.

CLINICAL PRESENTATION

The patient is a 71-year-old man with small cell lung cancer and known brain metastases who presents with new onset of right-sided weakness and sensory disturbances. His symptoms began approximately 2 to 3 weeks ago and have been getting progressively worse. He describes weakness on his right side, mainly involving his right hand and proximal right leg. He also notes numbness on his entire right side, involving his face, arm, trunk, and leg. His weakness has progressed to the point where he has difficulty writing, holding a pen or fork, and he has had three falls in the past 3 weeks because of gait instability. He has started using a walker to prevent falling. He denies having any bowel or bladder incontinence. He has developed headaches in the past 3 weeks, which he describes as dull in nature and frontal in location.

IMAGING PRESENTATION

Magnetic resonance (MR) imaging reveals an enhancing intramedullary mass in the cord from C5 to C7 level. Above this level is diffuse cord enlargement secondary to edema that extends into the lower brainstem (medulla). Findings are consistent with intramedullary spinal cord metastasis (*Figs. 70-1 to 70-3*).

DISCUSSION

Intramedullary spinal cord metastasis is a rare tumor, occurring in less than 2% of autopsied cancer patients.[1] Intramedullary metastases represent only 1% to 3% of spinal cord metastases.[1-3] An intramedullary metastasis may arise anywhere in the spinal cord but more frequently occurs in the cervical cord (see Figs. 70-1 to 70-3), followed by the thoracic cord (*Figs. 70-4 and 70-5*), conus medullaris (*Figs. 70-6 and 70-7*), and cauda equina.[4] Any primary malignant neoplasm can metastasize to the spinal cord, but lung carcinoma (especially small cell lung carcinoma) is by far the most common primary tumor to metastasize to the cord,[3,5-8] followed by breast carcinoma,[4] melanoma,[4,8] renal cell carcinoma,[9,10] colorectal carcinoma,[3] lymphoma,[11] and rarely other primary tumors.[4,12-14] These primary tumors are believed to spread to the spinal cord hematogenously, but retroperitoneal tumors can spread via Batson's plexus or perineural lymphatics.[1] Central nervous system (CNS) malignancies, such as glioblastoma multiforme, ependymoma, primitive neuroectodermal tumor (e.g,. medulloblastoma),

and rarely other intracranial tumors, can metastasize to the spinal cord by spreading within the cerebrospinal fluid (CSF).[4,15] These primary tumors usually deposit along the leptomeningeal surface of the spinal cord or cauda equina, rather than depositing in the cord centrum.

Uncommonly, intramedullary metastases may hemorrhage, and the resulting blood may extend into the CSF surrounding the cord, causing a subarachnoid hemorrhage. Rarely, a syrinx cavity develops adjacent to an intramedullary metastasis.[10]

Nearly all patients with intramedullary metastases present with myelopathy, more than 90% of patients having a motor deficit,[8,13] either acute onset of weakness or rapidly progressive paraparesis over a few weeks; 70% of patients present with back pain, but paresthesias and bladder and/or bowel dysfunction are also common, depending on the location of the tumor.[4] The patient may present with Brown-Séquard syndrome.[6,9,13,16]

IMAGING FEATURES

MRI is the imaging procedure of choice for diagnosing and assessing the extent of spinal cord metastases (see Figs. 70-1 to 70-7).[17,18] In the initial workup of these patients, a lumbar puncture is usually performed to examine the CSF for positive cytology.[18] Fluorine-18 fluorodeoxyglucose positron emission tomography (FDG-PET) scanning has also been shown to be sensitive for detection and assessing the extent of intramedullary and leptomeningeal metastases.[7,19,20] Imaging abnormalities of cord metastasis are usually not visible on radiographs or by plain computed tomography (CT). Fusiform enlargement of the cord, if present, is visible at myelography, but this fusiform enlargement is nonspecific, occurring with intramedullary tumors, vascular anomalies, and syringohydromyelia. Most intramedullary metastases are solitary, with an average cephalocaudal extent of two to three vertebral segments.[4]

Unenhanced, T1-weighted MR images may be normal but frequently show fusiform cord enlargement or may demonstrate a subtle region of T1 hypointensity in the cord, which can be confused with an intramedullary syrinx (see Fig. 70-2). True syrinx cavities rarely coexist with an intramedullary metastasis. The intramedullary metastasis and adjacent edema are T2 hyperintense, unless hemorrhage is present, which may be T2 hypointense, hyperintense, or of mixed intensity. There is often a considerable amount of edema in the cord adjacent to an intramedullary metastasis (see Fig. 70-1). Occasionally, the intramedullary metastasis

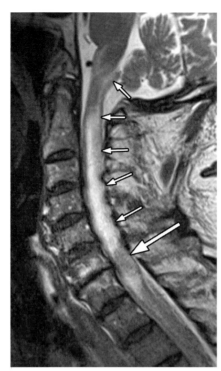

Figure 70-1 ▶ **Spinal Cord Metastasis C6-7 Level.** Sagittal T2-weighted MR image. A subtle ovoid region of T2 hypointensity is demonstrated in the cord at the C6-7 level (*long arrow*). There is diffuse cervical cord enlargement and T2 hyperintensity in the cord above this level extending into the lower brainstem consistent with edema (*short arrows*).

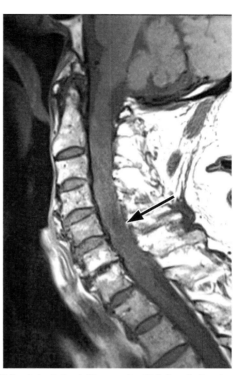

Figure 70-2 ▶ **Spinal Cord Metastasis C6-7 Level.** Unenhanced sagittal T1-weighted image, in same patient as in Figure 70-1, shows diffuse cervical cord enlargement with subtle region of T1 hypointensity in the cord at the C5-6 level (*arrow*), which is above the intramedullary mass.

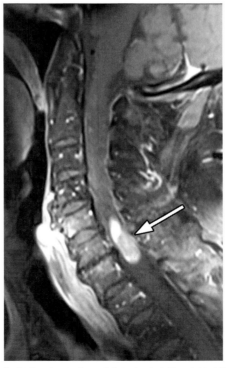

Figure 70-3 ▶ **Spinal Cord Metastasis C6-7 Level.** Sagittal contrast-enhanced, fat-saturated, T1-weighted MR image in same patient as in Figures 70-1 and 70-2. An enhancing mass (*arrow*) is located in the cord at the C6-7 level with diffuse cord enlargement above this level.

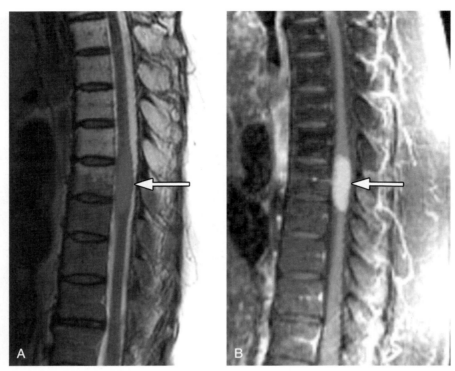

Figure 70-4 ▶ **Intramedullary Spinal Cord Metastasis at T8 Level from Small Cell Lung Carcinoma Primary Tumor.** Patient with existing brain metastases presented with new-onset difficulty with walking. On sagittal T2-weighted image **A**, the spinal cord metastasis is only slightly T2 hyperintense and causes slight cord enlargement (*arrow*). No adjacent cord edema. On contrast-enhanced, sagittal T1-weighted image **B**, the metastasis (*arrow*) enhances intensely and homogeneously.

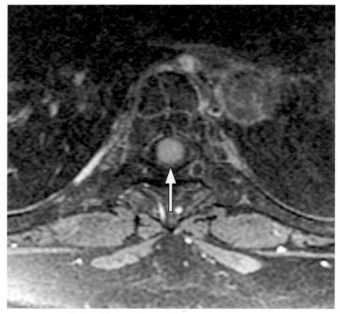

Figure 70-5 ▶ **Intramedullary Metastasis T8 Level from Lung Carcinoma Primary Tumor.** Axial fat-saturated T1-weighted image, in same patient as in Figure 70-4, reveals homogeneous enhancement of the intramedullary mass (*arrow*) causing mild cord enlargement.

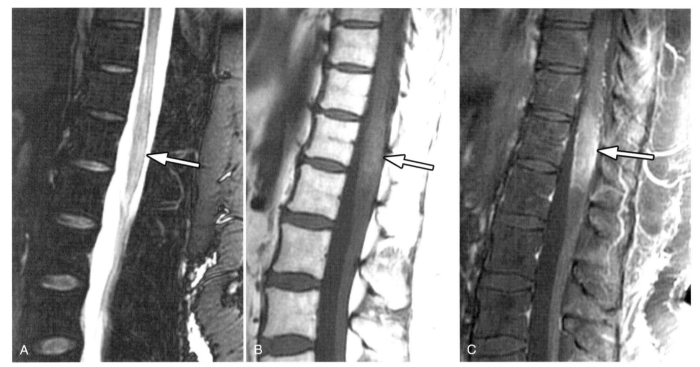

Figure 70-6 ▶ Intramedullary Metastasis at T12 Level from Intracranial Glioblastoma Multiforme. The intramedullary tumor is slightly hyperintense (*arrow*) on sagittal T2-weighted image **A** and causes slightly fusiform cord enlargement (*arrow*) on sagittal T1-weighted image **B**. There is mild to moderate heterogeneous enhancement of the intramedullary mass (*arrow*) on contrast-enhanced, fat-saturated, T1-weighted image **C**. Note prominent enhancing blood vessels along the anterior and posterior cord margins at and above the level of the tumor.

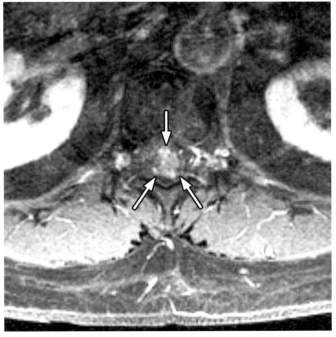

Figure 70-7 ▶ Intramedullary Metastasis T12 Level. (In same patient as in Fig. 70-6.) Axial contrast-enhanced, fat-saturated, T1-weighted image reveals slight cord enlargement and heterogeneous enhancement of the cord tumor (*arrows*). There are prominent enhancing vessels along the anterior and posterior margins of the cord.

may appear only slightly T2 hyperintense with little or no adjacent edema (see Figs. 70-4 and 70-6). The cord edema, when present, may be relatively localized or extend over a long cephalocaudal distance. The typical intramedullary metastasis enhances intensely, but the pattern of enhancement may be homogeneous or heterogeneous (see Figs. 70-3, 70-4, 70-6, and 70-7).[4,21] The enhancing portion of the intramedullary lesion is usually one to three vertebra in cephalocaudal length, and tends to be relatively small in comparison with the amount of associated cord edema, when edema is present (see Fig. 70-3).[22] Uncommonly, the cord metastasis enhances in a ringlike fashion.[14,19]

If an intramedullary metastasis is discovered with MR imaging, whole body F-18 FDG-PET scanning is recommended to exclude other metastases within and outside of the CNS, because there is a high incidence of other metastases in patients presenting with an intramedullary metastasis. Approximately 75% of patients with an intramedullary metastasis have systemic metastases, and 35% have CNS metastases elsewhere.[8]

DIFFERENTIAL DIAGNOSIS

1. **Intramedullary glioma** *(Fig. 70-8)*: These patients usually present with a slow onset of symptoms. An ependymoma or astrocytoma can have an imaging appearance similar to intramedullary metastasis. Astrocytomas may or may not enhance, but when enhancement occurs, it is usually heterogeneous and tends to involve the cord over several segments. The presence of a true syrinx cavity in the cord is much more commonly associated with intramedullary gliomas than with intramedullary metastasis. The presence of associated hemorrhage in the cord is much more common with ependymoma (see Fig. 70-8).

2. **Hemangioblastoma:** An hemangioblastoma may arise on the surface of the cord or within the cord and can simulate an intramedullary cord metastasis *(Fig. 70-9)*. Indeed, hemangioblastomas often recur as multicentric lesions along the pial surface of the cord, even though they are histologically benign tumors. They are commonly associated with syringomyelia formation in the cord.

3. **Neuromyelitis optica (Devic's disease):** In this condition, an acute demyelinating process causes swelling and a heterogeneous enhancement of the cervical cord *(Fig. 70-10)*. The patient classically has a coexistent visual disturbance secondary to acute optic neuritis.

4. **Sarcoidosis of the cord:** This commonly enhances with contrast. The enhancement tends to be heterogeneous and often extends over two vertebra in length. The imaging appearance closely resembles that seen in neuromyelitis optica.

5. **Lymphoma:** Rarely lymphoma manifest as an enhancing intramedullary mass.

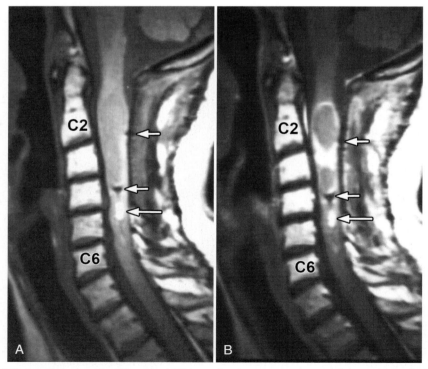

Figure 70-8 ▶ **Cervical Cord Ependymoma.** In sagittal T1-weighted MR image **A**, a heterogeneous intramedullary mass causes fusiform enlargement of the cervical spinal cord from C1-2 to the C5-6 level. In sagittal contrast-enhanced, T1-weighted MR image **B**, the intramedullary tumor enhances heterogeneously from the C1-2 to C5-6 level. A small ovoid area of T1 hyperintensity (*long arrow* in images **A** and **B**) in the cord at the C4-5 level represents subacute to chronic hemorrhage in the caudal aspect of the tumor. Hypointense regions (*short arrows* in images **A** and **B**) represent ferromagnetic artifact related to prior cord biopsy. *C2*, C2 vertebral body; *C6*, C6 vertebral body.

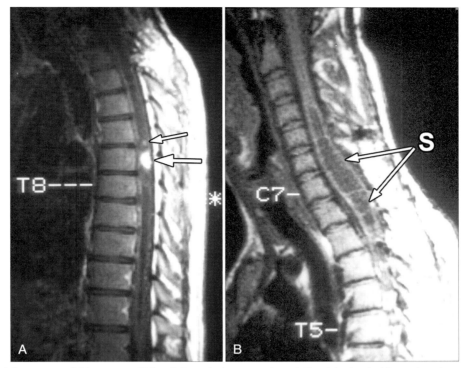

Figure 70-9 ► **Intramedullary Hemangioblastoma at T7 Level.** On sagittal contrast-enhanced, T1-weighted sagittal image **A**, an intense homogeneously enhancing intramedullary mass (*large arrow*) is demonstrated at the mid T7 level. A tiny enhancing intramedullary satellite mass (*small arrow*) is present at the T6-7 level. Associated syrinx cavity is located above and below the enhancing cord tumors in the thoracic spinal cord. The syrinx (*S*) is larger in the cervicothoracic region, as demonstrated on sagittal T1-weighted image **B**.

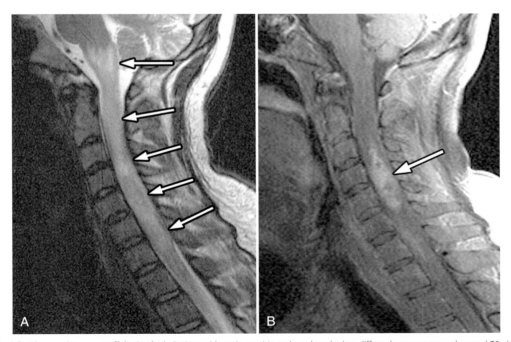

Figure 70-10 ► **Devic's Disease (Neuromyelitis Optica).** Patient with optic neuritis and myelopathy has diffuse, heterogeneous abnormal T2 signal intensity (*arrows*) that involves the medulla and cervical spinal cord on sagittal T2-weighted image **A**. On sagittal T1-weighted image **B**, a heterogeneously enhancing flame-shaped intramedullary lesion (*arrow*) extends from the C3 to the C6 level, which represents disruption of the blood-neural barrier in the cord secondary to active demyelination.

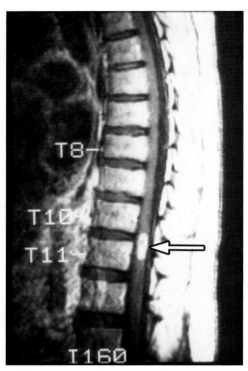

Figure 70-11 ▸ Transverse Myelitis at the T10-11 Level. Contrast-enhanced, T1-weighted image. Intense well-defined ovoid enhancing inflammatory lesion (*arrow*) in the cord mimics an intramedullary metastasis.

6. **Transverse myelitis:** This is a nonspecific myelitis that could be secondary to any of a number of viral or bacterial pathogens. This often is associated with localized cord enhancement *(Fig. 70-11)* and usually adjacent cord edema.

7. **HIV myelitis:** HIV can cause a unique form of myelitis, sometimes referred to as *vacuolar myelopathy,* that can predominantly involve the posterior white matter columns of the spinal cord, which can simulate the MR appearance of subacute combined degeneration (vitamin B_{12} deficiency) on T2-weighted images *(Fig. 70-12)*.[23-25]

8. **Spinal cord abscess** *(Fig. 70-13)*: Intramedullary cord abscess is a rare devastating complication of an infection elsewhere, often secondary to osteomyelitis in the nearby spine or sepsis. This could be mistaken for an intramedullary metastasis. With cord abscess, an intense ring-enhancing lesion is present in the cord. Typically with cord abscess, a large amount of edema is present in the cord extending over several levels, which closely resembles that which may be seen in intramedullary cord metastasis.

9. **Spinal cord tuberculoma:** This may have an imaging appearance similar to intramedullary metastasis.[26]

10. **Paraneoplastic necrotizing myelopathy (PNM):** This is a rare autoimmune condition that can have an imaging appearance very similar to intramedullary metastasis. PNM classically occurs in the thoracic spinal cord. Patients with PNM usually lack back pain, which is very common with cord metastasis. PNM patients usually have non-neoplastic cerebellar symptoms related to the paraneoplastic syndrome.[8]

11. **Vascular malformation:** Malformation within the cord manifests with an intramedullary nidus of small vessels with flow voids *(Fig. 70-14)*. Usually, associated edema is minimal or lacking. Cord atrioventricular (AV) malformations usually do not enhance appreciably.

12. **Cavernous angioma (cavernoma):** Cavernous angioma in the cord usually enhances minimally or not at all and has a characteristic peripherally T2 hypointense rim of hemosiderin. The intramedullary cavernoma is usually not confused with an intramedullary metastasis.

PROGNOSIS AND TREATMENT

Patients with spinal cord metastasis have an extremely poor prognosis, the majority of patients die in less than 6 months.[4,7,8] In cases with widespread metastases, treatment is usually supportive and conservative.

1. **Steroids:** Steroids are usually administered to reduce cord edema, which can alleviate the patient's symptoms dramatically.[13]

2. **Radiotherapy:** Radiotherapy along with steroids is often administered for treatment of a spinal cord metastasis, if the tumor is radiosensitive.[12] For a solitary intramedullary metastasis, localized radiotherapy is preferred over whole spine radiation.[13]

3. **Chemotherapy:** Systemic or intrathecal chemotherapy is used if the tumor is not radiosensitive or if there is concomitant leptomeningeal disease.[13]

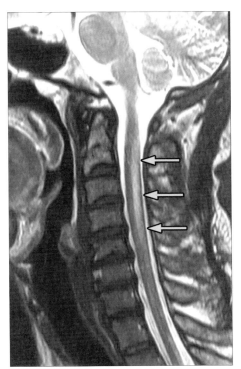

Figure 70-12 ► **Vacuolar Myelopathy (Myelitis) in an AIDS Patient.** Diffuse T2 signal hyperintensity (*arrows*) is visible in the posterior portion of the cervical cord from the C2 to C5 level on sagittal T2-weighted image obtained through the cervical spine. This lesion did not enhance after IV contrast administration. Subacute combined degeneration (vitamin B_{12} deficiency) has a similar MR appearance.

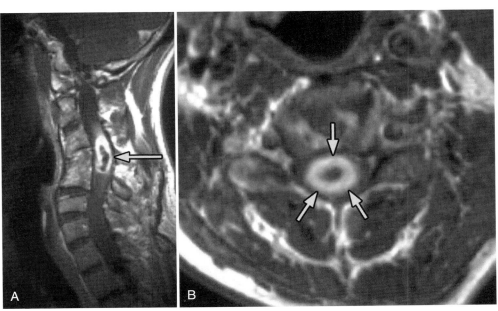

Figure 70-13 ► **Spinal Cord Abscess.** Tuberculous abscess with superinfection by *Staphylococcus aureus* occurred several weeks after anterior cervical fusion procedure. Contrast-enhanced, T1-weighted sagittal image **A** shows a peripheral rim-enhancing abscess (*arrows*) in the cord extending from the C3 to C5 level. On axial contrast-enhanced, T1-weighted MR image **B**, the enhancing abscess has a doughnut configuration (*arrows*). A necrotic intramedullary spinal cord neoplasm could have a similar appearance.

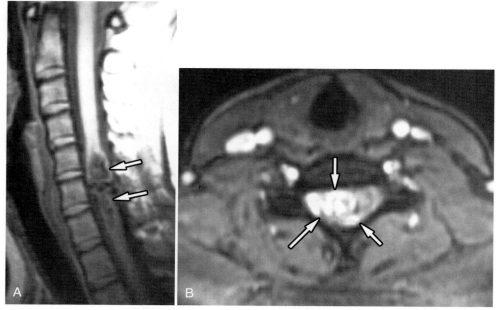

Figure 70-14 ► **Cervical Cord Atrioventricular (AV) Malformation.** Abnormal cluster of vessels within the expanded cord from C5 to C7 level display signal voids (*arrows*) on T1-weighted sagittal image **A**. The cluster of vessels (*arrows*) is hyperintense on axial gradient echo image **B**; these vessels have the same hyperintense signal as other blood vessels in the neck.

4. Surgery: Few surgeons consider aggressive surgery in these patients.[8] Surgical resection, using microsurgical techniques, can be attempted if the cord metastasis is the patient's only metastasis, or in an attempt to improve the patient's quality of life.[3,12] However, often there are metastases elsewhere.[8] The surgical risk versus benefit must be carefully considered, because adjacent normal spinal cord tissue may be damaged by surgery.

References

1. Costigan DA, Winkelman MD. Intramedullary spinal cord metastasis: A clinicopathological study of 13 cases. *J Neurosurg.* 1985;62(2):227-233.
2. Lee SS, Kim MK, Sym SJ, et al. Intramedullary spinal cord metastases: A single-institution experience. *J Neurooncol.* 2007;84(1):85-89.
3. Grasso G, Meli F, Patti R, et al. Intramedullary spinal cord tumor presenting as the initial manifestation of metastatic colon cancer: Case report and review of the literature. *Spinal Cord.* 2007;45(12):793-796.
4. Koeller KK, Rosenblum RS, Morrison AL. Neoplasms of the spinal cord and filum terminale: Radiologic-pathologic correlation. *Radiographics.* 2000; 20(6):1721-1749.
5. Nikolaou M, Koumpou M, Mylonakis N, et al. Intramedullary spinal cord metastases from atypical small cell lung cancer: A case report and literature review. *Cancer Invest.* 2006;24(1):46-49.
6. Aryan HE, Farin A, Nakaji P, et al. Intramedullary spinal cord metastasis of lung adenocarcinoma presenting as Brown-Séquard syndrome. *Surg Neurol.* 2004;61(1):72-76.
7. Komori T, Delbeke D. Leptomeningeal carcinomatosis and intramedullary spinal cord metastases from lung cancer: Detection with FDG positron emission tomography. *Clin Nucl Med.* 2001;26(11):905-907.
8. Connolly ES, Jr, Winfree CJ, McCormick PC, et al. Intramedullary spinal cord metastasis: Report of three cases and review of the literature. *Surg Neurol.* 1996;46(4):329-337; discussion 37-38.
9. Donovan DJ, Freeman JH. Solitary intramedullary spinal cord tumor presenting as the initial manifestation of metastatic renal cell carcinoma: Case report. *Spine.* 2006;31(14):E460-E463.
10. Keung YK, Cobos E, Whitehead RP, Roberson GH. Secondary syringomyelia due to intramedullary spinal cord metastasis: Case report and review of literature. *Am J Clin Oncol.* 1997;20(6):577-579.
11. Mathur S, Law AJ, Hung N. Late intramedullary spinal cord metastasis in a patient with lymphoblastic lymphoma: Case report. *J Clin Neurosci.* 2000;7(3):264-268.
12. Findlay JM, Bernstein M, Vanderlinden RG, Resch L. Microsurgical resection of solitary intramedullary spinal cord metastases. *Neurosurgery.* 1987;21(6):911-915.
13. Schiff D, O'Neill BP. Intramedullary spinal cord metastases: Clinical features and treatment outcome. *Neurology.* 1996;47(4):906-912.
14. Amin R. Intramedullary spinal cord metastasis from carcinoma of the cervix. *Br J Radiol.* 1999;72(853):89-91.
15. Taniura S, Taniguchi M, Mizutani T, Takahashi H. Metastatic hemangiopericytoma to the cauda equina: A case report. *Spine J.* 2007;7(3):371-373.
16. Wada H, Ieki R, Ota T, et al. Intramedullary spinal cord metastasis of lung adenocarcinoma causing Brown-Séquard Syndrome. *Nihon Kokyuki Gakkai Zasshi.* 2001;39(8):590-594.
17. Post MJ, Quencer RM, Green BA, et al. Intramedullary spinal cord metastases, mainly of nonneurogenic origin. *AJR Am J Roentgenol.* 1987;148(5): 1015-1022.
18. Heinz R, Wiener D, Friedman H, Tien R. Detection of cerebrospinal fluid metastasis: CT myelography or MR? *AJNR Am J Neuroradiol.* 1995;16(5): 1147-1151.
19. Poggi MM, Patronas N, Buttman JA, et al. Intramedullary spinal cord metastasis from renal cell carcinoma: Detection by positron emission tomography. *Clin Nucl Med.* 2001;26(10):837-839.
20. Jayasundera MV, Thompson JF, Fulham MJ. Intramedullary spinal cord metastasis from carcinoma of the lung: Detection by positron emission tomography. *Eur J Cancer.* 1997;33(3):508-509.
21. Scollato A, Buccoliero AM, Di Rita A, et al. Intramedullary spinal cord metastasis from synovial sarcoma: Case illustration. *J Neurosurg Spine.* 2008;8(4):400.

22. Sze G, Krol G, Zimmerman RD, Deck MD. Intramedullary disease of the spine: Diagnosis using gadolinium-DTPA-enhanced MR imaging. *AJR Am J Roentgenol.* 1988;151(6):1193-1204.

23. Sartoretti-Schefer S, Blattler T, Wichmann W. Spinal MRI in vacuolar myelopathy, and correlation with histopathological findings. *Neuroradiology.* 1997;39(12):865-869.

24. Miller RF, Sweeney B, Harrison MJ, Lucas SB. Spinal cord disease due to vacuolar myelopathy in AIDS. *Genitourin Med.* 1994;70(3):222-227.

25. Petito CK, Navia BA, Cho ES, et al. Vacuolar myelopathy pathologically resembling subacute combined degeneration in patients with the acquired immunodeficiency syndrome. *N Engl J Med.* 1985;312(14): 874-879.

26. Melhem ER, Wang H. Intramedullary spinal cord tuberculoma in a patient with AIDS. *AJNR Am J Neuroradiol.* 1992;13(3):986-988.

SPINAL STENOSIS—CERVICAL

Douglas S. Fenton, M.D.

CLINICAL PRESENTATION

The patient is a 60-year-old woman complaining of headache, imbalance, lightheadedness, and left-leg numbness. She also complains of increasing numbness in her hands with some hand discoordination. She has had significant neck and bilateral shoulder pain, possibly somewhat worse on the left side. On examination, she demonstrates −1 paresis of the biceps, triceps, wrist extensors, wrist flexors, and interossei musculature. Her grasp is diminished, particularly on the right.

IMAGING PRESENTATION

Sagittal T2-weighted and axial fat-saturated, T2-weighted magnetic resonance (MR) images were obtained and demonstrate a long segment region of decreased signal intensity along the posterior aspect of the vertebral bodies from C3-C5, which is greatest at the C3-4 level. The findings represent a disc herniation at C3-4 in a patient with ossification of the posterior longitudinal ligament. There is severe spinal stenosis at C3-4 and a long segment region of abnormal increased T2 signal intensity in the cervical spinal cord from mid C3 to the C5-6 level compatible with spinal cord ischemia and/or myelomalacia (*Fig. 71-1*).

DISCUSSION

Cervical spinal stenosis can be defined as any narrowing of the spinal canal that causes compression of the contents of the spinal canal because of a mismatch between the available space in the spinal canal and its contents. If the stenosis becomes severe enough, myelopathic symptoms can arise. Cervical myelopathy is the most serious condition that can arise from cervical spinal stenosis. The signs and symptoms of this condition depend on which part of the cervical cord is compressed.

Cervical spinal stenosis can be divided into congenital, developmental, and acquired causes. Congenital cervical stenosis often affects the craniovertebral junction. Patients with malformation of the dens or achondroplasia or who have Down syndrome or Klippel-Feil syndrome can present with cervical spinal stenosis.[1-4] Developmental stenosis is usually caused by short pedicles. As a person ages, degenerative changes ensue. Normally, a person would not be symptomatic from degenerative changes until they were moderate or severe. However, with short pedicles, one tends

to see symptoms with much milder degenerative changes because the available spinal canal space is already diminished in anterior-posterior diameter and area. Therefore, patients with developmental stenosis tend to have symptoms at a younger age. Acquired stenosis is much more common than congenital or developmental stenosis. Degenerative stenosis is the most common type of acquired stenosis. Other causes of acquired cervical spine stenosis include ossification of the posterior longitudinal ligament, ossification/thickening of the ligamentum flavum, rheumatoid arthritis with pannus formation, ankylosing spondylitis, Paget's disease with basilar impression, and metastatic disease.[5,6]

Disc degeneration and the degenerative cascade that follows is the most common cause of acquired cervical spinal stenosis. Generally, the midcervical region is most affected. In healthy individuals, the cervical intervertebral disc is similar to the lumbar intervertebral disc, consisting of an annulus fibrosis and nucleus pulposus. In the first and second decades of life, lateral tears occur in the annulus fibrosis.[7] These tears, over time, enlarge and extend toward the medial aspect of the disc. As we age, the degenerating disc cannot bear or transfer load because of annular fissuring, disappearance of the nucleus pulposus, and dehydration of the disc.[8] There is increased load upon the uncovertebral joints, which become flattened to accept the additional load. This then puts greater stress on the vertebral endplates. Osteophytes develop because of periosteal irritation at the vertebral margins in order to increase the weight-bearing surface of the endplates, stabilizing the adjacent vertebra.[9] The osteophytes can become quite large, bringing the degenerated disc material along with them. The intervertebral disc may calcify to further stabilize the vertebral motion segment.[8] The ligamentum flavum may hypertrophy and buckle into the spinal canal. The combination of the osteophyte/disc complex and thickened ligamentum flavum causes narrowing of the central spinal canal. The combination of the flattened, degenerated uncovertebral joints and facet joint hypertrophy can cause neural foraminal narrowing. Vertebral subluxations, secondary to facet degeneration and ligamentous laxity, can further contribute to spinal stenosis and foraminal narrowing.

Ossification of the posterior longitudinal ligament (OPLL) is a condition in which there is pathologic ossification of this ligament in the cervical and/or thoracic spine. When this ossification occupies enough of the spinal canal, it will result in cervical spinal stenosis, which can lead to myelopathy and/or radiculopathy secondary to chronic pressure on the spinal cord and nerve roots.[10] The posterior longitudinal ligament (PLL) is a band of collagen and elastin fibers that extends along a line along the posterior

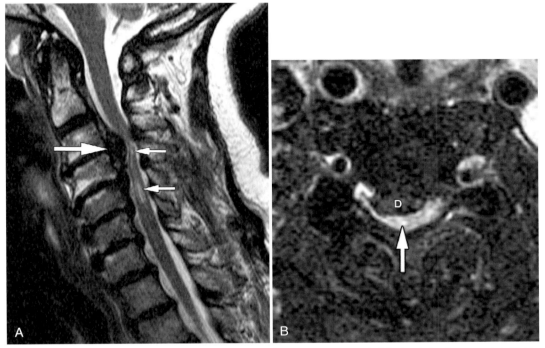

Figure 71-1 ▶ Cervical Spinal Stenosis Due to Large Disc Herniation. Sagittal T2 image **A**. Large cervical disc herniation (*large arrow*) at C3-4 in a patient that also has ossification of the posterior longitudinal ligament. Abnormal increased T2 signal in the cervical cord (*small arrows*) consistent with cord ischemia and/or myelomalacia due to chronic compressive changes. Axial T2 image **B** demonstrates a moderate disc herniation (*D*) with severe central spinal canal stenosis and the same T2 signal abnormality (*arrow*).

margins of the vertebral bodies from the atlas to the sacrum. The PLL is narrower and weaker than the anterior longitudinal ligament (ALL), which extends along the anterior margins of the vertebral bodies, also from the atlas to the sacrum. The fibers of both of these ligaments are firmly attached to the annulus of the intervertebral discs and the corner of the vertebral bodies.[11] The ligament is widest at the disc spaces and narrowest at the mid-vertebral levels. The ligament is also thicker centrally and progressively thins out laterally. OPLL usually occurs in patients over 40 years of age and is very rare until the third decade. OPLL has been well studied in East Asian countries with an incidence of 2% to 4%.[12] The prevalence of OPLL in other countries has not been well studied. OPLL has been estimated to have a prevalence of 0.12% in a radiology review.[13] One quarter of North Americans and Japanese patients with cervical myelopathy exhibit OPLL.[14] Most often, OPLL is found in the upper cervical spine (70%, C2-C4) and less often in the upper thoracic spine (15%, T1-T4). Cervical OPLL occurs twice as often in males as in females.[15]

Ossification of the ligamentum flavum (OLF) is more common in the lumbar and thoracic regions; however, it may occur at the atlantoaxial region as well.[16,17] OLF is common in the Japanese population, affecting up to 20% of Japanese patients greater than 65 years of age, with rare reports in Caucasians and people of African descent.[18-20] Neck pain and arm weakness are the most common symptoms; however, with greater spinal stenosis, bowel and bladder dysfunction can occur.

Cervical stenosis can be a dynamic process. Typical computed tomography (CT) and magnetic resonance imaging (MRI) demonstrate static abnormalities that can cause cervical stenosis. However, the size and shape of the available space in the central spinal canal can change with motion, particularly flexion and extension. Chen and colleagues[21] measured these changes in human cadavers and discovered that from flexion to extension, disc bulging decreased the spinal canal diameter by 10.8% and ligamentum flavum bulging decreased the spinal canal diameter by 24.3%. Similar changes were seen with axial loading on the cervical spine.

Upper cervical spinal stenosis, often due to congenital abnormalities, may cause neck pain and restricted movement. With greater stenosis, these patients can suffer from respiratory paralysis or even sudden death. Developmental stenosis secondary to short pedicles can have myelopathic symptoms and/or radicular pain. Acquired degenerative cervical spinal stenosis may have myelopathic symptoms such as weakness in the arms and hands; a staggering, wide gait; and interosseous atrophy.[22] With foraminal and lateral recess narrowing, shoulder and arm pain can appear.

IMAGING FEATURES

The role of imaging is not only to define whether spinal stenosis is present but also to determine what the cause is and what the relative contribution of bony versus soft tissue spinal stenosis is. Plain radiographs are often not useful. Although radiographs can demonstrate changes of disc space narrowing and osteophytes, the relative contribution of these abnormalities to spinal stenosis is not evident. Myelography has been used in the past but has been supplanted by less invasive cross-sectional imaging. Myelography indirectly demonstrates spinal stenosis as a narrowing of the contrast-filled thecal sac *(Fig. 71-2)*. One then needs to deduce whether the narrowing is caused by soft tissue and/or a bony substance. Myelography is very insensitive to abnormalities outside of the central canal and does not allow for visualization of abnormalities lateral to the midneural foramen. A combination of

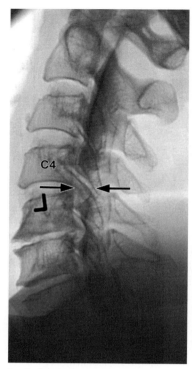

Figure 71-2 ► **Cervical Spinal Stenosis, Myelography.** Lateral view from cervical myelography demonstrates a negative filling defect on the ventral surface of the thecal sac (*between arrows*). The cause of the negative defect is unknown from myelography alone.

myelography followed by CT can improve visualization of both the bony detail and nerve root compression (*Fig. 71-3*), but because myelography is invasive and requires an intrathecal injection of contrast material, MRI and plain CT are the imaging modalities of choice for spinal stenosis.

Both CT and MRI can demonstrate the presence of spinal stenosis. CT has a clear advantage in the evaluation of the bony contribution to spinal stenosis (osteophytes, facet degeneration) (*Fig. 71-4*), whereas MRI has the advantage of soft tissue contributions to spinal stenosis (disc bulge/herniation, ligamentous hypertrophy, synovial cysts). Whether by CT or MR imaging, the imaging characteristics of spinal stenosis show a change in shape of the spinal canal from its rounded or oval shape to a more irregular or flattened appearance (*Fig. 71-5*). There may be displacement or obliteration of the epidural fat adjacent to the thecal sac or in the neural foramen (*Fig. 71-6*). With MRI, there may be loss of cerebrospinal fluid (CSF) around the nerve roots on T2-weighted sequences.[23] If stenosis is severe enough, there may be increased T2 signal intensity within the cervical cord compatible with cord ischemia, which could lead to cord infarction (*Fig. 71-7*). Foraminal narrowing can be evaluated on the sagittal MR images (which tends to overestimate foraminal narrowing) or from reformatted sagittal images from the CT axial data.

Most evaluation of spinal stenosis is subjective rather than objective and relies upon the experience of the interpreter. Various studies have shown moderate to poor interobserver results in agreement as to the presence or absence of stenosis, the degree of stenosis, and the cause of the stenosis.[24,25] Furthermore, spinal stenosis is a dynamic process, and imaging is a static process. If a patient is never symptomatic lying supine, then imaging studies performed in a supine position may not reveal the abnormality or may minimize the abnormality. Therefore, if one has high clinical suspicion of spinal stenosis that is not explained by cross-sectional

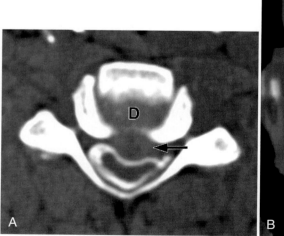

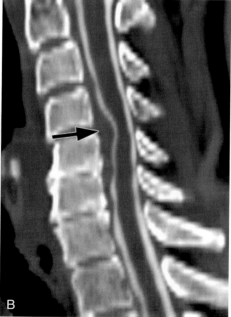

Figure 71-3 ► **Cervical Spinal Stenosis, Post-Myelogram CT.** Same patient as in Figure 71-2. Axial image **A** and reformatted sagittal image **B** post-myelography. The negative defect on myelography represents a left paramidline disc herniation (*arrow*). The disc herniation has the same density as the parent disc (*D*).

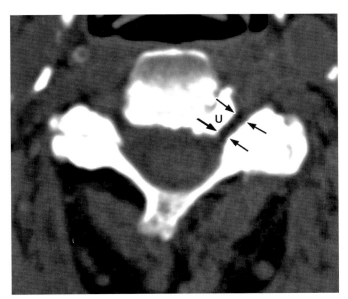

Figure 71-4 ▸ Uncovertebral Joint Spur. Axial CT of the cervical spine. Prominent left uncovertebral joint spur (*U*) causes moderate narrowing of the neural foramen (*bounded by arrows*).

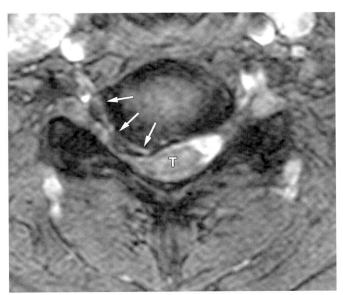

Figure 71-5 ▸ Large Right Posterolateral Osteophyte. Axial gradient recall image. Distorted shape of the thecal sac (*T*) secondary to a large right posterolateral osteophyte/disc complex (*arrows*).

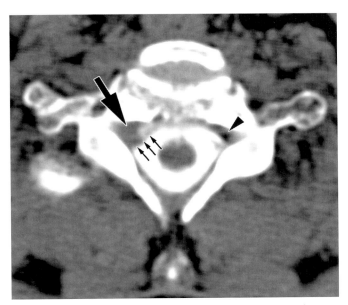

Figure 71-6 ▸ Subtle Cervical Disc Herniation. Postmyelogram axial CT. Loss of normal ventrolateral epidural fat (*large arrow*) with flattening of the right ventrolateral thecal sac (*small arrows*) caused by a subtle disc herniation. Note the normal ventrolateral epidural fat density on the left (*arrowhead*).

imaging, it may be prudent to perform a diagnostic study with axial loading (myelography, upright MRI or CT) and/or dynamic maneuvers of flexion/extension and lateral bending (myelography). Lastly, the importance of scanning angle cannot be emphasized enough. An accurate measurement of spinal stenosis must include an evaluation of the disc level parallel to the disc. If scanning is not parallel to the affected disc levels, one could easily underestimate or overestimate stenosis. With new imaging software, reformatted corrections of the angles can be made to give a more accurate evaluation of spinal stenosis.

Studies have defined some average cervical spinal measurements. The mean anteroposterior (AP) diameter of the cervical spinal canal is approximately 17 to 18 mm between C3-C7.[26] There have been several methods of measuring devised to evaluate for cervical spinal stenosis. Plain lateral radiographs were used to measure the distance from the middle of the posterior surface of a vertebral body to the spinolaminar line (*Fig. 71-8*). This measurement is known as the *developmental segmental sagittal diameter* and is not altered by degenerative changes because those occur at the disc level. The segmental sagittal diameter is a measure of congenital narrowing and can be used to identify whether a person is congenitally at risk for neurologic injuries and has been used in athletes. Patients with a segmental sagittal diameter of less than 13 mm are at a high risk for developing signs and symptoms of cervical myelopathy.[27] A canal AP diameter of less than 10 mm is considered absolutely stenotic. However, this measurement relies on the distance at which the image was obtained because there can be wide variations in the measurement as a result of magnification.[28]

The spinal canal-to-vertebral body ratio,[29] *Torg ratio*, was made to adjust for magnification error. The Torg ratio is made by dividing the sagittal diameter of the spinal canal (the developmental segmental sagittal diameter) by the sagittal diameter of the vertebral body at the same level (*Fig. 71-9*). These measurements are also performed at the mid vertebral body level and have been used to measure the risk of neurologic injury due to congenital cervical narrowing. A ratio of 1.0 is considered normal and a ratio of 0.82 or less was said to represent stenosis in 92% of cases with a 6% false-positive rate.[29] However, this ratio does not account for persons that may have larger vertebral bodies rendering a low Torg ratio in the face of no significant spinal stenosis.

The *compression ratio* is correlated with prognosis for recovery after decompression.[30] The compression ratio is obtained by dividing the smallest AP measurement of the spinal cord by the transverse measurement of the spinal cord at the same level (*Fig. 71-10*). A ratio of less than 0.4 has a poor prognosis for recovery.

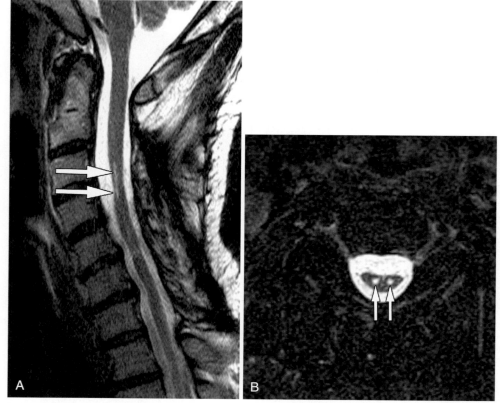

Figure 71-7 ► Spinal Cord Myelomalacia. Sagittal T2 image **A** and axial T2 image **B** after C3-C7 laminectomies for severe spinal stenosis. There is no evidence of residual central spinal canal stenosis; however, there is abnormal increased T2 signal intensity in both halves of the cervical cord, sometimes called snake eyes or owl eyes (*arrows*), compatible with spinal cord myelomalacia in the central gray matter.

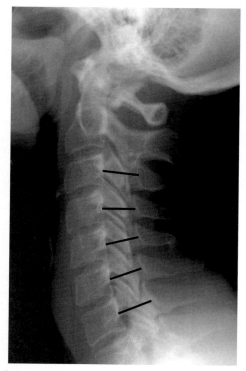

Figure 71-8 ► Developmental Segmental Sagittal Diameter. Straight line measurements taken from a cervical lateral radiograph. Distance from the posterior surface of the mid vertebral body to the mid portion of the spinolamellar line at the same level. Patients with a segmental sagittal diameter of less than 13 mm are at a high risk for developing signs and symptoms of cervical myelopathy. This measurement can be falsely positive or negative based on differences in magnification when the image is obtained.

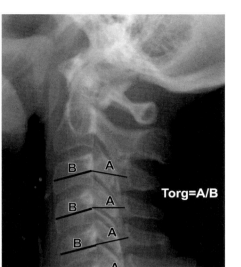

Figure 71-9 ▶ Torg Ratio. Also called the *spinal canal-to-vertebral body ratio*, the Torg ratio was made to adjust for magnification error. The Torg ratio is determined by dividing the sagittal diameter of the spinal canal (the developmental segmental sagittal diameter) by the sagittal diameter of the vertebral body at the same level. A ratio of 1.0 is considered normal and a ratio of 0.82 or less was said to represent stenosis in 92% of cases with a 6% false-positive rate. However, this ratio does not account for persons who may have larger vertebral bodies that would render a low Torg ratio in the face of no significant spinal stenosis.

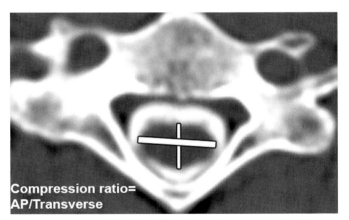

Figure 71-10 ▶ Compression Ratio. The compression ratio is obtained by dividing the smallest anteroposterior (AP) measurement of the spinal cord by the transverse measurement of the spinal cord at the same level. The compression ratio is correlated with prognosis for recovery after decompression. A ratio of less than 0.4 has a poor prognosis for recovery.

To date, there are no studies that give standardized measurements at the level of the disc in patients with cervical spondylosis.

DIFFERENTIAL DIAGNOSIS

1. **Epidural abscess/phlegmon:** Typically there is enhancement of an epidural phlegmon and peripheral enhancement of an epidural abscess *(Fig. 71-11)*. Laboratory evaluation

including white blood cell count, sedimentation rate, and C-reactive protein is often abnormal.
2. **Epidural hemorrhage:** Classically, epidural hemorrhage manifests with abrupt symptoms as opposed to the gradual and progressive symptomatology of spinal stenosis. It is often posterior to the cervical spinal cord and demonstrates variable signal intensity. Blood sensitive MRI sequences can assist in the diagnosis *(Fig. 71-12)*.
3. **Metastatic disease:** Many times, patients with metastatic disease have a known primary tumor. Metastatic disease that

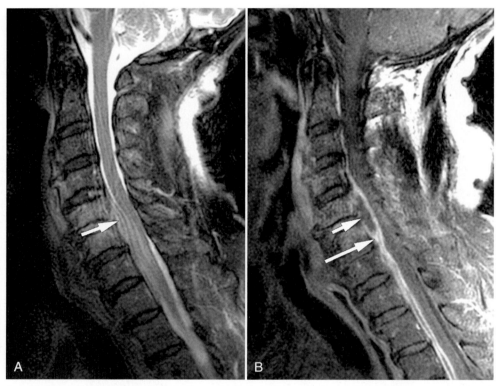

Figure 71-11 ▶ Cervical Discitis with Abscess Formation. Abnormal mixed signal intensity in the ventral epidural space spanning the C5 and C6 vertebral segments (*arrow*) as well as abnormal signal intensity within these vertebral bodies on sagittal T2 image **A**. Post-contrast T1 image **B** shows a nonenhancing abscess cavity (*short arrow*) with surrounding enhancing phlegmon (*long arrow*).

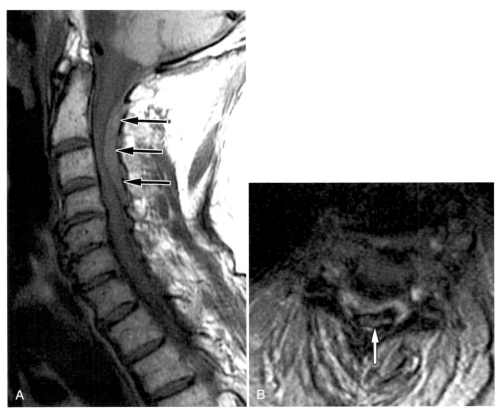

Figure 71-12 ▶ Spontaneous Cervical Epidural Hematoma. Dorsal intermediate T1 intensity epidural mass extending from the skull base to the C4-5 level (*arrows*) causing mass effect with ventral displacement of the cervical spinal cord. Blood-sensitive axial gradient image **B** confirms the mass as hemorrhage (*arrow*).

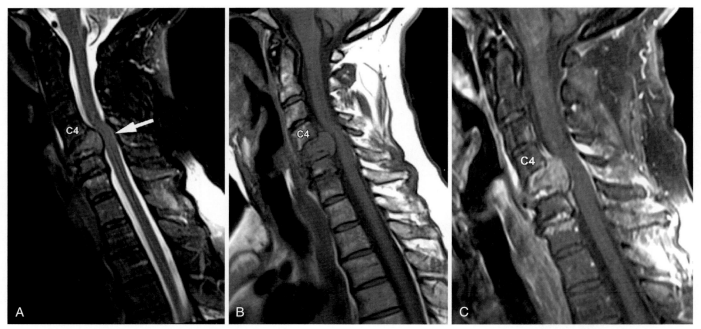

Figure 71-13 ► **Metastatic Disease with Pathologic Fracture.** Sagittal T2 image **A**, sagittal Tl image **B** and sagittal post-contrast T1 image **C**. Complete replacement of a partially collapsed C5 vertebral body with retropulsion of pathologic bone into the spinal canal causing stenosis. Increased T2 signal intensity within the cervical cord (*arrow*, image **A**) from the C4-5 to CS-6 level compatible with cord ischemia.

causes spinal stenosis has typical imaging findings of a soft tissue mass involving bone that enhances *(Fig. 71-13)*.

TREATMENT

1. **Nonoperative management of pain:** Typically managed with acetaminophen, nonsteroidal anti-inflammatory drugs (NSAIDs), and/or muscle relaxants. If these medications do not control the pain, then a mild oral narcotic can be prescribed. The patient's neck may need to be immobilized in a firm cervical orthosis. Physical therapy with isometric muscle strengthening and symptomatic measures such as heat, ice, and massage can be performed.[31] Injection therapy with corticosteroids can be used for pain flare-ups if it is felt to be inflammatory-mediated. An interlaminar injection can be performed if the pain is mainly in the neck. If there is lateralization of the pain to a single side or evidence of radicular pain, a transforaminal epidural injection can be performed. These injections can be quite beneficial not only in pain relief but also in allowing the patient to participate more in exercise therapy.

2. **Surgery:** Surgical treatment of symptomatic spinal stenosis (central canal, foraminal, or lateral recess) is performed to reestablish sufficient space for the thecal sac and its contents, as well as the traversing and exiting nerve roots. Surgical treatment depends on the site of compression and levels of abnormality. Decompression may be achieved with an anterior, posterior, or combined approach.

References

1. Michie I, Clark M. Neurological syndromes associated with cervical and craniocervical anomalies. *Arch Neurol.* 1968;18:241-247.

2. Gulati DR, Rout D. Atlantoaxial dislocation with quadriparesis in achondroplasia. *J Neurosurg.* 1974;40:394-396.
3. Curtis BH, Blank S, Fisher RL. Atlantoaxial dislocation in Downs syndrome: Report of two patients requiring surgical correction. *JAMA.* 1968;205:464-465.
4. Ramsey J, Bliznack J. Klippel-Feil syndrome with renal agenesis and other anomalies. *Am J Roentgenol.* 1971;113:460-463.
5. de Andrade R, MacNab I. Anterior occipitocervical fusion in rheumatoid arthritis. *Arthritis Rheum.* 1969;12:423-426.
6. Epstein BS, Epstein JA. The association of cerebellar tonsillar herniation with basilar impression incident to Paget's disease. *AJR Am J Roentgenol.* 1969;107:535.
7. Mercer S, Bogduk N. The ligaments and annulus fibrosis of human adult cervical intervertebral discs. *Spine.* 1999;24:619-626.
8. Baptiste DC, Fehlings MG. Pathophysiology of cervical myelopathy. *Spine J.* 2006;6:190S-197S.
9. Carette S, Fehlings MG. Clinical practice: Cervical radiculopathy. *N Engl J Med.* 2005;353:392-399.
10. Schmidt MH, Quinones-Hinojosa A, Rosenberg WS. Cervical myelopathy associated with degenerative spine disease and ossification of the posterior longitudinal ligament. *Semin Neurol.* 2002;212:143-148.
11. Ehara S, Shimamura T, Nakamura R, Yamazaki K. Paravertebral ligamentous ossification: DISH, OPLL and OLF. *Eur J Radiol.* 1998;27:196-205.
12. Matsunga S, Yamaguchi M, Hayashi K, Sakou T. Genetic analysis of ossification of the posterior longitudinal ligament. *Spine.* 1999;24:937-939.
13. Resnick D. *Diagnosis of Bone and Joint Disorders.* London: Saunders; 1994:1496-1507.
14. Epstein NE. The surgical management of ossification of the posterior longitudinal ligament in 43 North Americans. *Spine.* 1994;19:664-672.
15. Epstein NE. Ossification of the posterior longitudinal ligament: Diagnosis and surgical management. *Neurosurg Quart.* 1992;2:223-241.
16. Mak KH, Mak KL, Gwi-Mak E. Ossification of the ligamentum flavum in the cervicothoracic junction: Case report on ossification found on both sides of the lamina. *Spine.* 2002;27:E11-14.
17. Nadkarni TD, Menon RK, Desai KI, Goel A. Ossified ligamentum flavum of the atlantoaxial region. *J Clin Neurosci.* 2005;12:486-489.
18. Shenoi RM, Duong TT, Brega KE, Gaido LB. Ossification of the ligamentum flavum causing thoracic myelopathy: A case report. *Am J Phys Med Rehabil.* 1997;76:68-72.

19. Yamashita Y, Takahashi M, Matsuno Y, et al. Spinal cord compression due to ossification of ligaments: MR imaging. *Radiology.* 1990;175:843-848.

20. van Oostenbrugge RJ, Herpers MJ, de Kruijk JR. Spinal cord compression caused by unusual location and extension of ossified ligamenta flava in a Caucasian male: A case report and literature review. *Spine.* 1999;24:486-488.

21. Chen IH, Vasavada A, Panjabi MM. Kinematics of the cervical spine canal: Changes with sagittal plane loads. *J Spinal Disord.* 1994;7:93-101.

22. Epstein BS, Epstein JA, Jones MD. Cervical spinal stenosis. *Radiol Clin North Am.* 1977;15:215-226

23. Postacchini F, Amatruda A, Morace GB, Perugia D. Magnetic resonance imaging in the diagnosis of lumbar spinal canal stenosis. *Ital J Orthop Traumtol.* 1991;17:327-337.

24. Stafira JS, Sonnad JR, Yuh WTC, et al. Qualitative assessment of cervical spinal stenosis: Observer variability on CT and MR images. *AJNR Am J Neuroradiol.* 2003;24:766-769.

25. Drew B, Bhandari M, Kulkarni A, et al. Reliability in grading the severity of lumbar spinal stenosis. *J Spinal Disord.* 2000;13:253-258.

26. Murone I. The importance of the sagittal diameters of the cervical spinal canal in relation to spondylosis and myelopathy. *J Bone Joint Surg Br.* 1974; 56:30-36.

27. Arnold JG. The clinical manifestations of spondylochondrosis (spondylosis) of the cervical spine. *Ann Surg.* 1955;141:872-889.

28. Herzog RJ, Wiens JJ, Dillingham MF, Sontag MJ. Normal cervical spine morphometry and cervical spinal stenosis in asymptomatic professional football players: Plain film radiography, multiplanar computed tomography, and magnetic resonance imaging. *Spine.* 1991;16:178-186.

29. Pavlov H, Torg JS, Robie B, Jahre C. Cervical spinal stenosis: Determination with vertebral body ratio method. *Radiology.* 1987;164:771-775.

30. Fujiwara K, Yonenobu K, Ebara S, et al. The prognosis of surgery for cervical compression myelopathy: An analysis of the factors involved. *J Bone Joint Surg Br.* 1989;71:393-398.

31. Law MD, Bernhardt M, White AA. Cervical spondylotic myelopathy: A review of surgical indications and decision making. *Yale J Biol Med.* 1993; 66:165-177.

SPINAL STENOSIS—LUMBAR

Douglas S. Fenton, M.D.

CLINICAL PRESENTATION

The patient is a 77-year-old man who presented with chronic low back pain. The patient has had progressive low back pain with radiation into both hips and buttocks over the last 5 years. The pain is made worse with movements and transitions from sitting to standing. He cannot walk more than 50 yards before he begins to feel deep low back aching. He states that he has to lean forward on a shopping cart to support himself while he does his grocery shopping. He also states that this forward flexed position tends to diminish his pain. The patient denies any bowel or bladder symptoms. On examination, straight leg raising maneuvers were negative. The patient was able to flex at the waist 90 degrees but extend only 10 degrees.

IMAGING PRESENTATION

Sagittal T1-weighted and T2-weighted magnetic resonance (MR) images demonstrate a long segment of narrowing of the central spinal canal without evidence of disc herniation, discogenic degenerative changes, or prominence of the epidural fat. The patient's underlying abnormality is congenital narrowing of the lumbar spinal canal secondary to short pedicles. This patient is at a disadvantage because his small disc bulges at L2-3, L3-4, and L4-5 has converted him from asymptomatic to severely symptomatic (*Fig. 72-1*).

DISCUSSION

Lumbar spinal stenosis can be defined as any narrowing of the spinal canal that causes compression of its contents because of a mismatch between the available space in the spinal canal and its contents. There are three categories of lumbar spinal stenosis: congenital, developmental, and acquired. Most clinicians combine congenital and developmental stenosis. Congenital/developmental stenosis is usually caused by short pedicles. As a person ages, degenerative changes ensue. Normally, a person would not be symptomatic from degenerative changes until they were moderate or severe. However, with short pedicles, one tends to see symptoms with much milder degenerative changes because the available spinal canal space is already smaller in anterior-posterior diameter and area. Therefore, symptoms in patients with congenital/developmental stenosis tend to occur at a younger age; in the third to fifth decades of life.[1]

Acquired stenosis is much more common than congenital/developmental stenosis. Degenerative stenosis is the most common type of acquired stenosis. Degenerative arthritis often becomes symptomatic after the fifth decade of life.[2] It is often due to arthritic changes of the intervertebral disc, facet joints, and surrounding ligaments. First, there is loss of disc height with bulging of the disc annulus and thickening/redundancy of the ligamentum flavum. Disc bulging then leads to ventral compression of the thecal sac. The ligamentous redundancy causes posterior/posterolateral compression of the thecal sac. Loss of disc height leads to foraminal compromise. This then leads to osteoarthritis and hypertrophy of the zygapophyseal joints with thickening of the joint capsule. Osteophytes form in order to stabilize the degenerating level, giving it more surface area. Osteophyte formation of the inferior articular processes results in posterolateral compression of the thecal sac.[3] Osteophyte formation from the superior articular processes can result in stenosis of the lateral recesses or foraminal narrowing causing radicular pain. With severe facet joint arthritis, synovial-lined cysts can arise and protrude into the spinal canal, foramen, or lateral recess (*Fig. 72-2*).[1,3]

Other causes of acquired spinal stenosis include stenosis related to a degenerative spondylolisthesis (*Fig. 72-3*), spondylolisthesis associated with a spondylolysis (*Fig. 72-4*) or at a level adjacent to a spinal fusion, increased intraspinal fat secondary to endogenous or exogenous steroids (*Fig. 72-5*), Paget's disease (*Fig. 72-6*), epidural mass from metastatic disease (*Fig. 72-7*) and acromegaly.[1] Another very common cause of acquired stenosis is a disc herniation (*Fig. 72-8*).

The classic symptoms of lumbar spinal stenosis are those of neurogenic claudication: pain during walking, numbness, tingling, weakness, and pain that radiates from the lower back, frequently into the thighs and lower legs.[1,4] The symptoms are exacerbated with lumbar extension and improved with lumbar flexion, felt to be secondary to the increase in cross-sectional area of the lumbar spinal canal in flexion.[5] Patients can commonly ride a bike or walk uphill because these movements require being in lumbar flexion, but have difficulty walking downhill because of the required lumbar extension.[3] Radicular symptoms are caused by foraminal or lateral recess stenosis.

IMAGING FEATURES

The role of imaging is not only to define whether spinal stenosis is present but also to determine the cause and the

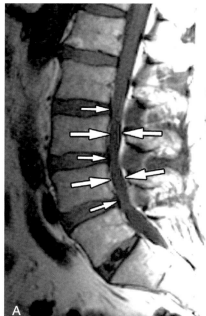
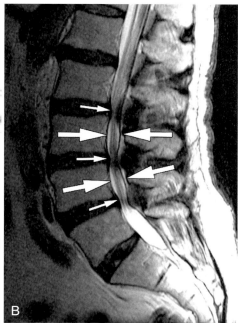

Figure 72-1 ▶ Congenital Central Spinal Canal Stenosis. Sagittal T1 image **A** and sagittal T2 image **B** in a patient with diffuse spinal stenosis most pronounced at the L3 and L4 levels (*between large arrows*). There is no evidence of discogenic degeneration (*short arrows*) as the cause of the narrowing. This patient's narrowing is secondary to congenital short pedicles.

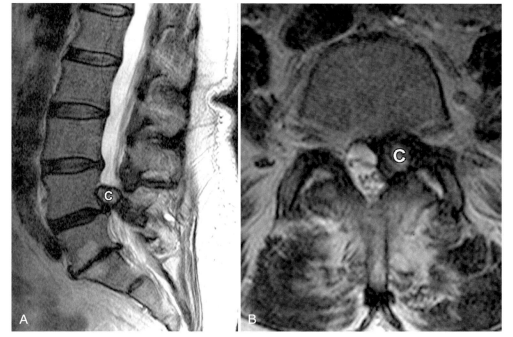

Figure 72-2 ▶ Synovial Cyst. Sagittal T2-weighted image **A** and axial T2-weighted image **B** demonstrate a large ovoid mass (*C*) contiguous with and ventromedial to a degenerated facet joint and compressing the left ventrolateral aspect of the thecal sac.

relative contribution of bony versus soft tissue spinal stenosis. Plain radiographs are often not useful because although they can demonstrate changes of disc space narrowing and osteophytes, the relative contribution of these abnormalities to spinal stenosis is not evident. Myelography has been used in the past but has been supplanted by less invasive cross-sectional imaging. Myelography indirectly demonstrates spinal stenosis as a narrowing of the contrast-filled thecal sac *(Fig. 72-9)*. One then needs to deduce whether the narrowing is caused by soft tissue and/or bony causes.

Myelography is very insensitive to abnormalities outside of the central canal and does not allow for visualization of abnormalities lateral to the midneural foramen. A combination of myelography and computed tomography (CT) can improve visualization of both the bony detail and nerve root compression *(Fig. 72-10)*, but is invasive because myelography requires an intrathecal injection of contrast material.

Magnetic resonance imaging (MRI) and plain CT are the imaging modalities of choice for spinal stenosis. Both CT and

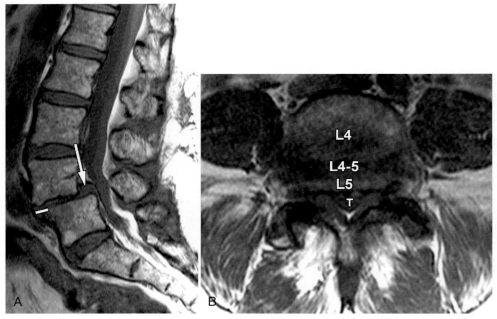

Figure 72-3 ▶ Degenerative Spondylolisthesis. Sagittal T1-weighted image **A** shows anterior subluxation of L4 with respect to L5 (*short line*) with uncovering of the posterior L4-5 disc (*arrow*). Axial T1-weighted image **B** reveals severe narrowing of the thecal sac (*T*) secondary to the anterolisthesis and facet degenerative changes. Note the typical appearance of axial imaging of spondylolisthesis in the lower lumbar spine that is not performed angled to the disc. One can see both the posterior margin of the L4 and L5 vertebral bodies and a portion of the intervening disc.

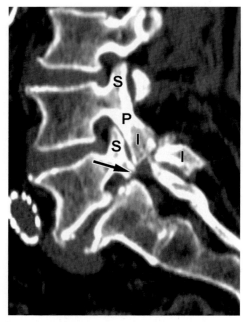

Figure 72-4 ▶ Spondylolysis. Off-midline sagittal reformatted CT. Break and separation of the superior articular process (*S*) and inferior articular process (*I*) of L5 at the level of the pars interarticularis (*arrow*). Normal appearance of the superior articular process, pars interarticularis (*P*) and inferior articular process of L4.

MRI can demonstrate the presence of spinal stenosis. CT has a clear advantage in the evaluation of the bony contribution to spinal stenosis (osteophytes, facet degeneration), whereas MRI has the advantage of depicting soft tissue contributions to spinal stenosis (disc bulge/herniation, ligamentous hypertrophy, synovial cysts). Whether by CT or MR imaging, the imaging characteristics of spinal stenosis is a change in the shape of the spinal canal from its rounded or oval shape to a more irregular or flattened appearance (*Figs. 72-11 and 72-12*). There may be displacement or obliteration of the epidural fat adjacent to the thecal sac or in the neural foramen. There may be obliteration or displacement of the thecal sac. With MRI, there may be loss of cerebrospinal fluid (CSF) around the nerve roots on T2-weighted sequences (*Fig. 72-13*).[6] The spinal canal may have a trefoil appearance secondary to bone proliferation or ligamentous thickening or may have an asymmetric appearance (*Fig. 72-14*). Foraminal narrowing can be evaluated on the sagittal MR images or from reformatted sagittal images from the CT axial data (see Fig. 72-4).

Most evaluation of spinal stenosis is subjective rather than objective and relies on the experience of the interpreter. It is important to realize that although the sensitivities of CT and MRI in depicting spinal stenosis exceed 70%, more than 20% of people greater than 60 years of age have imaging findings of spinal stenosis without symptoms or functional limitations.[4] Furthermore, spinal stenosis is a dynamic process and imaging is a static process. If a patient is never symptomatic lying supine, then imaging studies performed in a supine position may not reveal the abnormality or may minimize the abnormality. One study demonstrated a mean underestimation of 16% in the diameter of the thecal sac when supine myelography/CT was compared with extension myelography/CT. This underestimation was greater than 30% in over 15% of the levels measured.[7] Therefore, if one has high clinical suspicion of spinal stenosis that is not explained by cross-sectional imaging, it may be prudent to perform a diagnostic study with axial loading (myelography, upright MRI or CT) and/or dynamic maneuvers of flexion/extension and lateral bending (myelography). Lastly, the importance of the scanning angle cannot be emphasized enough. An accurate measurement of spinal stenosis

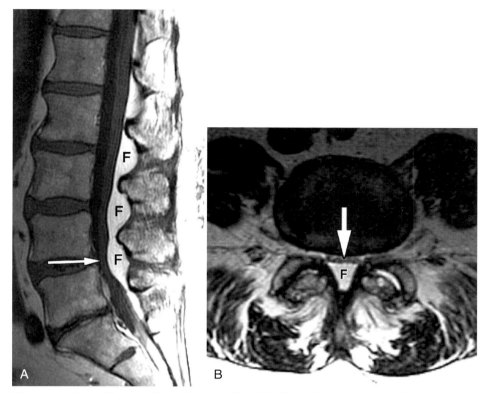

Figure 72-5 ▸ Epidural Lipomatosis. Sagittal T1-weighted image **A** and axial T2-weighted image **B**. Increased quantity of the posterior epidural fat (*F*) with significant compression and narrowing of the thecal sac (*arrow*).

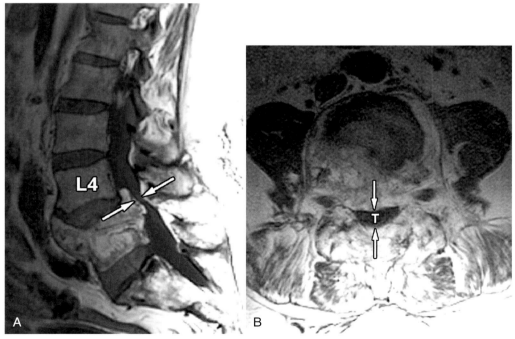

Figure 72-6 ▸ Paget Disease. Sagittal T1-weighted image **A** and axial T1-weighted image **B**. Overgrowth and squaring of the L5 vertebral body. Excessive overgrowth of the posterior superior L5 vertebral body causes severe narrowing of the central spinal canal (*between arrows*) and thecal sac (*T*).

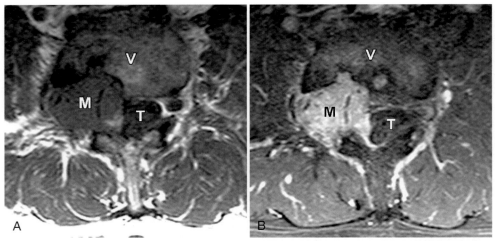

Figure 72-7 ▶ Metastatic Disease. Axial T1-weighted image **A** and post-contrast T1-weighted image **B**. Large enhancing mass (*M*) in the right neural foramen eroding the right posterior vertebral body (*V*) and displacing the thecal sac (*T*) to the left.

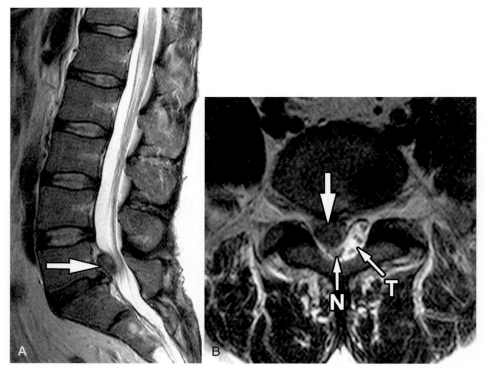

Figure 72-8 ▶ Disc Herniation. Sagittal T2-weighted image **A** and axial T2-weighted image **B**. Large right L5-S1 disc herniation extruded superiorly behind the L5 vertebral body (*arrow*) with preferential compression of the right ventral thecal sac (*T*) and posterior displacement of the intrathecal nerve roots (*N*).

must include an evaluation of the disc level parallel to the disc. Patients are routinely imaged in the supine position with axial scanning perpendicular to the floor. This often gives fairly parallel to the disc imaging from L1-2 to L3-4. However, scanning may be far from parallel at the L4-5 and L5-S1 levels and could easily underestimate or overestimate stenosis. With new imaging software, reformatted corrections of the angles can be made to give a more accurate evaluation of spinal stenosis.

To date, there are no grading systems to evaluate lumbar spinal stenosis. It has been demonstrated that intraobserver and interobserver agreement in evaluating the degree of spinal stenosis is only fair.[8] This could mean that there are patients who are being graded higher or lower than their actual stenosis, which may significantly alter the patients' treatment. It is likely best practice to use a combination of a good history and physical combined with imaging that is read by someone with great experience in spine imaging.

Studies have defined some average lumbar spinal measurements. An anterior-posterior (AP) maximum lumbar spinal canal dimension of 15 or more mm and an interpedicular distance of 25 or greater mm is considered to be normal. Interpedicular distance increases slightly from L3 to L5. The cross-sectional areas from L3

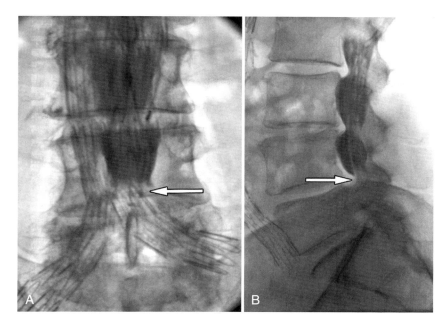

Figure 72-9 ▶ Myelographic Block Due to Spinal Stenosis. Frontal **A** and lateral **B** lumbar myelogram images. Near complete obliteration of the contrast-filled spinal canal at the L4-S disc level from unknown etiology (*arrow*).

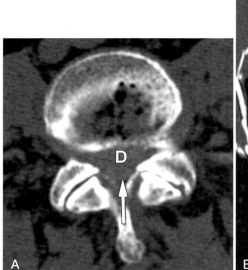

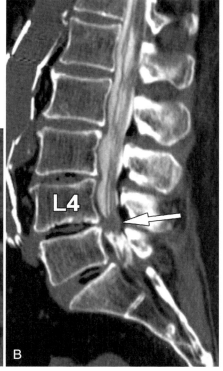

Figure 72-10 ▶ Severe Spinal Stenosis, Post-Myelogram CT. Same patient as in Figure 72-9. Axial **A** and reformatted sagittal **B**. Near complete obliteration of the contrast-filled spinal canal and thecal sac (*arrow*) at the L4-S disc level is now seen to be due to a disc herniation (*D*).

to L5 increase from 277 mm² to 386 mm².[9] These values can be used as a general guideline in measuring spinal canal stenosis. Verbeist[10] identified two subgroups of patients with spinal stenosis: absolute stenosis (those with AP diameters of 10 mm or less) and relative stenosis (those with AP diameters between 10 and 12 mm). More recent studies have decreased the importance of any one dimension in the evaluation of spinal stenosis and now regard the cross-sectional area to be the preferred method in evaluating spinal stenosis. In one study, a cross-sectional area of less than 100 mm² was highly associated with neurogenic claudication.[11]

Congenital spinal canal narrowing is due to short pedicles. Lumbar pedicle length was seen to average between 5 and 6 mm in those with congenital narrowing versus approximately 9 mm in the normal patient.[12] The cross-sectional area was also significantly less in asymptomatic patients with congenitally short pedicles (L2-L5:176 mm²-213 mm² vs. L2-L5: 259 mm²-323 mm²).[12] No difference was noted when comparing the AP diameter of the vertebral body, the vertebral body height, spinal width, and pedicle width between those with congenitally short pedicles and the norm.[12]

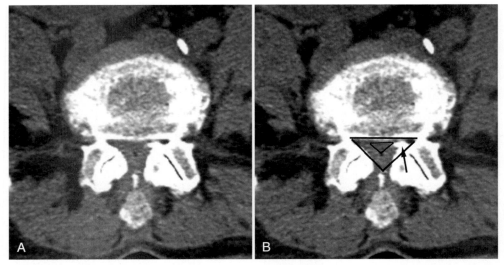

Figure 72-11 ▸ **Central Spinal Stenosis.** Identical axial CT images. Outer triangle (image **B**) demonstrates the change in shape from the spinal canal's normal rounded shape to a more triangular shape secondary to posterior vertebral spurring and facet joint degeneration. Inner triangle is the additional narrowing of the thecal sac and its contents due to outer triangle abnormalities and thickening of the ligamentum flavum. Facet joint spur (*arrow*) severely narrows the lateral recess.

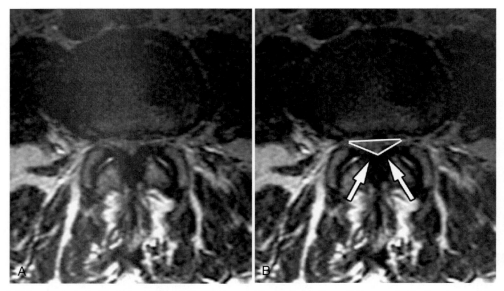

Figure 72-12 ▸ **Central Spinal Stenosis.** Identical axial T2-weighted MR images. Triangle depicts the available room for the thecal sac and its contents. Thickened ligamentum flavum (*arrows*).

DIFFERENTIAL DIAGNOSIS

Clinical Differential

1. **Hip osteoarthritis:** One must clinically distinguish the pain of lumbar spinal stenosis from that of hip osteoarthritis. With hip osteoarthritis the pain is typically in the groin, which is provoked with internal rotation of the hip.
2. **Trochanteric bursitis:** This entity has tenderness to palpation over the greater trochanter.
3. **Vascular claudication:** The pain with vascular claudication is usually not influenced with lumbar extension, flexion, or by standing up. It is exacerbated by walking, especially uphill, unlike neurogenic claudication, which is worse in extension and with walking downhill.

Imaging Differential

1. **Epidural abscess/phlegmon:** Typically there is enhancement of an epidural phlegmon and peripheral enhancement of an epidural abscess *(Fig. 72-15)*: Laboratory evaluation including white blood cell count, sedimentation rate, and C-reactive protein is often abnormal.
2. **Epidural hemorrhage *(Fig. 72-16)*:** An epidural hemorrhage classically has abrupt symptoms as opposed to the gradual and progressive symptomatology of spinal stenosis. The hematoma can have variable imaging characteristics depending on its age.
3. **Primary or metastatic disease** (see Fig. 72-7): Primary or metastatic disease that causes spinal stenosis has typical imaging findings of a soft tissue mass involving bone.

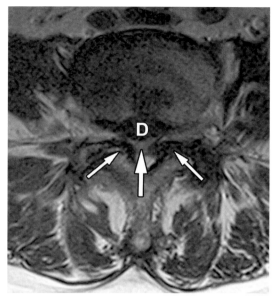

Figure 72-13 ▶ Spinal Stenosis with Loss of Normal Intrathecal CSF Signal. Axial T2-weighted image. When there is no spinal stenosis, there is typically increased T2 signal intensity CSF surrounding the individual intrathecal nerve roots. In this patient, there is absence of CSF signal intensity within the thecal sac (*large arrow*) due to stenosis from a disc herniation (*D*) and facet joint spurring (*small arrows*).

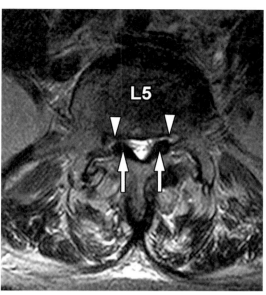

Figure 72-14 ▶ Spinal Stenosis, Trefoil Appearance. Axial T2-weighted image of the lumbar spine demonstrates a trefoil shape secondary to prominent thickening of the ligamentum flavum (*arrows*) causing severe narrowing of both lateral recesses (*arrowheads*).

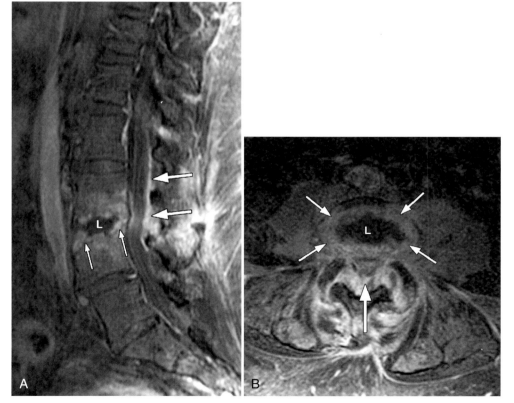

Figure 72-15 ▶ Discitis/Osteomyelitis with Epidural Phlegmon. Sagittal post-contrast, Tl-weighted image **A** and axial post-contrast, T1-weighted image **B**. Enhancement of the L4-5 intervertebral disc (*small arrows*), liquefaction of the central disc (*L*) and enhancement in the epidural space (*large arrows*) compatible with phlegmon. Phlegmon can have similar imaging characteristics to scar tissue; however, there should be no enhancement of the disc with scar tissue. Patients with an epidural phlegmon are typically ill, with elevated temperatures and white blood cell counts.

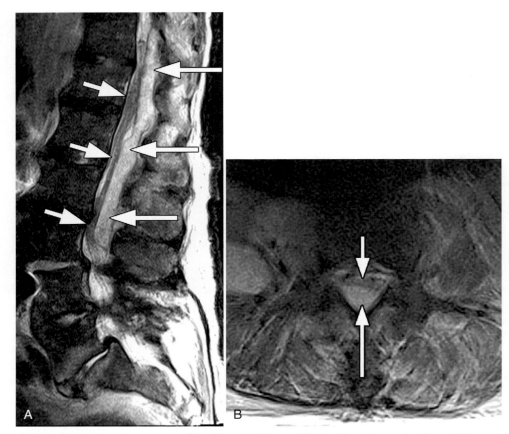

Figure 72-16 ▶ **Spinal Epidural Hematoma.** Long-segment region of intraspinal increased T2 signal intensity on sagittal image **A** (*long arrows*). The spinal cord and cauda equina (*short arrows*) is displaced anteriorly. Axial T2-weighted image **B** shows the hematoma posteriorly (*long arrow*) and the spinal cord ventrally (*short arrow*).

TREATMENT

Treatment of spinal stenosis includes both nonoperative and surgical management. However, in the case of symptomatic central canal stenosis, most patients treated nonoperatively demonstrate no substantial change over the course of 1 year.[13,14] Spontaneous improvement is also rare, making a treatment of rest and watchful waiting a poor strategy for symptomatic patients.[1] There have been no trials on most nonoperative strategies for lumbar spinal stenosis.

1. **Exercise therapy** that keeps the patient in lumbar flexion (bicycling) is better tolerated than walking.
2. **Weight loss and abdominal musculature strengthening** may help the patient have less extension posturing, thus reducing symptoms.
3. **Lumbar corsets** may also help patients maintain a more favorable posture.[1]
4. **Medications** such as acetaminophen or nonsteroidal anti-inflammatory drugs (NSAIDs) are typically used to manage pain. If these medications do not control the pain, then a mild oral narcotic can be prescribed. Injection therapy with corticosteroids can be used for pain flare-ups if it is felt to be inflammatory mediated. An interlaminar injection can be performed if the pain is mainly in the low back and hips. If there is lateralization of the pain to a single side or evidence of radicular pain, a transforaminal epidural injection can be performed. These injections can be quite beneficial not only in pain relief but also in allowing the patient to participate more in exercise therapy.

5. **Surgical treatment** of symptomatic spinal stenosis (central canal, foraminal, or lateral recess) is performed to reestablish sufficient space for the thecal sac and its contents as well as the traversing and exiting nerve roots. Traditionally, this is performed with a decompressive laminectomy and partial facetectomy. If there are radicular symptoms due to foraminal narrowing, then a foraminotomy is performed. There is controversy as to whether the decompression should be supplemented with a fusion. Data suggest that a decompression with fusion is more effective than decompression alone in patients with spinal stenosis secondary to a spondylolisthesis but not in patients without a spondylolisthesis.[15,16] However, other studies indicate that removal of as little as 30% of the facet joint can cause lumbar instability and that fusion may be necessary to counteract this instability.[17] It is also uncertain whether instrumentation (pedicle screws) or biologic agents (bone morphogenic protein) should be used to assist in fusion. Although these help with the technical fusion, it is unknown whether they are associated with improved clinical outcomes.[1] More recently, intradiscal metallic implants have been placed to restore disc height and, more importantly, to increase the craniocaudal dimension of the neural foramen allowing more room for the exiting nerve root. Overall, 80% of patients having surgery for spinal stenoses have some degree of symptomatic relief; however, within 7 to 10 years, one third have

recurrent or new back pain.[18] The re-operation rate is 10% to 23% within 7 to 10 years of the initial operation.[18] The mortality rate for spinal stenosis surgery is less than 1%.[19] Another, more recent, surgical alternative to decompressive laminectomy is called *interspinous distraction* (X STOP). During this surgical procedure, an implant is placed between the spinous processes of the affected level, forcing that segment into lumbar flexion. This procedure has been shown to give greater pain relief than nonoperative therapy; however, there are no long-term data.[20]

References

1. Katz JN, Harris MB. Lumbar spinal stenosis. *N Engl J Med*. 2008;358:818-825.
2. Epstein NE, Maldonado VC, Cusick JF. Symptomatic lumbar spinal stenosis. *Surg Neurol*. 1998;50:3-10.
3. Saifuddin A. The imaging of lumbar spinal stenosis. *Clin Radiol*. 2000;55:581-594.
4. de Graaf I, Prak A, Bierma-Zeinstra S, et al. Diagnosis of lumbar spinal stenosis: A systematic review of the accuracy of diagnostic tests. *Spine*. 2006;31:1168-1176.
5. Willen J, Danielson B, Gaulitz A, et al. Dynamic effects of the lumbar spinal canal. *Spine*. 1997;22:2968-2976.
6. Postacchini F, Amatruda A, Morace GB, Perugia D. Magnetic resonance imaging in the diagnosis of lumbar spinal canal stenosis. *Ital J Orthop Traumtol*. 1991;17:327-337.
7. Danielson BI, Willen J, Gaulitz A, et al. Axial loading of the spine during CT and MR in patients with suspected lumbar spinal stenosis. *Acta Radiol*. 1998;39:604-611.
8. Speciale AC, Pietrobon R, Urban CW, et al. Observer variability in assessing lumbar spinal stenosis severity on magnetic resonance imaging in this relation to cross-sectional spinal canal area. *Spine*. 2002;27:1082-1086.
9. Rapala K, Chaberek S, Truszczynska A, et al. Assessment of lumbar spinal canal morphology with digital computed tomography. *Ortop Traumatol Rehabil*. 2009;11:156-163.
10. Verbeist H. Results of surgical treatment of idiopathic developmental stenosis of the lumbar vertebral canal: A review of twenty-seven years' experience. *J Bone Joint Surg Br*. 1977;59:181-188.
11. Hamanishi C, Matukura N, Fujita M, et al. Cross-sectional area of the stenotic lumbar dural tube measured from the transverse views of magnetic resonance imaging. *J Spinal Disord*. 1994;7:388-393.
12. Singh K, Samartzis D, Vaccaro AR, et al. Congenital lumbar spinal stenosis: a prospective, control-matched, cohort radiographic analysis. *Spine J*. 2005;5:615-622.
13. Atlas SJ, Keller RB, Robson D, et al. Surgical and nonsurgical management of lumbar spinal stenosis: Four-year outcomes from the Maine Lumbar Spine Study. *Spine*. 2000;25:556-562.
14. Simotas AC, Dorey FJ, Hansraj KK, Cammisa F. Nonoperative treatment for lumbar spinal stenosis: Clinical and outcome results and a 3-year survivorship analysis. *Spine*. 2000;25:197-204.
15. Herkowitz HN, Kurz LT. Degenerative lumbar spondylolisthesis with spinal stenosis: A prospective study comparing decompression with decompression and intertransverse process arthrodesis. *J Bone Joint Surg Am*. 1991;73:802-808.
16. Grob D, Humke T, Dvorak J. Significance of simultaneous fusion and surgical decompression in lumbar spinal stenosis. *Orthopade*. 1993;22:243-249 (German translation).
17. Selby DK, Gill K, Blumenthal SL, et al: Fusion of the lumbar spine. In: Youmans JR, ed. *Neurological Surgery*. 3rd. ed. Philadelphia: Saunders; 1990:2785-2804.
18. Katz JN, Lipson SJ, Chang LC, et al. Seven- to 10- year outcome of decompressive surgery for degenerative lumbar spinal stenosis. *Spine*. 1996;21:92-98.
19. Deyo RA, Cherkin DC, Loeser JD, et al. Morbidity and mortality in association with operations on the lumbar spine: The influence of age, diagnosis, and procedure. *J Bone Joint Surg Am*. 1992;74:536-543.
20. Zucherman JF, Hsu KY, Hartjen CA, et al. A multicenter, prospective, randomized trial evaluating the X STOP interspinous process decompression system for the treatment of neurogenic intermittent claudication: Two-year follow-up results. *Spine*. 2005;30:1351-1358.

SPONDYLOLISTHESIS

Douglas S. Fenton, M.D.

CLINICAL PRESENTATION

The patient is a 73-year-old woman with a chief complaint of low back pain. The patient states that the pain began 3 years ago with some back spasms that started while she was sitting down. There was no significant trauma at that time. The frequency of her pain progressed and for the past year she feels it has been present daily. The pain is of a deep, aching quality, severe at times, in the midline in the lower back. It is relieved by heating pads and a mild oral narcotic and made worse with attempts at dressing and when she wears low-heeled shoes. The patient is worse when sitting and somewhat better walking and standing. There is also relief when she leans over the cart at the grocery store. The pain is not intensified by coughing, sneezing, or bearing down. The patient also complains of pain in the lower extremities, slightly greater on the left side. She describes the pain as being at the lateral aspect of the thigh and the lateral aspect of the leg. The character of her leg pain is burning and sharp. There is no bowel or bladder dysfunction.

IMAGING PRESENTATION

Sagittal and axial T1-weighted images demonstrate anterior subluxation of L4 relative to L5 with severe spinal stenosis secondary to the pseudo broad-based disc bulging from the anterolisthesis and facet degenerative changes. There is approximately 25% uncovering of the L4-5 disc compatible with a grade 1 spondylolisthesis (*Fig. 73-1*).

DISCUSSION

Degenerative spondylolisthesis is defined as the slipping of one vertebral body with respect to an adjacent vertebral body with an intact neural arch. Generally, the direction of slip is defined as the more cephalad vertebral body in relation to the adjacent, inferior vertebral body. *Anterolisthesis* is defined as anterior slipping of the cephalad vertebral body in relation to the inferior one. *Retrolisthesis* is posterior slipping of the cephalad vertebral body in relation to the inferior one. One may also refer to *lateral listhesis* when there is slippage of a vertebral body left or right compared with the inferior vertebral body, which is readily seen with coronal reformatted images.

The various types of spondylolisthesis are divided into six subgroups: degenerative, isthmic, congenital/dysplastic, traumatic, pathologic, and iatrogenic.[1,2] The isthmic lytic lesion of the pars interarticularis is the most common cause of spondylolisthesis and is called *spondylolysis*. The pars defect is what differentiates degenerative spondylolisthesis from isthmic spondylolisthesis/ spondylolysis. See Chapter 69 for further discussion of spondylolysis.

Spondylolisthesis is a condition unique to humans. It is thought that spondylolisthesis developed in response to man's ability to maintain an erect posture and the development of the lumbar lordosis. The lumbar lordosis is unique to human beings.[3,4]

Degenerative spondylolisthesis usually affects people over 50 years of age.[5] An autopsy study demonstrated the incidence of degenerative spondylolisthesis to be 4.1%, with the most affected level being L4-5,[6] which differs from spondylolysis in which the L5-S1 level is most affected from an L5 pars defect. Most studies demonstrate a female predominance of degenerative spondylolisthesis, which has been postulated to be caused by the increased ligamentous laxity in women compared with that in men.[7] Other potential risk factors include pregnancy, African-American ethnicity, sagittally oriented facet joints, and hyperlordosis.[8] Degenerative spondylolisthesis can also occur in the cervical spine and has been reported in the thoracic spine as well.[9,10]

Degenerative slippage occurs because of disc degenerative changes leading to facet arthritis, laxity of the paravertebral ligaments, and ineffective paravertebral muscular stabilization.[8] The typical signs and symptoms of degenerative spondylolisthesis are often related to the degenerated and subluxed facet joints, the instability of the facet joint capsule from the ligamentous laxity, and spinal stenosis and/or neural foraminal stenosis from the slippage.[8] Therefore, the patients often present with back/neck pain and/or radicular pain. Given that L4-5 is the most affected level, low back pain along with pain in the L5 distribution (pain in the hips with radiation down the posterolateral legs) is commonly found. The pain may be unilateral or bilateral, and the patients will often describe pain that shifts from one extremity to the other. Another common pain presentation is that of neurogenic claudication from the spinal stenosis.[8] Spinal stenosis symptoms are present in 42% to 82% of patients who seek help because of their spondylolisthesis.[8] Other complaints include cold feet, altered gait, and drop episodes (where the patient unexpectedly falls while walking).[11] Like any of the conditions that cause stenosis, pain relief is often achieved by the patient with spinal flexion. This is thought to be due to an increase in the anteroposterior dimension of the spinal canal that occurs during flexion.

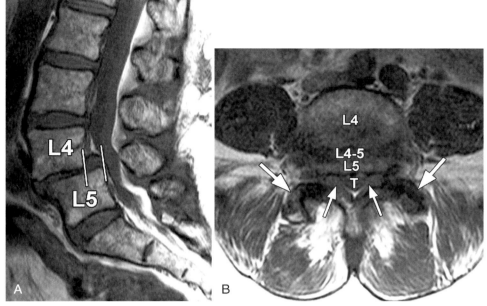

Figure 73-1 ► Degenerative Spondylolisthesis. Sagittal T1-weighted MRI **A**. There is anterior subluxation of L4 with respect to L5 with approximately 25% uncovering of the L4-5 disc and central spinal canal stenosis (*white lines*). Axial T1-weighted image **B** better demonstrates the degree of spinal canal narrowing secondary to the antero-listhesis, facet degenerative changes (*large arrows*), and thickening of the ligamentum flavum (*small arrows*). A portion of the L4 vertebral body, L4-5 disc, and L5 vertebral body is seen on the axial image because of straight axial imaging rather than axial imaging parallel to the disc.

The natural history of degenerative spondylolisthesis has a favorable prognosis. In a 10-year follow-up study,[12] 34% of patients who presented with degenerative spondylolisthesis had further slipping at the abnormal segment. However, 76% of patients that had degenerative spondylolisthesis without neurologic deficit remained without neurologic deficit. Eighty-three percent of the patients who had a neurologic deficit at the presentation of their degenerative spondylolisthesis and refused surgery had progression of their deficit. These patients had a poor prognosis. Overall, only 10% to 15% of patients with degenerative spondylolisthesis eventually require surgery.[12]

IMAGING FEATURES

Spondylolisthesis can be readily visualized with plain radiographs. The lateral radiograph is most important and demonstrates anterior or posterior displacement of one vertebral body in comparison to an adjacent vertebral body *(Fig. 73-2)*. Oblique radiographs can often identify an intact par interarticularis (the portion of bone that connects the superior and inferior articular processes of a vertebral segment) *(Fig. 73-3)*. Lateral flexion and extension radiographs are important to evaluate for any dynamic motion of the abnormal segment and to evaluate for reduction of the spondylolisthesis. With degenerative spondylolisthesis, there may be narrowing of the disc space, hypertrophic facet degeneration, osteophytes, vacuum disc phenomenon, and/or endplate sclerosis. Computed tomography (CT) using a bone window or bone algorithm is more sensitive in evaluating the cause of the slip, in evaluating the degenerative changes, and to exclude a pars interarticularis defect *(Fig. 73-4)*. With soft tissue algorithm CT, one is better able to evaluate the effect of the slip in relation to spinal canal narrowing, neural foraminal impingement, and lateral recess stenosis *(Fig. 73-5)*. Magnetic resonance imaging (MRI) has

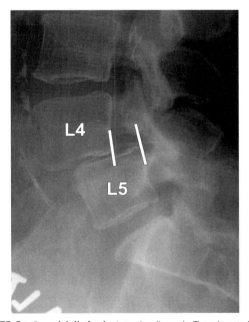

Figure 73-2 ► Spondylolisthesis. Lateral radiograph. There is anterior subluxation of the L4 vertebral body relative to the L5 vertebral body by approximately 50% of the anteroposterior distance of the superior L5 vertebral endplate compatible with a grade 2 anterolisthesis.

largely replaced CT in the evaluation of neurologic symptoms related to the spine.[8] MRI is more sensitive than CT in evaluating the spinal cord and cauda equina, but is less sensitive in the evaluation of the osteolytic defect of spondylolysis. In larger patients, MRI may be able to assess central canal and foraminal

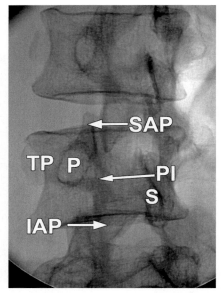

Figure 73-3 ▶ Scotty Dog with Intact Pars Interarticularis. Oblique radiograph of the lumbar spine. This view demonstrates the normal "Scotty dog" with an intact pars interarticularis (*PI*, neck of the dog) connecting the superior articular process (*SAP*, ear of the dog) and inferior articular process (*IAP*, front leg of the dog) of a single vertebral level. *P* = Pedicle (eye of the dog); *TP* = transverse process (nose of the dog); *S* = spinous process (tail and back leg of the dog).

stenosis better than CT due to limitations of CT in large patients, particularly in the lower lumbar spine (*Figs. 73-1 and 73-6*).

The degree of spondylolisthesis is quantified by one of two methods. The Meyerding method[13,14] divides the superior endplate of the inferior vertebral body into quarters and assigns a grade of I to IV if the slip falls within each of the quarters. The second method is described by Taillard.[14,15] Taillard's method is a more specific grading system and measures the degree of anterior or posterior slippage as a percentage of the anterior-posterior diameter of the inferior vertebra. Therefore a Meyerding grade I equals 1% to 25% of slippage (*Fig. 73-7*), grade II equals 26% to 50% slippage (*Fig. 73-8*), grade III equals 51% to 75% slippage, and grade IV equals 76% to 99% slippage. A complete slip of one vertebra relative to another is termed *spondyloptosis* (*Fig. 73-9*). The majority of degenerative spondylolistheses have slippages of 25% or less due to the facet joints limiting the slippage.

DIFFERENTIAL DIAGNOSIS

1. **Isthmic spondylolisthesis:** This is also termed *spondylolysis with spondylolisthesis*. This has a similar appearance to spondylolisthesis except that a break in the pars interarticularis is identified with spondylolysis (*Fig. 73-10*). There is also widening of the anteroposterior canal diameter with spondylolysis as opposed to the narrowing seen with degenerative spondylolisthesis.
2. **Traumatic spondylolisthesis:** Evaluate for antecedent trauma.
3. **Pathologic spondylolisthesis:** Evaluate for infectious/neoplastic history.
4. **Congenital spondylolisthesis:** Evaluate for dysplastic pedicles.

5. **Iatrogenic spondylolisthesis:** Evaluate for history of spinal surgery.
6. **Physiologic subluxation:** Small subluxations can normally be seen in young patients, particularly in the cervical spine.

TREATMENT

Most patients with degenerative spondylolisthesis will never require surgery. Nonoperative therapy is the primary mode of treatment, not only for degenerative spondylolisthesis but also for anyone with low back pain.

1. **Rest and anti-inflammatory medications:** Treatment may begin with rest and a short course of anti-inflammatory medications.
2. **Physical therapy:** If symptoms persist, then physical therapy should be instituted. The stationary bicycle is ideal for patients with spinal stenosis secondary to spondylolisthesis because it promotes spine flexion, which increases the anteroposterior diameter of the spinal canal allowing the patient to exercise longer by delaying the onset of their neurogenic claudication.
3. **Injection therapy:** If physical therapy fails after a 4- to 6-week period, a short course of injection therapy (epidural, selective nerve block) could be performed.[16]
4. **Surgery:** Surgical intervention should be performed if there is a progressive neurologic deficit or cauda equina syndrome. Surgery can be considered if there are persistent symptoms after conservative treatment or loss of quality of life.[16] There are several different surgical approaches, each with different indications including decompression alone, laminectomy and posterior spinal fusion without interpedicled instrumentation, decompression with posterolateral instrumented fusion, or decompression with anterior and posterior spinal fusion.[16]

Text continued on page 565

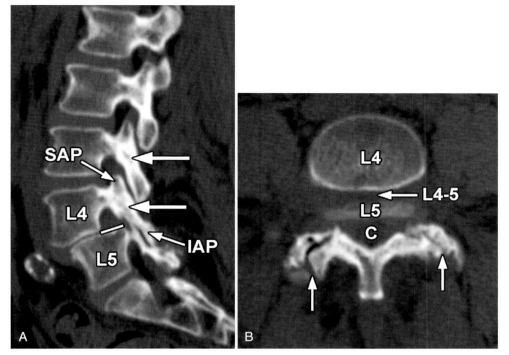

Figure 73-4 ▸ Degenerative Spondylolisthesis. Same patient as in Figure 73-1. Sagittal CT bone window image **A** demonstrates anterior subluxation of L4 relative to L5 (*white line*). The pars interarticularis (*arrows*) are intact, connecting the superior articular processes (*SAP*) to the inferior articular processes (*IAP*). Axial bone window image **B** reveals the severe degree of central spinal canal stenosis (*C*) secondary to the anterolisthesis and facet degenerative changes (*arrows*). A portion of the L4 vertebral body, L4-5 disc, and L5 vertebral body is seen on the axial image because of straight axial imaging rather than axial imaging parallel to the disc.

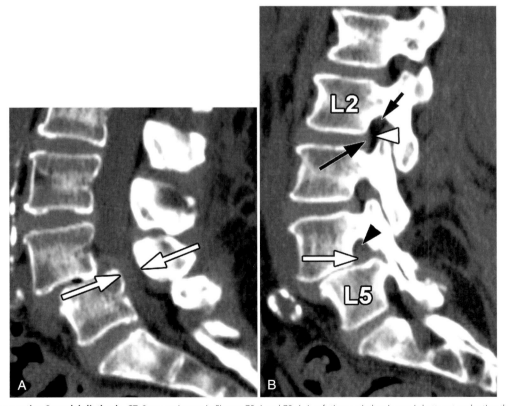

Figure 73-5 ▸ Degenerative Spondylolisthesis, CT. Same patient as in Figures 73-1 and 73-4. A soft tissue window image is better at evaluating the degree of soft tissue spinal stenosis and/or foraminal narrowing. Midline sagittal CT image **A** shows the central spinal canal stenosis related to the anterolisthesis (*between arrows*). Off-midline sagittal CT image **B** demonstrates the normal keyhole appearance of the L2-3 neural foramen with fat density in the inferior aspect (*white arrowhead*) and the exiting nerve root in the superior aspect (*short black arrow*). The L2-3 disc is at the posterior margin of the vertebral bodies (*long black arrow*). The L4-5 neural foramen is narrowed secondary to anterolisthesis of L4 relative to L5 with loss of the epidural fat because of disc material (*white arrow*) and compression of the exiting L4 nerve root (*black arrowhead*).

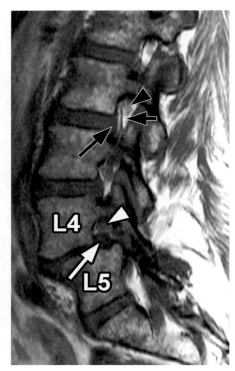

Figure 73-6 ► **Degenerative Spondylolisthesis, MRI.** Same patient as in Figures 73-1, 73-4, and 73-5. Off midline sagittal T1-weighted MR demonstrates the normal keyhole appearance of the L2-3 neural foramen with fat signal intensity in the inferior aspect (*short black arrow*) and the exiting nerve root in the superior aspect (*black arrowhead*). The L2-3 disc is at the posterior margin of the vertebral bodies (*long black arrow*). The L4-5 neural foramen is narrowed secondary to anterolisthesis of L4 relative to L5 with loss of the epidural fat because of disc material (*white arrow*) and compression of the exiting L4 nerve root (*white arrowhea*d).

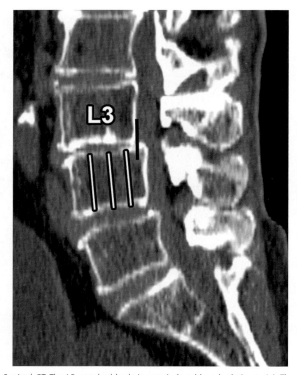

Figure 73-7 ► **Grade 1 Spondylolisthesis.** Sagittal CT. The L3 vertebral body is anteriorly subluxed relative to L4. The superior endplate of L4 is divided into four equal parts (*white vertical lines*). A *black line* drawn along the posterior aspect of L3 falls between the posterior L4 vertebral body and posterior-most vertical line compatible with less than 25% subluxation.

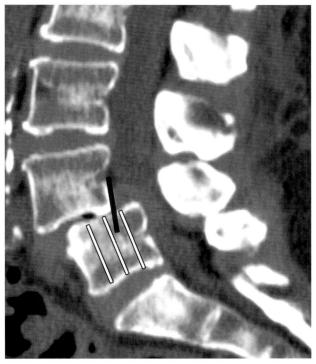

Figure 73-8 ▶ Grade 2 Spondylolisthesis. Sagittal CT. The L4 vertebral body is anteriorly subluxed relative to L5. The superior endplate of L5 is divided into four equal parts (*white vertical lines*). A black line drawn along the posterior aspect of L5 falls between the middle and posterior vertical white lines compatible with 25% to 50% subluxation.

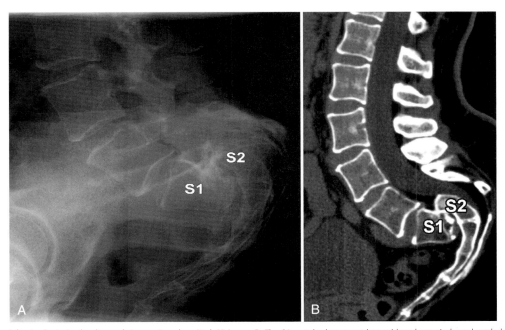

Figure 73-9 ▶ Spondyloptosis. Lateral radiograph image **A** and sagittal CT image **B**. The S1 vertebral segment has subluxed anteriorly and settled directly anterior to the S2 segment compatible with spondyloptosis.

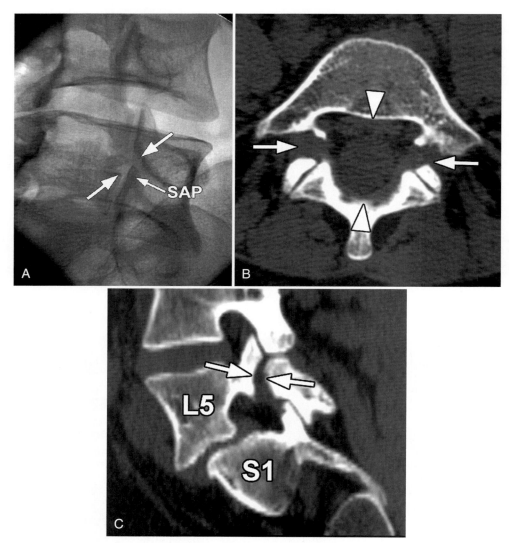

Figure 73-10 ► **Spondylolysis.** Oblique radiograph image **A**, axial CT image **B** and off midline sagittal CT image **C**. Break in the pars interarticularis on all images (*between arrows*). The oblique radiograph demonstrates that the superior articular process (*SAP*) of Si is more cranial than normal and is narrowing the region where the exiting L5 nerve root will pass. The axial CT reveals overall widening of the anterior-posterior dimension of the central spinal canal (*between arrowheads*), which is typical of spondylolysis. Typically, there is a decrease in the anterior-posterior dimension with degenerative spondylolisthesis.

References

1. Wiltse LL, Newman PH, Macnab I. Classification of spondylolysis and spondylolisthesis. *Clin Orthop.* 1976;117:23-29.
2. Newman PH. The etiology of spondylolisthesis. *J Bone Joint Surg Br.* 1963; 75:39-59.
3. Rowe GG, Roche MB. The etiology of separate neural arch. *J Bone Joint Surg Am.* 1953;35:102-110.
4. Wynne-Davies R, Scott JH. Inheritance and spondylolisthesis: A radiographic family survey. *J Bone Joint Surg Br.* 1979;61:301-305.
5. Vilbert BT, Sliva CD, Herkowitz HN. Treatment of instability and spondylolithesis: Surgical versus nonsurgical treatment. *Clin Orthop Relat Res.* 2006;443:222-227.
6. Farfan HF. The pathologic anatomy of degenerative spondylolisthesis: A cadaver study. *Spine.* 1980;5:412-418.
7. Bird HA, Eastmond CJ, Hudson A, Wright V. Is generalized ligamentous joint laxity a factor in spondylolisthesis? *Scand J Rheumatol.* 1980;9:203-205.
8. Kalichman L, Hunter DJ. Diagnosis and conservative management of degenerative lumbar spondylolisthesis. *Eur Spine J.* 2008;17:327-335.
9. Dean CL, Gabriel JP, Cassinelli EH, et al. Degenerative spondylolisthesis of the cervical spine: Analysis of 58 patients treated with anterior cervical decompression and fusion. *Spine J.* 2009;9:439-446.
10. Shimada Y, Kasukawa Y, Miyakoshi N, et al. Spondylolisthesis of the thoracic spine. *J Neurosurg Spine.* 2006;4:415-418.
11. Frymoyer JW. Degenerative spondylolisthesis: Diagnosis and treatment. *J Am Acad Orthop Surg.* 1994;2:9-15.
12. Matsunaga S, Ijiri K, Hayashi K. Nonsurgically managed patients with degenerative spondylolisthesis: A 10- to 18-year follow-up study. *J Neurosurg.* 2000;93:194-198.
13. Meyerding HW. Spondyloptosis. *Surg Gynaecol Obstet.* 1932;54:371-377.
14. Wiltse LL, Winter RB. Terminology and measurement of spondylolisthesis. *J Bone Joint Surg.* 1983;65A:768-772.
15. Taillard W. Le spondylolisthesis chez l'enfant et L'adolescent. *Acta Orthop Scand.* 1954;24:115-144.
16. Vibert BT, Sliva CD, Herkowitz HN. Treatment of instability and spondylolisthesis: Surgical versus nonsurgical treatment. *Clin Orthop and Rel Research.* 2006;443:222-227.

CHAPTER
74

SPONDYLOLYSIS

Douglas S. Fenton, M.D.

CLINICAL PRESENTATION

The patient is a 75-year-old man who presented with 4 weeks of low back pain and bilateral lower extremity pain. He states he was lifting some sand and felt pain in his lower back and hips. He states that he fell off a ladder while climbing 4 weeks ago. He has had a total of five falls, and states that he has no warning, but simply collapses. This is preceded immediately by a sharp pain in his back. He occasionally gets this same pain when he turns in bed or bends forward. He has problems when he is coughing while sitting down, but no problems when coughing if he is lying supine or standing up. On physical examination, there is no neurologic deficit. Straight leg raise was negative. Reflexes were symmetric bilaterally in the lower extremities. He is otherwise without problems. No specific gait abnormality is appreciated.

IMAGING PRESENTATION

Sagittal and axial T1-weighted images demonstrate anterior subluxation of L5 relative to S1 with approximately 40% uncovering of the disc compatible with a grade 2 spondylolisthesis. There is widening of the spinal canal, which is seen with subluxations secondary to defects in the pars interarticularis/spondylolysis. Typically, there is spinal stenosis with degenerative spondylolisthesis and usually no greater than a grade 1 subluxation, because the intact pars interarticularis limits the amount of movement of one vertebral body relative to the next *(Fig. 74-1)*.

DISCUSSION

Spondylolisthesis is defined as the slipping of one vertebral body with respect to an adjacent vertebral body. Generally, the direction of slip is defined as the more cephalad vertebral body in relation to the adjacent, inferior vertebral body. *Anterolisthesis* is defined as anterior slipping of the cephalad vertebral body in relation to the inferior one. *Retrolisthesis* is posterior slipping of the cephalad vertebral body in relation to the inferior one. One may also refer to *lateral listhesis* when there is slippage of a vertebral body left or right compared with the inferior vertebral body, which is readily seen with coronal reformatted images.

The various types of spondylolisthesis are divided into six subgroups; degenerative, isthmic, congenital/dysplastic, traumatic, pathologic, and iatrogenic.[1,2] The isthmic lytic lesion of the pars interarticularis is the most common cause of spondylolisthesis and is called *spondylolysis*. The pars defect is what differentiates degenerative spondylolisthesis from isthmic spondylolisthesis.

The pars interarticularis, also known as the *isthmus*, is that portion of the neural arch that connects the spinal lamina with the pedicle, facet joints, and transverse process.[3] Roughly, on oblique views, it is midway between the superior and inferior articular process *(Fig. 74-2)*. Because of its shape and location, the pars interarticularis is subject to the greatest force of any structure in the lumbar spine, but unfortunately may be the weakest part of the neural arch.[4]

Spondylolytic spondylolisthesis is the most common cause of spondylolisthesis. The incidence of spondylolysis ranges from 4.4% to 5.8% and that of isthmic spondylolisthesis ranges from 2.6% to 4.4%.[5,6] In other words, 50% to 81% of patients with spondylolysis have spondylolisthesis. Isthmic spondylolisthesis occurs twice as often in males as females, however, females are four times more likely to have progression of the slippage.[3] Spondylolysis appears to be multifactorial in origin with mechanical, congenital, and potentially hormonal factors. Spondylolysis is commonly seen with athletic participation, particularly in gymnasts, football linemen, weightlifters, wrestlers, and divers.[7,8] Spondylolysis is the most common cause of low back pain in young athletes and is seen in 47% of young athletes complaining of low back pain.[9] It has been postulated that the repetitive forces of flexion, hyperextension, and rotation required in these sports results in stress fractures of the pars.[10] Inheritance studies have shown a high incidence of spondylolysis with spondylolisthesis in near relatives with the same process. Although the incidence of spondylolysis ranges from approximately 4% to 6% in the general population, the incidence in near relatives is approximately 25% to 30%.[2,11,12] Progression of vertebral slippage has been noted during adolescence, which could imply hormonal influences or growth factors in the development of spondylolisthesis.[11,12]

The most common level of a pars defect is L5. The L5 level is involved in 70% to 95% of cases, the L4 level in 5% to 20% of cases, and other areas throughout the spine in the remaining cases.[12,13]

Pain is the typical manifesting symptom in patients with isthmic spondylolisthesis. This may be low back pain and/or radicular pain. The pain is often a deep ache that is localized to the lumbar area, which may radiate to the buttocks or posterior thighs. Weight bearing and lifting exacerbate the symptoms, whereas rest and recumbency relieve it.[14] Radicular pain is often in the L5 distribution, either unilateral or bilateral. With higher grade subluxations, the cauda equina can be stretched over the sacrum, which can lead

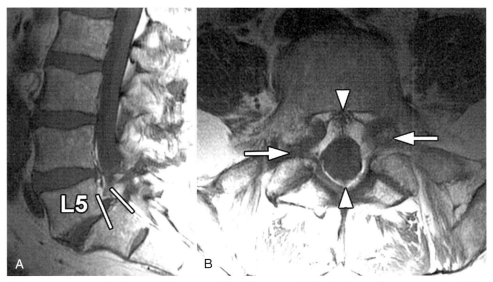

Figure 74-1 ▸ Spondylolysis. Sagittal T1-weighted image **A**. There is ventral slip of the L5 vertebral body relative to the S1 segment. Vertical lines drawn along the dorsal aspect of these vertebral bodies do not align compatible with listhesis. Axial T1-weighted image **B** shows widening of the spinal canal in its anterior-posterior dimension (*between arrowheads*) and breaks in the pars interarticularis bilaterally (*white arrows*). Patients with spondylolysis can have foraminal narrowing without spinal stenosis, and those with degenerative spondylolisthesis can have both spinal stenosis and foraminal stenosis.

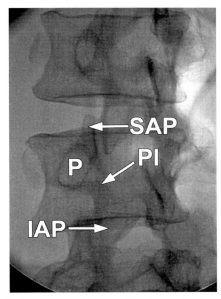

Figure 74-2 ▸ Scotty Dog with Intact Pars Interarticularis. Oblique radiograph of the lumbar spine. "Scotty dog." The pars interarticularis (*PI*) is the bone between the superior articulating process (*SAP*) and inferior articulating process (*IAP*) at the same level. P = Pedicle.

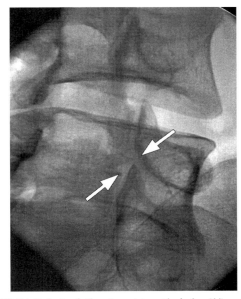

Figure 74-3 ▸ Defect of the Pars Interarticularis. Oblique radiograph. Congenital break in the pars interarticularis (*between arrows*).

to signs and symptoms of cauda equina syndrome, including perineal numbness, sphincter disturbances, and S1-related symptoms.[3]

IMAGING FEATURES

Spondylolysis can often be visualized with plain radiographs. The oblique radiograph can identify the defect of the par interarticularis (also known as the collar of the "Scottie Dog") (*Fig.*

74-3). The lateral radiograph demonstrates anterior or posterior displacement of one vertebral body in comparison to an adjacent vertebral body. One can see widening of the spinal canal when there is spondylolysis associated with spondylolisthesis (*Fig. 74-4*). This is in contrast to the narrowing of the anteroposterior diameter of the spinal canal seen with degenerative spondylolisthesis. Lateral flexion and extension radiographs are important to evaluate for any dynamic motion of the abnormal segment and to evaluate for reduction of the spondylolisthesis. Computed tomography (CT) is more sensitive in evaluating the cause of the slip and can readily demonstrate a spondylolytic defect (*Fig. 74-5*). With

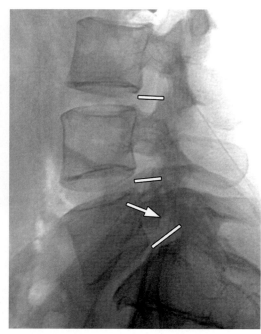

Figure 74-4 ► **Spondylolysis with Widening of the Central Spinal Canal.** Same patient as in Figure 74-3. Lateral radiograph. Break in the pars interarticularis of L5 (*arrow*). *White lines* depict anterior-posterior spinal canal width at the L3-4, L4-5 and L5-S1 disc levels. There is widening of the spinal canal in anterior-posterior dimension at L5-S1.

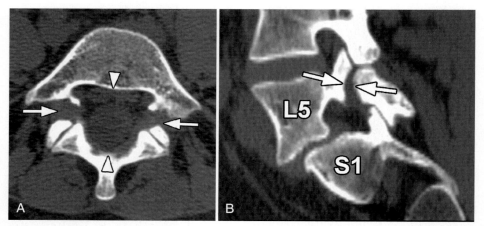

Figure 74-5 ► **Spondylolytic Defect.** Axial CT image **A** and sagittal CT image **B**. Ventral subluxation of L5 relative to S1 with breaks in the L5 pars interarticularis bilaterally (*arrows*) and widening of the spinal canal in-anterior-posterior dimension (*between arrowheads*).

CT, one is better able to evaluate the effect of the slippage in relation to neural foraminal impingement and lateral recess stenosis. CT with sagittal reformatted images best demonstrate the elongation of the affected neural foramen and the degree of nerve root compromise *(Fig. 74-6)*.

Magnetic resonance imaging (MRI) has largely replaced CT in the evaluation of neurologic symptoms related to the spine.[15] MRI is more sensitive than CT in evaluating the spinal cord and cauda equina, but is less sensitive in the evaluation of the osteolytic defect of spondylolysis. In larger patients, MRI may be able to assess foraminal narrowing better than CT because of the limitations of CT in large patients, particularly in the lower lumbar spine

(Fig. 74-7). MRI using short tau inversion recovery (STIR), fat-saturated, T2-weighted or post-contrast T1-weighted sequences can demonstrate edema and/or inflammation in and/or around the pars defect *(Fig. 74-8)*. We have found that this abnormality responds favorably to anesthetic/steroid injection therapy. A nuclear medicine bone scan can be helpful to evaluate for activity within and around the pars defects. Increased activity often corresponds to an active problem with acute pain, which will typically respond to injection therapy. However, the absence of radiotracer uptake does not mean that injection therapy will not be helpful because there may be a greater soft tissue inflammatory component with an active spondylolysis that cannot be seen with a bone scan.

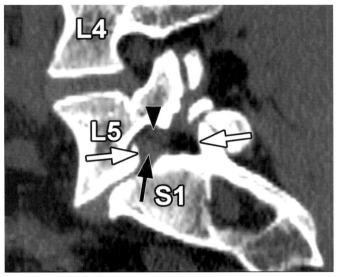

Figure 74-6 ▶ **Spondylolysis with Elongation of the Neural Foramen.** Sagittal CT. Elongation of the L5-S1 neural foramen (*between white arrows*) compared with the normal neural foramen above at L4-5. The anterolisthesis of L5 on S1 causes the posterior L5-S1 disc (*black arrow*) to extend into the neural foramen and impinge on the exiting L5 nerve root (*arrowhead*).

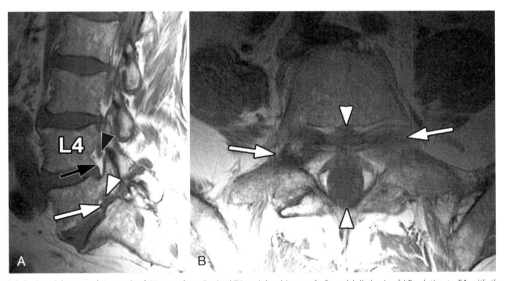

Figure 74-7 ▶ **Spondylolysis with Neural Foraminal Narrowing.** Sagittal T1-weighted image **A**. Spondylolisthesis of L5 relative to S1 with the uncovered disc (*white arrow*) severely narrowing the elongated neural foramen and impinging on the exiting L5 nerve root (*white arrowhead*). Normal posterior disc (*black arrow*), neural foramen and exiting L4 nerve root (*black arrowhead*) at the L4-5 level. Axial T1-weighted image **B** demonstrates breaks in the pars bilaterally (*arrows*) and widening of the anterior-posterior dimension of the spinal canal (*between arrowheads*).

The degree of spondylolisthesis is quantified by one of two methods. The Meyerding method[12,16] divides the superior endplate of the inferior vertebral body into quarters and assigns a grade of I to IV if the slip falls within each of the quarters. The second method is described by Taillard.[12,17] Taillard's method is a more specific grading system and measures the degree of anterior or posterior slippage as a percentage of the anterior-posterior diameter of the inferior vertebra. Therefore a Meyerding grade I equals 1% to 25%

of slippage (*Fig. 74-9*), grade II equals 26% to 50% slippage (*Fig. 74-10*), grade III equals 51% to 75% slippage, and grade IV equals 76% to 99% slippage. A complete slip of one vertebra relative to another is termed *spondyloptosis* (*Fig. 74-11*). If one identifies slippage of greater than 25%, it is usually due to isthmic spondylolisthesis as opposed to degenerative spondylolisthesis. The majority of degenerative spondylolistheses have slippage of 25% or less because of the facet joints limiting the slippage.

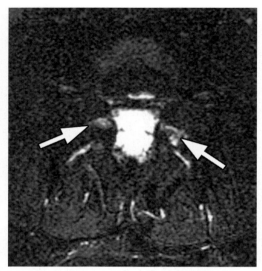

Figure 74-8 ▶ Edema/Inflamation in the Pars Defect. Same patient as in Figure 74-7. Axial fat-saturated, T2-weighted image. Increased signal intensity in the pars defects bilaterally (*arrows*) compatible with fluid, edema, and/or inflammation.

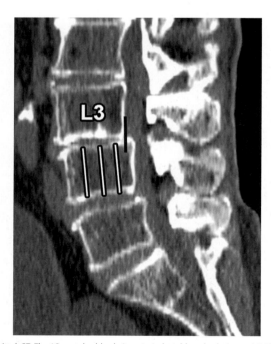

Figure 74-9 ▶ Grade I Spondylolisthesis. Sagittal CT. The L3 vertebral body is anteriorly subluxed relative to L4. The superior endplate of L4 is divided into four equal parts (*white vertical lines*). A black line drawn along the posterior aspect of L3 falls between the posterior L4 vertebral body and posterior-most vertical line compatible with less than 25% subluxation.

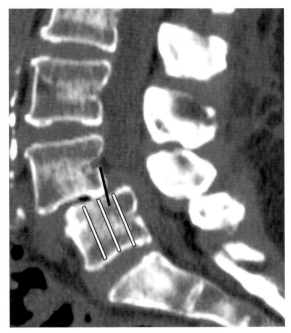

Figure 74-10 ► **Grade II Spondylolisthesis.** Sagittal CT. The L4 vertebral body is anteriorly subluxed relative to L5. The superior endplate of L5 is divided into four equal parts (*white vertical lines*). A *black line* drawn along the posterior aspect of L5 falls between the middle and posterior vertical white lines compatible with 25% to 50% subluxation.

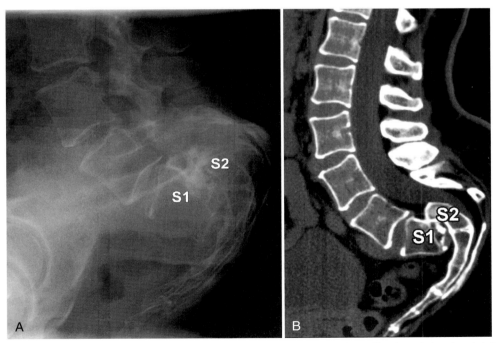

Figure 74-11 ► **Spondyloptosis.** Lateral radiograph image **A** and CT image **B**. The S1 vertebral segment has subluxed anteriorly and settled directly anterior to the S2 segment compatible with spondyloptosis.

DIFFERENTIAL DIAGNOSIS

1. **Degenerative spondylolisthesis**: This has an appearance similar to spondylolysis except that the neural arch (pars interarticularis) is intact with degenerative spondylolisthesis. There is generally narrowing of the anteroposterior canal diameter with degenerative spondylolisthesis as opposed to the widening seen with spondylolysis with spondylolisthesis (*Fig. 74-12*).
2. **Traumatic spondylolisthesis**: Evaluate for antecedent trauma.
3. **Pathologic spondylolisthesis**: Evaluate for infectious/neoplastic history.
4. **Congenital spondylolisthesis**: Evaluate for dysplastic pedicles.
5. **Iatrogenic spondylolisthesis**: Evaluate for history of spinal surgery.
6. **Physiologic subluxation**: Small subluxations can normally be seen in young patients, particularly in the cervical spine.

TREATMENT

Nonoperative management

Most patients with spondylolysis and/or spondylolisthesis are asymptomatic. If symptoms do arise, conservative, nonoperative treatment is successful in the majority of patients.

1. **Rest and anti-inflammatory medications**: Treatment may begin with rest and a short course of anti-inflammatory medications.
2. **Physical therapy**: If symptoms persist, then physical therapy should be instituted.
3. **Infection therapy**: If a 4- to 6-week course of physical therapy fails, a short course of injection therapy (facet injections, pars injection, epidural, selective nerve block) could be performed.[18] We find, in the majority of cases, that a direct pars injection is unnecessary. Rather, an injection of the facet joint related to the pars (L5-S1 facet joint for an L5 pars) connects with the pars. In one study, 70% of patients with grade I or II subluxations improved after conservative therapies.[19]

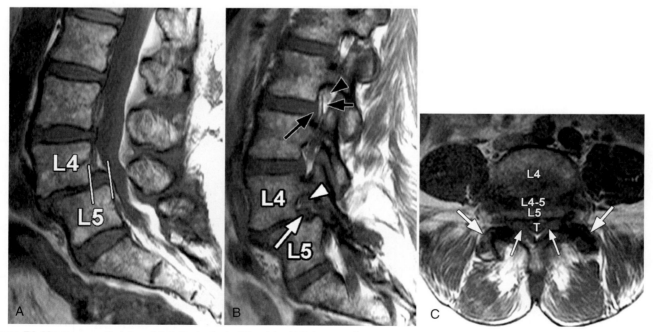

Figure 74-12 ▶ Degenerative Spondylolisthesis. Sagittal T1-weighted MR image **A**. There is anterior subluxation of L4 with respect to L5 with approximately 25% uncovering of the L4-5 disc and central spinal canal stenosis (*white lines*). Off-midline sagittal T1-weighted MR image **B** demonstrates the normal keyhole appearance of the L2-3 neural foramen with fat signal intensity in the inferior aspect (*short black arrow*) and the exiting nerve root in the superior aspect (*black arrowhead*). The L2-3 disc is at the posterior margin of the vertebral bodies (*long black arrow*). The L4-5 neural foramen is narrowed secondary to anterolisthesis of L4 relative to L5 with loss of the epidural fat due to disc material (*white arrow*) and compression of the exiting L4 nerve root (*white arrowhead*). Axial T1-weighted image **C** better demonstrates the degree of spinal canal narrowing secondary to the anterolisthesis, facet degenerative changes (*large arrows*), and thickening of the ligamentum flavum (*small arrows*). A portion of the L4 vertebral body, L4-5 disc, and L5 vertebral body is seen on the axial image because of straight axial imaging rather than axial imaging parallel to the disc.

4. **Surgery:** Only a minority of patients need surgical intervention. Indications for surgical intervention include "the persistence of pain or neurologic symptoms despite an adequate course of nonoperative treatment, progression of slippage greater than 30%, presentation with greater than grade II subluxation, and cosmetic deformity secondary to postural and gait difficulties."[3,20,21] Surgical interventions include decompression, bone fusion, instrument-assisted fusion, and reduction surgery.[3]

References

1. Wiltse LL, Newman PH, Macnab I. Classification of spondylolysis and spondylolisthesis. *Clin Orthop.* 1976;117:23-29.
2. Newman PH. The etiology of spondylolisthesis. *J Bone Joint Surg Br.* 1963;75:39-59.
3. Ganju A. Isthmic spondylolisthesis. *Neurosurg Focus.* 2002;13:E1.
4. Hutton WC, Cyron BM. Spondylolysis. The role of the posterior elements in resisting the intervertebral compressive force. *Acta Orthop Scand.* 1978;49:604-609.
5. Lauerman WC, Cain JE. Isthmic spondylolisthesis in the adult. *J Am Acad Orthop Surg.* 1996;4:201-208.
6. Fredrickson BE, Baker D, McHolick WJ, et al. The natural history of spondylolysis and spondylolisthesis. *J Bone Joint Surg Am.* 1984;66:699-707.
7. Harvey CV. Spinal surgery patient care. *Orthopaedic Nursing.* 2005;24:426-440.
8. Hodge B. Common spinal injuries in athletes. *Nurs Clin North Amer.* 1991;26:211-219.
9. Micheli L, Wood R. Back pain in young athletes: Significant differences from adults in causes and patterns. *Arch Pediatr Adolesc Med.* 1995;149:15-18.
10. Jackson DW, Wiltse LL, Cirincione RJ. Spondylolysis in the female gymnast. *Clin Orthop.* 1976;117:68-73.
11. Wiltse LL, Rothman SLG. Spondylolisthesis: Classification, diagnosis, and natural history. *Semin Spine Surg.* 1989;1:78-94.
12. Wiltse LL, Winter RB. Terminology and measurement of spondylolisthesis. *J Bone Joint Surg Am.* 1983;65:768-772.
13. Iwamoto J, Takeda T, Wakano K. Returning athletes with severe low back pain and spondylolysis to original sporting activities with conservative treatment. *Scand J Med Sci Sports.* 2004;14:346-351.
14. McPhee B. Spondylolisthesis and spondylolysis. In: Youmans JR, ed. *Neurological Surgery: A Comprehensive Reference Guide to the Diagnosis and Management of Neurosurgical Problems.* 3rd. ed. Vol 4. Philadelphia: Saunders; 1990:2749-2784.
15. Kalichman L, Hunter DJ. Diagnosis and conservative management of degenerative lumbar spondylolisthesis. *Eur Spine J.* 2008;17:327-335.
16. Meyerding HW. Spondyloptosis. *Surg Gynaecol Obstet.* 1932;54:371-377.
17. Taillard W. Le spondylolisthesis chez l'enfant et L'adolescent. *Acta Orthop Scand.* 1954;24:115-144.
18. Vibert BT, Sliva CD, Herkowitz HN. Treatment of instability and spondylolisthesis: Surgical versus nonsurgical treatment. *Clin Orthop and Rel Research.* 2006;443:222-227.
19. Pizzutillo PD, Hummer CD III. Nonoperative treatment for painful adolescent spondylolysis or spondylolisthesis. *J Pediatr Orthop.* 1989;9:538-540.
20. Bradford DF. Spondylolysis and spondylolisthesis, In: Chou SN, Seljeskog EL, eds. *Spinal Deformities and Neurological Dysfunction.* New York: Raven Press; 1978:175-198.
21. Harvell JC Jr, Hanley EN Jr. Spondylolysis and spondylolisthesis, In: Pang D, ed. *Disorders of the Pediatric Spine.* New York: Raven Press; 1995:561-574.

SYNOVIAL CYST

Leo F. Czervionke, M.D.

CLINICAL PRESENTATION

The patient is a 58-year-old man with 4- to 6-week history of low back pain, bilateral buttock pain, right lower extremity pain, numbness of both feet, and difficulty walking. He has weakness in both hip extensors, both hip abductors, and bilateral weakness of the foot, right greater than left. Clinical findings are consistent with multilevel radiculopathy and neurogenic claudication.

IMAGING PRESENTATION

Magnetic resonance (MR) imaging of the lumbar spine reveals a large, lobulated synovial cyst arising from the anteromedial aspect of the right L4-5 facet joint. The cyst encroaches upon the medial aspect of the right L4-5 neural foramen and causes marked compression and displacement of the thecal sac from right to left (*Figs. 75-1 to 75-6*).

DISCUSSION

Synovial cysts are synovial-lined cystic outpouchings that communicate with the facet joint. Synovial cysts arise within thickened, redundant synovium and facet capsular tissue. Synovial cysts most commonly arise in the setting of facet joint osteoarthritis, as a result of chronic inflammation and facet degeneration, but can arise secondary to acute or repeated trauma, rheumatoid arthritis, or calcium pyrophosphate deposition disease (CPPD).[1,2]

Most synovial cysts arise in the lower lumbar region, likely secondary to mechanical stress. These cysts contain gelatinous liquid or synovial fluid. Hypermobility of the facet joint (facet subluxation) is considered an important predisposing factor in synovial cyst formation.[3] There is an increased incidence of symptomatic synovial cyst formation in patients with facet joint mobility or spondylolisthesis.[4] In the lumbar region, the greatest mobility is at the L4-5 level, and the majority (80%) of lumbar synovial cysts arise at the L4-5 level,[3] more frequently occurring on the right side, for reasons unknown. Tiny (less than 5 mm diameter) synovial cystic outpouchings from the posterior-inferior facet joint capsule are very common and usually asymptomatic. Synovial cysts that project from the facet joint medially extend into the spinal canal where they may cause significant compression of the lateral aspect of the thecal sac (see Figs. 75-4 to 75-6). Most of these cysts are less than 1.5 cm in diameter, but they can be larger. Some medial projecting synovial cysts extend into the potential space between the lamina and ligamentum flavum, displacing the ligamentum flavum medially; these cysts communicate with the facet joint (*Fig. 75-7*). These cysts may be confused with nonsynovial-lined *flavum cysts* that are attached to or embedded within the ligamentum flavum that do not communicate with the facet joint (*Figs. 75-8 and 75-9*).[1,5] Synovial cysts may also project from the anterosuperior margin of the facet joint into the neural foramina (*Figs. 75-10 and 75-11*), where they may be confused for nerve sheath cysts that also occur in the neural foramen.

Some cysts located adjacent to the facet joint are not lined by synovium and do not communicate with the facet joint. The nature of these nonsynovial-lined parafacetal cysts has been a subject of debate in the literature.[6,7] The terminology used to describe these cysts varies, sometimes referred to as *pseudocysts, juxtafacet cysts,* or *ganglion cysts*.[1,5,8,9] Some believe that these cysts originated from synovial cysts that became walled-off, no longer communicating with the facet joint, but their precise etiology is unknown.[10] Parafacetal pseudocysts usually contain tan or yellow gelatinous or mucoid liquid. Hemosiderin, secondary to previous intracystic hemorrhage, may be present in synovial cysts and parafacetal pseudocysts.[5]

Patients with synovial cysts most commonly present with chronic low back pain with or without radicular symptoms. Synovial cysts can be associated with hypesthesia or dysesthesias.[3] These symptoms can be secondary to mechanical compression of adjacent structures or inflammation surrounding the cyst.[11] Depending on their size and location, synovial cysts can contribute to central canal stenosis or neural foraminal stenosis (see Figs. 75-8 to 75-11). Large synovial cysts can cause cauda equina syndrome in the lumbar region or myelopathy if located in the thoracic or cervical region. Synovial cysts occur less frequently in the thoracic and cervical regions and in these locations tend to be relatively small in size, but some thoracic synovial cysts can be quite large and cause cord compression or radiculopathy.[12]

IMAGING FEATURES

There is nearly always degeneration of the adjacent facet joint in patients with synovial cysts or juxtafacet (ganglion) cysts.[13] Facet joint degeneration is manifested on radiographs, computed tomography (CT), or magnetic resonance (MR) imaging as articular facet hypertrophy/overgrowth, commonly joint space narrowing

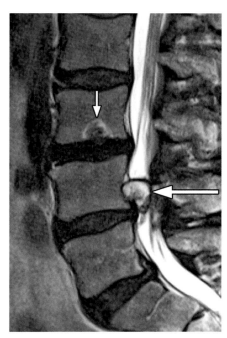

Figure 75-1 ▶ **Large Synovial Cyst, L4 Level.** Right parasagittal T2-weighted MRI. A large fluid-filled synovial cyst (*long arrow*) is positioned above the L4-5 intervertebral disc level in the spinal canal posterior to the L4 vertebral body. Noted is a Schmorl's node (*short arrow*) in L3 vertebral body inferiorly.

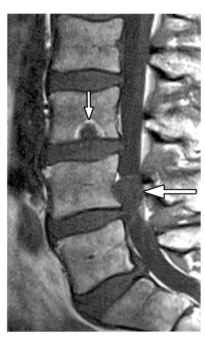

Figure 75-2 ▶ **Large Synovial Cyst, L4 Level.** Same patient as in Figure 75-1. Corresponding right parasagittal T1-weighted MRI. The synovial cyst (*long arrow*) is nearly isointense relative to intrathecal CSF. Noted is Schmorl's node (*short arrow*) in L3 vertebral body inferiorly.

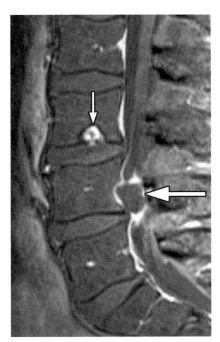

Figure 75-3 ▶ **Large Synovial Cyst, L4 Level.** Same patient as in Figures 75-1 and 75-2. Right parasagittal contrast-enhanced fat-saturated T1-weighted MRI. The synovial cyst contains fluid that is isointense relative to CSF. The margins of the cyst enhances intensely (*long arrow*). The L3 Schmorl's node (*short arrow*) enhances intensely.

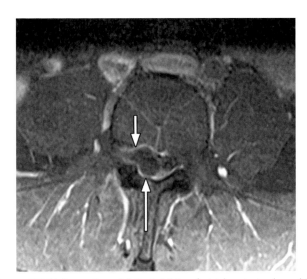

Figure 75-4 ▶ **Large Synovial Cyst, L4 Level.** Axial contrast-enhanced fat-saturated T1-weighted MRI obtained just above L4-5 intervertebral disc level in same patient as in Figures 75-1 to 75-3. The cyst margins (*arrows*) enhance with contrast, but fluid in the cyst does not enhance. The cyst extends into the medial aspect of the right L4-5 neural foramen (*short arrow*). A portion of the cyst is located in the spinal canal (*long arrow*) where it displaces the thecal sac to the left.

with subchondral cyst formation, intra-articular gas formation, and occasionally facet joint widening secondary to facet joint effusions. Synovial cysts are usually not visible on plain radiographs unless calcified. Synovial cyst calcification, when it occurs, is usually peripheral within the wall of the cyst and this is best shown with CT *(Fig. 75-12)*. More extensive calcification of the synovial cyst may occur in cysts that arise in patients with CPPD.[2] Synovial cysts may not calcify at all. These are usually of nearly homogeneous density and isodense or slightly hyperdense relative to the cerebrospinal fluid (CSF). The synovial cyst may contain gas if there is gaseous degeneration of the adjacent facet joint, which is in communication with the cyst.[11]

MR imaging is the modality of choice for detecting synovial cysts and evaluating their relationship to adjacent structures.[11,13,14] On MR images, most synovial cysts are T1 hypointense and T2 hyperintense centrally relative to CSF (see Figs. 75-1, 75-2, 75-5, 75-6, 75-8, and 75-10).[11] If the cyst contains gas, blood, or inspissated material, it is usually T2 hypointense.[10] The cyst wall is T2 hypointense, composed of a fibrous capsule, often containing hemosiderin.[10] The cyst wall can be thin or thick *(Fig. 75-13)*. The wall of the cyst often enhances after IV contrast administration, and this enhancement may be visible on enhanced CT or MR images, but is more conspicuous on contrast enhanced MR (see Figs. 75-3, 75-8, and 75-11). Occasionally, there is considerable inflammatory tissue adjacent to the synovial cyst that enhances with contrast (see Figs. 75-8 and 75-11). Occasionally, bilateral synovial cysts occur at a given lumbar level, which can cause significant side-to-side compression of the thecal sac and cauda equina *(Figs. 75-12 and 75-14)*.

DIFFERENTIAL DIAGNOSIS

1. **Parafacetal pseudocyst**: Also called a *juxtafacet cyst* or *ganglion cyst*, these cysts are not lined by synovium and do not communicate with the facet joint.[1,5] Commonly, these cysts arise adjacent to the ligamentum flavum (see *Figs. 75-8, 75-9, and 75-15*). Juxtafacet cysts may also arise within the posterior longitudinal ligament.[1] It is usually not possible to differentiate a parafacetal pseudocyst from a synovial cyst with MRI or CT. If a parafacetal cyst opacifies when contrast is injected into the adjacent facet joint, this is considered a synovial cyst. Cysts that are located adjacent to the ligamentum flavum that communicate with the joint space are considered synovial cysts (see Fig. 75-7).

2. **Epidural cyst**: These may occur in the anterior or posterior epidural space.[1] The posteriorly located epidural cyst is usually positioned between the leaves of the ligamentum flavum within the posterior epidural fat pad.

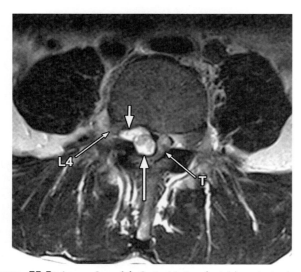

Figure 75-5 ► **Large Synovial Cyst, L4 Level.** Axial contrast-enhanced T2-weighted MRI obtained just above L4-5 intervertebral disc level in same patient as in Figure 75-4. The cyst (*arrows*) is lobulated and contains T2 hyperintense fluid. The infrapedicular portion of the cyst (*short arrow*) extends into the medial aspect of the right L4-5 neural foramen where it encroaches upon the right L4 nerve root (*L4*). The portion of the cyst in the spinal canal (*long allow*) compresses and displaces the thecal sac (*T*) toward the left.

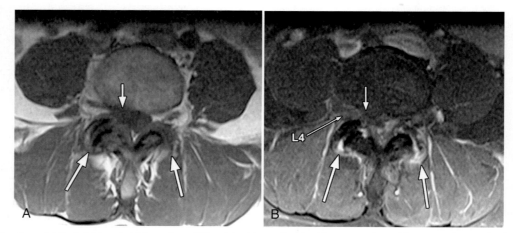

Figure 75-6 ► **Large Synovial Cyst, L4 Level.** Axial unenhanced T1-weighted image **A** and axial contrast-enhanced fat-saturated T1-weighted MR image **B**, obtained at the L4-5 facet level, in same patient as in Figures 75-1 to 75-5. The synovial cyst (*short arrow in* **A** *and* **B**) obscures the fat in the medial aspect of the right L4-5 neural foramen. The facets (*long arrows in image* **A**) are hypertrophic secondary to osteoarthritis. The posterior facets and facet capsules (*long arrows in* **B**) enhance following IV contrast compatible with active inflammatory facet arthropathy. L4 = right L4 nerve root in lateral aspect of right L4-5 neural foramen.

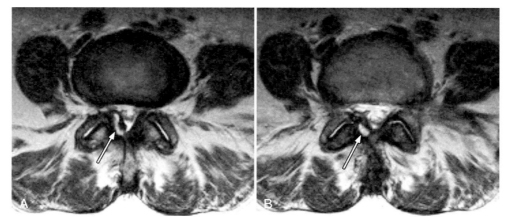

Figure 75-7 ▶ L4-5 Subligamentous Synovial Cyst. Contiguous axial T2-weighted MR images **A** and **B**, obtained at the L4-5 intervertebral disc level. Demonstrated is a synovial cyst arising along the medial margin of the right L4-5 facet joint. The cyst (*arrow in images* **A** and **B**) is positioned posterior to the right ligamentum flavum and displaces the right ligamentum flavum anteriorly.

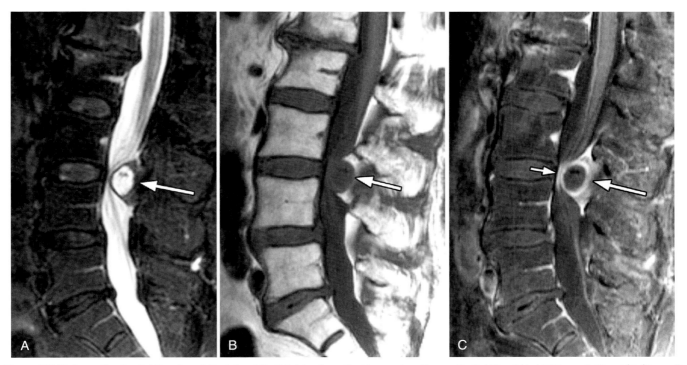

Figure 75-8 ▶ Large Parafacetal Pseudocyst (Juxtafacet Cyst) Arising from the Ligamentum Flavum. Sagittal T2-weighted MR image **A**. T1-weighted image **B**, and contrast-enhanced fat-saturated T1-weighted MR image **C**. A large cyst (*arrow*) causes anterior displacement of the thecal sac and compresses the cauda equina. The cyst (*arrow*) is T2 hyperintense centrally on image **A** and is T1 isointense relative to CSF on image **B**. In image **C**, the cyst fluid centrally does not enhance but the margins of the cyst enhance intensely, including the ligamentum flavum (*long arrow*). The thecal sac is displaced anteriorly. Adjacent compressed cauda equina nerve roots also enhance (*short arrow in image* **C**).

3. **Tarlov cyst:** A synovial cyst or parafacetal pseudocyst located in the neural foramen can have an appearance similar to an intraforaminal root sheath (Tarlov) cyst.

4. **Post-inflammatory paraspinous cysts**: Inflammation of the interspinous ligaments (Baastrup's disease) may result in cystic dilation of paraspinous bursa.[1] These bursae may communicate with the posterior facet joint capsules (see Chapter 39 for detailed description of interspinous bursitis).

5. **Facet joint capsular/synovial proliferation:** Thickened, redundant T2 hypointense capsular or synovial tissue, which does not contain fluid, may project into the spinal canal or neural foramen. This redundant facet capsular tissue can contribute to thecal sac deformity in the setting of central canal stenosis.

6. **Herniated disc:** Disc extrusions are typically T2 hypointense and slightly T1 hyperintense relative to the CSF. Proliferative

capsular/synovial tissue may be T2 hypointense. The posterior margin of a chronic herniated disc fragment or sequestered disc fragment rarely contains a small T2 hyperintense cystic region, which may represent cystic degeneration within the disc fragment or liquefaction of a small paradiscal hematoma.[1]

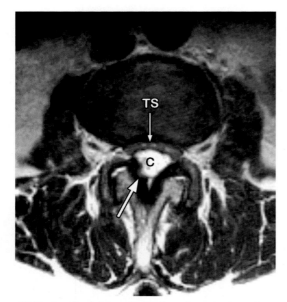

Figure 75-9 ▶ Parafacetal Pseudocyst (Juxtafacet Cyst). Axial T2-weighted MRI in same patient as in Figure 75-8. A large cyst (*C*) is positioned between the ligamentum flava. The cyst likely originates from the right ligamentum flavum where a small notch (*arrow*) is seen in the ligamentum flavum. The thecal sac (*TS*) and contained cauda equina nerve roots are compressed and displaced anteriorly along the posterior margin of the L3-4 intervertebral disc.

TREATMENT

A minority of synovial cysts will involute spontaneously.[15] Back pain or radicular pain can be managed conservatively by administering oral nonsteroidal anti-inflammatory agents or with short-term systemic steroid therapy. Invasive therapy for treatment of synovial cysts includes the following:

1. **Epidural steroid injection:** Interlaminar or transforaminal steroid injections can provide temporary relief of pain for symptomatic synovial cysts, but this is of limited long-term benefit in our experience. This may reduce inflammation surrounding the cyst but does not usually result in reduction in cyst volume in our experience.

2. **Facet joint steroid injection:** Injection at the level adjacent to the synovial cyst may provide temporary relief and sometimes long-term relief of symptoms.[16,17] Without accompanying cyst decompression, we have not found this technique to provide long-term benefit in our patient population.

3. **Direct synovial cyst puncture:** This procedure is performed by inserting a needle directly into the synovial cyst using fluoroscopic or CT guidance.[18] Needle positioning is confirmed by injecting a tiny amount of iodinated contrast agent into the cyst. A mixture of anesthetic and steroid is then injected directly into the cyst. This technique alone does not usually result in lasting symptomatic relief unless the cyst wall ruptures. Furthermore, it is difficult to cause a sizeable rent in the cyst by direct injection into the cyst alone, because the facet joint acts to decompress the pressure when the cyst fills with the injected contrast agent and/or anesthetic-steroid mixture.

4. **Synovial cyst injection and decompression via percutaneous facet joint injection.** This procedure is readily performed in an outpatient setting and not significantly more involved than facet joint epidural injection alone. This can be performed

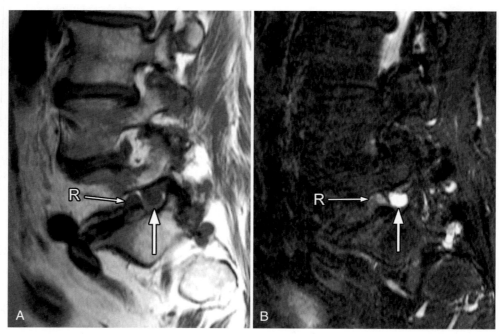

Figure 75-10 ▶ L5-S1 Foraminal Synovial Cyst. On left parasagittal T1-weighted MR image **A**, a T1 hypointense synovial cyst (*arrow*) in the left L5-S1 neural foramen is located posterior to the left L5 dorsal root ganglion/nerve root (*R*). On fat-saturated T2-weighted image **B**, the cyst (*arrow*) is hyperintense relative to the slightly less intense L5 nerve root (*R*).

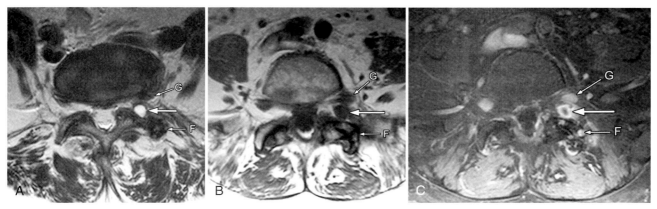

Figure 75-11 ▶ L5-S1 Foraminal Synovial Cyst. Axial T2-weighted MR image **A**, T1-weighted image **B**, and contrast-enhanced fat-saturated T1-weighted MR image **C**, in same patient as n Figure 75-10. The cyst is T2 hyperintense (*arrow in* **A**) and T1 hypointense (*arrow in* **B**) relative to the intraforaminal fat. In image **C**, the outer margin of the cyst (*arrow*) enhances intensely. The cyst is positioned between the dorsal root ganglion (*G*) anteriorly and the hypertrophic superior articular facet (*F*) posteriorly. Note enhancing tissue in subchondral erosions or tiny geodes within the facets.

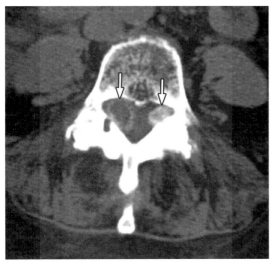

Figure 75-12 ▶ Bilateral Synovial Cysts in L4 Lateral Recesses. Axial CT image at L4 level shows bilateral peripherally calcified synovial cysts (*arrows*) within both lateral recesses of L4. The cysts arise from bilateral osteoarthritic L4-5 facet joints and cause bilateral compression of the thecal sac.

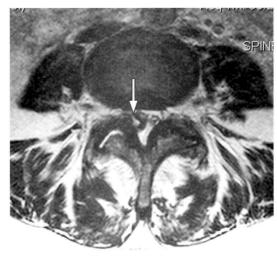

Figure 75-13 ▶ Thick-Walled Synovial Cyst on Right at L4-5 Level. Axial T2-weighted MR image. The synovial cyst (*arrow*) contains a small amount of T2 hyperintense fluid. Note small facet joint effusion on right and severe facet hypertrophy on left.

under CT or fluoroscopic guidance.[19] This is the initial procedure of choice for treating symptomatic synovial cysts at our institution, where we routinely perform this procedure using fluoroscopic guidance. The goal of the procedure is to decompress the cyst by producing a defect or rent in the cyst wall. A facet joint injection is first performed by inserting a needle into the facet joint communicating with the synovial cyst. A syringe filled with iodinated contrast agent is attached to the needle via a connecting tube. Under fluoroscopic visualization, the contrast agent is rapidly and forcibly injected by hand injection into the facet joint with the goal of distending and rupturing the cyst (*Fig. 75-16*). The patient usually experiences an accentuation of the usual pain as the cyst distends, and then immediate pain relief occurs when the cyst wall ruptures. As the cyst ruptures, the contrast agent will be seen extending into the epidural space. A mixture of normal saline, steroid, and anesthetic agent is then injected into the facet

joint, filling the facet joint as well as the ruptured synovial cyst, and extending into the epidural space. A high percentage of patients experience pain relief with or without cyst regression using this technique.[19] Approximately 50% to 60% of patients, who undergo "successful" percutaneous cyst decompression, using this technique, will reaccumulate liquid in the cyst after 3 to 4 months. These patients may be treated with repeat percutaneous synovial cyst decompression using this same technique. If this procedure fails to reduce the size of the cyst and symptoms do not improve or recur after three percutaneous cyst injection procedures, surgical excision of the synovial cyst should be considered.

5. **Combined percutaneous approach:** If the cyst cannot be ruptured by percutaneous injection into the facet joint, we have found a combined approach often is successful. With the needle in the facet joint, as described above in treatment 4, a second needle is inserted directly into the synovial cyst, using

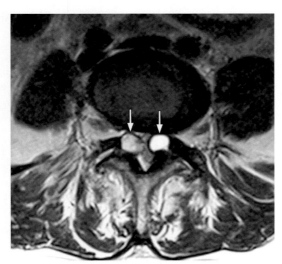

Figure 75-14 ▶ Bilateral L4-5 Synovial Cysts. Bilateral "kissing" synovial cysts (*arrows*) shown on axial T2-weighted MRI. The cysts arise from the medial aspect of the L4-5 facet joint bilaterally. The cysts cause marked side to side compression of the thecal sac and required decompressive laminectomy and bilateral facetectomies for treatment.

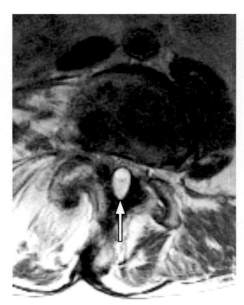

Figure 75-15 ▶ Parafacetal Pseudocyst (Juxtafacet Cyst). The cyst likely originates from ligamentum flavum at L3-4 level. The cyst (*arrow*) is hyperintense on this axial T2-weighted MR image. The fluid-filled cyst (*arrow*) does not communicate with the facet joints. The cyst causes compression and anterior displacement of the thecal sac.

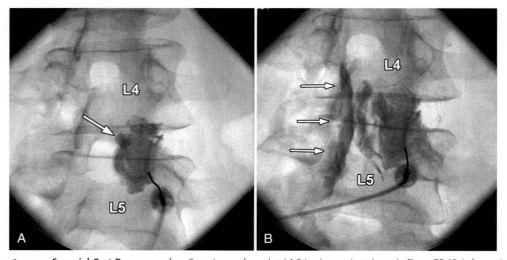

Figure 75-16 ▶ Percutaneous Synovial Cyst Decompression. Procedure performed at L4-5 level on patient shown in Figure 75-13. Left anterior oblique (LAO) radiographic images **A** and **B**. In image **A**, the facet joint capsule is distended with contrast agent just prior to rupture. The small fluid filled portion of the synovial cyst is indicated by the arrow in image **A**. In image **B**, obtained immediately following rupture of the cyst, the contrast agent has extended from the ruptured cyst into the epidural space (*arrows*). L4 = L4 vertebral body. L5 = L5 vertebral body.

fluoroscopic or CT guidance. A contrast-filled syringe is then connected via a connecting tube to each needle and the cyst is distended by simultaneous forcible hand injection of each syringe. This causes rapid distention of the cyst and usually results in rupture of the cyst wall. When the contrast agent is seen in the epidural space, a mixture of normal saline, anesthetic, and steroid is injected into the facet joint, which passes into the cyst and then into the epidural space.

6. **Surgical excision of synovial cyst:** Surgical excision has the highest success rate for treatment of synovial cysts. Laminectomy, removal of the ligamentum flavum, and surgical

excision of the synovial cyst is the definitive therapy for treating symptomatic synovial cysts if other treatment methods fail to provide long-term relief.[4] Sometimes medial facetectomy is performed to prevent recurrence of the cyst. However, extensive surgery carries the risk of developing spinal instability. Microsurgical cyst excision with limited decompression can be effective.[20]

References

1. Khalatbari K, Ansari H. MRI of degenerative cysts of the lumbar spine. *Clin Radiol.* 2008;63(3):322-328.

2. Gadgil AA, Eisenstein SM, Darby A, Cassar Pullicino V. Bilateral symptomatic synovial cysts of the lumbar spine caused by calcium pyrophosphate deposition disease: A case report. *Spine*. 2002;27(19):E428-E431.

3. Trummer M, Flaschka G, Tillich M, et al. Diagnosis and surgical management of intraspinal synovial cysts: Report of 19 cases. *J Neurol Neurosurg Psychiatry*. 2001;70(1):74-77.

4. Tillich M, Trummer M, Lindbichler F, Flaschka G. Symptomatic intraspinal synovial cysts of the lumbar spine: Correlation of MR and surgical findings. *Neuroradiology*. 2001;43(12):1070-1075.

5. Christophis P, Asamoto S, Kuchelmeister K, Schachenmayr W. "Juxtafacet cysts", a misleading name for cystic formations of mobile spine (CYFMOS). *Eur Spine J*. 2007;16(9):1499-1505.

6. Banning CS, Thorell WE, Leibrock LG. Patient outcome after resection of lumbar juxtafacet cysts. *Spine*. 2001;26(8):969-972.

7. Hsu KY, Zucherman JF, Shea WJ, Jeffrey RA. Lumbar intraspinal synovial and ganglion cysts (facet cysts): Ten-year experience in evaluation and treatment. *Spine*. 1995;20(1):80-89.

8. Kao CC, Winkler SS, Turner JH. Synovial cyst of spinal facet. Case report. *J Neurosurg*. 1974;41(3):372-376.

9. Kao CC, Uihlein A, Bickel WH, Soule EH. Lumbar intraspinal extradural ganglion cyst. *J Neurosurg*. 1968;29(2):168-172.

10. Jackson DE Jr, Atlas SW, Mani JR, Norman D. Intraspinal synovial cysts: MR imaging. *Radiology*. 1989;170(2):527-530.

11. Apostolaki E, Davies AM, Evans N, Cassar-Pullicino VN. MR imaging of lumbar facet joint synovial cysts. *Eur Radiol*. 2000;10(4):615-623.

12. Fritz RC, Kaiser JA, White AH, et al. Magnetic resonance imaging of a thoracic intraspinal synovial cyst. *Spine*. 1994;19(4):487-490.

13. Liu SS, Williams KD, Drayer BP, et al. Synovial cysts of the lumbosacral spine: Diagnosis by MR imaging. *AJR Am J Roentgenol*. 1990;154(1):163-166.

14. Davis R, Iliya A, Roque C, Pampati M. The advantage of magnetic resonance imaging in diagnosis of a lumbar synovial cyst. *Spine*. 1990;15(3):244-246.

15. Swartz PG, Murtagh FR. Spontaneous resolution of an intraspinal synovial cyst. *AJNR Am J Neuroradiol*. 2003;24(6):1261-1263.

16. Parlier-Cuau C, Wybier M, Nizard R, et al. Symptomatic lumbar facet joint synovial cysts: Clinical assessment of facet joint steroid injection after 1 and 6 months and long-term follow-up in 30 patients. *Radiology*. 1999;210(2):509-513.

17. Bjorkengren AG, Kurz LT, Resnick D, et al. Symptomatic intraspinal synovial cysts: opacification and treatment by percutaneous injection. *AJR Am J Roentgenol*. 1987;149(1):105-107.

18. Melfi RS, Aprill CN. Percutaneous puncture of zygapophysial joint synovial cyst with fluoroscopic guidance. *Pain Med*. 2005;6(2):122-128.

19. Bureau NJ, Kaplan PA, Dussault RG. Lumbar facet joint synovial cyst: Percutaneous treatment with steroid injections and distention—clinical and imaging follow-up in 12 patients. *Radiology*. 2001;221(1):179-185.

20. Shah RV, Lutz GE. Lumbar intraspinal synovial cysts: Conservative management and review of the world's literature. *Spine J*. 2003;3(6):479-488.

SYRINGOMYELIA

Leo F. Czervionke, M.D.

CLINICAL PRESENTATION

The patient is a 73-year-old woman with a history of old fracture of the T12 vertebra secondary to prior motor vehicle accident. Patient was treated at the time of the fracture with thoracolumbar laminectomy and posterior fusion. The patient complains of progressive low back pain, lower extremity weakness, numbness, and pain. She has no bladder or bowel dysfunction. Upon examination, lower thoracic kyphosis is evident. She has mild to moderate motor weakness in both lower extremities proximally.

IMAGING PRESENTATION

Magnetic resonance (MR) imaging obtained reveals kyphotic deformity of the spine at the T11-12 level and an old compression fracture of the T12 vertebral body with retropulsion of the T12 vertebral body impinging upon the ventral cord surface. Spinal cord syringomyelia extends from the T10 to the T12 level (*Figs. 76-1 and 76-2*).

DISCUSSION

Hydromyelia (sometimes called *primary cord syrinx*) refers to dilation of the ependymal-lined central canal of the spinal cord. *Syringomyelia* (or *secondary cord syrinx*) is the term used to indicate a glial-lined cavity in the cord parenchyma without involvement of the central canal of the cord. The term *syringohydromyelia* encompasses both syringomyelia and hydromyelia and is used to include both cavitations occurring in the cord parenchyma and/or dilation of the central canal or an unspecified cavity in the cord. If the syrinx extends into the brainstem, this is referred to as *syringobulbia*.

Hydromyelia usually manifests in younger patients and is often associated with a developmental anomaly such as Chiari type 1 malformation, Chiari type 2 malformation (also called *Arnold-Chiari malformation*), meningomyelocele, diastematomyelia, tethered cord, congenital scoliosis, basilar invagination, or hydrocephalus.[1-3] In approximately 50% of patients with Chiari type 1 malformation, a hydromyelic cavity develops in the spinal cord. The hydromyelia may be of variable size, configuration, and length (*Figs. 76-3 and 76-4*). The hydromyelia may extend over a few vertebral levels or may extend the entire length of the spinal cord. Posterior fossa tumors can also cause dilation of the central canal of the spinal cord by obstruction of the obex or altered

cerebrospinal fluid (CSF) flow dynamics near the foramen magnum region. Hydromyelia is believed to be due to interference in CSF flow in the spinal cord secondary to a mass, adhesions, or obstructing process in the posterior fossa interfering with CSF flow at the obex, foramen magnum, or C2-3 level.[4] One theory suggests that when an obstructing or partially obstructing process exists at or near the foramen magnum level, caudal motion of the spinal cord, cerebellar tonsils, and brainstem, generates a piston-like effect that results in pulse-pressure abnormalities that drive the CSF downward into the central canal forming the hydromyelic cavity, assuming the central canal still communicates with the fourth ventricle.[5] If the central canal does not communicate with the fourth ventricle, it is possible that exaggerated spinal pulse pressures may lead to increased transmedullary pressure gradients between the spinal subarachnoid space and the extracellular space within the cord, forcing CSF into the spinal cord via perivascular spaces and eventually leading to cord cavitation.[5,6]

Syringomyelia is widely believed to be an acquired condition that is often idiopathic, but can be seen following trauma, spinal cord infarction, cord infection, noninfectious myelitis, arachnoiditis, or scoliosis, or can be associated with intramedullary tumors such as hemangioblastoma or ependymoma (*Figs. 76-5 and 76-6*). In these cases, the syrinx may form because of actual destruction of the cord parenchyma by the trauma, infection, or tumor. Alternatively, the syrinx cavity may form secondarily by underlying pathologic process interfering with the blood supply of the cord resulting in degeneration of spinal cord tissue and eventual cavitation. Uncommonly, a syrinx may develop adjacent to a large spondylitic ridge or large herniated disc compressing the spinal cord. However, in such cases, it is not known whether the cord compression is responsible for the syrinx formation or merely is a coexistent finding (*Figs. 76-7, 76-8, and 76-9*).

The etiology of "idiopathic" syringomyelic cavity formation is controversial. One possibility is that an abnormal process in the subarachnoid space such as a tumor, inflammation, or hemorrhage causes a pressure buildup in the subarachnoid space that forces CSF into the spinal cord parenchyma via the perivascular spaces resulting in intramedullary cavitation.[6-8] Others believe that the spinal cord normally possesses a positive extracellular fluid balance such that fluid passes via the perivascular spaces into the subarachnoid space surrounding the cord.[9,10] If this is true, then it is possible that some cases of idiopathic syringomyelia develop as a primary cystic process in the cord, because of obstruction of the cord perivascular spaces, which prevents

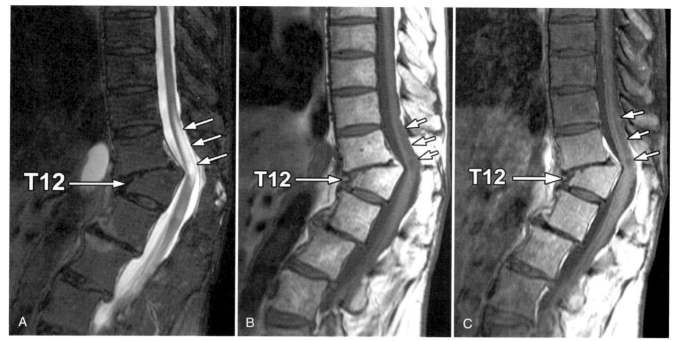

Figure 76-1 ▶ Post-traumatic Syringomyelia. Old T12 compression fracture with resulting kyphotic deformity at the T11-12 level viewed on sagittal T2-weighted image **A**, T1-weighted image **B**, and contrast enhanced image **C**. There has been retropulsion of the posterosuperior vertebral body margin which impinges upon the ventral aspect of the thecal sac and spinal cord at the T1 2 level. A T2 hyperintense and T1 hypointense syrinx cavity (*arrows*) extends from the T12 level superiorly to mid T10 level. The substance of the cord is very thin posterior to the syringomyelic cavity (*arrows*). There is no abnormal contrast enhancement of the spinal cord as shown on image **C**.

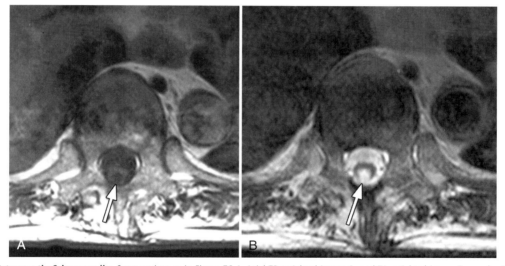

Figure 76-2 ▶ Post-traumatic Sringomyelia. Same patient as in Figure 76-1. Axial T2-weighted image **A**, and T1-weighted image **B** reveal a T1 hypointense and T2 hyperintense syrinx (*arrow in images* **A** *and* **B**) within the cord at the T11 level. Note marked thinning of posterior spinal cord substance posterior to the syrinx cavity.

normal interstitial fluid in the cord from flowing into the spinal subarachnoid space.[11]

Whatever the etiology, symptoms secondary to syringohydromyelia are likely produced by increased pressure upon the spinal cord neurons or from interference with the spinal cord vascular supply resulting in compromise of the microvascular integrity of the cord, followed by infarction, tissue necrosis, and eventual cavitation.

Post-traumatic spinal cord syringomyelia occurs in up to 22% of patients with spinal cord injury.[12,13] Initially after cord trauma,

the cord becomes edematous causing mass effect on adjacent neurons and compromise of the cord microcirculation.[14] Later, macrophages infiltrate into this region of the cord, followed by capillary proliferation and gliosis. A myelomalacic core is believed to develop at the site of post-traumatic cord infarction, microhemorrhage, or as a result of direct cord injury).[12,14] Another theory suggests that intracellular excitatory amino acids are released into the extracellular space of the injured cord tissues, initiating a cytotoxic cascade leading to cell death and subsequent tissue necrosis.[13] Regardless of the precise mechanism, the post-traumatic syrinx

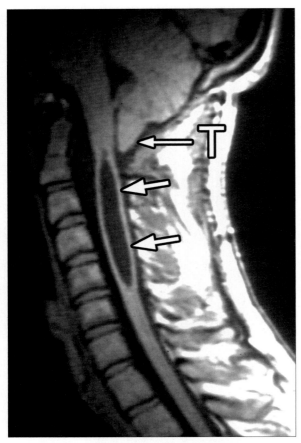

Figure 76-3 ▶ Chiari Type 1 Malformation with Hydromyelia. Sagittal TI-weighted MRI shows malformed, inferiorly pointed cerebellar tonsil (*T*). A moderated sized "unilocular" intramedullary hydromyelic cavity (*arrow*) causes fusiform enlargement of the spinal cord.

develops within a *myelomalacic core* that is consistently located either in the base of the dorsal column or at the junction of the dorsal column and posterior gray matter horn.[12] This region of the cord is a watershed zone between the anterior and posterior spinal arteries.

Patients with syringohydromyelia classically present with slow, progressive loss of pain and temperature sensation (lateral white matter column affected) usually with preservation of dorsal column function (pain, proprioception, touch). Distal upper extremity weakness, gait disturbance, back pain, radicular pain, and spastic paraparesis may also be present. Long tract findings may also be present with syringomyelia, depending on the position of the cavity. Symptoms usually improve after decompression of the syrinx cavity but often do not resolve completely. Sensory symptoms usually show a greater degree of improvement than motor symptoms. Cervical syringomyelia is the most common cause of a neuropathic shoulder joint.[15]

IMAGING FEATURES

Syringomyelia sometimes, but not always, causes fusiform enlargement of the spinal cord, which may be visible on myelography or post-myelogram computed tomography (CT) images, where the fusiform enlargement may resemble that of an intramedullary

mass. If the syrinx cavity is very large, resulting in marked fusiform cord expansion, the spinal canal may be expanded from bone remodeling. This is rarely observed today, because syringomyelia is usually detected with magnetic resonance (MR) imaging before significant cord expansion occurs.

MR imaging is the modality of choice for diagnosing and assessing the extent of the syrinx cavity. Incidental slitlike dilation of the central canal or segments of the central canal are commonly seen on routine MRI studies of the thoracic spine. More pronounced dilation of the central canal is seen in conditions that alter CSF flow dynamics in the spinal cord such as hydromyelia in patients with Chiari type 1 malformation (see Figs. 76-1 to 76-4). It has been shown that in some cases with Chiari type 1 malformation, prior to actual syrinx cavity formation, a potentially reversible *pre-syrinx state* may exist secondary to disturbance in CSF flow dynamics near the foramen magnum level, and during this time abnormal T2 signal hyperintensity can be demonstrated in the upper cervical spinal cord.[6]

In patients with syringomyelia, a noncavitary region of T2 signal hyperintensity may also be observed caudal or rostral to the actual syrinx cavity. This pre-syrinx zone may represent cord edema and/or myelomalacia adjacent to the advancing margin of the syrinx, which may predispose to eventual cavitation.[16] This situation is commonly seen with syringomyelia associated with spinal cord tumors (see Fig. 76-6). This region of noncavitary signal disturbance is potentially reversible after removal of the tumors or decompression of syrinx cavity.[16]

Smaller syringohydromyelic cavities tend to have more uniform diameters (see Figs. 76-3 and 76-7). Larger cavities tend to have a multiloculated or septated appearance (see Fig. 76-4). These apparent loculations are actually pseudoloculations, because they are partially but not completely septated. These loculated syrinx cavities have a configuration resembling colonic haustrations rather than being discrete walled off compartments because adjacent loculations nearly always communicate. The size and configuration of the syrinx cavity may vary considerably in different portions of the spinal cord.

With MR imaging, the syrinx cavity is isointense relative to CSF on all imaging sequences (see Figs. 76-1 to 76-4 and 76-8). With syringomyelic cavities associated with spinal cord tumors, such as ependymoma, astrocytoma, or hemangioblastoma, the cavity may be isointense relative to CSF or can be slightly hyperintense relative to CSF on T1- and T2-weighted images presumably because of proteinaceous fluid in the cavity (see Figs. 76-5 and 76-6).

IV contrast-enhanced images should be obtained if a syrinx is detected on unenhanced MR images to exclude associated cord neoplasm. The margins of the typical simple, uncomplicated, syringomyelic or hydromyelic cavity do not enhance after IV contrast (see Figs. 76-1 and 76-4). The presence of marginal or nodular enhancement adjacent to the syrinx usually indicates that an inflammatory or neoplastic process is the cause of the syrinx (***Figs.** 76-5, 76-6, and **76-10**).

In patients with syringohydromyelia, intracystic velocities and velocities in the adjacent subarachnoid space can be measured using velocity phase encoding MRI techniques.[17,18] In one study, higher systolic and diastolic cyst velocities were seen in larger cysts and in patients with relatively poor clinical status.[17] Intracystic systolic and diastolic velocities should diminish, whereas the velocity in the adjacent subarachnoid space should increase after successful surgery. If the diastolic CSF velocity remains the same or increases after surgery, this is an indicator of a poor prognosis.[17]

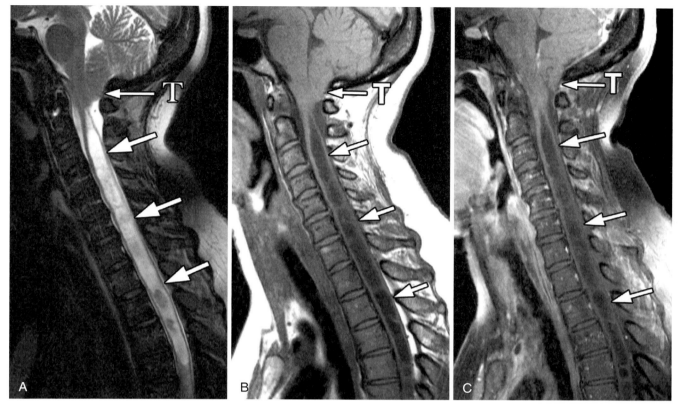

Figure 76-4 ▶ Chiari Type 1 Malformation with Hydromyelia. Sagittal T2-weighted MR image **A**, T1-weighted image **B**, and contrast enhanced fat saturated image **C**. The cerebellar tonsils (*T*) are pointed inferiorly and are low lying, extending inferiorly to the level of the posterior arch of C1. A large T1 hypointense, T2 hyperintense "mulitlocular-appearing" or "haustrated" hydromyelic intramedullary cavity (*arrows in images* **A** *and* **B**) causes diffuse enlargement of the spinal cord. Heterogeneous flow artifacts are noted in the cavity on T2-weighted image **A**. No abnormal contrast enhancement is visible in the spinal cord tissue adjacent to the intramedullary cavity.

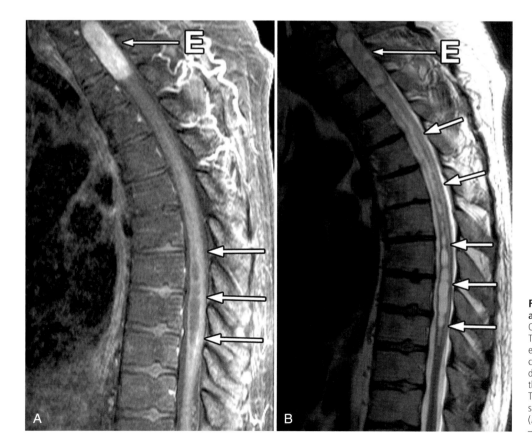

Figure 76-5 ▶ Ependymoma Aassociated with Spinal Cord Syringomyelia. On sagittal contrast enhanced fat-saturated T1-weighted MR image **A**, the intramedullary ependymoma (*E*) is located within the spinal cord from C7 to T2 level. Syringomyelia is demonstrated in the mid-thoracic lower-thoracic spinal cord (*arrows*) on sagittal T2-weighted image **B**, the full extent of the syrinx cavity (*arrows*) below the ependymoma (*E*) is defined to better advantage.

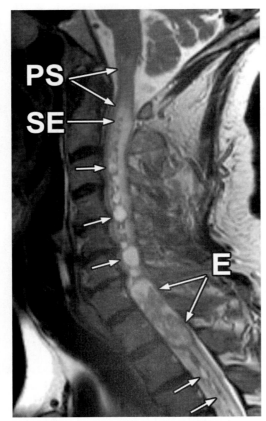

Figure 76-6 ▶ Ependymoma Associated with Spinal Cord Syringomyelia. Same patient as in Figure 76-5. Sagittal T2-weighted MRI of the cervical spinal cord. A multiloculated syrinx cavity (*short arrows*) extends above the intramedullary ependymoma (*E*). The superior extent (*SE*) of the syrinx is at the C2 level. There is a vague region of T2 hyperintensity, likely representing cord edema and/or myelomalacia, in the spinal cord adjacent to the syrinx and also in the lower portion of the medulla. The region above the syrinx is considered a "pre-syrinx" zone (*PS*), where additional cord cavitation may eventually occur.

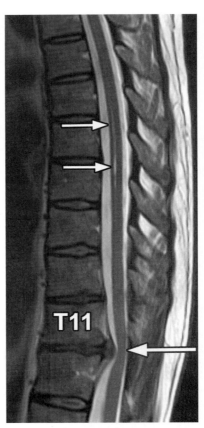

Figure 76-7 ▶ Herniated Disc Causing Cord Compression and Coexistent Syringomyelia. On sagittal T2-weighted MRI, a herniated disc at the T11-12 level causes cord compression (*long arrow*). A small diameter syrinx (*short arrows*) is located within the cord from T6 to T8 level.

DIFFERENTIAL DIAGNOSIS

1. **Tumor-related syrinx:** Intramedullary tumors including ependymoma, hemangioblastoma, astrocytoma, and metastasis may cause cord cavitation resulting in syrinx formation (see Figs. 76-5, 76-6, and 76-10). Fluid in the tumoral syrinx cavity is often, but not always, slightly more hyperintense than CSF on T2-weighted images.
2. **Cord edema or cord myelomalacia extending over several vertebral levels:** This may be confused with a syrinx. The signal intensity of the edematous or myelomalacic cord is slightly T1 hypointense and T2 hyperintense. The T1 signal intensity of the simple, uncomplicated syringohydromyelic cavity has the same intensity as CSF.
3. **Slitlike dilations of the central canal of the spinal cord:** These are routinely observed on routine MR imaging studies of the spine. These tiny slitlike cavities may be localized to a few vertebrae in length or can be discontinuous, tiny multisegmental cavities. These are most commonly located in the lower thoracic spinal cord but can be located anywhere in the spinal cord (*Figs. 76-11*). These are nearly always asymptomatic.

4. **Persistent ventriculus terminalis (terminal ventricle):** During embryogenesis, the ventriculus terminalis is normally located in the caudal aspect of the spinal cord; this usually regresses a few weeks after birth. If this persists, a small cystic cavity, approximately 1 cm in length and 2 to 4 mm in diameter, remains in the conus medullaris (*Fig. 76-12*). This condition is a normal anatomic variant and is asymptomatic.[3]

TREATMENT

1. **Surgical correction of congenital or developmental anomalies:** If an underlying congenital or developmental condition is responsible for the hydromyelia, this condition should be surgically corrected first, if possible. For example, this would include shunting patients with hydrocephalus, correction of congenital scoliosis,[2] surgery to release a tethered cord or diastematomyelia, repair of a meningomyelocele, or decompression of the foramen magnum region in patients with Chiari malformations.
2. **Decompression of the syrinx:** In symptomatic syringomyelic cavities, surgical decompression of the syrinx by insertion of an indwelling drainage catheter can be effective in some patients. Syringoperitoneal or syringosubarachnoid shunts can be effective.[19,20]

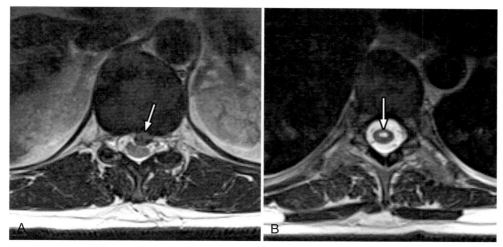

Figure 76-8 ▶ Herniated Disc Causing Cord Compression and Coexistent Syringomyelia. Same patient as in Figure 76-7. Axial T2-weighted image **A**, obtained at T11-12 level, reveals a herniated disc (*arrow*) compressing the anterior aspect of the spinal cord on the left. Axial T2-weighted image **B**, obtained at the T7 level, shows T2 hyperintense syrinx cavity in the cord (*arrow*).

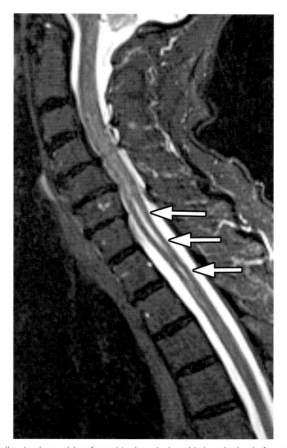

Figure 76-9 ▶ Cervicothoracic Syrinx. A small syrinx (*arrows*) has formed in the spinal cord below the level of several bulging cervical discs and spondylitic ridges as demonstrated on this sagittal T2-weighted MRI.

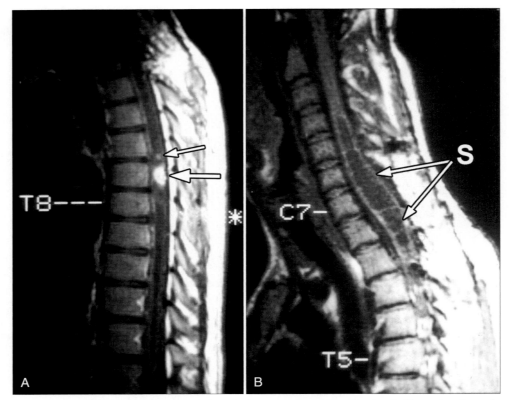

Figure 76-10 ▶ Intramedullary Hemangioblastoma at T7 Level. On sagittal contrast enhanced T1-weighted sagittal image **A**, an intense homogeneously enhancing intramedullary mass (*large arrow*) is demonstrated in the spinal cord at the mid T7 level. A tiny enhancing intramedullary satellite hemangioblastoma (*small arrow*) is present at the T6-7 level and other tiny enhancing lesions are located along the pial surface of the lower thoracic cord. Associated syringomyelic cavity is located above and below the level of the T7 intramedullary tumor. On sagittal T1-weighted image **B**, centered at the cervicothoracic junction, the syrinx (*S*) is larger in diameter than in the thoracic spinal cord more inferiorly.

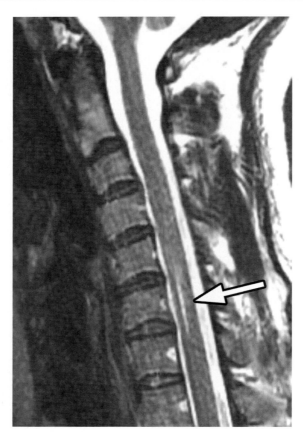

Figure 76-11 ▶ Minimal Localized Hydromyelia. Slit-like dilattion of the central canal of the spinal cord (*arrow*) is shown at the C6 level on this sagittal T2-weighted MRI. Minimal dilattion of the central canal of the cord is commonly encountered on routine MR imaging studies.

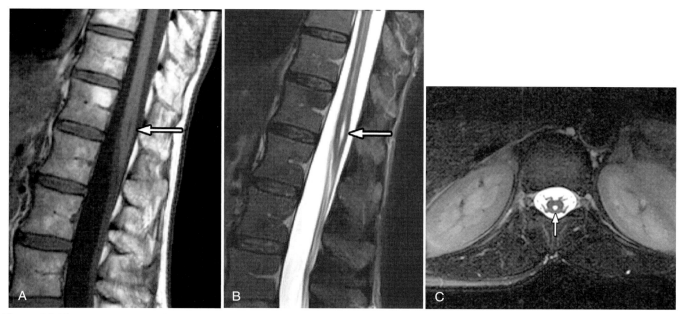

Figure 76-12 ► Persistent Ventriculus Terminalis. A small terminal ventricle is seen as a small intramedullary cavity (*arrow*) in the conus on sagittal T1-weighted MR image **A** and T2-weighted image **B**. On axial fat saturated T2-weighted image **C**, obtained at the level of the conus medullaris, the tiny T2 hyperintense intramedullary cavity is located slightly posterior to cord center.

3. **Tumor removal:** If a spinal cord tumor is present, removal of the tumor can result in decompression of the syrinx. In some cases, a catheter must also be inserted into the syrinx for drainage.[21]

4. **Surgical lysis of adhesions:** If the syrinx is secondary to arachnoiditis, surgical lysis of arachnoidal adhesions can be performed, if adhesions or arachnoidal loculations can be demonstrated.[8] Intraoperative sonography is valuable to identify these adhesions at time of surgery.

References

1. Ozerdemoglu RA, Denis F, Transfeldt EE. Scoliosis associated with syringomyelia: Clinical and radiologic correlation. *Spine.* 2003;28(13): 1410-1417.

2. Eule JM, Erickson MA, O'Brien MF, Handler M. Chiari I malformation associated with syringomyelia and scoliosis: A twenty-year review of surgical and nonsurgical treatment in a pediatric population. *Spine.* 2002;27(13): 1451-1455.

3. Unsinn KM, Geley T, Freund MC, Gassner I. US of the spinal cord in newborns: Spectrum of normal findings, variants, congenital anomalies, and acquired diseases. *Radiographics.* 2000;20(4):923-938.

4. Wolpert SM. In Re: The Presyrinx state: a reversible myelopathic condition that may precede syringomyelia. *AJNR Am J Neuroradiol.* 2000;21(5): 984-985.

5. Levy LM. Toward an understanding of syringomyelia: MR imaging of CSF flow and neuraxis motion. *AJNR Am J Neuroradiol.* 2000;21(1): 45-46.

6. Fischbein NJ, Dillon WP, Cobbs C, Weinstein PR. The "presyrinx" state: A reversible myelopathic condition that may precede syringomyelia. *AJNR Am J Neuroradiol.* 1999;20(1):7-20.

7. Levy LM. MR identification of Chiari pathophysiology by using spatial and temporal CSF flow indices and implications for syringomyelia. *AJNR Am J Neuroradiol.* 2003;24(2):165-166.

8. Brodbelt AR, Stoodley MA. Syringomyelia and the arachnoid web. *Acta Neurochir (Wien).* 2003;145(8):707-711; discussion 11.

9. Sato O, Asai T, Amano Y, et al. Extraventricular origin of the cerebrospinal fluid: Formation rate quantitatively measured in the spinal subarachnoid space of dogs. *J Neurosurg.* 1972;36(3):276-282.

10. Olivero WC. Pathogenesis of syringomyelia. *AJNR Am J Neuroradiol.* 1999;20(10):2024-2045.

11. Castillo M. Further explanations for the formation of syringomyelia: Back to the drawing table. *AJNR Am J Neuroradiol.* 2000;21(10):1778-1779.

12. Squier MV, Lehr RP. Post-traumatic syringomyelia. *J Neurol Neurosurg Psychiatry.* 1994;57(9):1095-1098.

13. Yezierski RP, Santana M, Park SH, Madsen PW. Neuronal degeneration and spinal cavitation following intraspinal injections of quisqualic acid in the rat. *J Neurotrauma.* 1993;10(4):445-456.

14. Carroll AM, Brackenridge P. Post-traumatic syringomyelia: A review of the cases presenting in a regional spinal injuries unit in the north east of England over a 5-year period. *Spine.* 2005;30(10):1206-1210.

15. Jones EA, Manaster BJ, May DA, Disler DG. Neuropathic osteoarthropathy: Diagnostic dilemmas and differential diagnosis. *Radiographics.* 2000;20 Spec No:S279-S293.

16. Jinkins JR, Reddy S, Leite CC, et al. MR of parenchymal spinal cord signal change as a sign of active advancement in clinically progressive posttraumatic syringomyelia. *AJNR Am J Neuroradiol.* 1998;19(1):177-182.

17. Brugieres P, Idy-Peretti I, Iffenecker C, et al. CSF flow measurement in syringomyelia. *AJNR Am J Neuroradiol.* 2000;21(10):1785-1792.

18. Bhadelia RA, Bogdan AR, Wolpert SM, et al. Cerebrospinal fluid flow waveforms: Analysis in patients with Chiari I malformation by means of gated phase-contrast MR imaging velocity measurements. *Radiology.* 1995; 196(1):195-202.

19. Asano M, Fujiwara K, Yonenobu K, Hiroshima K. Post-traumatic syringomyelia. *Spine.* 1996;21(12):1446-1453.

20. Barbaro NM, Wilson CB, Gutin PH, Edwards MS. Surgical treatment of syringomyelia: Favorable results with syringoperitoneal shunting. *J Neurosurg.* 1984;61(3):531-538.

21. Cusick JF, Bernardi R. Syringomyelia after removal of benign spinal extramedullary neoplasms. *Spine.* 1995;20(11):1289-1293; discussion 93-94.

CHAPTER 77

TARLOV CYST

Douglas S. Fenton, M.D.

CLINICAL PRESENTATION

The patient is an 81-year-old woman who has a long history of intermittent low back pain for more than 15 years. She states that she has developed difficulty when walking over the last 18 months. In particular, she can walk up to a quarter mile but then feels like she is "walking in water" with a heavy feeling in her posterior thighs extending down to the knees, right greater than left. If she continues to walk past this point, she develops a "back ache" and further heaviness in her legs. Her leg symptoms also occur when standing for any long period of time. She is not symptomatic when sitting or lying down. She does have occasional aching pain in her posterior thighs, particularly when sitting for long periods. The pain is described as aching in quality. It is 2/10 on average, 8/10 at worst when walking or standing, and 0/10 when lying down or sitting still.

IMAGING PRESENTATION

Axial T1-weighted and fat-saturated T2-weighted images demonstrate a large cerebrospinal fluid–filled region in the right S1 lateral recess. The right S1 sacral foramen is enlarged compared with the left secondary to chronic pressure erosion from this large Tarlov cyst (*Fig. 77-1*).

DISCUSSION

Tarlov cysts, also known as *nerve root cysts, perineurial cysts,* or *perineural cysts,* are cerebrospinal fluid–filled cysts that occur at the junction of the posterior root and dorsal root ganglion.[1-3] These cysts were originally described by Tarlov in 1938 at autopsy.[1] The cysts are located between the perineurium and endoneurium. They are typically found in the sacral region involving the S2 and S3 nerve roots, but have been found to occur anywhere in the cervical, thoracic, and lumbar spine.[4,5]

Tarlov went on to distinguish these cysts from meningeal cysts by three main findings.[1,2,6] First, the Tarlov cyst does not have an actual communication with the spinal subarachnoid space but rather a potential one. Meningeal cysts, on the other hand, have a direct communication. During myelography, the Tarlov cyst may have delayed filling, whereas the meningeal cyst fills immediately. This delayed filling was more prevalent with the use of oil-based myelographic contrast. Second, Tarlov cysts occur at or distal to

the junction of the posterior nerve root and dorsal root ganglion (DRG), whereas meningeal cysts occur proximal to the DRG. Lastly, Tarlov cysts have at least part of their wall composed of nerve fibers or ganglion cells, and meningeal cysts have an arachnoid-lined wall and do not contain nerve fibers. The first finding has been disputed and studies have shown that there is an actual communication between Tarlov cysts and the subarachnoid space.[7] It appears that the defining feature of Tarlov cysts is the presence of nerve fibers in the cyst wall or in the cyst itself.[1-3,6] Tarlov cysts have been classified as a Nabors type II cyst.[3] Nabors classification type I cysts are extradural meningeal cysts without spinal nerve root fibers.[3] Nabors classification type II cysts are extradural meningeal cysts with spinal nerve root fibers, and Nabors classification type III cysts are spinal intradural meningeal cysts.[3]

The pathogenesis of Tarlov cysts is unclear. Some have postulated that trauma with hemorrhage into the subarachnoid space impairs drainage of the veins of the perineurium and epineurium with resultant rupture of these veins and cyst formation.[2] Others postulate a congenital etiology with arachnoid proliferations within the nerve root sleeve and subsequent obstruction of normal cerebrospinal fluid flow and cyst formation.[8]

The prevalence of Tarlov cysts is estimated at 4.6% to 9%.[8,9] The majority of these cysts (greater than 80%) are asymptomatic; however, they can produce, depending on location, low back pain, radicular pain, perineal pain, coccygodynia, paresthesias, bowel/bladder dysfunction, angina-like symptoms, and headaches.[1-3,8,10] Symptomatic cysts cause predominantly sensory symptoms because of the proximity of the cysts to the dorsal roots and dorsal root ganglion. The patient may describe worsening symptoms on standing, coughing, or other Valsalva maneuvers. These maneuvers force more cerebrospinal fluid (CSF) into the Tarlov cyst from the spinal subarachnoid space through a ball-valve communication into the Tarlov cyst[11,12] leading to transient compression and/or stretching of local nerve fibers. This ball-valve mechanism and pulsatile forces of CSF are considered to be the major contributing factors to the growth of these cysts.[13]

The difficulty is deciding whether or not a Tarlov cyst is the symptomatic lesion because there are often other radiographic findings, such as disc degeneration, disc protrusions/herniation, and facet degeneration that may be present at the same time. One cannot assume that the mere presence of a Tarlov cyst is the causative agent. Procedures such as image-guided percutaneous cyst drainage[8] usually yield only temporary relief; however, it can be an important diagnostic tool for the surgeon who can perform a more

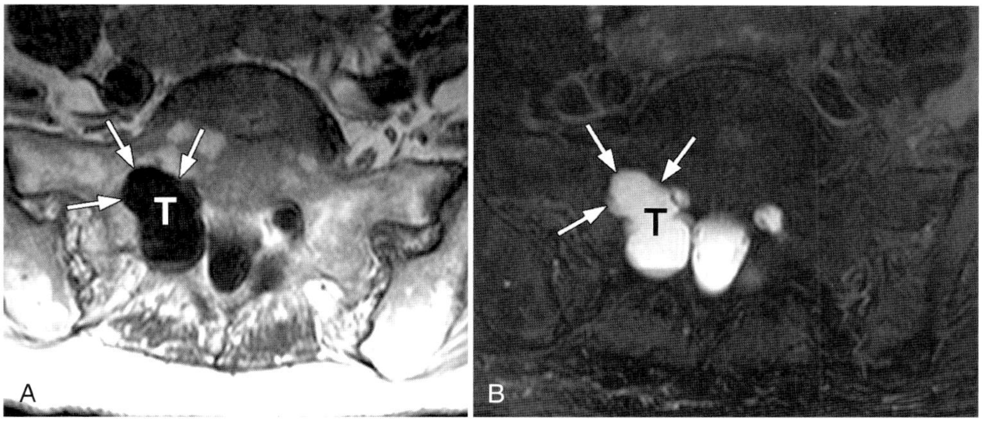

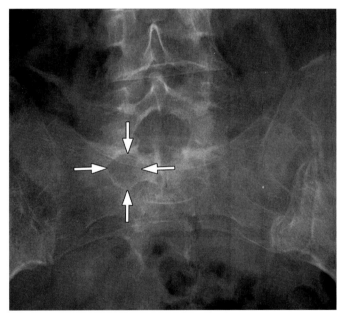

Figure 77-1 ▶ **Tarlov Cyst.** Axial T1-weighted image **A** and fat-saturated T2-weighted image **B** at the level of the S1 lateral recesses. There is a large T1 hypointense/T2 hyperintense region (T) occupying the right S1 lateral recess/foramen with smooth expansion of the right S1 lateral recess/foramen (arrows) compatible with a perineural/Tarlov cyst.

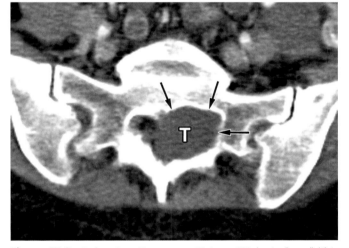

Figure 77-2 ▶ **Tarlov Cyst.** Frontal radiograph. Smooth expansion of the right S1 sacral foramen (arrows).

Figure 77-3 ▶ **Tarlov Cyst, Noncontast CT.** Large CSF density "mass" (T) in the left S1 foramen and lateral recess with smooth expansion of the left S1 foramen (arrows).

definitive procedure. Some have added fibrin glue after the aspiration to prevent recurrence of the cyst; however, 75% of these patients had aseptic meningitis after the procedure.[14] Others have used high-volume lumbar punctures to attempt to decrease the hydrostatic pressure and thus lessen flow into the cyst thus ameliorating symptoms, although this is more a temporary therapeutic procedure rather than a diagnostic procedure.[13]

IMAGING FEATURES

Plain film radiographs may demonstrate long-standing smooth expansile changes of a sacral foramen (*Fig. 77-2*), a widened spinal canal, and/or thinned pedicles; however, this is neither sensitive nor specific to a Tarlov cyst or a sacral nerve root. Furthermore, plain radiographs are unable to detect bone changes in the

remainder of the spine. On noncontrast computed tomography (CT), Tarlov cysts are isodense to CSF (*Fig. 77-3*). The typical bone scalloping is readily identified by CT. Tarlov cysts can be seen to fill with myelographic contrast (*Fig. 77-4*). In the past, when oil-based contrasts such as Pantopaque were used, the Tarlov cyst frequently showed delayed filling from hours to weeks. However, with the newer water-soluble agents, a Tarlov cyst may fill as fast as the intrathecal subarachnoid space and appear as a contrast-filled elongation of the nerve root sleeve. Magnetic resonance (MR) imaging is considered to be the preferred imaging method for Tarlov cysts. With MRI, one can readily see the cyst as a rounded structure of decreased T1-signal intensity, increased T2-signal intensity without enhancement (*Fig. 77-5*). The nerve is often seen eccentrically located within the cyst on T2-weighted images. MRI is also useful to demonstrate the relationship of the cyst to the neural structures and the volume of the cyst.

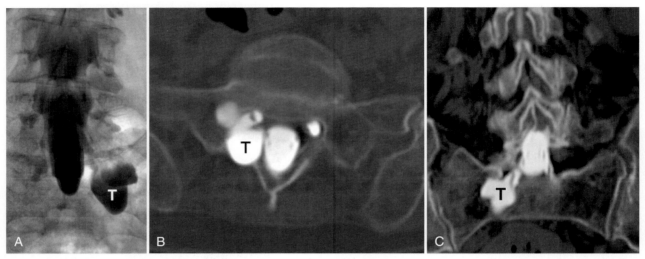

Figure 77-4 ► **Tarlov Cyst, Myelogram and Post-Myelogram CT. A**, Frontal radiograph during a lumbar myelogram. Axial post-myelogram CT image **B**, and coronal reformatted CT image **C**. This Tarlov cyst (*T*) readily fills with myelographic contrast.

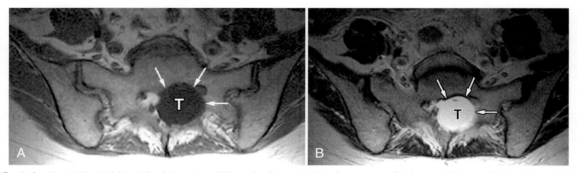

Figure 77-5 ► **Tarlov Cyst, MR.** Axial T1-weighted image **A** and T2-weighted image **B**. Typical appearance of Tarlov cyst (*T*) having CSF signal characteristics (decreased T1/increased T2). There is smooth expansion of the left S1 neural foramen (*arrows*) and posterior neural arch.

DIFFERENTIAL DIAGNOSIS

1. **Facet joint synovial cyst**: The joint cyst has similar imaging characteristics but is seen abutting a degenerated facet joint *(Fig. 77-6)*. The cyst is separate from the nerves.
2. **Meningocele**: Meningoceles have imaging characteristics similar to Tarlov cysts. One needs to evaluate for an anterior or posterior sacral defect with meningoceles that are not present with Tarlov cysts.
3. **Nerve sheath tumor**: The nerve sheath tumor can have cystic features and scallop the adjacent bone; however, it demonstrates intense enhancement *(Fig. 77-7)*.
4. **Spinal nerve root avulsion**: There is a definite history of trauma with nerve root avulsion. Nerve root avulsions are more commonly seen in the cervical and upper thoracic regions. At myelography, the nerve root avulsion fills immediately, and no bone erosion is identified. Nervous tissue is not identified within the CSF-filled avulsion *(Fig. 77-8)*.

TREATMENT

1. **Nonoperative management**: Nonoperative management includes lumbar drainage to decrease hydrostatic pressure, cyst-subarachnoid shunt, and direct cyst puncture and drainage with possible fibrin glue injection. The nonsurgical treatments have proven to give great relief; however, such treatment is only temporary. It is felt that these nonsurgical treatments are best used as a diagnostic tool prior to surgical intervention.
2. **Surgery**: Surgical treatments include complete cyst removal including the posterior root and ganglion, partial excision with or without fat or muscle graft, cyst fenestration and imbrication, and cyst shrinkage using bipolar cautery. Simple decompressive laminectomy has been attempted but with a very low success rate.[11,13,15] One study suggests that patients with cysts greater than 1.5 cm in diameter with associated radicular pain or bowel/bladder dysfunction have the best surgical outcomes.[16]

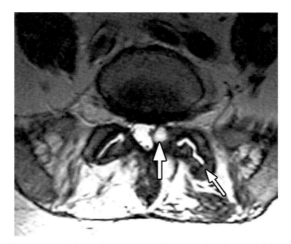

Figure 77-6 ▶ Synovial Cyst. Axial T2-weighted MR image. Fluid signal intensity cyst (*large arrow*) within the left lateral spinal canal displacing the thecal sac to the left. This cyst is associated with a degenerated facet joint (*small arrow*).

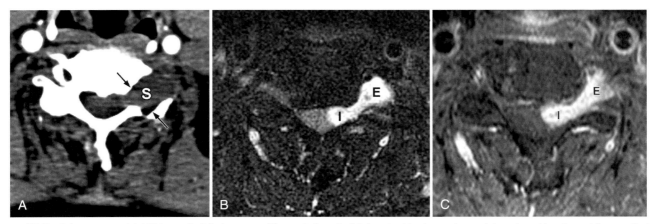

Figure 77-7 ▶ Schwannoma. Axial CT image **A**. Soft tissue mass (*S*) extends from the left lateral epidural space into and through a widened neural foramen (*between arrows*). Axial fat-saturated, T2-weighted image **B** and fat-saturated, post-contrast, T1-weighted image **C**. Dumbbell-shaped mass extending through the neural foramen having both intraspinal (*I*) and extraforaminal (*E*) components. The thecal sac is compressed and displaced to the left.

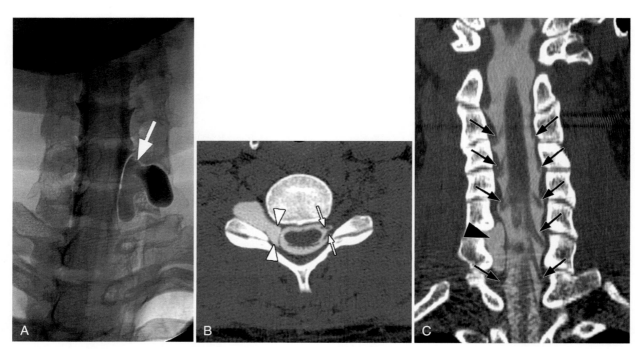

Figure 77-8 ▶ Pseudomeningocele. A, Radiograph of the cervical spine during myelography. There is a large right paravertebral collection of contrast that is centered upon the right C6-7 neural foramen (*arrow*). Axial post-myelogram image **B** reveals the large fluid collection within and extending through the right neural foramen. No nervous tissue is seen within the intraspinal portion of this fluid collection (*arrowheads*) compared with normal ventral and dorsal nerve roots on the opposite side (*arrows*). Coronal reformatted CT image C demonstrates normal traversing nerve roots at all levels (*arrows*) except for the right C7 nerve root, which has been avulsed. Fluid-containing pseudomeningocele is seen centered on the right C6-7 neural foramen (*arrowhead*).

References

1. Tarlov IM. Perineural cysts of the spinal nerve roots. *Arch neurol Psychiatry.* 1938;40:1067-1074.
2. Tarlov IM. Spinal perineurial and meningeal cysts. *J Neurol Neurosurg Psychiatry.* 1970;33:833-843.
3. Nabors MW, Pait TG, Byrd EB, et al. Updated assessment and current classification of spinal meningeal cysts. *J Neurosurg.* 1988;68:366-377.
4. Gortavi P. Extradural cysts of the spinal canal. *J Neurol Neurosurg Psychiatry.* 1963;26:223-230.
5. Lombardi G, Morello G. Congenital cysts of the spinal membranes and roots. *Br J Radiol.* 1963;36:197-205.
6. Tarlov IM. Cyst of the sacral nerve roots: Clinical significance and pathogenesis. *Arch Neurol Psychiatry.* 1952;68:94-108.
7. Acosta FL, Quinones-Hinojosa A, Schmidt MH, Weinstein PR. Diagnosis and management of sacral Tarlov cysts: Case report and review of the literature. *Neurosurg Focus.* 2003;15:E15.
8. Paulsen RD, Call GA, Murtagh FR. Prevalence and percutaneous drainage of cysts of the sacral nerve root sheath (Tarlov cysts). *AJNR Am J Neuroradiol.* 1994;15:293-297.
9. Smith DT. Cystic formations associated with human spinal nerve roots. *J Neurosurg.* 1961;18:654-660.
10. Kumar K, Malik S, Schulte PA. Symptomatic spinal arachnoid cysts: Report of two cases with review of literature. *Spine.* 2003;28:25-29.
11. Mummaneni PV, Pitts LH, McCormack BM, et al. Microsurgical treatment of symptomatic sacral Tarlov cysts. *Neurosurgery.* 2000;47:74-78.
12. Strully KJ, Heiser S. Lumbar and sacral cysts of meningeal origin. *Radiology.* 1954;62:544-549.
13. Bartels RH, an Overbeeke JJ. Lumbar cerebrospinal fluid drainage for symptomatic sacral nerve root cysts: An adjuvant diagnostic procedure and/or alternative treatment? Technical case report. *Neurosurgery.* 1997;40:861-864.
14. Patel MR, Louie W, Rachlin J. Percutaneous fibrin glue therapy of meningeal cysts of the sacral spine. *AJR Am J Radiol.* 1997;168:367-370.
15. Caspar W, Papavero L, Nabhan A, et al. Microsurgical excision of symptomatic sacral perineurial cysts: A study of 15 cases. *Surg Neurol.* 2003;59:101-105.
16. Voyadzis JM, Bhargava P, Henderson FC. Tarlov cysts: A study of 10 cases with review of the literature. *J Neurosurg.* 2001;95:25-32.

TETHERED SPINAL CORD

Douglas S. Fenton, M.D.

CLINICAL PRESENTATION

The patient is a 42-year-old man who over the course of the past year has been aware of increasing difficulty with bladder control. He describes marked urgency and frequency of micturition and on some occasions has been incontinent. He has also, at times, noticed that voiding may be imperfect and he may struggle to initiate micturition. There is also a long history of episodic fecal incontinence. This dates to childhood and the incontinence tends to occur only when he has diarrhea. There is also a long history of back pain. More recently, he describes episodic sensory symptoms. There are times when he has noticed a feeling of the outer aspects of the feet "going to sleep." He has not been aware of atrophy of leg muscles but has always noticed that his calve musculature has been poorly developed, this more obvious on the right side. Leg weakness has not been a prominent feature, although his gait appears to have deteriorated over time, this attributed to unequal length of his legs. There are no symptoms in his upper limbs.

IMAGING PRESENTATION

Sagittal T1-weighted and fat-saturated, T2-weighted images demonstrate a low-lying spinal cord terminating and tethered into a large region of increased T1 signal intensity/decreased fat-saturated T2 signal intensity compatible with fat (*Fig. 78-1*).

DISCUSSION

The tethered cord syndrome (TCS), also known as *tight filum terminale syndrome* is a clinical entity by which signs and symptoms are caused by excessive tension on the spinal cord. The majority of cases of tethered cord are related to spinal dysraphism. The concept of the tethered cord has been around for over 150 years; however, it was not until 1953 when Garceau[1] attributed the orthopedic spinal deformities and neurologic dysfunction of three patients to tension on the conus medullaris from a thickened filum terminale, which was found at surgery. All three patients had good clinical results after sectioning of the filum terminale. In 1976, Hoffman[2] coined the phrase *tethered spinal cord* in patients with an abnormally low conus medullaris and a filum terminale of 2 mm or more in diameter.

The spinal cord forms through three complex processes: neurulation, canalization, and retrogressive differentiation. Retrograde differentiation results in the formation of the filum terminale, cauda equina, and the relative ascension of the conus medullaris in relation to the vertebra column.[3] As the conus *ascends* because of disproportionate vertebral column to spinal cord growth, the filum terminale elongates and the nerve roots that must exit inferior to the conus elongate in order to pass through their respective foramen, thus forming the cauda equina.[3] There has been debate as to what is considered the normal level of the conus medullaris and when it attains that position. Barson[4] demonstrated in an anatomic study that the conus medullaris is at approximately the L2-L3 interspace at full-term birth and ascends to the L1-L2 level by approximately 2 months of age. Beek and colleagues[5] demonstrated, using ultrasound, that the conus lies at L1-L2 by 40 weeks of gestation. Other investigators have the conus terminating between the T10-T11 interspace and mid-body of L4, with all studies accepting that a conus at or above the L2-L3 level is normal. Kesler and colleagues[6] evaluated the level of the conus medullaris in 100 children after whole-spine magnetic resonance (MR) imaging. This was the first study to count vertebral levels from C2. All other studies counted from the lumbosacral junction up and therefore did not account for transitional vertebrae and did not assess rib-bearing vertebrae. Kesler's study demonstrated that the conus medullaris terminates most commonly at the L1-L2 interspace and in the absence of cord tethering, never ends below the mid-body of L2.

The filum terminale's functions are believed to be to fixate, stabilize, and buffer the distal spinal cord from both normal and abnormal cephalic and caudal traction.[7] The filum terminale is a viscoelastic band that allows slight upward and downward movement of the conus medullaris during flexion and extension of the spine. Mechanical causes of cord tethering can arise from thickening of the filum terminale attached to the spinal cord or any other inelastic structures including a fatty filum terminale, lipomas (see Fig. 78-1), epidermoid tumors, myelomeningoceles (*Fig. 78-2*), lipomyelomeningoceles, granulation tissue, or osseous or fibrous septum (*Fig. 78-3*).[8] It is further believed that the inelasticity of the filum terminale causes failure of "ascension" of the conus medullaris to its normal position. The hypothesis is that if there is loss of the viscoelastic properties of the filum terminale, that caudal tension and traction can cause undue stress on the conus medullaris, resulting in TCS. Yamada and colleagues[9] demonstrated that in patients with TCS, the filum terminale elongated by only 10% when stretched, and in those without TCS, the filum terminale elongated by more than 50%. This shows that there is less reserve in patients with TCS and that their spinal cords are

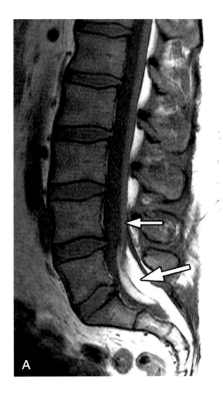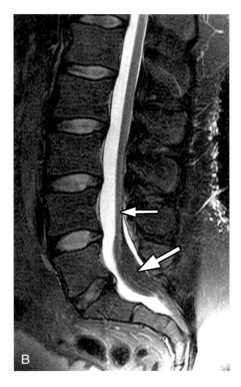

Figure 78-1 ▶ Tethered Cord. Sagittal T1-weighted image **A** and fat-saturated image **B**. The distal spinal cord is abnormally low (*small arrow*), terminating at the L4-5 level. The spinal cord terminates into a globular region of soft tissue beginning at L5 (*large arrow*) that is of increased T1 signal intensity and is of homogeneous decreased signal intensity on the fat-saturated sequence and is compatible with a fat.

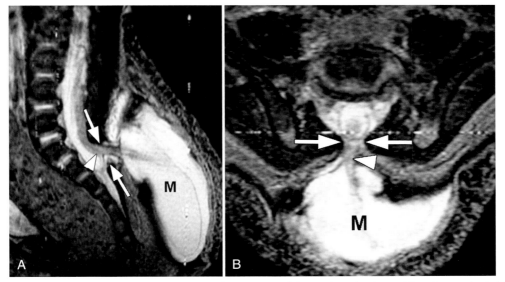

Figure 78-2 ▶ Myelomeningocele. Sagittal T2-weighted image **A** and axial image **B**. Neural elements (*arrowhead*) extend through a neural arch defect in the upper sacral region (*between arrows*) and into a large fluid-filled sac (*M*) compatible with a myelomeningocele.

preloaded with additional tension so that minor additional stretching can cause severe and permanent damage.[10,11] Furthermore, Yamada and colleagues[10] demonstrated that caudal traction of the distal cord caused impairment in oxidative metabolism with a corresponding reduction in spinal cord blood flow resulting in hypoxia. There are clinicians who believe that the TCS can occur in patients with normally located distal cords and that the tethering element may still restrict movement and cause traction on the conus.[12]

The clinical presentation of patients with TCS varies by age. In neonates and infants, cutaneous manifestations of a spinal dysraphism such as hairy tufts, hemangiomas, and nevi may suggest an underlying tethered cord.[3] An orthopedic malformation (foot deformity, limb-length discrepancy, leg malformations, gluteal asymmetry) and vertebral abnormalities (butterfly vertebrae, hemivertebrae, segmentation errors, scoliosis) may be present.[7] Toddlers and early adolescents show motor and sensory dysfunction.[3] There may be difficulties with gait or running. There may be

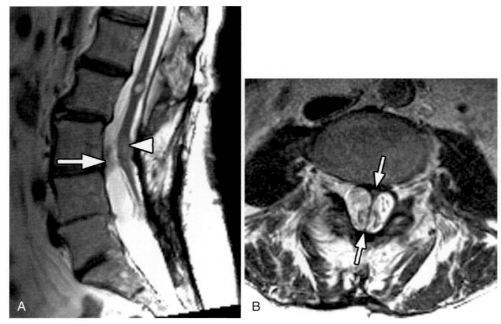

Figure 78-3 ▶ **Fibrous Septum of Diastematomyelia.** Sagittal T2-weighted image **A**. There is a small region of intermediate signal posterior to the L3 vertebral body (*arrow*), and apparent increased signal intensity in the conus medullaris (*arrowhead*). Axial image **B** demonstrates the fibrous septum (*between arrows*) separating the thecal sac into two halves. The arrow in image **A** is partial averaging with the septum, and the apparent signal in the distal cord is CSF between the split cord.

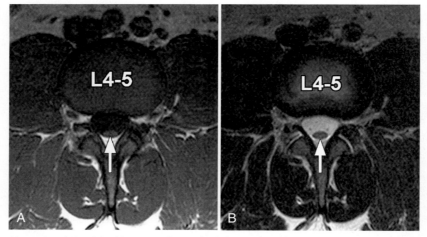

Figure 78-4 ▶ Axial T1-weighted image **A** and T2-weighted image **B** at the L4-5 level. The spinal cord (*arrow*) should not normally be visualized at the L4-5 level, but rather the nerve roots of the cauda equina.

regressive changes in bowel or bladder habits. Occasionally, there may be pain in the back or lower extremities. Teenagers and many adults present with scoliosis, lower extremity deformities, pain, and sphincter dysfunction.[3] Scoliosis is felt to develop as a functional adjustment of the paraspinal muscles to bend the spine into a curvature that allows for the shortest course of the spinal cord along the inner curvature so as to reduce tension on the cord.[8] The most common manifesting complaint in approximately two thirds of adults with TCS is pain.[13] Pain can be present in the pediatric population too; however, it is more difficult to identify because the pain often manifests as irritability. The pain may be in the anorectal or perineal region. Leg pain is often bilateral, diffuse, and nondermatomal.[13] Electric-like pain can radiate down both legs and extend cephalad into the interscapular region during forward spinal flexion.[13] Bilateral lower extremity weakness may be present. Upper and lower motor neuron deficits can result in bladder abnormalities with urgency, frequency, and stress incontinence.[13]

IMAGING FEATURES

Magnetic resonance imaging (MRI) is the modality of choice in evaluating TCS. Routine sagittal and axial T1- and T2-weighted images through the lumbosacral spine should be obtained. The

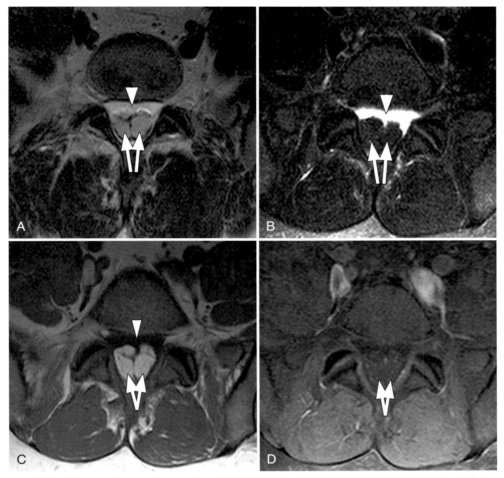

Figure 78-5 ► **Fibrolipoma of the Filum Terminale and the Imaging of Fat.** MRI techniques can be used to distinguish fat from other soft tissues by using fat-saturation (also referred to as fat suppression) techniques. Axial T2-weighted image **A** performed without fat saturation demonstrates a lobular high signal intensity intradural: mass (*arrows*) with increased signal intensity ventrally (*arrowhead*). Axial T2-weighted image **B** is performed using fat saturation, which turns the high signal intensity mass homogeneously dark (*arrows*) compatible with fat, whereas the intradural CSF (*arrowhead*) remains bright. Similarly, axial T1-weighted image **C** without fat saturation shows the fat to be of increased signal intensity (*arrows*) with low T1 signal intensity CSF (*arrowhead*). The addition of fat saturation to a T1-weighted acquisition with contrast (image **D**) makes the nonenhancing fat turn dark (*arrows*).

level of the conus medullaris in relation to the vertebral level is readily identified and also quantifies the thickness of the filum terminale (*Figs.* 78-1 and *78-4*). The conus medullaris normally terminates at or above the L2-3 level. The filum terminale, excluding fatty infiltration, should not be any thicker than 2 mm on axial imaging. Fibrolipomas of the filum terminale are seen as increased T1 and T2 signal intensity that can be further confirmed using a fat-suppression technique rendering the adipose structures dark (*Fig. 78-5*). Other fat-containing tethering masses such as a lipomyelomeningocele or dermoid can be identified with MRI. Arachnoid adhesions can be seen as clumping of nerve roots and/or intermediate to low signal intensity intrathecal masses. The nerve roots can be clumped into a solitary mass or be adhesed to the walls of the thecal sac (*Fig. 78-6*). Although split cord malformations can be diagnosed with MRI, computed tomography (CT) is particularly useful in demonstrating bony anatomy and the nature of the septum (bony vs. fibrous) with diastematomyelia (*Fig. 78-7*). Ultrasonography can be useful in young infants to obtain a dynamic view of the spinal cord without having to submit them to radiation and/or sedation; however, the acoustic window usually closes by 4 to 5 months of age and images can be difficult

to interpret and are subject to operator skill. Plain radiographs are not useful in the confirmatory diagnosis of TCS; however, they can demonstrate bone abnormalities (scoliosis, vertebral anomalies) that may suggest underlying pathology.

DIFFERENTIAL DIAGNOSIS

1. **Normal low-lying conus medullaris**: The conus medullaris can, in some patients, extend below the L2-L3 level. These patients are asymptomatic and have a normal thickness filum terminale. These patients should be followed because this finding could be found incidentally in patients with TCS when they are asymptomatic.
2. **Postoperative low-lying conus medullaris**: Patients who have had sectioning of the filum terminale will still have a low-lying conus medullaris, although it is no longer tethered. If this type of patient is returning for imaging secondary to new symptoms, then retethering should be considered.

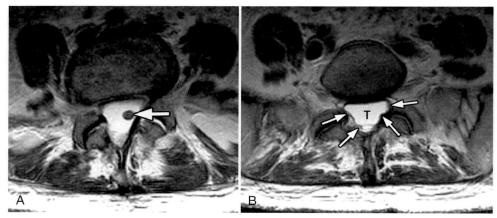

Figure 78-6 ▶ Adhesions. Axial T2-weighted images **A** and **B**. Two different appearances of adhesions. The cauda equina is clumped into a solitary mass (*arrow*) in image **A**. The intrathecal nerve roots (*arrows*) in image **B** are adhesed to the periphery of the thecal sac (*T*). In both presentations, the thecal sac has a featureless appearance.

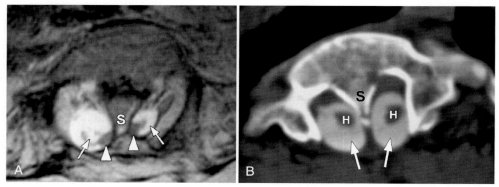

Figure 78-7 ▶ Diastematomyelia, Bony Septum. Axial T2-weighted image **A**. Osseous spur (*S*) separates the thecal sac into two asymmetric halves (*arrows*) and the spinal cord into equal halves (*arrowheads*). Axial CT lumbar spine image **B**. Osteocartilaginous spur (*S*) inserts between paired thecal sacs (*arrows*) and hemicords (*H*).

TREATMENT

1. **Conservative therapy:** Conservative therapy of TCS is limited to the management of symptoms and consists of physical therapy, muscle relaxants, and analgesics.[3] Patients should avoid vigorous exercise, heavy lifting, and repetitive flexion/extension of the lumbosacral spine.

2. **Surgical management:** Most clinicians agree that surgical untethering through sectioning of the filum terminale is the treatment of choice for symptomatic or progressive neurologic and/or mechanical symptoms. The goal of untethering surgery is to remove tension on the spinal cord, to stabilize deficits in the symptomatic patient, and to prevent future deficits in the asymptomatic patient.[3,7] In the case of a low-lying conus medullaris with a thickened filum, a sectioning of the filum terminale through a laminectomy defect is performed. Surgical untethering related to a more complex etiology is beyond the scope of this section. Of the various symptoms that patients with TCS can have, the one most likely to improve after surgical untethering is pain. Success rates range from 75% in adult studies to 100% in pediatric studies.[14,15] Stabilization or improvement in neurologic function is seen in pediatric and adult series in 80% to 90% of patients.[15,16] It appears that the earlier the surgical intervention from the onset of symptoms, the greater the recovery of neurologic function, with many making full recoveries. Rates of improvement in bowel and bladder function after surgical untethering range from 16% to 67%, with greater improvement in the pediatric population.[3,7] Approximately one half of patients with scoliotic curves of less than 40 degrees have stabilization or improvement in their deformity. Nearly all patients with curves greater than 40 degrees do not stabilize and require fusion.[17,18] When tethering is simply caused by a thickened filum terminale, postsurgical retethering is extremely rare. In the more complex cases, retethering can occur and has been reported in 5% to 50% of cases.[19,20] Repeat surgery can be performed with similar success rates as the initial surgery.[19,20]

3. **Postsurgical complications:** Complications of untethering surgery have been estimated at 9.5%.[21] The primary complications were postoperative hematoma (2.3%), renal complications (2.2%), neurologic complications (1.6%), and infection (1.1%). Cerebrospinal fluid leak has also been frequently cited as a surgical complication.

References

1. Garceau GJ. The filum terminale syndrome (the corde-traction syndrome). *J Bone Joint Surg Am.* 1953;35:711-716.

2. Hoffman HJ, Hendrick EB, Humphreys RP. The tethered spinal cord: Its protean manifestations, diagnosis and surgical correction. *Childs Brain.* 1976;2:145-155.

3. Lew SM, Kothbauer KF. Tethered cord syndrome: An updated review. *Pediatr Neurosurg.* 2007;43:236-248.

4. Barson AJ. The vertebral level of termination of the spinal cord during normal and abnormal development. *J Anat.* 1970;106:489-497.

5. Beek FJ, de Vries LS, Gerards LJ, Mali WP. Sonographic determination of the position of the conus medullaris in premature and term infants. *Neuroradiology.* 1996;38:S174-S177.

6. Kesler H, Dias MS, Kalapos P. Termination of the normal conus medullaris in children: A whole-spine magnetic resonance imaging study. *Neurosurg Focus.* 2007;23:E7.

7. Bui CJ, Tubbs RS, Oakes WJ. Tethered cord syndrome in children: A review. *Neurosurg Focus.* 2007;23:E2.

8. Yamada S, Won DJ, Yamada SM. Pathophysiology of tethered cord syndrome: Correlation with symptomatology. *Neurosurg Focus.* 2004;16: Article 6.

9. Yamada S, Won DJ, Pezeshkpour G, et al. Pathophysiology of tethered cord syndrome and similar complex disorders. *Neurosurg Focus.* 2007;23:E6.

10. Yamada S, Zinke DE, Sanders D. Pathophysiology of "tethered cord syndrome." *J Neurosurg.* 1981;54:494-503.

11. Tani S, Yamada S, Knighton RS. Extensibility of the lumbar and sacral cord: Pathophysiology of the tethered spinal cord in cats. *J Neurosurg.* 1987;66: 116-123.

12. Selden NR. Minimal tethered cord syndrome: What's necessary to justify a new surgical indication? *Neurosurg Focus.* 2007;23:E1.

13. Pang D, Wilberger JE. Tethered cord syndrome in adults. *J Neurosurg.* 1982;57:32-47.

14. Sarwark JF, Weber DT, Gabrielie AP, et al. Tethered cord syndrome in low motor level children with myelomeningocele. *Pediatr Neurosurg.* 1996;25: 295-301.

15. van Leeuwen R, Notermans NC, Vandertop WP. Surgery in adults with tethered cord syndrome: Outcome study with independent clinical review. *J Neurosurg.* 2001;94:205-209.

16. Byrne RW, Hayes EA, George TM, McLone DG. Operative resection of 100 spinal lipomas in infants less than 1 year of age. *Pediatr Neurosurg.* 1995;23: 182-186.

17. Pierz K, Bantga J, Thomson J, et al. The effect of tethered cord release on scoliosis in myelomeningocele. *J Pediatr Orthop.* 2000;20:362-365.

18. McLone DG, Herman JM, Gabrieli AP, Dias L. Tethered cord as a cause of scoliosis in children with a myelomeningocele. *Pediatr Neurosurg.* 1990; 16:8-13.

19. Archibeck MJ, Smith JT, Carroll KL, et al. Surgical relearse of tethered spinal cord: Survivorship analysis and orthopedic outcome. *J Pediatr Orthop.* 1997;17:773-776.

20. Herman JM, McLone DG, Storrs BB, Dauser RC. Analysis of 153 patients with myelomeningocele or spinal lipoma reoperated upon for a tethered cord: Presentation, management and outcome. *Pediatr Neurosurg.* 1993;19:243-249.

21. Lad SP, Patil CG, Ho C, et al. Tethered cord syndrome: Nationwide inpatient complications and outcomes. *Neurosurg Focus.* 2007;23:E3.

VERTEBRAL OSTEOPHYTOSIS (SPONDYLOSIS DEFORMANS)

Douglas S. Fenton, M.D.

CLINICAL PRESENTATION

The patient is a 68-year-old man who presented with back and leg pain. Patient has a history of two L1-L2 lumbar diskectomies. He did not have much improvement of his preoperative back and leg pain. The leg pain involved the right lower extremity. He has had progressive symptoms since. The pain originates in the right paraspinal area, in the mid to upper lumbar spine, and radiates to the buttock and anterolateral thigh. It does not go past the knee. The back pain is much worse than the buttock and leg pain and can reach 7 out of 10 on the pain scale. There is no left lower extremity pain. There is no numbness or weakness in the left upper and lower extremity.

IMAGING PRESENTATION

Axial T1-weighted image and fat-saturated, post-contrast, T1-weighted image reveal a rind of soft tissue along the ventral and right lateral aspect of the vertebral body that extends posteriorly to the lateral aspect of the pedicle in the region of the right lumbar trunk. Similar signal intensity is seen within the right ventral vertebral body. There is an osteophyte projecting from the right ventral vertebral body. The findings are thought to represent inflammation related to the osteophyte formation (*Fig. 79-1*).

DISCUSSION

Vertebral osteophytes are a characteristic of disc degeneration. By definition, an osteophyte is an overgrowth of bone tissue. It is commonly referred to as a *bone spur*. Osteophytes can occur anywhere in the body, but they are most commonly found along the spine. As we age, the intervertebral discs become more desiccated and less compliant. The intervertebral disc acts as a cushion between a motion segment, preventing trauma to the adjacent vertebral bodies while allowing smooth movement in multiple directions. Degeneration of the annulus fibrosis of the disc renders it unable to withstand the stresses of axial loading, causing it to bulge outward.[1] Over time, this bulging of the annulus on the vertebral edge leads to formation of an osteophyte at the osseous site of attachment to the annulus (Sharpey's fibers). The osteophytes can be small and parallel to the endplate (*traction osteophyte*) or be larger, curved, and even bridging two adjacent vertebra (*claw osteophyte*) (*Fig. 79-2*). Some believe that claw osteophytes are a natural progression from traction osteophytes. They believe that traction osteophytes are the initial stage of an ossification process at an unstable level, and that their conversion to claw osteophytes indicates an attempt to increase stability by ossification of annular fibers.[2]

Osteophytes are often found in the aging spine; however, there is an increased frequency of vertebral osteophytes in athletes and those involved with chronic heavy physical activity. Osteophytes are found in approximately 80% of men and 60% of women by age 50 and 95% in both genders by age 70.[3] The study of lumbar osteophytes conducted by Shao and colleagues[4] demonstrated that men had a greater prevalence of osteophytes when compared with women throughout all ages, although the gap narrows after the age of 70. The study also demonstrated that the most prevalent site for a lumbar osteophyte in men was at the L4 level and for women at the L3 level.[4] A study of a population of South-African black and white people by Taitz[5] demonstrated a significantly lower incidence of cervical osteophytosis in the black population of both genders as compared with the white population. Furthermore, in the white population, there was a combination of same level vertebral osteophyte and facet osteophyte as opposed to the black population that demonstrated osteophyte formation at either the vertebral level or facet level. The white population also demonstrated a greater degree of facet osteophytosis compared to the black population. The distribution of osteophytes within the spine is greatest at T9-10 and L3-4, which is intuitive because these levels are at or near the sites of maximum sagittal thoracic and lumbar curvature.[2,6,7] Many studies show positive correlation between intervertebral disc degeneration and osteophyte formation with heavy activity.[8,9] Other studies show obesity as a risk factor for osteophyte formation because of the mechanical factors involved in the additional stress on the skeletal system.[10,11]

It is traditionally thought that osteophytes are not painful themselves, but can cause low back pain because of compression of the spinal canal, neural foramen, and/or lateral recess. Osteophytes, along with associated disc height loss, disc bulging, and facet joint degeneration, are frequently a contributing factor in neural foraminal narrowing, which may lead to radicular symptoms. Cervical vertebral osteophytes and disc degeneration as well as apophyseal joint osteoarthrosis can progress to involve the nerve root and cause neck and/or radicular pain,[12] as can posterolateral osteophytes in the lumbar spine. A study by Matsumoto and colleagues[13] reported several cases of patients with L5 radicular pain related to entrapment of the extraforaminal L5 nerve root between an L5 osteophyte and the sacral ala.

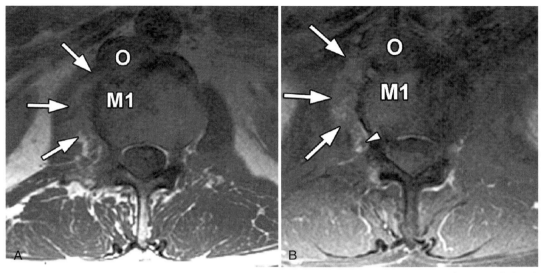

Figure 79-1 ▶ Osteophyte Formation. Axial T1-weighted image **A** and fat-saturated, post-contrast, T1-weighted image **B**. Right paravertebral rind of intermediate T1 signal intensity and enhancement (*arrows*) displaying the same imaging characteristics as the Modic type 1 degenerative changes (*M1*) in the vertebral body. Note enhancement surrounding the right lumbar trunk (*arrowhead*, image **B**). An osteophyte (*O*) projects from the right ventral vertebral body.

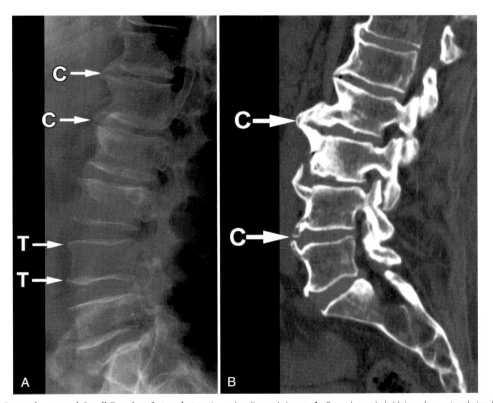

Figure 79-2 ▶ Claw Osteophytes and Small Traction Osteophytes. Lateral radiograph image **A**. Curved, nearly bridging claw osteophytes (*C*) at T12-L1 and L1-2. Small traction osteophytes (*T*) projecting from the anterior-superior and anterior-inferior margins of L4. Sagittal CT image **B**. Claw osteophytes (*C*) projecting from the anterior margins of T12-L1 through L4-5.

Recently, a hypothesis that painful stimuli could arise directly from an osteophyte has been proposed.[14] Five patients were described with degenerative spine arthritis and large vertebral osteophytes. Each had undergone a traditional therapeutic regimen of nonsteroidal anti-inflammatory drugs (NSAIDs), oral narcotics, epidural and facet injections, and physical therapy that did not result in any significant pain relief. All five patients received percutaneous injections of anesthetic and steroid around the margin of the osteophyte (*Fig. 79-3*), and all patients had postinjection pain scores that decreased by 50% or more. All patients had return of their pain, with some patients having relief for 3 to 4 months. There is likely an inflammatory

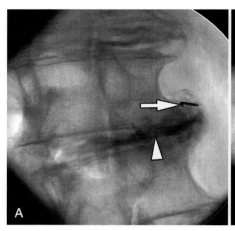
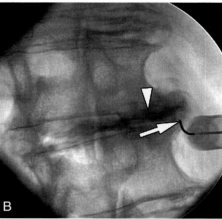

Figure 79-3 ▶ **Osteophyte Injection.** Left anterior oblique images **A** and **B**. Injection of a potential *inflammatory osteophyte* along its superior margin (*arrow*, **A**) and its inferior margin (*arrow*, **B**). Contrast is seen within the disc (*arrowhead*) from discography, which demonstrated positivity at this level.

component with some vertebral osteophytes. It may be that an inflammatory reaction occurs around a vertebral osteophyte as it grows/enlarges and that the inflammatory reaction quiesces when the osteophyte is dormant. It is well known that patients may have no pain in a region of severe foraminal narrowing, and yet others may have pain with very mild narrowing. Neural compression alone is not the only factor in the cause of pain. There is often an inflammatory reaction that envelops or is adjacent to the spinal nerve root or its branches that is the immediate cause of the pain and is what is being treated with steroid injections (see Fig. 79-1). This type of pain generation may be similar to what one sees with inflammatory facet joint arthopathy (facet synovitis).[15]

IMAGING FEATURES

Plain radiographs are sufficient to diagnose osteophytes. Osteophytes are seen as horizontal, often triangular, radioopaque projections from the margin of the vertebral endplate (see Fig. 79-2). However, computed tomography (CT) or magnetic resonance imaging (MRI) is necessary to demonstrate the relationship of an osteophyte to the neural structures. CT, given its superior detail for bone imaging, best demonstrates the degree of spinal canal, neural foraminal, or lateral recess narrowing. An osteophyte will appear as a hyperdense projection from the vertebral endplate cortex. There is no evidence of continuity with the vertebral medullary cavity. There can be sclerosis and/or thickening of the vertebral cortex adjacent to an osteophyte *(Fig. 79-4)*. This sclerosis and thickening may be a reactive change secondary to abnormal stress at that segment.

It has been reported that MRI has relatively low specificity for the detection of foraminal lesions, and that MRI cannot accurately differentiate disc herniations from osteophytes.[16] The advantage of MRI is that one is able to see the signal characteristics of the spinal cord and whether a posterior cervical or thoracic osteophyte is affecting the spinal cord. Another advantage of MRI is its lack of ionizing radiation. The MR imaging characteristics of an osteophyte is the same as bone. Noninflammatory osteophytes are often of low T1- and T2-weighted signal intensity *(Fig. 79-5)*. In the case of an inflammatory osteophyte, one may see variable T2 signal intensity within and increased T2 signal intensity around the osteophyte and often within the adjacent vertebral cortex and

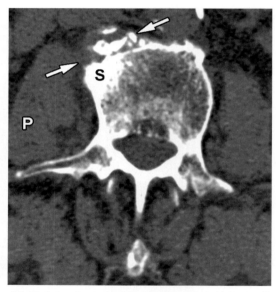

Figure 79-4 ▶ **Osteophyte with Adjacent Sclerosis.** Axial CT. Mixed bone and soft tissue density osteophyte (*between arrows*) with adjacent region of sclerosis (*S*). Note that the right psoas muscle (*P*) appears to be twice as large as the left psoas muscle.

marrow (see Fig. 79-5). This is thought to be related to edema and/or inflammatory changes. This signal change becomes even more evident if one uses a fat-saturation technique. The addition of contrast and the use of a T1-weighted, fat-saturated sequence will enhance the areas of inflammation, distinguishing these areas from regions of edema.

DIFFERENTIAL DIAGNOSIS

1. **Vertebral endplate compression**: These can have an appearance similar to osteophytes; however, one should evaluate for loss of vertebral height *(Fig. 79-6)*. One also does not see reactive changes on MRI in the adjacent vertebral cortex with chronic compression deformities *(Fig. 79-7)*.

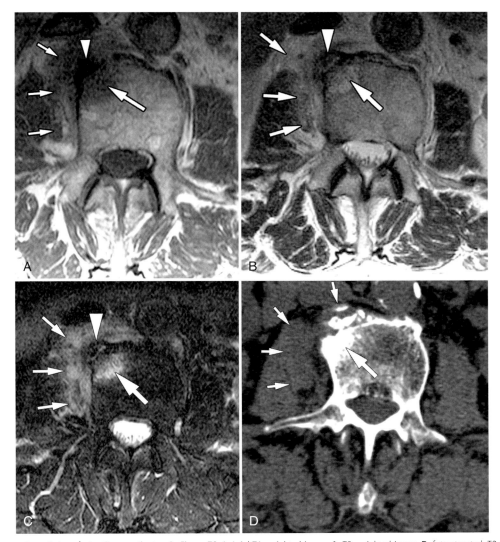

Figure 79-5 ► Inflammatory Osteophyte. Same patient as in Figure 79-4. Axial T1-weighted image **A**, T2-weighted image **B**, fat-saturated, T2-weighted image **C**, and axial CT image **D**. The small right ventrolateral osteophyte (*arrowhead*) demonstrates decreased T1 signal intensity and mixed T2 signal intensity. There is a thick rind of decreased T1, increased T2 signal intensity surrounding the osteophyte and along the right lateral vertebral body (*small arrows*). Note that the region of sclerosis on CT (*large arrow*) demonstrates identical signal intensity as the paravertebral rind of tissue and is compatible with a Modic type 1 inflammatory change. One can also see that the assumed enlargement of the psoas muscle on CT is actually a combination of the muscle laterally and the inflammatory tissue (*bounded by small arrows*) medially.

2. **Calcified disc herniation**: Calcification is associated with the disc and not the vertebral endplate *(Fig. 79-8)*.
3. **Osteochondroma**: An osteochondroma has corticomedullary continuity that can be readily discerned on CT or MR imaging *(Fig. 79-9)*.

TREATMENT

1. **Rest:** The treatment of an osteophyte either directly or indirectly causing pain often begins with rest.
2. **Drug therapy:** A trial of nonsteroidal anti-inflammatory drugs (NSAIDs) or a mild narcotic drug can be prescribed.
3. **Physical therapy:** Physical therapy can be used as an adjunct to increase range of motion.

4. **Steroid injections:** An interlaminar or transforaminal steroid injection can be performed to lessen symptoms thought to be inflammatory in nature; however, if the symptoms are believed to be due to compression, then the injection will have only very short-term effect. If the symptoms are inflammatory; either caused by a traumatic (possibly mild and unknown to the patient) injury in the face of narrowing from an osteophyte or directly related to an inflammatory osteophyte, then a transforaminal injection of steroid or a periosteophyte injection of steroid may give the patient relief. It is the hope, in these patients, that the inflammatory reaction will dissipate, knowing that otherwise pain symptoms may return.
5. **Surgical management:** If diagnostic/therapeutic injections have demonstrated that an osteophyte is the cause of the patient's pain, the osteophyte can be surgically removed.

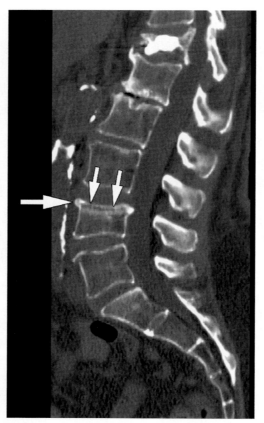

Figure 79-6 ▶ **Vertebral Endplate Compression.** Sagittal CT. Small ventral (*large arrow*) and posterior projections from the superior aspect of the L4 vertebral body are not osteophytes but are the sequela of compression of the vertebral body (*small arrows*).

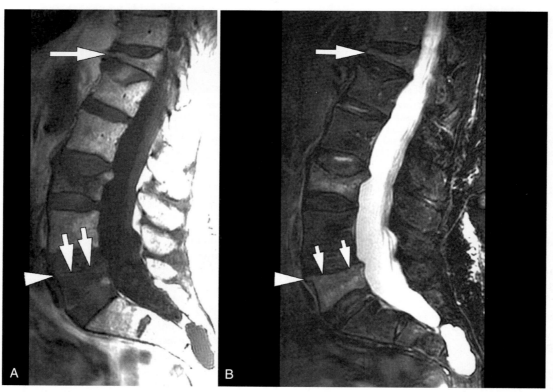

Figure 79-7 ▶ **Compression Deformities.** Sagittal T1-weighted image **A** and fat-saturated, T2-weighted image **B**. Small anterior projection of bone from the superior aspect of the L5 vertebral body (*arrowhead*) is secondary to compression of the superior endplate (*short arrows*). Diffuse abnormal decreased T1 and increased T2 signal intensity in the L3 and L5 vertebral bodies are consistent with more recent fractures. The severe compression deformity of T12 (*long arrow*) displays normal signal intensity on T1- and T2-weighted images compatible with a chronic fracture.

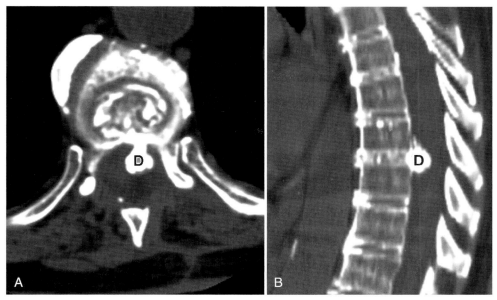

Figure 79-8 ▶ Calcified Disc Herniation. Axial CT image **A** and sagittal CT image **B** demonstrate a dense calcification (*D*) that is associated with the disc level and not the vertebral endplate.

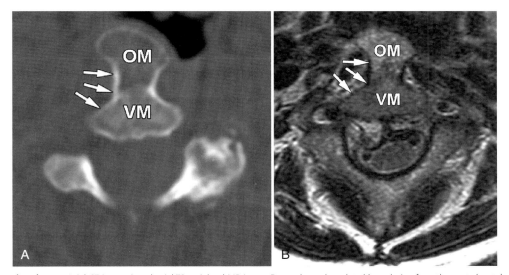

Figure 79-9 ▶ Osteochondroma. Axial CT image **A** and axial T2-weighted MR image **B** reveal a pedunculated bone lesion from the ventral vertebral body. The medullary cavities of the vertebral body (*VM*) and bone lesion (*OM*) are in continuity, as are their cortices (*arrows*), which are the pathognomonic findings of an osteochondroma.

References

1. Miller TT. Imaging of disk disease and degenerative spondylosis of the lumbar spine. *Semin Ultrasound CT MRI.* 2004;25:506-522.
2. Pate D, Goober J, Resnick D, et al. Traction osteophytes of the lumbar spine: Radiographic-pathologic correlation. *Radiology.* 1988;166:843-846.
3. O'Neill T, McCloskey EV, Kanis JA, et al. The distribution, determinants, and clinical correlates of vertebral osteophytosis: A population based survey. *J Rheumatol.* 1999;26:842-848.
4. Shao Z, Rompe G, Schiltenwolf M. Radiographic changes in the lumbar intervertebral discs and lumbar vertebrae with age. *Spine.* 2002;27:263-268.
5. Taitz C. Osteophytosis of the cervical spine in South African blacks and whites. *Clin Anat.* 1999;12:103-109.
6. Nathan H. Osteophytes of the vertebral column. *J Bone Joint Surg Br.* 1962;44:243-268.
7. Shore LR. Polyspondylitis marginalis osteophytica. *Br J Surg.* 1935;22:850-863.
8. Biering-Soensen F, Hansen FR, Schroll M, Runeborg O. The relation of spinal x-ray to low back pain and physical activity among 60 year old men and women. *Spine.* 1985;10:445-451.
9. Lawrence JS. Disc degeneration: Its frequency and relationship to symptoms. *Ann Rheum Dis.* 1969;28:121-138.
10. van Sasse JLCM, Vandenbroucke JP, van Romunde LKJ, Walkenburg HA. Osteoarthritis and obesity in the general population: A relationship calling for an explanation. *J Rheumatol.* 1988;15:1152-1158.
11. Egger P, Frith S, Duggleby S, et al. Obesity, occupational activity and osteoarthritis of the spine. *Br J Rheumatol.* 1995;34:35.

12. Kelsey JL. Epidemiology of radiculopathies. *Adv Neurol*. 1978;19:385-398.

13. Matsumoto M, Chiba K, Nojiri K, et al. Extraforaminal entrapment of the fifth lumbar spinal nerve by osteophytes of the lumbosacral spine. *Spine*. 2002;27:169-173.

14. Lamer TJ. Lumbar spine pain originating from vertebral osteophytes. *Reg Anesth Pain Med*. 1999;24:347-351.

15. Czervionke LF, Fenton DS. Fat-saturated MR imaging in the detection of inflammatory facet arthropathy (facet synovitis) in the lumbar spine. *Pain Med*. 2008;9:400-406.

16. van de Kleft E, van Vyve M. Diagnostic imaging algorithm for cervical soft disc herniation. *J Neurol Neurosurg Psychiatry*. 1994;57:724-728.

INDEX

Page numbers followed by "f" indicate figures, "t" indicate tables.